ACUTE RENAL FAILURE

ACUTE RENAL FAILURE

Pathophysiology, Prevention, and Treatment

edited by

Vittorio E. Andreucci

Martinus Nijhoff Publishing
a member of the Kluwer Academic Publishers Group

BOSTON   THE HAGUE   DORDRECHT   LANCASTER

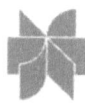

Distributors:

for North America
Kluwer Academic Publishers
190 Old Derby Street
Hingham, MA 02043

for all other countries
Kluwer Academic Publishers Group
Distribution Centre
P.O. Box 322
3300 AH Dordrecht
The Netherlands

Library of Congress Cataloging in Publication Data
Main entry under title:

Acute renal failure.

  1. Renal insufficiency, Acute.   I.   Andreucci,
Vittorio E.   [DNLM: 1.   Kidney failure, Acute. WJ
342 A1896]
RC918.R4A347   1984   616.6'14   83-23837

ISBN-13:978-1-4612-9794-9   e-ISBN-13:978-1-4613-2841-4
DOI: 10.1007/978-1-4613-2841-4

To my dear wife Gabriella, *and to my beautiful children* Michele *and* Maria Vittoria, *who were patient enough to allow my editing work even during weekends and holidays.*

CONTENTS

CONTRIBUTING AUTHORS

Vittorio E. Andreucci
Professor of Nephrology and Chairman
Department of Nephrology
Second Faculty of Medicine
University of Naples
80131 Naples
ITALY

Jean-Jacques Béraud
Praticien du Cadre Hospitalier
Division of Metabolic Diseases and Endocrinology
Montpellier University Hospital
34059 Montpellier Cedex
FRANCE

Gérard Bochereau
Service de Néphrologie et Réanimation Polyvalente
Centre Hospitalier
56 Boulevard de la Boissière
93105 Montreuil
FRANCE

J. Steward Cameron
Clinical Science Laboratories
Guy's Hospital Medical School
17th Floor Guy's Tower
London SE1 9RT
UNITED KINGDOM

Alfredo Capuano
Department of Nephrology
Second Faculty of Medicine
University of Naples
80131 Naples
ITALY

Paul Chauveau
Service de Néphrologie et Reanimation Polyvalente
Centre Hospitalier
56 Boulevard de la Boissière
93105 Montreuil
FRANCE

Bruno Cianciaruso
Department of Nephrology
Second Faculty of Medicine
University of Naples
80131 Naples
ITALY

Luigi Cirillo
Department of Radiology
Second Faculty of Medicine
University of Naples
80131 Naples
ITALY

Antonio Dal Canton
Department of Nephrology
Second Faculty of Medicine
University of Naples
80131 Naples
ITALY

Stefano Federico
Department of Nephrology
Second Faculty of Medicine
University of Naples
80131 Naples
ITALY

Carlos A. Gianantonio
Head, Department of Pediatrics
Hospital Italiano
Gascon 450
(1181) Buenos Aires
ARGENTINA

Joel A. Gordon
Assistant Professor of Medicine
Renal and Electrolyte Division
The Milton S. Hershey Medical Center
The Pennsylvania State University
P.O. Box 850
Hershey, Pennsylvania 17033
USA

George B. Haycock
Evelina Children's Department
Guy's Hospital
St. Thomas Street
London SE1 9RT
UNITED KINGDOM

Vittorio Iaccarino
Department of Radiology
Second Faculty of Medicine
University of Naples
80131 Naples
ITALY

Alain Kanfer
Service de Néphrologie
Hopital Bichat
Paris
FRANCE

Arthur Kennedy
Muirhead Professor of Medicine
University Department of Medicine
Royal Infirmary, Phase I
10, Alexandra Parade
Glasgow G31 2ER
UNITED KINGDOM

Dieter Kleinknecht
Service de Néphrologie et Réanimation Polyvalente
Centre Hospitalier
56 Boulevard de la Boissiére
93105 Montreuil
FRANCE

Franciszek Kokot
Department of Nephrology
Silesian School of Medicine
ul. Francuska 20
40-027 Katowice
POLAND

Joel D. Kopple
Professor of Medicine and Public Health Chief
Division of Nephrology and Hypertension
Harbor-UCLA Medical Center
1000 Carson Street
Torrance, California 90509
USA

Olivier Kourilsky
Centre Hospitalier Louise Michel
Quartier du Canal
Courcouronnes
91014 Évry Cedex
FRANCE

Bruno Memoli
Department of Nephrology
Second Faculty of Medicine
University of Naples
80131 Naples
ITALY

Charles M. Mion
Professor of Nephrology
Head, Division of Nephrology
Montpellier Medical School
University Hospital Saint-Charles
34059 Montpellier Cedex
FRANCE

Liliane Morel-Maroger
Hôpital Tenon and INSERM U64
4, rue de la Chine
75970 Paris Cedex 20
FRANCE

Steen Olsen
Professor of Pathology
University Institute of Pathology
DK-8000 Aarhus C
DENMARK

Solomon Papper
Distinguished Professor and Head
Department of Medicine
University of Oklahoma Health Sciences Center and
the Veterans Administration Medical Center
Oklahoma City, Oklahoma 73190
USA

Victor Parsons
Director, Renal Unit
King's College Hospital
Dulwich Hospital
East Dulwich Grove
London SE22 8PT
UNITED KINGDOM

Gabriel Richet
Hôpital Tenon and INSERM U64
4, rue de la Chine
75970 Paris Cedex 20
FRANCE

Brian H.B. Robinson
Consultant Physician and Director
Department of Renal Medicine
East Birmingham Hospital
Bordesley Green East
Birmingham B9 5ST
UNITED KINGDOM

Robert W. Schrier
Professor and Chairman
Department of Medicine, B-178
University of Colorado Health Sciences Center
Denver, Colorado 80262
USA

Visith Sitprija
Professor of Medicine and Associate Dean
Department of Medicine
Chulalongkorn Hospital Medical School
Bangkok
THAILAND

Jean-Daniel Sraer
Service de Néphrologie
Hôpital Tenon
4, rue de la Chine
75970 Paris Cedex 20
FRANCE

Mario Usberti
Department of Nephrology
Second Faculty of Medicine
University of Naples
80131 Naples
ITALY

PREFACE

Acute renal failure is undoubtedly one of the most interesting and frequent syndromes observed by clinicians. A great number of factors may acutely impair renal function, but the pathogenetic mechanism by which this occurs is frequently unknown. Even the pathophysiology of ischaemic/toxic forms of acute renal failure remains controversial despite the huge number of experimental and clinical studies.

Medical management of patients with acute renal failure has greatly improved in recent years, particularly with the use of different types of dialytic treatment. However mortality remains high. Further studies are necessary for improving our knowledge of the syndrome, for providing a better management of patients with acute impairment of renal function, for suggesting adequate prevention of renal shutdown, particularly with the increasing use of potentially nephrotoxic drugs.

It appears therefore evident why clinicians involved in the treatment of acute renal failure should be frequently updated on this important topic. For this reason I have accepted with enthusiasm to edit a book on acute renal failure. The aim was to summarize in one volume the recent advances on pathophysiology of acute renal failure, the clinical aspects of the various forms (even those which have been disregarded in other surveys), the diagnostic tests available today in our clinical practice, the general and specific therapeutic measures and (very important, indeed), some useful suggestions for prevention.

The contributors have provided clear, complete and up-to-date chapters. I am deeply grateful to them all.

I like to express my sincere thanks to Dr. A.J. Wing (St. Thomas' Hospital, London, U.K.), for his great help in editing the language in the chapters of non English-speaking authors (my chapters included). This arduous, very important task had to be performed, in my opinion, by an English nephrologist. Dr. Wing was so kind as to do it very quickly.

Special thanks to Martinus Nijhoff Publishing for their patience and for the excellent and rapid publication of this volume.

Napoli, Vittorio E. Andreucci

LIST OF ABBREVIATIONS USED IN THE BOOK

ACN: acute (bilateral) cortical necrosis
ACTH: adrenocorticotropin hormone
ADH: antidiuretic hormone; vasopressin
ADP: adenosine diphosphate
AI and AII: angiotensin I and angiotensin II
AIN: acute interstitial nephritis
ALG: antilymphocyte globulin
AMP: adenosine monophosphate
ARF: acute renal failure
ATN: acute tubular necrosis
ATP: adenosine triphosphate

BAL: mercaprol
β_2M: beta 2 microglobulin
BUN: blood urea nitrogen
BUO: bilateral ureteral obstruction

cAMP: cyclic $3',5'$-adenosine monophosphate
CAPD: continuous ambulatory peritoneal dialysis
CAVH: continuous arterio-venous hemofiltration
CEPD: continuous equilibration peritoneal dialysis
C_{H_2O}: positive free-water clearance
CMV: cytomegalovirus
CPK: creatine phosphokinase
CRF: chronic renal failure
CT: calcitonin
CT: computerized tomography
C_{UA}/C_{Cr}: uric acid clearance to creatinine clearance ratio
CVS: cardiovascular system
CyA: cyclosporin A

DDP: cis-diammine dichloroplatinum
DIC: disseminated intravascular coagulation
DIP: drip infusion pyelography
DNA: desoxyribonucleic acid
DPN: diphosphopyridine nucleotide
DSA: digital subtraction angiography

ECV: extracellular fluid volume
EFP: effective glomerular filtration pressure

FDP: fibrin/fibrinogen degradation products
FE_{Na}: fractional excretion of sodium
FSH: follicle-stimulating hormone
FT_4I: free T_4 index

GBM: glomerular basement membrane

GCP: glomerular capillary hydrostatic pressure
GFR: glomerular filtration rate
GOT: glutamic oxaloacetic transaminase

HCG: human chorionic gonadotropin
HD: haemodialysis
HGH: growth hormone
HRS: hepatorenal syndrome
HUS: Haemolytic uraemic syndrome

IC: intravascular coagulation
IPD: intermittent (periodic) peritoneal dialysis
IRI: immunoreactive insulin
ITP: intratubular hydrostatic pressure
IVP: intravenous pyelography

JGA: juxtaglomerular apparatus

K_f: glomerular capillary ultrafiltration coefficient

LDH: lactic dehydrogenase
LH: luteinizing hormone
LH-RH: luliberin
LtH: lactogenic hormone, prolactin
LVEDP: left ventricular end diastolic pressure
LVFP: left ventricular filling pressure

NE: norepinephrine
NSAID: nonsteroidal anti-inflammatory drugs

P_{cr}: plasma concentration of creatinine
PD: peritoneal dialysis
PG: prostaglandin
P_G: glomerular capillary hydrostatic pressure
PGI_2: prostacyclin
P_{Na}: plasma sodium concentration
PP: pancreatin polypeptide
PRA: Plasma renin activity
PTH: parathyroid hormone
PVS: peritoneal jugular venous shunt

RAS: renin-angiotensin system
RBC: red blood cells
RBF: renal blood flow
RCN: renal cortical necrosis
RDT: regular dialysis treatment
RES: reticulo-endothelial system
RFI: renal failure index
RNA: ribonucleic acid

RPF: renal plasma flow

rT$_3$: reverse T$_3$

SA: body surface area

S$_{Cr}$: serum concentration of creatinine

SLE: systemic lupus erythematosus

SNGFR: glomerular filtration rate in single nephron

SUN: serum urea nitrogen

SW: stroke work

TBG: throxine-binding globulin

TBM: tubular basement membrane

TBW: total body water

TGF: tubuloglomerular feedback

T$_{H_2O}^c$: negative free-water clearance

TPN: total parenteral nitrogen

TRH: thyroliberin

TSH: thyrotropin

TxA$_2$: thromboxane A$_2$

T$_3$: triiodothyronine

T$_3$I: T$_3$ binding index

T$_4$: thyroxine

UA: uranyl acetate

UAN: uric acid nephropathy

U$_{Cr}$: urinary concentration of creatinine

UN: uranyl nitrate

UNA: urea nitrogen appearance

U$_{Na}$: urinary sodium concentration

U$_{Osm}$: urine osmolality

U/P$_{Cr}$: urine to plasma creatinine ratio

U/P$_{Osm}$: urine to plasma osmolality ratio

U/P UN: urine to plasma urea nitrogen ratio

UUO: unilateral ureteral obstruction

VDM: vasodilator material

VIP: vasoactive intestinal polypeptide

ACUTE RENAL FAILURE

1. PATHOPHYSIOLOGY OF ISCHEMIC/TOXIC ACUTE RENAL FAILURE

Vittorio E. Andreucci

1 Introduction

An adequate blood flow through the renal cortex and sufficient hemodynamic pressure in the glomerular capillaries are both critical prerequisites for normal glomerular filtration. If either a fall in systemic blood pressure or circulatory failure (due to acute myocardial infarction or other heart disease) or reduction of blood volume (due to volume depletion secondary to hemorrhage or fluid loss from burns, vomiting, diarrhea, excessive sweating, etc.) occurs, renal perfusion is reduced and glomerular filtration decreased. Homeostatic mechanisms of body fluid conservation are then activated with an increase in antidiuretic hormone and aldosterone secretion and enhancement of reabsorptive activity of renal tubular epithelium. Reduction in urine output results, while the fall in the urinary excretion of nitrogenous end products increases plasma concentrations of urea and creatinine. In this "functional" phase of acute renal failure (ARF) [1] or extrarenal failure or renal functional insufficiency [2] (the so-called "prerenal azotemia" or "prerenal ARF"), the kidney is not damaged and tubular integrity is preserved: tubules, in fact, retain sodium avidly and concentrate urine; thus, urine becomes hypertonic, with low sodium concentration and with a markedly reduced fractional excretion of sodium (FE_{Na}). If volume depletion or blood pressure or cardiac output is restored to normal values, renal function rapidly returns to normal. If the reduction in renal perfusion (due to hypotension, sustained circulatory failure, or hypovolemia) is maintained or even worsened, an "organic" damage in the kidney ensues (the so-called "acute tubular necrosis," ATN, or "intrinsic ARF") in which oligo-anuria is associated with a reduction in the reabsorptive ability of tubular epithelium, resulting in isoosmotic urine and increased fractional excretion of filtered sodium ($FE_{Na} > 1\%$). If the patient survives (with the help of dialysis) despite the loss of renal function, a recovery phase ensues with an increase in urine volume, which usually occurs within 10 to 15 days, but sometimes 30 days or even more after the onset of oligo-anuria [3].

Hence, on the basis of our clinical experience, ARF may be considered a three-phase disease: (a) the initial functional phase ("functional ARF," improperly called "prerenal azotemia"), which is readily reversible; (b) the following irreversible phase of organic damage ("organic ARF", improperly defined as ATN); and (c) a phase of recovery of renal function. Nephrotoxic drugs (such as aminoglycoside antibiotics) may cause immediate organic damage (ATN) through a direct toxic effect on renal tubular epithelium.

In contrast with agreement on the above clinical observations, there is still controversy on the pathophysiology of ARF. Many theories in recent years have been usually seen as mutually exclusive. Even the terminology has been a matter of debate. Scientists who believe that tubular mechanisms play a primary role in the pathogenesis of ARF define the ARF due to ischemic or toxic factors as "acute tubular necrosis" (ATN); those who believe that vascular mechanisms are predominant define ARF as "vasomotor nephropathy" [4]. Actually, as we will describe later, vascular and tubular mechanisms are both involved in the pathogenesis of ARF.

Most of our knowledge of ARF derives from experimental studies in animals. Clinical studies of ARF are inadequate for understanding the fine mechanisms involved in the pathogenesis of the renal function shutdown. It is impossible, in fact, to follow in humans in a prospective trial the predisposing factors and the initiating stage of ARF, since usually physicians will face the problem when the failure is already established. Furthermore, many studies cannot be performed because they are unsuitable for human beings (e.g., micropuncture techniques, radioactive microsphere methods) or because for ethical reasons the patients cannot be exposed to unnecessary risks.

Thus, the experimental models of ARF appear to be very important because they reproduce the human forms and can be adequately studied.

Unfortunately, conflicting results have been obtained quite frequently not only from different models, but even from the same experimental model of ARF. Many reasons may account for this discrepancy in experimental data [5]:

a. Too many different nephrotoxins or ischemic methods have been employed, and the observation of similar renal abnormalities obtained by different means does not necessarily imply a similar pathogenetic mechanism.
b. The doses of nephrotoxin or the durations of the ischemic insult were frequently different so that resulting renal damage might differ.
c. The observation time intervals following the toxic or ischemic challenge were quite variable, while it is well known that factors responsible for the initiation stage of ARF are usually different from those responsible for the maintenance stage and for recovery.
d. The route of nephrotoxin administration was not always the same, the same toxin having been given intravenously, intramuscularly, or subcutaneously; this might

make the time course of the renal insult very different.
e. Different techniques, which are not always comparable, have been used to measure total and regional renal blood flow (RBF).
f. Changes in renal hemodynamics may be either the cause or the consequence of the renal insult, or may even be unrelated to the fall in glomerular filtration rate (GFR).
g. Species difference may exist as far as the sensitivity to nephrotoxins is concerned.

2   Heavy Metal-Induced ARF

Three major experimental models of ARF have been induced in animals by the use of heavy metals.

2.1   URANYL NITRATE-INDUCED ARF

The administration of uranyl nitrate (UN) in experimental animals (usually rats and dogs) intravenously, intraperitoneally, or subcutaneously, in doses ranging from 5 to 25 mg/kg b.w., usually leads to a polyuric ARF. A non-oliguric ARF has been similarly induced in rabbits by i.v. injection of uranyl acetate (UA) [6].

The fall in GFR and the increase in urine output and salt excretion observed both after UN [7] and UA [6] clearly demonstrate a depression in tubular reabsorption caused by uranyl ions, suggesting a functional impairment of tubular epithelium soon after uranium salt administration. The increase in urine output and in salt excretion occurred in association with a reduction in PAH extraction and was observed much earlier than the occurrence of tubular necrosis [6].

The uranyl cation of the uranium salts is responsible for renal injury at the tubular epithelial cell level. It seems that uranyl ions complex with phosphoryl, carboxyl, and sulphydryl groups of surface cell membranes without penetrating the cells.

Early after UN administration, minimal epithelial lesions are observed in proximal tubules in the form of cell swelling, vacuolation and mitochondrial degeneration. Only after 48 hours the proximal tubules exhibit, almost uniformly, a cell necrosis in the "pars recta" with shedding of epithelial cell cytoplasm into the tubular lumen [8, 9]. The convoluted portion of proximal tubules shows, at this stage, degenerative changes with swelling and granularity of the epithelial cytoplasm [9]. Many casts are seen in the proximal and distal tubules. In a similar fashion, when ARF was induced in rabbits by i.v. UA (mg/kg b.w.), minor lesions were observed in tubular cells even 24 hours following UA; only after three days were tubular necrosis and intratubular casts and debris seen by light and electron microscopy [6].

2.1.1 Renal Blood Flow (RBF) and Glomerular Filtration Rate (GFR)

Experiments in rats [10] and in dogs [8, 11, 12] have demonstrated that early (i.e., already in the first hour and throughout the first six hours) after the administration of UN, parallel falls in RBF and in GFR occur. Subsequently, 48 hours after UN, further decrements both in RBF and in GFR have been observed in rats [10] but not in dogs [12].

When the distribution of renal blood flow was studied in UN-treated dogs by Xenon 133 washout or Strontium 85-labeled microsphere techniques, a preferential cortical ischemia appeared to be the main contributor to the fall in RBF [8, 9, 13].

Since the course of ARF in dogs was not modified by the intrarenal infusion of PGE_2 (a vasodilator prostaglandin) and the fall in GFR occurred despite normalization of RBF [14], renal vasoconstriction has not been regarded as the main factor in initiating the impairment of renal function in this model of ARF [15]. In the experiments with PGE_2 [14], however, a low dose of UN (5 mg/kg b.w.) was used, so that the RBF even in the control (non-PGE_2-injected) kidney was not significantly decreased, as observed with greater doses (10 mg/kg b.w.) [8, 11]; but GFR fell anyhow, and this fall may be accounted for by factors other than changes in renal hemodynamics.

When renal vasodilation was induced in dogs treated with greater doses of UN (10 mg/kg b.w.), by the association dopamine + furosemide, an attenuation of the fall in GFR was obtained [16].

2.1.2 The Glomerular Capillary Ultrafiltration Coefficient (K_f)

The glomerular capillary ultrafiltration coefficient (K_f) is given by the product of glomerular permeability and the effective filtering surface area. Thus, a reduction in glomerular permeability and/or in the filtering area may decrease K_f. In rats with ARF secondary to UN administration (15 and 25 mg/kg b.w. i.v.), K_f is reduced within two hours of UN administration; and this reduction is proportional to the dose of administered UN [17].

A reduction in both diameter and density of endothelial fenestrae was observed, by scanning electron microscopy, within two hours of UN administration in rats [18]; this observation may well account for the decrease in K_f. A further progressive reduction in the endothelial fenestrae was detected with time (up to 17 hours after UN) and directly correlated with the progressive fall in GFR [18]. Loss of endothelial fenestrae associated with a decrease in K_f has also been observed in rats in vitro, in isolated glomeruli, 36 to 48 hours after UN administration [19].

Glomerular epithelial cells were normal two to six hours following UN (i.e., when ARF was already established). Changes of podocytes (swelling of foot processes; wide areas with primary, secondary, and foot processes no longer distinguishable) were initially observed 7 hours following UN and appeared more marked after 17 hours [18] and after 48 hours [9, 12]. It is possible that alteration in both endothelial and epithelial cells may lead to a greater reduction in the glomerular filtration area [18], thus contributing to the decrease in K_f in the maintenance stage of this model of ARF.

The demonstrated increase in intrarenal angiotensin II (AII) early (six hours) after UN administration [7, 20] may well account for the fall in K_f; possibly through the reduction in the endothelial fenestrae area. AII, in fact, is known to reduce K_f [21]. In favor of this hypothesis is the observation that salt-loaded rats (in which renal renin is suppressed) were protected against renal function impairment following UN administration; in these rats, the endothelial cell morphology was normal with a normal area of endothelial fenestrae. In salt-depleted rats (in which the renin-angiotensin system is markedly activated), GFR was greatly reduced; in these rats, a severe reduction in the area of endothelial fenestrae was observed [18].

2.1.3 Role of Tubular Obstruction in the Pathogenesis of UN-Induced ARF Early (six hours) in the course of UN-induced ARF, intratubular hydrostatic pressure (ITP) was not increased [10] (as expected behind a tubular obstruction), and no intratubular casts (obstructing tubular lumina) have been observed in histopathologic specimens [8, 22]. These observations argue against an early tubular obstruction in this model.

Obstruction of proximal and distal tubules by eosinophilic casts occurred 24 hours after UN administration, when widespread damage of tubular epithelium was present, with cell necrosis, mainly in the "pars recta" of the proximal tubules; these observations suggest an important role of tubular obstruction in maintaining rather than initiating UN-induced ARF [15].

It should be noted that values of ITP significantly lower than control, 8 to 24 hours after 10 mg/kg b.w. of UN, and not different from control 24 to 33 hours after 15 mg/kg b.w. of UN have been observed in rats [23]. Similarly, near normal values of ITP in the maintenance stage of UN-induced ARF have been reported in dogs [9]. These observations, however, do not rule out the possibility of an important role of tubular obstruction in maintaining ARF, since the concomitant fall in GFR may well account for normalization of ITP despite obstruction [24].

2.1.4 Role of the Backleak of Filtrate in the Pathogenesis of UN-Induced ARF Microinjection studies in rats with UN-induced ARF have given conflicting results. Thus, the microinjection of radioactive inulin into proximal convoluted tubules of superficial nephrons two to six hours after subcutaneous injection of 10 mg/kg b.w. of UN was followed by a complete recovery of the inulin from the urine of the microinjected kidney, exactly as it occurred in control normal animals [25]. A substantial recovery of microinjected radioactive inulin and mannitol from the urine of the contralateral

kidney has been reported, instead, at similar intervals but with 25 mg/kg b.w. of UN administered intravenously, suggesting an important leak of tubular fluid from the microinjected nephrons [17]. The site of the leak of inulin and tubular fluid was located beyond the superficial portion of the proximal tubules (pars recta?) since values of GFR measured in single nephrons (SNGFR) by micropuncture of early and late loops of proximal convoluted tubules were identical [17]. Since the tubular cell damage after UN administration has been shown to be proportionally increased with increasing doses [22], the described discrepancy in the microinjection studies is presumably related to the different severity of tubular damage [25]. Since ARF occurred with a relatively low dose of UN (10 mg/kg b.w.) and leak of inulin was not observed at this dosage, backleak of filtrate cannot be regarded as one of the predominant factors in promoting the ARF, as suggested by some authors [15]. Backleak may be important in the maintenance stage of ARF; thus 48 hours after UN administration (5 to 10 mg/kg b.w.) in dogs, only an average of 14% (against 97% observed in normal dogs) of microinjected inulin was recovered from the urine of the microinjected kidney [12].

2.1.5 Role of the Renin-Angiotensin System (RAS) in UN-Induced ARF Early (six hours) after UN administration in rats, significant increases in (a) plasma renin activity (PRA) [7, 20, 25, 26], (b) renin activity in the juxtaglomerular apparatus (JGA) of single superficial nephrons associated with a greater sodium chloride concentration in the distal tubule at the macula densa level [20, 25, 26], and (c) intrarenal AII [7, 20] have been demonstrated, reflecting activation of the RAS. When salt depletion secondary to the UN-induced natriuresis was prevented by oral sodium chloride replacement, PRA and intrarenal renin were not different from control values, and the animals were protected against ARF (i.e., creatinine clearance remained normal) despite a minor but still significant increase in intrarenal AII (attributed either to a direct effect of UN or to minor degrees of volume depletion) [7].

These observations suggest that (a) volume depletion has a critical role in the development of UN-induced ARF; (b) neither PRA nor intrarenal renin reflects the activity of the intrarenal RAS [20]. Changes in PRA and in intrarenal renin are, in fact, dissociated from those in intrarenal AII [20].

2.1.6 Summary

According to Hostetter et al. [15], reduction in K_f and backleak of filtrate are the predominant factors in promoting the fall in GFR in UN-induced ARF. While we may agree on the important promoting role of the fall in K_f, it is unlikely that passive backflow of filtrate can occur in early stages of this model since the fall in GFR precedes the tubular necrosis; the latter, in fact, occurs 48 to 72 hours after UN or UA administration [6, 13]. On the other hand, the backleak of filtrate has been demonstrated at an early stage, only with high doses of UN [17]; it also occurred in late stages of ARF induced by relatively low doses [12].

In my opinion the bulk of evidence in recent studies favors the view that renal vasoconstriction and reduction in K_f play prominent roles in initiating ARF secondary to the administration of uranium salts. Tubular obstruction and backleak of filtrate represent the prominent factors in maintaining this model of ARF.

2.2 MERCURIC CHLORIDE-INDUCED ARF

ARF may be induced in experimental animals (usually rats and dogs) following intravenous, intramuscular, or subcutaneous injection of mercuric chloride ($HgCl_2$). The doses used by different authors may vary greatly, ranging between 4 mg/kg b.w. [27, 28] and 12 mg/kg b.w. [29] in rats, and between 0.5 mg/kg b.w. [30] and 30 mg/kg b.w. [31] in dogs.

Low doses of $HgCl_2$ usually cause nonoliguric ARF, with an increase in urine output and in fractional excretion of sodium. It may become anuric with time, unless the animals are pretreated with beta-adrenergic blocking agents [32]. Anuric ARF may occur with large doses of $HgCl_2$.

$HgCl_2$ has a great affinity for protein-containing sulphydryl groups so that it interferes with both surface and intracellular enzyme ac-

tivities, thus affecting many cellular processes [33]. Furthermore, the formation of mercaptide with sulphydryl groups of plasma membrane proteins leads to alteration in cell permeability [34]. These lesions may lead to cell death.

Following $HgCl_2$ injection in rats, Hg^{++} deposition has been observed initially in endothelial cells of peritubular capillaries, then in glomerular capillaries and in epithelial cells of proximal tubules [35] with the highest concentration in the pars recta [28].

2.2.1 Ultrastructural and Histochemical Changes of the Proximal Tubules

When enzyme activities of the proximal tubules were studied histochemically in rat kidneys at different time intervals following subcutaneous injection of 4 mg/kg b.w. of $HgCl_2$ and data were related to ultrastructural changes, the following interesting observations were obtained [27, 28]. A decreased activity of alkaline phosphatase and 5'-nucleotidase of the brush border throughout the proximal tubule was observed within 15 minutes of $HgCl_2$ [27], when no morphological alterations were detectable by light and electron microscopy in any proximal tubular segment [28]; 15 minutes later the acid phosphatase activity was also reduced, both in the "pars convoluta" and in the "pars recta" of proximal tubules, suggesting incorporation of Hg^{++} into the lysosomes within the cells [27]. At this time and up to three hours following $HgCl_2$ injection, only slight ultrastructural changes were observed, affecting all portions of proximal tubules: dispersion of cytoplasmic ribosomes, mitochondrial matrix condensation, and, in the distal part, some increased endocytotic activity [28]. Not until 6 hours did severe morphological changes occur, but they were limited to the "pars recta": focal loss of brush border, swelling of mitochondria, dilatation of endoplasmic reticulum [28]. At this stage, the impairment of enzyme activities also included malic dehydrogenase, α-glycerophosphate dehydrogenase, and succynic dehydrogenase (expression of altered mitochondrial membrane function) but was again extended to all portions of proximal tubules [27]. After 24 hours, cell necrosis was finally observed, limited to the "pars recta" [28], while enzyme activities were severely reduced or even abolished in the "pars convoluta" [27].

Taken together these results show clearly that, in this model, cell necrosis does not begin, in the "pars recta," until long after six hours following $HgCl_2$ injection, i.e., when ARF is already initiated (see below), suggesting that necrosis in the "pars recta" is a relatively late event (possibly due to further accumulation of Hg^{++}), dissociable from the pathogenetic mechanism of ARF [28].

2.2.2 RBF and GRF

RBF has been found to be significantly decreased (by 20 to 40% from control values), both in rats [36] and in dogs [37], within the first three hours after $HgCl_2$ administration. A decrease in outer cortical blood flow parallel to the fall in total RBF has been found in rats [36] but not in dogs [37].

Changes in systemic hemodynamics have been invoked as responsible for the impairment in renal perfusion following $HgCl_2$ administration [38]. Thus, the decrease in RBF observed early after $HgCl_2$ has been attributed to the decrease in cardiac output because of the cardiotoxic action of $HgCl_2$ [39]. Since volume expansion by plasma has been shown to reverse both systemic and renal hemodynamic changes although plasma volume was not reduced, it has been postulated that following the reduction in cardiac output, reflex sympathetic changes occur with a consequent renal vasoconstriction [38, 39]. Hence, a fall in GFR might result both from the fall in cardiac output and from the resulting reflex vasoconstriction.

GFR does fall significantly early after $HgCl_2$ injection [36, 37, 40]. Its fall is actually more marked than that of RBF, suggesting that the impairment in renal function, in the early stage of this model of AFR, cannot be accounted for solely by the decrease in RBF [36]. When the decrease in RBF in dogs was, in fact, prevented by sustained renal vasodilation (by plasma volume expander plus phentolamine), GFR was still observed to fall following $HgCl_2$ i.v. injection [37].

RBF has been found to be normalized completely in rats 24 and 48 hours after $HgCl_2$, when GFR was still severely reduced [29, 36, 39]. In dogs, in contrast, RBF remained low, with a clear cortical ischemia, 48 hours after 2 mg/kg b.w. $HgCl_2$; but the normalization of RBF by extracellular volume (ECV) expansion did not modify the reduced GFR [41]. These observations suggest that renal functional impairment, even in the maintenance stage of this model, does not depend on the reduced perfusion of the kidney. Two possible mechanisms may account for the fall in GFR at this stage: First, a rise in preglomerular resistance may be accompanied by a fall in postglomerular resistance to such an extent as to keep total vascular resistance constant [29, 42]; this condition (not yet proven) would maintain RBF but would decrease the effective glomerular filtration pressure (EFP) [43], accounting for the fall in GFR. Changes in segmental vascular resistance due to the increased blood viscosity secondary to the rise in plasma fibrinogen levels, as demonstrated 24 hours after $HgCl_2$ injection in rats, have been proposed as the possible mechanism of this dissociated behavior of RBF and GFR [44]. Second, a reduction in K_f of glomerular capillaries may decrease GFR without affecting RBF.

2.2.3 Reduction in K_f

Some authors [37, 41] have proposed that a reduction in K_f plays a possible role in initiating $HgCl_2$-induced ARF, but this has not yet been investigated. A moderate, clear swelling of the glomerular epithelial structures, which has been observed by scanning electron microscopy early in the course of this model in dogs [37], is consistent with a reduction in K_f, as has been documented, for instance, in other models of heavy-metal-induced ARF (e.g., UN-induced ARF). Recent "in vitro" studies have demonstrated that $HgCl_2$ stimulates PGE_2 synthesis by isolated glomeruli and, even more notably, by rat glomerular cells in culture (both mesangial and epithelial cells) [45]. PGE_2 is known to decrease K_f [46] even though this effect seems to be mediated by AII [47].

A clear fall in K_f associated with loss of endothelial fenestrae on scanning electron microscopy has been observed "in vitro" in isolated rat glomeruli 36 to 48 hours after the administration of 10 mg/kg b.w. $HgCl_2$; K_f was normal after 4 mg/kg b.w. despite the occurrence of ARF [19].

2.2.4 Tubular Obstruction

The direct toxic effects of $HgCl_2$ on tubular epithelia [48] and the accumulation of cellular debris in the tubular lumen have suggested an important role for tubular obstruction in the pathogenesis of $HgCl_2$-induced ARF.

Intratubular casts, however, were not observed early after $HgCl_2$ injection [37]. Furthermore, i.m. injection of 12 mg/kg b.w. of $HgCl_2$ in rats was followed by normal ITP for 8 hours [40]; 3 to 10 hours [23] and 24 hours [49] after 4.7 mg/kg b.w. of $HgCl_2$ subcutaneously, the ITP was not significantly different from control values. With the decrease in urine flow, intratubular debris sometimes coalesced into potentially occlusive masses, but ITP remained normal; with tubular microperfusion at pressure only slightly higher than control ITP, these debris were seen floating free through the lumina of the distal tubular segment [49].

These observations appear to support the view that tubular obstruction is more a result rather than a cause of the decrease in GFR [4]; if it is playing any role, it is in maintaining rather than in initiating this model of ARF.

2.2.5 Backleak of Filtrate

The backleak of filtrate has been proposed, since 1929 [50], as the most important factor in inducing ARF by $HgCl_2$. Constant values of GFR in single nephron (SNGFR) measured in early and late superficial loops of proximal convoluted tubules [51] and no reabsorption of saline during split-droplet studies in superficial proximal convolutions [40] do not rule out the possibility of "leakage" of filtrate, since this "leakage" may occur more distally, for instance in the "pars recta," which is inaccessible to micropuncture [43]. The "pars recta" is actually the site where cell necrosis is observed following $HgCl_2$. It is, however, improbable that backleak of filtrate occurs in the early stage of this model since tubular necrosis of the "pars recta" was not seen until at least six hours after $HgCl_2$ [28].

The only reports with clear evidence of back-

leak of filtrate refer to microinjection studies performed 24 hours after mercury poisoning of rats: a significant recovery of radioactive inulin microinjected into superficial proximal tubules was obtained from the contralateral kidney, clearly suggesting a "leakage" of inulin through the damaged walls of microinjected tubules [52]. However, microinjection studies performed early (up to 12 hours) after 4.7 mg/kg b.w. subcutaneous injection of $HgCl_2$ in the rat exhibited a complete recovery of microinjected ^{14}C-inulin from the ureteral urine of the microinjected kidney [53].

Despite all these observations, some authors [15] still suggest that "backleak" of filtrate is the primary factor in inducing ARF. In my opinion, leakage of filtrate through the damaged tubular wall may play a role, if any, in maintaining rather than in initiating the $HgCl_2$-induced ARF.

2.3 CIS-DIAMINE DICHLOROPLATINUM (CISPLATINUM)-INDUCED ARF

A new experimental model of ARF in rats has recently been obtained by the intraperitoneal injection of 10 mg/kg b.w. of cis-diamine dichloroplatinum (cisplatinum) [54].

Serum creatinine increased significantly 72 hours after the injection, reaching a peak value after 6 days; ARF appeared well established at 96 hours.

In the maintenance phase of this model, urine output is not decreased (it is a nonoliguric form of ARF). Urine osmolality and U/P creatinine ratio are decreased, and FE_{Na} is significantly increased [54].

2.3.1 Urinary Excretion of Cisplatinum and Cell Toxicity

Cisplatinum, given intravenously, is excreted by the kidney; 76% of the administered dose (3mg/kg b.w.) in dogs is excreted within 48 hours; this percentage has been shown to increase to 95% in well-hydrated dogs and in dogs treated with mannitol [55]. Cisplatinum accumulates in the liver and in the kidney, the greatest renal content having been found in the corticomedullary junction [56].

The cellular mechanism of renal toxicity is not known. A decrease in sulphydryl groups has been reported in rat kidneys treated with cisplatinum, especially in the cytosol and mitochondrial fractions, that is, the fractions with the highest concentration of platinum [57]. Mercury and cisplatinum have similar effects on renal SH groups; the former, however, bind directly to sulphydryl groups, whereas cisplatinum has shown no direct interaction with SH of renal homogenates [57]. The fall in renal SH by cisplatinum has been suggested to be secondary to inhibition of oxidative metabolism [58].

2.3.2 RBF and GFR

Currently, there are no studies on the RBF in the initiation phase of cisplatinum-induced ARF, which occurs, in this model, prior to 48 hours after cisplatinum [59, 60]. Experimental studies on acute nephrotoxicity of other heavy metals ($HgCl_2$ and UN), however, suggest that a fall in RBF may occur in the initiating phase [61]. GFR is already decreased at 24 to 48 hours. [59, 60].

In the maintenance phase (96 hours post-cisplatinum), SNGFR in superficial nephrons is decreased by 38% from control while total kidney-GFR is decreased by 88%; a significant backleak of filtrate in the pars recta of the proximal tubules can clearly account for this disproportionate fall in total kidney GFR [54]. But the fall in SNGFR, measured by micronpuncture technique in tubular segments proximal to the sites of cell injury and backleak, suggests a primary fall in glomerular filtration that may be due to either a decrease in RBF or to a reduction in K_f or to both. The observed intravascular volume depletion 96 hours after cisplatinum, presumably secondary to subnormal fluid intake, diarrhea, and high urine output, could not account for the fall in superficial SNGFR, since ECV expansion by Ringer's solution reversed this depletion but did not affect the fall in SNGFR [54].

2.3.3 Reduction in K_f

K_f has not been measured in this experimental model. It may be presumably reduced in the maintenance phase, as mentioned, and possibly in the early phase as well.

2.3.4 Tubular Obstruction

Morphologic and microinjection studies appear in favor of some pathogenetic role of tubular obstruction in the maintenance stage of cisplatinum-induced ARF [59]. Morphologic studies have, in fact, demonstrated foamy casts, composed of cell debris, in proximal and also in distal tubules [54]. Microinjection studies gave a significantly reduced (40.2%) overall recovery of microinjected H^3-inulin from both kidneys (the recovery in control rats was 98.9%) [54], demonstrating a sequestration of the marker in the obstructed tubules.

2.3.5 Backleak of Filtrate

A great body of evidence has been gathered in favor of a primary role for a backleak of filtrate in maintaining the cisplatinum induced ARF:

a. Lissamine green (the dye commonly used in micropuncture to localize successive segments of proximal and distal tubules) [43] never appeared in the distal tubules when injected into the proximal tubules or intravenously, suggesting a transepithelial back-diffusion of the dye [54];

b. When H^3-inulin was microinjected into proximal convoluted tubules 96 hours post-cisplatinum, 26.3% (against 97.6% in control animals) was recovered from the ipsilateral kidney, and 13.9% (against 1.4% in control rats) from the contralateral kidney [54];

c. Morphologic studies, by light microscopy, transmission, and scanning electron microscopy, revealed only slight lesions at 6 to 24 hours, but severe cell injury and necrosis in the S_3 segments ("pars recta") (see note 1 on page 40 for an explanation of cell types) of the proximal tubules three to five days post-cisplatinum; they consisted of loss of brush border, cell swelling, mitochondria condensation, loss of intercellular junctional complexes, focal areas of tubular necrosis with tubular cell sloughing into the lumen, and, five days after cisplatinum, widespread tubular necrosis in the S_3 segments [54, 62]. This appeared to be the morphologic basis for the transtubular back-diffusion of glomerular filtrate, which occurs in the "pars recta" of proximal tubules, since S_1 and S_2 segments of proximal tubules did not show any morphologic abnormality [54, 62].

2.3.6 Summary Taken together, the available data on this model of ARF suggest an impairment of renal function that precedes the development of tubular necrosis. Only in the maintenance phase, with the widespread tubular necrosis of the "pars recta" of proximal tubules, may tubular obstruction by necrotic debris and backleak of filtrate across the damaged tubular epithelium account for the impairment of renal function [59].

Recent studies have demonstrated that rats made diabetic by streptozotocin injection exhibited complete functional and morphologic protection from cisplatinum-induced nephrotoxicity [60]. The mechanism of this protection is not known.

3   Gentamicin-Induced ARF

It is well established that aminoglycosides are nephrotoxic antibiotics. Most studies on aminoglycoside nephrotoxicity have been performed with gentamicin, usually in rats, but also in dogs. Thus, a model of experimental ARF has been created. It is a nonoliguric form when induced by the usual dose (40 mg/kg b.w./day i.p. for ten days), being oliguric only with very high dosages (200 mg/kg b.w./day for three days by subcutaneous injections) [63]. Actually, on a weight basis, the usual dose of gentamicin necessary to produce ARF in rats and dogs is many times greater than that employed clinically in human patients, but the difference is greatly reduced when the dose is referred to the body area [64].

Decrease in urine-concentrating capacity, increase in urine output and sodium excretion, tubular proteinuria, lysosomal enzymuria, alterations (early stimulation followed by depression) in organic acid transport by the proximal tubule—all precede the decrease in GFR [65], suggesting an early effect of the drug on tubular function.

3.1   FACTORS POTENTIATING AMINOGLYCOSIDE NEPHROTOXICITY

While the addition of cephalosporins increases the nephrotoxicity of aminoglycosides in human subjects, this does not occur in rats [66, 67], nor in rabbits [68]. Several reports even suggest a protection of rats by cephalosporins

(cephaloridine, cefazolin, and cephalothin) against aminoglycoside nephrotoxicity, presumably through a reduced concentration of the aminoglycoside in renal tissue [66, 67, 69–71].

Methoxyflurane anesthesia [72], salt depletion [73], dehydration [63], furosemide [63, 74] or indomethacin [75] administration, metabolic acidosis [76], and potassium deficiency [73, 77] have all been found to increase gentamicin toxicity.

The potentiating effect of salt depletion, dehydration, and furosemide on gentamicin nephrotoxicity has been attributed to the vasoconstriction secondary to contraction of extracellular fluid volume, which may be mediated by the RAS [63].

3.2   RENAL HANDLING OF GENTAMICIN

Gentamicin accumulates in renal tissue, mainly in the cortex, especially in animals maintained on a low sodium diet [73]. Its renal concentration is much greater than that attained in serum [78–80] and may become extremely high after repeated injections [81]. A significant renal concentration of the unchanged drug may persist for weeks after the end of the therapy despite morphological and functional recovery of gentamicin-induced renal lesions [63, 82]; detectable amounts of gentamicin have been demonstrated in the renal cortex even three months after treatment [80]. Thus, urinary excretion of aminoglycosides continues long after (up to three weeks) discontinuation of therapy [79, 80, 83].

Gentamicin is excreted, virtually unchanged, almost entirely by glomerular ultrafiltration [82]. It is undoubtedly also transported across the epithelium of the proximal tubules [84–86]. Recent studies by micropuncture techniques have, in fact, demonstrated that gentamicin undergoes net reabsorption in the proximal tubules of superficial nephrons and net secretion in the proximal tubules of juxtamedullary nephrons [86]; this may account for the proximal tubule cell damage commonly observed in gentamicin-induced ARF [63, 83, 87, 88].

Autoradiography of microdissected nephrons has demonstrated that gentamicin distribution within the kidney is limited to the proximal tubules, with increasing concentration going from the early part toward the "pars recta," where the largest amount of tritiated gentamicin was detected [89]. This observation seems to contrast with morphological studies of Schor et al. [90], who found only minor lesions in the "pars recta," the main lesions being located in the "pars convoluta" (see below).

It has been clearly demonstrated that in the proximal tubular epithelium the drug is not distributed throughout the cell, but accumulates within the lysosomes from which it is released by disruption of the lysosomal membrane [91].

The expansion of extracellular fluid volume with isotonic sodium chloride or sodium bicarbonate results in an increased excretion of gentamicin in the urine [85].

3.3 TUBULAR LESIONS

Ultrastructure studies in gentamicin-treated rats have shown tubular cell necrosis in the proximal tubules ("pars convoluta" and "pars recta") [83, 87].

Early lesions include an increase in number and size and degeneration of lysosomes (phagolysosomes) containing myeloid bodies (structures made of electron-dense, concentrically arranged membranes), cytoplasmic vacuolization, swelling of mitochondria, and focal losses of brush border [65, 81, 83, 87, 88]. Recent studies by Schor et al. [90] have shown that the mentioned tubular lesions were similar with gentamicin and with tobramycin and were limited to S_1 and S_2 segments of the proximal tubules while the S_3 segment (i.e., the straight segment of the proximal tubules) showed only an occasional focal increase in number of lysosomes. These tubular changes may then progress to focal or diffuse cell necrosis, depending on dose schedules and other predisposing factors, such as duration of treatment or salt depletion. Thus, while no tubular necrosis was observed in normal rats treated with 40 mg/kg b.w./day for 10 days [88, 90], focal necrosis in proximal convoluted tubules occurred with longer periods of treatment [92] or in salt-depleted rats treated with the same dosage [73] and in normal rats treated for three days with subcutaneous injection of doses as high as 200

mg/kg b.w./day [63]. In the latter study tubular necrosis was markedly increased in extent by 48-hour dehydration or by continuous i.v. infusion of furosemide (10 mg daily).

These and other experiments show clearly that the threshold for aminoglycoside nephrotoxicity in experimental animals is much greater (up to 60 fold) than in humans; but once the threshold is exceeded, both functional and morphological lesions in the kidneys are the same in men and in animals [65].

When epithelial necrosis has occurred, in the maintenance stage of gentamicin-induced ARF, tubular obstruction by cellular debris and backleak of filtrate through the damaged tubular wall may be expected. The occurrence of tubular obstruction has been demonstrated by the observed slight but significant increase in ITP in rats treated with 40 mg/kg b.w./day of gentamicin for 10 days [88] and in rats treated with 200 mg/kg b.w./day for 3 days [63]. The recent histopathologic findings of tubular occlusion by cellular debris in gentamicin-treated rats [92] appear to be in agreement with these functional data.

In rats, in contrast, no backleak of filtrate has been demonstrated with gentamicin-induced ARF using the microinjection technique [43]; in fact, the radioactive inulin microinjected into the proximal tubules was completely recovered from the urine of the microinjected kidney after treatment with 40 mg/kg b.w./day for 10 days [88].

3.4 PATHOGENESIS OF TUBULAR LESIONS

The reabsorption of aminoglycosides in proximal tubules and the toxic effect of these drugs on tubular epithelium seem to occur as follows. Aminoglycosides enter the tubular cells by adsorptive pinocytosis; that is, they bind to phospholipid receptors of the brush border membrane [93] and are then included into the cytoplasmic vacuoles arising from the pericellular membrane; they fuse with lysosomes and interfere with lysosomal digestion by inhibiting one or more lysosomal enzymes; this will result in impairment of the degradation of complex polar lipids and accumulation of phospholipids in the form of myeloid bodies [65, 91].

But lysosomes also contain enzymes capable of catalyzing cytoplasmic degradation; it has been demonstrated that aminoglycosides alter the permeability or cause disruption of lysosomal membrane so that liberation of both lysosomal enzymes and aminoglycosides occurs, which is responsible for the lysis of the cells [80]. These experimental observations may well account for the tubular cell injury and death observed after high doses of gentamicin. An inhibitory influence of gentamicin on mitochondrial respiration has also been demonstrated in "in vitro" experiments using mitochondria isolated from the renal cortex and from liver [80].

Interestingly, the phospholipid receptors of the brush border also represent a binding site for reabsorption of cationic proteins, amino acids, etc.; it is expected that the infusion of a basic amino acid, such as lysine, would competitively block aminoglycoside accumulation in the renal cortex [94]. This has been demonstrated in dogs treated with lysine intravenously: lysine reduced the renal cortical concentrations of both gentamicin and tobramycin [95]. It was therefore surprising to observe that i.v. infusion of lysine increases the toxicity of gentamicin in Fisher rats [94] and that a single dose of aminoglycoside, which is not toxic when given alone, becomes severely nephrotoxic when associated with lysine [94, 96]. More recently, experimental studies in rabbits and rats have clearly demonstrated that amino acid solutions infused intravenously during gentamicin or tobramycin treatment increase the severity and rapidity of onset of aminoglycoside-induced ARF [97]. Although these observations do not seem to deal with the possible beneficial effect of amino acids on recovery of patients with already established ARF, they have raised some concern about the possible hazard of parenteral nutrition with amino acids in patients under treatment with aminoglycosides [94].

A very strange and fascinating feature of gentamicin-induced ARF in experimental animals is the regeneration of tubular epithelium coexisting with tubular cell necrosis [65, 87, 98] and the recovery of renal function despite continuous administration of toxic doses of the drug [99, 100]. Even pretreatment with tobramycin [64], mercuric chloride [101], or dichromate [64] will protect renal function in rats against the nephrotoxicity of gentamicin, with only minor changes in GFR. These observations suggest that more susceptible tubular cells will experience cellular necrosis early in treatment with gentamicin; if the administration of the drug is continued, while more tubular cells will experience the necrosis, cellular regeneration will begin; for unknown reasons, however, the regenerating tubular epithelium, whatever the cause of tubular necrosis, has a much lower susceptibility to the toxic effects of gentamicin [64, 65]. Thus, the risk factor of advanced age in aminoglycoside nephrotoxicity [102] may be accounted for by the different susceptibility of tubular cells, in relation to their age, to the toxic injury of these drugs. Similarly, the relative tolerance of neonates to the nephrotoxic effects of gentamicin (nephrotoxicity of aminoglycosides in newborn infants is rarely described) may be due to a lower susceptibility of the young tubular cells to these drugs. A recent report, however, has suggested that this tolerance may be attributed to the prevalent distribution of RBF to the juxtamedullary cortex at birth; this will prevent gentamicin accumulation in the outer cortex and will spare the superficial and more numerous nephrons from gentamicin toxicity [103].

3.5 REDUCTION IN K_f

A significant fall in total kidney GFR as well as in SNGFR was observed at low dose (4 mg/kg b.w./day i.p. for 10 days) of gentamicin in rats when glomerular blood flow was still normal; the fall in SNGFR was accounted for by the reduction in K_f [88]. With a higher dose of gentamicin or tobramycin (40 mg/kg b.w./day i.p. for 10 days), total kidney GFR, SNGFR, glomerular plasma flow rate, and K_f were all reduced with a clear increase in the afferent and efferent glomerular arteriolar resistance [90]. There is still controversy as to whether the fall in K_f is accounted for by ultrastructural alterations in the endothelium of glomerular capillaries. Thus, in rats treated with different doses (4, 20, 40 and 120 mg/kg b.w.) of gentamicin for 10 days, a critical reduction in diameter, density, and area of endothelial fenestrae has been observed by scanning electron microscopy, the severity of which was proportional to the dosage [104, 105]; these alterations improved "pari passu" with recovery in renal function. Many authors, however, have denied such glomerular changes [87, 88, 90]. Conditions of tissue fixation and selection of photographic field have been implicated to account for the discrepancy in these observations [94].

But the decrease in K_f, as well as the decline in glomerular plasma flow and the attendant rise in arteriolar resistances, might be the result of the activation of RAS [90] since AII has been shown to induce these vascular effects [21, 106]. Even the observed alterations in glomerular endothelial cells may well be accounted for by the activation of RAS [104]. In favor of this hypothesis was the original observation that the chronic administration of the oral angiotensin I- (AI) converting enzyme inhibitor captopril for three days prior to and for ten days of gentamicin treatment was successful in offsetting the alterations in GFR, K_f, and glomerular plasma flow; the rats were protected against ARF, despite a persisting aminoglycoside-induced proximal tubular damage [90]. It has been suggested [90] that the beneficial effect of captopril might be due to its ability to increase the renal accumulation of bradykinin [107], the potent endogenous renal vasodilator and stimulator of intrarenal PG synthesis; it is known, in fact, that AI-converting enzyme is identical with kininase II, the enzyme which inactivates kinins.

However, the protective effect of captopril against gentamicin nephrotoxicity has not been confirmed in a more recent study [108]. In rats treated for 10 days with gentamicin, 80 mg/kg b.w./day, the association of oral intake of captopril in doses that appeared effective in suppressing AI-converting enzyme failed to ameliorate the fall in GFR, the tubular lesions, and even the glomerular changes due to gentamicin nephrotoxicity; the reduction of endothelial fenestral area after 10 days of gentamicin + captopril was, in fact, indistinguishable from that observed in animals receiving gentamicin alone [108].

It is possible that the crucial point for protection (which may account for conflicting reports of the effects of captopril) is to inhibit AI-converting enzyme activity prior to and not only during the gentamicin insult; once established, glomerular lesions may be relatively irreversible.

3.6 PROTECTION AGAINST AMINOGLYCOSIDE NEPHROTOXICITY

Taken together, the above observations suggest that the first toxic effect of aminoglycosides is a functional impairment of proximal tubules. Proximal tubular reabsorption is reduced, with the consequent increase in urine output and in natriuresis [109]. Reduction in K_f and renal vasoconstriction represent the factors directly responsible for inducing ARF; the occurrence of epithelial necrosis in proximal tubules will then cause tubular obstruction by cellular debris, which may maintain the ARF.

High salt intake and possibly captopril administration may afford partial functional protection without any amelioration in the proximal tubular damage [90]. This observation appears to support a role of RAS in the pathogenesis of the initiating phase of gentamicin-induced ARF, even though other systems seem to be involved; inhibition of the PG system by indomethacin, in fact, enhances impairment of renal function by gentamicin [75]; lower values of plasma and urinary kallikrein have been found in gentamicin-treated rats, suggesting an additional role for the kallikrein-kinin system [75, 105].

Functional protection was also surprisingly observed in diabetes insipidus rats with chronic high-rate water diuresis; this protection has been attributed to the prevention of tubular obstruction by the high tubular flow rate; on renal histopathology of these rats, in fact, tubular lumina were dilated without the tubular casts or debris detected in rats without diabetes insipidus similarly treated with gentamicin [92]. Complete protection against gentamicin nephrotoxicity was reported in rats with streptozotocin-induced diabetes mellitus, which was independent of the duration of the diabetic condition: both functional and morphological integrities were preserved, with very low renal cortical gentamicin content, after moderate and high doses of gentamicin [60, 92]; a clearly diminished toxicity was evident after massive dosage of the antibiotic [60]. This observation suggested an inhibition of the early cellular uptake of gentamicin in the proximal tubules of diabetic rats either because of the diabetes-induced osmotic diuresis (but this rate of osmotic diuresis does not protect against gentamicin nephrotoxicity) [110] or because of the enhanced glucose transport in the proximal tubules, which may somehow prevent gentamicin uptake (but saturation of proximal tubular glucose transport by i.v. infusion of glucose in dogs treated with gentamicin did not influence the renal cortical concentration of the antibiotic) [95], or because of an alteration in the phospholipid receptors of the brush border membrane [60, 92], which are necessary for gentamicin reabsorption [93].

4 Post-Ischemic ARF

Post-ischemic ARF has been induced in experimental animals (mainly rats and dogs) either by intrarenal arterial infusion of norepinephrine (NE) or by clamping of the renal artery. The resulting model of experimental ARF is analogous to human post-ischemic ARF, as observed, for instance, during circulatory shock or following renal transplantation. Both procedures, in fact, cause temporary interruption of blood flow through the involved kidney. When blood flow is restored, renal functional impairment persists; GFR is reduced and tubular reabsorption of the remaining filtrate is clearly decreased [111, 112].

Renal ischemia in rats for a duration of 25 minutes caused readily reversible renal damage [113]; when the ischemia lasted 60 minutes in rats [114] and 40 minutes in dogs [115], severe renal damage occurred and remained reversible after a few weeks; with two hours of ischemia in dogs, the renal damage was irreversible [115, 116]. Recovery from unilateral post-ischemic ARF produced by one hour of complete renal artery occlusion in rats has been improved by removal of the contralateral normally functioning kidney [117].

4.1 EFFECTS OF RENAL ISCHEMIA ON RBF AND GFR

4.1.1 Effects on RBF   Following the relief of 60 minutes renal artery clamping in rats, RBF has been found to be reduced to 40 to 50% of control because of an increase in intrarenal vascular resistance that lasted a day or two [118]. Soon after (1 to 2 hours), 30, 60, or even 120 minutes of intrarenal NE infusion (0.75 μg/kg b.w./min) in unilaterally nephrectomized dogs, RBF was reduced to only 75 to 80% of control values; the reduction was not statistically significant [111]. In two-kidney dogs, on the other hand, the NE infusion into one renal artery for 40 minutes decreased RBF to 40% of control at one hour after the infusion; RBF then recovered to 67% of control values by two to three hours [111, 119].

4.1.2 Effects on GFR   In rats anesthetized with inactin, GFR was reduced to 20 to 25% of control values after 60 minutes of renal artery clamping when measured 60 minutes following reperfusion [112, 120]. The fall in GFR was much greater (2% of the control) when using pentobarbital for anesthetizing the rats. This observation suggests that the choice and/or the dosage of the anesthetic agent may modify the renal response to the ischemic insult [120].

In unilaterally nephrectomized dogs, two hours after intrarenal NE infusion, creatinine clearance was reduced to 50% of the preinfusion levels following 30 minute-infusion, to 13% and 2% of the preinfusion levels following 60 and 120 minutes of NE infusion, respectively [111]. In two-kidney dogs, on the other hand, inulin clearance was reduced to 2 to 9% of control values one hour after 40 minute-NE infusion into one renal artery, remaining then unmodified up to 24 hours following the infusion [119, 121]. In the contralateral kidney, GFR was normal and remained unchanged throughout the study [119, 121]. The difference in RBF and in GFR between one-kidney and two-kidney dogs with unilateral NE-induced ARF may be attributed to the functional recruitment of nephrons in mononephrectomized animals, which would have become atrophic in two-kidney animals [117].

4.2 PATHOGENESIS OF RENAL PERFUSION IMPAIRMENT FOLLOWING RENAL ISCHEMIA

The reduction in RBF in post-ischemic ARF has been attributed (a) to endothelial cell swelling, (b) to afferent arteriolar constriction, and (c) to compression of peritubular capillaries by distended tubules.

According to the first theory, the endothelial cell swelling that is produced by ischemia would mechanically prevent the normal resumption of circulation in rats on relief of clamping (no-reflow phenomenon) [122]. This hypothesis was proven to be unreasonable because (a) the cell swelling has been observed as prevailing in tubular epithelia rather than in vascular endothelia [113]; (b) the hypoxic damage has appeared to be not self-perpetuating, as was predicted by the "no-reflow" hypothesis, a large fraction of RBF being, in fact, rapidly re-established with relief of clamping [123]; and (c) the "no-reflow" phenomenon does not occur in dogs [124].

A second theory has attributed the fall in RBF to afferent arteriole constriction. This constriction may be secondary to the activation of the RAS; in favor of this hypothesis is the increase of both plasma and intrarenal renin activities observed after renal artery clamping [125] and the effectiveness of beta-adrenergic blockade in reducing the severity of post-ischemic ARF [126]. Several experimental data, however, argue against this activation of RAS: (a) 45 minutes of renal ischemia significantly reduces GFR (to 24% of control) without activating renal renin [127]; (b) the chronic suppression of renal renin content in rats does not prevent the fall in GFR that follows the 45 minute-ischemia [127]; (c) restoration of RBF does not restore GFR [118, 121, 128]—in dogs with unilateral NE-induced ARF, in fact, the intrarenal acetylcholine infusion prior to NE resulted in complete normalization of RBF in three hours, but GFR remained drastically reduced (13% of control values) [121]. Intrarenal infusion of PGE prior to and during NE administration has a significant protective effect on renal function even though it does not prevent the early fall in RBF [14].

Despite these observations, it remains possible that renal vasoconstriction, whatever the cause, contributes to the fall in GFR. A near absence of net glomerular ultrafiltration pressure has been, in fact, observed three hours after NE infusion into a renal artery in two-kidney dogs [119]. Since a dramatic fall in GFR was already evident one hour after the infusion of NE—when ITP was normal and RBF was only 39% of control values and since lessening of renal vasoconstriction by mannitol was followed by increase in RBF, in GFR (despite the rise in ITP), and in glomerular capillary pressure (GCP)—a decrease in GCP seems to play a primary role in unilateral NE-induced ARF in two-kidney dogs[119]. It has been recently postulated that the increase in cytosolic calcium concentration in the smooth muscle cells of the afferent arterioles occurring in ischemic ARF may favor afferent arteriole vasoconstriction; and pretreatment with mannitol has been shown to prevent the increase in calcium content of mitochondria from renal cortex of dogs receiving 40 minutes of unilateral infusion of NE [129].

According to the third theory, the compression of peritubular capillaries by distended tubules of obstructed nephrons is the factor responsible for the fall in RBF. On the basis of direct simultaneous measurements of the both ITP and diameter of adjacent peritubular capillaries, in fact, an inverse relationship has been found between these two parameters in rat kidneys [130]. Thus, it has been suggested that tubular obstruction will increase ITP and cause dilatation of proximal tubules with the consequent mechanical compression of adjacent peritubular capillaries, thereby contributing to maintaining a reduced RBF in the post-ischemic kidney [120]. Blood flow in peritubular capillaries adjacent to dilated tubules with elevated ITP was, in fact, absent at the direct observation of the kidney surface in rats with post-ischemic ARF; it appeared resumed when ITP was reduced by aspiration of tubular fluid by a micropipette, to disappear again upon reintroduction of fluid within the obstructed tubule [120]. In favor of this theory is the observation that any maneuver that prevents or relieves tubular obstruction will accelerate recovery; and in clinical practice the nonoliguric type of ARF, which has presumably less tubular obstruction, has a better prognosis [120].

4.3 EFFECT OF RENAL ISCHEMIA ON K_f

The greater reduction in GFR than in RBF observed by many authors in post-ischemic ARF [111, 118, 119, 121, 131, 132] suggests that factors other than reduced renal perfusion may contribute to the post-ischemic renal function impairment.

A reduction in K_f may play an important role in post-ischemic ARF as observed in nephrotoxic ARF.

Changes in podocyte morphology (flattening of cell body and spreading of cytoplasma on glomerular capillaries with diffuse loss of foot processes) have been observed by scanning electron microscopy one hour after the vascular anastomosis in those transplanted human kidneys, which then exhibited post-ischemic ARF [133]. Similar shapes were obtained in rabbits following one-hour clamping of the renal artery [133, 134] and in two-kidney dogs following two hours of unilateral intrarenal NE infusion [116]. These changes, which could be reversed (rather than prevented) by clonidine by a still undefined mechanism [134], may represent the morphologic counterpart of a decrease in K_f.

K_f has not been determined "in vivo" as yet in post-ischemic ARF. It has been measured in isolated dog glomeruli following 90 minutes of renal pedicle clamping [135]; no significant change was noted at clamp release or one hour later, when RBF and GFR were both found significantly decreased; 24 hours after the acute ischemia, however, when RBF had returned to normal but GFR was still very low, K_f was significantly reduced. This suggests that a decrease in K_f may play an important role in maintaining a low GFR in ARF [135].

4.4 EFFECTS OF RENAL ISCHEMIA ON TUBULAR STRUCTURES

Following 20 minutes of ischemia (renal artery clamping) in rats and before relief of clamping, proximal tubules are collapsed, but distal and collecting tubules are patent; when renal ischemia is prolonged to 60 minutes, most distal tubules are also collapsed [112]. Upon relief of the clamping, proximal tubules reopen in two

minutes [112], clearly demonstrating a prompt resumption of glomerular filtration; furthermore, a dramatic reduction of tubular reabsorption occurs, even after only 20 minutes of renal ischemia, as demonstrated by the clear fall in urine-to-plasma inulin ratio [112].

4.4.1 Intracellular Effects of Renal Ischemia
When electrolyte concentrations in single proximal tubular cells were measured by electron microprobe, the intracellular concentrations of sodium and chlorine have been found significantly increased and the intracellular concentrations of potassium and phosphorus significantly decreased following 20-minute ischemia, and even more following 60-minute ischemia [112]. Similar effects, but much milder in degree (almost nil following 20-minute ischemia) were observed in single distal tubular cells [112]. On restoration of blood flow to the kidney, intracellular electrolyte composition rapidly returned to normal, being completely normalized within 60 minutes in proximal tubular cells and within 20 minutes in distal cells (following 60-minute ischemia) [112].

A severe intracellular acidosis has also been demonstrated in post-ischemic ARF [136–138]. A fall in intracellular pH occurs in rat kidney following as little as 5 minutes of ischemia, as demonstrated, in vivo, by ^{31}phosphorus nuclear magnetic resonance [137, 138]. The critical pathogenetic role played by the low intracellular pH was demonstrated by the progressive inhibition of tubular reabsorption and by the proportional fall in GFR in isolated kidneys perfused with solutions at decreasing pH (from 7.4 to 6.0): renal function was completely abolished with a 20-minute perfusion at pH 6.5, which is the pH observed in vivo in ischemic ARF [136] to be restored to normal upon reperfusion at pH 7.4 [137]. The degree of renal function impairment appeared correlated both with duration of exposure to acidosis and with severity of acidosis itself [138].

4.4.2 Morphologic Changes of Tubular Epithelium
Studies by light and electron microscopy have similarly demonstrated progressive epithelial damage in the proximal tubules with the increase in duration of ischemia, whether in-

duced by renal artery clamping [113, 139] or by intrarenal infusion of NE [111]. Thus, after 25 minutes of renal artery clamping in rats, the microvilli of the brush border are extensively lost by two mechanisms: (a) in most nephrons, by a coalescence of adjacent microvilli that are then incorporated into the cell cytoplasm; (b) in 10 to 25% of the nephrons, by their disintegration into fragments that are shed into the tubular lumen with intraluminal impaction of membrane-bound blebs; the latter will cause mild and transient tubular obstruction [113]. This 25-minute ischemia will cause a reversible injury in S_1 and S_2 cells, which recover completely within four hours; S_3 cells, however, undergo progressive irreversible cell damage and death with exfoliation into tubular lumina [113]. Following 60 minutes of renal ischemia, in the early reflow period, disintegration of microvilli and tubular obstruction by microvillar fragments and by extruded apical cytoplasm of epithelial cells occur, in nearly all nephrons, mainly in the "pars recta" of proximal tubules [139]. Cell necrosis will ensue, mainly in the "pars recta" of proximal tubules, which is more vulnerable to the ischemic injury [139], because of a greater susceptibility to ischemia of S_3 cells [113]; S_1 and S_2 cells, however, may also exhibit ischemic necrosis [139].

Similarly, in dogs, immediately after 30 minutes of intrarenal infusion of NE, proximal tubules (both "pars convoluta" and "pars recta") appear dilated, with their lumina containing eosinophilic granular material at light microscopy (a shape typical of human shock patients) and foamy blebs at electron microscopy [111, 139]. These features become more severe by increasing NE infusion time, with extension of dilatation to Bowman's space, which is filled with blebs and with appearance of cellular necrotic changes [111]. Two hours following NE infusion, the shape is identical but blebs are more numerous, extending also to distal nephrons [111].

Apparently, blebs in proximal tubules are formed in three ways: (a) extrusion of membrane-bounded cytoplasma into the tubular lumen followed by separation from the cell; (b) flux of cytoplasma into the brush border microvilli, which swell and then separate from the cells; and (c) intracellular formation of cytoplasmic bodies and their subsequent extrusion into the lumen [111].

All these experimental data clearly demonstrate the following points:

a. Twenty minutes of renal ischemia is sufficient to cause renal functional impairment, intracellular acidosis, and tubular cell depletion of adenosine triphosphate (ATP) with the consequent interruption of those cellular processes that require metabolic energy [112, 138]. In particular, since the low intracellular sodium concentration and the high intracellular potassium concentration are maintained by the energy-requiring Na/K pump located in the cell membrane, 20-minute ischemia will cause, in tubular epithelial cells a clear inhibition of Na/K pump with a consequent gain of Na^+ and loss of K^+ by tubular cells; an influx of extracellular fluid into the cells with cell swelling, increase in intracellular chloride, fall in phosphorus concentration, and decrease in dry weight fraction of the cells; intracellular acidosis; a significant decrease in the ability of tubular epithelium to reabsorb the tubular fluid [112, 140]. The reabsorptive capacity of proximal tubules has been found to be clearly depressed, with the Gertz split-droplet method [43] in experimental ARF [140].

b. A 25- to 30-minute ischemia is necessary to cause morphological aberrations in tubular epithelium, as observed by electron microscopy [111, 113, 139].

c. Impairment of tubular cell function appears to occur, after the ischemic insult, earlier than structural damage [140].

d. Proximal tubular cells are much more sensitive than distal cells to renal ischemia; almost no changes in cellular electrolyte composition or in epithelial morphology were, in fact, observed in distal tubules following 20- to 30-minute ischemia when significant changes were, on the other hand, evident in proximal tubules [112, 140].

e. Rapid and complete recovery occurs, upon restoration of RBF, both in cellular composition (in 60 minutes) [112] and in electron microscope appearance of tubular cells (in a few hours) [113].

f. Despite normalization of cellular composition after 60 minutes of reperfusion following 20- or 60-minute ischemia, tubular reabsorption is very low (low urine-to-plasma inulin ratio) [112].

It is also very interesting to note that following 18 hours of reperfusion after 60 minutes of renal ischemia, those disturbances in cellular electrolyte composition that had been normalized by 60-minute reperfusion appeared again in many tubular cells [112]. Similarly, morphologic studies have shown that while many tubular cells survive 60 minutes of renal ischemia [141], those irreversibly damaged cells appear necrotic only 12 to 24 hours following kidney reperfusion [142–145]. These observations have suggested that the partial reestablishment of RBF in the post-ischemic period (it remains approximately 50% of normal in the six hours following the ischemia) [118] is not enough to prevent the progression of the irreversible tubular cell damage [120]. On the other hand, impairment of mitochondrial respiratory activity (as mirrored by the failure of mitochondria from renal cortex of dogs with ARF to regulate cytosolic calcium concentration with a clear increase in their calcium content) was still evident after 24 hours of reperfusion following 40 minutes of intrarenal infusion of NE [129]. Mitochondria play an important role in producing the energy necessary for preventing influx into cells of those ions that are normally at greater concentration in the extracellular fluid and for maintaining cell volume, through the Na/K pump [129]. It has been postulated that the increase in cytosolic calcium content in tubular epithelial cells may contribute to cell necrosis [129].

4.5 TUBULAR OBSTRUCTION FOLLOWING RENAL ISCHEMIA

Morphologic and functional studies have given strong evidence in favor of an important role of tubular obstruction in the pathogenesis of post-ischemic ARF.

4.5.1 *Morphologic Studies*   As described above, after as little as 25 to 30 minutes of renal ischemia, swollen blebs may obstruct some proximal tubules [111, 113]. But 60 minutes of renal ischemia causes tubular obstruction in nearly all nephrons in the "pars recta" [139] or even in both the "pars recta" and the "pars convoluta" of proximal tubules [111].

It seems reasonable to conclude that in those nephrons in which the proximal tubular lumen is filled with swollen blebs, glomerular filtration no longer occurs, despite resumption and even normalization of RBF; in those nephrons in which filtration does not stop, blebs are flushed distally and may aggregate in the loop of Henle, distal tubule, and collecting duct, thus causing obstruction [111].

It has been observed that 24 hours after relief of renal artery clamping, luminal blebs in proximal tubules disappear, presumably because of autolytic processes; obstruction persists in distal nephrons [139] due to tubular casts made of cellular debris and Tam-Horsfall protein [112, 113]; on the other hand, Steinhausen and his associates [146] have directly observed, by stereoscopic microscope, the tubular obstruction caused by "proteinaceous material" in rat kidney with NE-induced ischemia.

4.5.2 *Behavior of Intratubular Pressure (ITP)* The ITP measured by micropuncture techniques in proximal tubules of rats has been found to be clearly increased up to 6 hours after 60 minutes of renal ischemia [23, 118, 131, 132, 147, 148], while microinjection of fluid into the proximal tubules required high pressures to flush out intraluminal obstructing casts [132].

In dogs with unilateral NE-induced ARF, ITP has been found normal one hour after NE infusion, presumably because of the severe fall in GCP [119]. When RBF increased, in fact, to 70% of normal values three hours after NE infusion, this recovery of RBF unmasked elevated levels of ITP [119]. Furthermore, microperfusion studies in these dogs at a tubular perfusion rate that does not modify ITP in normal dogs clearly increased ITP [119]. Both observations represent clear evidence of tubular obstruction.

It has been suggested that the beneficial effects on NE-induced ARF by maneuvers that increase urine flow and/or solute excretion (i.e., intrarenal infusion of PGE_2, bradykinin, furosemide, or mannitol) [14, 119, 121, 128, 149] may be due to flushing out of cellular debris and prevention of intratubular casts formation [15]. Thus, 30-minute pretreatment with 5% mannitol prevented the rise in ITP during microperfusion of tubules in dogs with unilateral post-ischemic kidney [119]. It is more difficult to explain the improvement in GFR obtained by pretreatment with propranolol in rats 1 to 3 hours after 60-minute renal artery clamping; since RBF did not increase, while ITP increased less than in unpretreated rats, it has been stated that attenuation of tubular obstruction by the drug (by a still unknown mechanism) may account for the partial protection against post-ischemic ARF [148].

From 22 to 24 hours after the acute ischemia, ITP in rats has been found again to be normal although GCP was reduced, suggesting afferent arteriole vasoconstriction. The acute ECV expansion with rat plasma or isotonic saline rapidly reversed this vasoconstriction, normalizing RBF and GCP; but oliguria persisted and the ITP increased again, clearly suggesting a key role for tubular obstruction in maintaining ARF [118].

ITP in proximal tubules was still greater than normal one week following 60 minutes of one renal artery clamping in rats, but was completely normal at two weeks [114].

4.5.3 Microinjection studies Microinjection studies in rats following 60-minute clamping of the renal artery have shown an overall 72% recovery from the urine of both kidneys of the inulin microinjected into proximal tubules of the ischemic kidney. Most of the missing inulin was recovered from the parenchyma of the injected ischemic kidney, clearly showing a sequestration of the marker in the obstructed tubules [139].

Similar results were obtained in dogs. While in normal animals, 94% of radiolabeled inulin was recovered from the microinjected kidney

within three minutes, in dogs with unilateral NE-induced ARF, three hours after NE infusion, 20 minutes were necessary for a 70% recovery of microinjected inulin from the ipsilateral kidney, while no radioactivity was detectable in the contralateral urine [119]. This delayed incomplete excretion of ^{3}H-inulin represents further evidence of tubular obstruction.

These observations clearly demonstrate that tubular obstruction must play a role in the pathophysiology of this model of ARF. But the occurrence of post-ischemic ARF in rats [23] and in dogs [119] with only 40 to 45 minutes of renal ischemia—when a significant fall in GFR (during the first few hours after the relief of the clamping in rats or the end of NE infusion in dogs) is associated with no significant change in ITP—clearly suggests that obstruction cannot be the primary initiating pathogenetic factor but may only contribute to renal failure already in existence [23, 119]. Tubular casts may accumulate when GFR is already low for other reasons.

4.6 EFFECT OF RENAL ISCHEMIA ON URINE OUTPUT

Actually, both a low (oliguric ARF) [118] and a high urine output (nonoliguric ARF) [23, 112, 131] have been reported after unilateral renal artery clamping in rats for 60 minutes. It has been suggested that this difference was due to the choice of the anesthetic agent, pentobarbital in the former study, inactin in the latter [120]. Thus, when the effects of these two anesthetic agents were evaluated in rats with post-ischemic ARF (60 minutes of renal artery clamping), the following results were obtained [120]: rats anesthetized with pentobarbital exhibited, in the post-ischemic period, very low RBF, GFR, and urine output (oliguric ARF); all tubules were obstructed, with very high ITP. Rats anesthetized with inactin, instead, exhibited minor reduction in RBF and in GFR with a dramatic increase in urine output (nonoliguric ARF); only two-thirds of proximal tubules were dilated, with elevated ITP; the remaining one-third had normal caliber with a maintained flow of tubular fluid. These observations suggest that inactin has a protective effect on tubular cells that reduces the number of nephrons with tubular obstruction; furthermore, there is an inverse relationship between the number of nephrons with tubular obstruction and the urine output.

4.7 BACKLEAK OF FILTRATE IN POST-ISCHEMIC ARF

Tubular lesions, as mentioned, already occur after 25-minute ischemia and their severity increases with the increase in ischemic time. Severe cellular damage may cause a back-diffusion of filtrate from the tubular lumen toward the peritubular capillaries. Thus, radioactive inulin microinjected into proximal tubules of post-ischemic rat kidney was recovered from the urine of the contralateral kidney [131, 139] in a proportion that increased progressively with the increase in duration of the ischemia; the recovery was in fact insignificant after 15 minutes of ischemia, modest (11%) after 25 minutes, and severe (35%) after one hour of complete ischemia [139]. When microperfusion with inulin solution was performed through micropipettes placed in proximal tubules of rats, inulin recovery from distal tubules and from ureteral catheter was significantly reduced one to four hours after clamping of a renal artery for 45 to 60 minutes [53].

The backleak of filtrate has also been visualized by histochemical studies. Thus, when horseradish peroxidase (m.w. 40,000) was injected intravenously or microinjected into proximal tubules in rats two hours after relief of the arterial occlusion, the marker was observed, by histochemical reaction, to diffuse through the plasma membranes and cytoplasm of damaged epithelial cells and enter the peritubular interstitium and capillaries; however adjacent cells in the same tubule were impermeable to horseradish peroxidase (as normally observed in kidneys not subjected to ischemia), indicating a difference in cell damage among cells of the same nephron as well as among nephrons of the same ischemic kidney [139].

Backleak of inulin has been demonstrated, by clearance technique, even in humans with ARF following open-heart surgery. Myers et al. [150–152] have, in fact, observed in these patients a fractional clearance of neutral dextran/

inulin greater than one. Since dextran molecules are larger than inulin molecules, these results have been regarded as a demonstration of a greater backleak of the smaller molecules (inulin) across the damaged tubular epithelium.

That tubules may become leaky after an ischemic insult has been demonstrated also by microperfusion studies "in vitro." Thus, microperfusion of isolated tubular segments dissected from kidneys of rabbits with post-ischemic ARF has shown (a) an impaired transport capacity, as measured by fluid reabsorption, mainly in the convoluted and straight proximal tubules, but also in the thick ascending limb of Henle's loops and (b) a clear inulin leak in proximal straight tubules of juxtamedullary nephrons. Furthermore, the microperfusion of the isolated ischemic segments frequently resulted in the formation of cellular debris in the lumen due to separation of surface epithelium from basement membrane during microperfusion [153].

Taken together, all these observations appear in favor of an important role for the backleak of filtrate in maintaining ARF once severe damage to the tubular epithelium has occurred.

4.8 RECOVERY FROM POST-ISCHEMIC ARF

It has been stated that renal vasoconstriction, tubular obstruction, and backleak of filtrate can be demonstrated for at least one week following ischemic insult [147].

When the pattern of recovery from post-ischemic ARF (60 minutes of one renal artery clamping in rats) was evaluated for as long as eight weeks, the following data were obtained [114]. One week following the ischemia, GFR was 2% of control, RBF 26% of control values; quite numerous intratubular casts were observed both in the cortex and in the renal papilla; ITP in proximal tubules was higher, GCP and afferent EFP much lower than normal; urine output was very low and urinary sodium concentration (U_{Na}) very high, with a fractional excretion of sodium (FE_{Na}) of 10%.

Two weeks following the ischemia, GFR was significantly increased from 2 to 22% of control values, while the rise in RBF was only slight (from 26 to 31%) and not significant; intratubular casts were greatly reduced in number; ITP was completely normalized while GCP remained unchanged (when compared to one week earlier) so that afferent EFP was increased, accounting for the increase in GFR. The tendency of a return to anatomical and functional integrity of tubular epithelium at this stage is further demonstrated by (a) the significant reduction of U_{Na} and FE_{Na}; (b) the normalization of urine output, and (c) the complete recovery from the ipsilateral final urine of ^{3}H-inulin microinjected in proximal tubules.

From the second to the eighth weeks, the rise in GFR was gradual and paralleled the increase in RBF and in GCP, the latter accounting for the rise in afferent EFP (ITP remaining normal); meanwhile U_{Na} and FE_{Na} completely normalized.

Taken together these data suggest a biphasic pattern in the recovery from post-ischemic ARF: in an early phase, relief of tubular obstruction and recovery of tubular integrity occur, thus accounting for a brisk improvement of renal function; in a later phase, the release of preglomerular vasoconstriction will allow the complete normalization of renal function [114].

5 Glycerol-Induced ARF

Quite frequently in clinical practice, massive intravascular hemolysis or extensive skeletal muscle necrosis has been found to be associated with ARF. This observance has led to the belief that either hemoglobin and myoglobin or their derivatives may be nephrotoxic—hence, the research for experimental models of myohemoglobinuric ARF.

ARF resulting from intravenous injection of methemoglobin in rats has been studied by some authors. But glycerol-induced ARF is undoubtedly the most widely used experimental model of ARF resembling the human form of pigment-induced ARF [33].

The intramuscular or subcutaneous injection of hypertonic (50%) glycerol solution (usually 10 ml/Kg b.w.) elicits a myohemoglobinuric ARF in rats, especially in conditions of dehydration [154], but also in chronically salt-loaded animals [155]. A half hour after glyc-

erol injection, the rats pass deep burgundy red urine containing both myoglobin and hemoglobin [154]. Urine volume is clearly increased three hours after the injection [7] and even more after 24 hours, at least in nondehydrated rats [154, 156].

It is well demonstrated that subcutaneous injection of glycerol in rats or rabbits causes intravascular hemolysis and hemoglobinuria. Intramuscular injection also causes muscle cell necrosis, local fluid accumulation contributing to the contraction of ECV, and myoglobinuria. Impairment of renal function may result with an initial ischemic component due to ECV contraction, in addition to the nephrotoxic effects leading to pathological lesions of acute tubular necrosis.

5.1 RBF AND GFR IN THE INITIATION STAGE OF GLYCEROL-INDUCED ARF

Within 10 minutes after i.m. injection of glycerol, RBF is already clearly decreased [157], and the microscopic observation of the kidney surface shows a significant decrease in peritubular capillary blood flow, virtual cessation of glomerular ultrafiltration, and tubular collapse [154, 158, 159]. Thereafter, the appearance of the kidney surface improves [158, 159], but RBF further decreases to reach very low values two to three hours following injection [157, 160, 161] with severe cortical ischemia [157, 160].

During these first hours of ARF, a decrease in cardiac output and an increase in systemic blood pressure [163–165], in total peripheral resistance [162–165] and in renal vascular resistance [162–165] have been reported. In sequential studies of glycerol-induced ARF in rats, a significant parallel fall in RBF and GRF two hours after glycerol administration has been observed; the i.v. infusion of Ringer solution, three to six hours after glycerol, normalized both RBF and GFR [166]. Similar salutary effects of saline combined with mannitol have also been reported [156, 159, 161]. In particular, on microscopic observation, the appearance of the kidney surface soon after glycerol injection in rats pretreated with mannitol, saline, or both mannitol and saline was quite different from that of unpretreated animals: the immediate decrease in peritubular capillary blood flow and the consequent pallor of the kidney surface were prevented, although peritubular circulation deteriorated one to two hours later [159].

These observations suggest that ECV expansion or prevention of ECV contraction may partially protect against glycerol-induced ARF.

5.1.1 Plasma Volume Reduction in plasma volume has been demonstrated in rats treated with glycerol [154, 167], and a reduced plasma volume (as it occurs after 24 hours of water deprivation) prior to glycerol injection has been proven to increase the severity of ARF [154]. Thus, not only saline infusion [156, 166] but even 1% saline (rather than water) drinking [167], during 24 hours after glycerol injection, was sufficient to greatly protect the rats against renal functional impairment; and this protection was coincident with and has been attributed to a normalization of plasma volume [167]. Failure of protection occurred when saline drinking was performed before rather than after the glycerol injection [168]. On the other hand, protection was obtained when saline drinking preceded *and* also followed glycerol insult; in this case cortical blood flow rapidly increased up to 85% of the control value within the first 10 hours, whereas it remained very low (one-fourth of control value) for as long as 24 hours after the injection, in water-drinking animals [160]. It has been suggested that the decrease in plasma volume, observed in the initial stage of glycerol-induced ARF, may cause a reduction in cardiac output [162, 163] (through a decreased venous return) and a reflex sympathetic change in peripheral resistance (including renal resistance). On the other hand, a severe volume depletion may also cause an increased release of vasopressin, since its plasma concentration has been found elevated in this model of ARF [164]. Vasopressin seems to play some role in causing renal vasoconstriction since glycerol injection in Brattleboro rats (with hypothalamic diabetes insipidus) was not followed by a marked rise in renal vascular resistance as in normal rats (although it did not prevent the subsequent occurrence of ARF) [169]. It must

be admitted, however, that a specific competitive antagonist of vascular effects of vasopressin has not prevented the increase in renal vascular resistance that followed glycerol injection in normal rats [165].

Reduction in cardiac output and renal vasoconstriction, therefore, seem to be responsible for the initial decrease in RBF [38], which is undoubtedly the primary cause of the fall in GFR in the initiation stage of this model of ARF. Plasma infusion, in fact, has been shown to significantly increase cardiac output and restore RBF [162].

Thus, the initiation stage of glycerol-induced ARF, which is partially reversible by ECV or plasma-volume expansion, appears as a "functional" ARF, with a marked reduction in plasma volume, [162] and in RBF. FE_{Na} has been found, in fact, far less than 1% [166], which is consistent with a "functional" phase of ARF (prerenal ARF).

The primary role of intrarenal hemodynamic changes in the pathogenesis of glycerol-induced ARF is further supported by the observation that recent (48 hours) uninephrectomy partially protects the rats against ARF [163, 170]. Thus, the fall in RBF and GFR and the increase in renal vascular resistance and in systemic blood pressure were much less pronounced in 48-hour uninephrectomized rats than in two-kidney sham-operated animals [163]. This protection was attributed to the increase in RBF and GFR that followed the previous reduction of renal mass [170].

5.1.2 Role of Renin-Angiotensin System (RAS) The observed decrease in RBF and increase in renal vascular resistance have been attributed, also in this model of ARF, to an activation of the RAS.

Some experimental data appeared to support this hypothesis. Thus, long-term salt loading, known to reduce cortical renin content, appeared to protect the rats against glycerol-induced ARF despite the occurrence of tubular necrosis [160, 171–174]. Conversely, dietary salt deprivation, known to increase intrarenal renin, appeared to increase the severity of this experimental model of ARF [172].

Recent studies, however, have failed to

demonstrate, directly and indirectly, an activation of the RAS in the glycerol-induced ARF:

a. Long-term (one to three months) saline loading (1% saline drinking or daily i.p. injection of 20 ml of 0.9% saline) has been shown not to protect rats against glycerol-induced ARF, although it decreased BUN by increasing urea clearance; inulin clearance was, in fact, severely reduced 24 and 48 hours after glycerol injection [155].
b. Immunization with antibodies against renin or AII [168, 173] and the use of converting enzyme inhibitors or AII blockers [175–177] have failed to protect the rats against the renal damage by glycerol.
c. If intrarenal RAS plays an important role in the development of glycerol-induced ARF, a kidney with high renin content is expected to be more susceptible to the development of ARF by glycerol. The Goldblatt model of renovascular hypertension provided an excellent example for such a situation: rats maintained for a limited time (17–23 days) with a partial clamping of one renal artery had, for at least 24 hours after clip removal, a renin content markedly increased in the previously clamped kidney and suppressed in the controlateral kidney; yet glycerol injection caused a functional impairment of comparable degree in both kidneys (reduction of GFR to 25% of control values 24 hours after glycerol injection). This experiment by itself, however, does not exclude an important role of intrarenal AII, since it has been demonstrated that unilateral renal artery clipping does not necessarily suppress intrarenal AII in the contralateral kidney even though kidney renin is suppressed [179].
d. Three hours following i.m. injection of hypertonic glycerol in rats, a myohemoglobinuric ARF is already established, with a GFR clearly decreased; yet plasma renin activity, kidney renin concentration, and intrarenal AII are all normal [7, 20, 180].
e. Intrarenal renin and intrarenal AI and AII have been found normal early (one to six hours) in the course of glycerol-induced

ARF in rats; an increase in their renal concentration occurred only 17 hours after glycerol injection, that is, much later than the fall in renal function [180].

Thus, even though the literature has shown some discrepancies on the behavior of both PRA and renal renin in glycerol-induced ARF, these observations, taken together, suggest that ARF may occur in rats without any evidence of activation of either circulating or intrarenal RAS [7]. An activation of RAS may probably only contribute to the vasoconstriction early in the course of glycerol-induced ARF; it is, however, not essential for the occurrence of ARF.

5.1.3 Role of Prostaglandins (PGs) It has been recently suggested that PGs may play a key role in the pathogenesis of glycerol-induced ARF. It is well demonstrated that the continuous i.v. infusion of PGE_2, begun just before [181] or immediately after [156] the subcutaneous injection of glycerol, reduces the severity of ARF in rats, presumably because of its vasodilator effect on the afferent arterioles. These findings are consistent with the observation that indomethacin exacerbates the glycerol-induced ARF, presumably through an inhibition of PG release [182]. But the important role of the PG system is due not only to vasodilator PGs—which may counterbalance the vasoconstricting effects of AII so that the minor release of the former may leave unopposed the vasoconstriction induced by the latter—but is also due to an increased production of vasoconstrictor PG, which may potentiate the effect of AII. Recent studies, in fact, have demonstrated that thromboxane A_2 (TxA_2) may play an important role in increasing the vascular resistance in this model of ARF [183, 184]. Thus, the kidneys of rabbits treated with subcutaneous glycerol exhibited, 24 hours after the injection, an increased capacity to produce TxA_2 [183]. These findings have suggested a possible alteration in the relative proportion of vasodilating and vasoconstricting PGs in glycerol-induced ARF in rabbits with a predominance of vasoconstrictor substances; hence, the protective effect observed with i.v. infusion of

PGE_2 [156, 181] may be due to a "normaliza-tion" of that proportion [183].

It has also been suggested that the protective effect of saline against this model of ARF is PGE_2-mediated since it is blunted by indo-methacin and restored by PGE_2 administration [156]. There are, indeed, some experimental data demonstrating that saline infusion induces release of PGs [185]; this may be the mecha-nism by which saline loading elicits partial protection on the initial "functional" stage of this model of ARF. But it remains to be estab-lished why indomethacin, which exacerbates glycerol-induced ARF [177] presumably through a reduction in PGE_2 release, does not reduce also TxA_2 production since the drug is, indeed, an inhibitor of cyclooxygenase. Thus, either TxA_2 is not the only vasoconstricting factor involved in glycerol-induced ARF (more probable hypothesis) or indomethacin does not inhibit PGE_2, PGI_2, and TxA_2 to the same extent [186]. Further studies using selective inhibition of different pathways of endoperox-ide metabolism are therefore necessary [183].

5.2 RENAL FUNCTIONAL IMPAIRMENT IN THE MAINTENANCE STAGE OF GLYCEROL-INDUCED ARF

When the experimental animals were treated with i.v. infusion of Ringer 12 to 18 hours after glycerol injection, RBF was normalized but GFR remained low [166]. Similarly, other authors have found that RBF is not signifi-cantly reduced in conscious rats during the maintenance phase of glycerol-induced ARF. Thus, the fall in RBF is important in initiating but not in maintaining ARF due to glycerol [162, 174].

Actually, 24 hours after glycerol injection in rats, while RBF is normal, GFR is reduced to approximately 25% of control values, and frac-tional excretion of water and salt is significantly increased [178, 187] with FE_{Na} much greater than 1% [155, 166], suggesting an "organic" ARF (ATN).

Other factors should therefore account for the low GFR in the maintenance phase: these may include increase in blood viscosity, de-crease in K_f, tubular obstruction, and backleak of filtrate.

5.3 EFFECT OF GLYCEROL ON BLOOD VISCOSITY

It has been demonstrated that blood viscosity is increased 24 hours after glycerol injection; this increase in blood viscosity has been attrib-uted to the observed higher concentration of plasma fibrinogen and may account for changes in GFR, despite normal RBF, through changes in segmental vascular resistance [44]. The marked increase in serum and urinary fi-brin(ogen) degradation products (FDP) ob-served in rats unprotected but not in those pro-tected (i.e., made refractory by prior ARF challenge) against glycerol-induced ARF [188] seems to support the theory of an essential role of fibrinogen utilization in the pathogenesis of this model of ARF. There is, however, the al-ternative possibility that it represents the result rather than the cause of ARF.

5.4 EFFECT OF GLYCEROL ON K_f

K_f has not been measured as yet in glycerol-induced ARF. The demonstrated elevation of plasma levels of arginin vasopressin in this model of ARF [164], however, and the capa-bility of arginin vasopressin for reducing K_f in normal animals [189] by triggering glomerular mesangial cell contraction suggest that K_f may be reduced.

Alterations in glomerular morphology may also indirectly suggest the existence of K_f changes early in the course of this model of ARF. Thus, swelling of both epithelial and mesangial cells has been observed by electron microscopy in rat glomeruli 30 minutes to 16 hours after glycerol injection, but not at 24 hours [190].

5.5 EFFECT OF GLYCEROL ON TUBULAR STRUCTURES

Twenty-four hours after i.m. injection of 10 ml/Kg b.w. 50% glycerol solution in rats, proximal tubular function is severely impaired (depression of glucose, bicarbonate, and phos-phate reabsorption, of PAH secretion and ex-traction, of the activities of Na-K-ATPase and other enzymes of the proximal tubules); at the same time severe tubular damage is observed on renal histology by light and electron mi-croscopy [191]. Tubular damage is more diffuse and severe in the proximal convoluted tubule of superficial and deep nephrons, has a patchy distribution in the "pars recta," and is minor in the thick ascending limb. Epithelial lesions in proximal tubules consist in loss of brush border, cytoplasmic vacuolization, and mitochondrial swelling [191]. Tubular cell debris and pigment casts are observed in the proximal convolution, in the "pars recta," in the loop of Henle, and even in the collecting tubules, which exhibit, however, an intact epithelium [190, 191].

5.6 TUBULAR OBSTRUCTION FOLLOWING GLYCEROL INJECTION

It has been stated that tubular obstruction by pigmented casts, as observed in histologic preparations, has to play an important pathogenetic role in the initiation stage of myohemoglobinuric ARF [15]. No experimental data, however, can support such a view. Thus, in the first three to four hours following glycerol injection, proximal tubules have been observed either completely collapsed or with such a low ITP as to make very difficult or even impossible any fluid collection by micropuncture technique [158, 159]. Similarly, even 18 to 26 hours after glycerol injection, 75% of proximal tubules had neither a visible lumen nor a detectable intraluminal flow, while in the remaining puncturable tubules, ITP was lower than normal [159]. When ITP was evaluated every day for as long as six days after glycerol injection in rats, the daily mean values were found constantly to be normal [192]. Elevated ITP values in dilated proximal tubules were found only in a minority of the nephrons in rats with methemoglobin-induced ARF.

Taken together these observations do not support the common belief that pigment-induced ARF is caused by tubular obstruction.

5.7 BACKLEAK OF FILTRATE FOLLOWING GLYCEROL INJECTION

No backleak of inulin was detected 30 minutes to 24 hours after glycerol administration in the rat [158]. Very slight backleak of inulin was observed, by microinjection experiments, in rats with methemoglobin-induced ARF [23]. These observations suggest that the role of backleak of filtrate, if any, should be minor in the pathogenesis of myohemoglobinuric ARF.

5.8 SUMMARY

Taken together, these experimental data suggest that hemodynamic changes are responsible for the initiation stage of glycerol-induced ARF, which appears as a "functional" failure secondary to volume contraction. Vasoconstriction of afferent arterioles due to sympathetic stimulation, AII, and/or TxA_2 secretion may well account for the fall in RBF and GFR constantly observed in the early stage. ARF is then maintained despite normalization of RBF. This may occur because of an increase in blood viscosity (proved), a decrease in K_f (unproved), tubular obstruction by cell debris and pigment casts observed on histologic preparations (but ITP has not been found elevated), and backleak of filtrate (if any, of minor importance). Further studies appear necessary for better understanding of the pathogenetic mechanism of the maintenance stage of this model of ARF.

6 Pathogenesis of Ischemic and Nephrotoxic Models of ARF

The present state of knowledge of ischemic and nephrotoxic models of ARF appears to support a primary role of both glomerular arteriolar vasoconstriction and reduction in K_f in the pathogenesis of the initiation phase of ARF, as well as a key role of both tubular obstruction and backleak of filtrate in the maintainance phase.

6.1 IMPAIRMENT IN PROXIMAL TUBULAR REABSORPTION IN INTRINSIC ARF (ATN)

If we consider nephrotoxic ARF, the demonstration of early histochemical changes in the brush border of the entire proximal tubules with inactivation of certain brush border enzymes following $HgCl_2$ administration in rats [27] suggests an early decrease in proximal sodium chloride reabsorption in heavy metal-induced ARF, which precedes any morphological aberration of epithelial cells. On the other hand, "in vitro" studies have shown that uranyl and mercuric ions inhibit active sodium transport across the frog skin [193] and across the urinary bladder of the freshwater turtle even without loss of structural membrane integrity [194]; this effect is reversed by dithiothreitol, a sulphydryl-reducing agent and heavy metal chelator [194]. These observations have suggested that toxic inhibition of proximal tubular reabsorption in rats treated with heavy metals may activate the tubuloglomerular feedback (TGF) mechanism through an increased delivery of filtrate to the macula densa [25].

In the ischemic models of ARF, tubular cell function is similarly impaired, after the ischemic insult, much before the clear occurrence of morphological lesions in tubular structures. Changes in intracellular electrolyte composition, cell depletion of ATP, and intracellular acidosis usually precede histologic damage to proximal tubules [112, 140]. These biochemical alterations are associated with a significant reduction in tubular reabsorption [113, 127], while microperfusion of isolated tubular segments dissected from kidneys of rabbits with post-ischemic ARF have exhibited an impaired transport capacity especially in proximal tubules [153]. Since O_2 consumption by the kidney is mostly due to tubular reabsorption of filtrate, it is not surprising that tubular epithelia are the renal structures most sensitive to the hypoxic insult and that the initiating event of ATN is the dramatic reduction in proximal tubular reabsorption [140]. The latter phenomenon may activate the TGF mechanism in a fashion quite similar to that postulated in nephrotoxic ARF.

6.2 GLOMERULAR HEMODYNAMICS; RBF AND GFR REGULATION

The main sites of resistance in the renal vasculature may be located in the afferent and efferent arterioles and, possibly, in the interlobular arteries. Changes in RBF are inversely related to the changes in overall intrarenal resistance. Changes in GFR, instead, may depend on the site and extent of single resistance change. Thus, increases and falls of afferent arteriolar resistance cause inverse changes of RBF and GFR. Changes in efferent arteriolar resistance will still induce inverse changes in RBF, but will elicit a biphasic response of GFR [195]. In a low resistance range, GFR will increase with increasing resistance because of the increase in glomerular capillary pressure (GCP); this rise in GFR, however, will be slight under conditions of filtration pressure equilibrium at the efferent end of the glomerular capillary tuft [196], but will be more marked in case of disequilibrium. In the high-resistance range, GFR will fall with increasing resistance because the decrease in RBF becomes predominant [195].

Undoubtedly, the afferent arteriole is the predominant site of the interaction of vasoconstrictor and vasodilator hormones. It has been stated that a similar interaction also occurs at the efferent arteriole level [195]. Andreucci and his associates [197], however have demonstrated that changes of pressure in the first order peritubular capillaries of superficial nephrons are merely secondary to changes in GCP and that superficial efferent arterioles behave as passive vessels; that is, they are unable to dilate and to constrict in response to neural and/or humoral stimuli [197].

6.3 THE TUBULOGLOMERULAR FEEDBACK (TGF) AND THE RENIN-ANGIOTENSIN SYSTEM (RAS)

A substantial body of evidence has been adduced that in normal kidneys a negative TGF mechanism is continuously operating in order to prevent salt depletion by adjusting the GFR of the single nephron to the reabsorptive capacity of its proximal tubule [196]. This rapidly acting, negative TGF mechanism has been demonstrated in rats, dogs, and even in the isolated human cadaver kidney [198] and appears to respond to flow-dependent changes in the composition of distal tubular fluid—that is, changes either in NaCl [199–202] or in total solute concentration [203, 204]. The altered tubular fluid composition is sensed by the macula densa cells, probably through an increase in receptor cell cytoplasmic calcium activity [204] and will induce a local AII generation [7, 205]. AII will cause afferent arteriole constriction [206] and the consequent fall in GFR through a decrease in GCP [207] and/or in glomerular blood flow [208] and in K_f [208]. Thus, GFR has been shown to decrease, for instance, following acetazolamide

[209] or benzolamide [210], carbonic anhydrase inhibitors that act primarily by decreasing reabsorption from proximal tubules; this fall in GFR has been attributed to activation of TGF.

Should ischemic or toxic factors cause a tubular dysfunction that restricts proximal tubular reabsorption, an increased delivery of filtrate to the macula densa will activate this TGF mechanism and elicit a great local production of AII with a consequent critical fall in blood flow and filtration rate in injured nephrons [211–213]. This pathophysiological mechanism of ARF has been proposed by Thurau's group as the key factor in initiating ARF.

The occurrence of an increased distal delivery of tubular fluid in ARF, that is in a condition of reduced GFR, is demonstrated by (a) the frequently high urine output, (b) the frequent increase in fractional excretion of sodium [6, 7, 127], and (c) the higher sodium chloride concentration in the tubular fluid obtained, by micropuncture, from distal tubules at the macula densa level [25, 26].

On the other hand, not only the increased distal delivery of salt (or solutes) but also the salt depletion—that may result from the initially high urine output and salt excretion both in ischemic and nephrotoxic models of ARF, as testified by the body weight loss observed after ischemia [123], uranyl nitrate [22], or $HgCl_2$ administration [41, 49]—may stimulate the RAS. It has been demonstrated, in fact, that intrarenal AII is significantly increased in rats in which sodium deficiency was induced by low-salt diet plus furosemide [214] (i.e., by the increased urinary excretion of salt in a condition of reduced intake).

Thus, both renal vasoconstriction and reduction in K_f observed in ischemic and toxic models of ARF may be attributed to AII and may well account for the initiation of ARF, when no morphological lesions can be detected as yet throughout the nephrons.

6.3.1 Observations Supporting a Key Role of RAS in the Pathogenesis of ARF According to many authors, in the mammalian kidney there are three main intrinsic mechanisms for renin release: (a) the renal baroreceptors, are located at the afferent arteriole level, which are sensitive to changes of either perfusion pressure or vascular wall tension; (b) the macula densa, which is sensitive to changes in distal delivery of either sodium chloride or total solutes; and (c) the sympathetic nervous system (that may be activated by systemic baroreceptors), which may act through the direct activation of beta-adrenergic receptors in the juxtaglomerular cells [215]. These mechanisms may act in concert, for instance, in conditions of hemorrhagic hypotension when renin release may increase because of (a) decrease in perfusion pressure, (b) increase in distal tubular delivery of NaCl (or total solutes), as a consequence of ischemic impairment in proximal tubular reabsorption, and (c) activation of the sympathetic nervous system secondary to the hypovolemia.

The role of RAS in ARF, however, is still a matter of debate. The following observations appear to support a key role for RAS in the pathogenesis of ARF:

a. The renin content in superficial glomeruli (outer cortex) is greater than in deep glomeruli [10, 25] (even though TGF mechanism has been recently shown to be operative also in juxtamedullary nephrons) [216]. This observation is consistent with the studies by arteriography [217], silicone rubber [13], and microspheres [116], which have demonstrated a preferential outer cortical hypoperfusion in ARF.

b. The magnitude of TGF response to different perfusion rates of distal tubules with Ringer's solution is directly proportional, in normal rats, to juxtaglomerular renin activity [213].

c. The TGF response to marked flow rate changes is significantly reduced in normal rats by i.v. infusion of either AII antagonist, Sar^1, Ala^8angiotensin II (Saralasin, which interferes with AII-receptor interaction) [218], or converting-enzyme inhibitor SQ 20,881, (which interferes with AII formation) [205, 219].

d. Sodium concentration has been found significantly increased in the early distal tubular fluid in rats after experimental renal ischemia [220] and in rats with UN-induced ARF [25, 26], suggesting an activation of TGF.

e. Renin activity has been found to be increased in individual JGAs of rats with either hemorrhagic hypotension or renal hypoperfusion due to aortic clamping [221], with post-ischemic ARF [125, 211], with glycerol-induced ARF [222], with UN-induced ARF [25, 26, 223], or with $HgCl_2$-induced ARF [223].

f. TGF mechanism is preserved and operative in many experimental models of ARF [127, 212, 213]; the magnitude of the feedback response is maintained directly proportional to the JGA's renin activity after 45-minutes ischemia, suggesting that the sensitivity of the mechanism is preserved by ischemia [127].

g. The TGF can be inhibited in experimental ARF by the presence of furosemide in the fluid perfusing the macula densa segment [208, 213, 214]. Since the ion initiating the TGF seems to be chloride, furosemide may act by inhibiting active chloride reabsorption at the macula densa level as it does in the thick ascending limb of the loop of Henle [201, 208, 211, 224]. This may account for the protective effect of furosemide in ARF despite the increased delivery of salt to the macula densa elicited by this diuretic agent.

h. A TGF response has been triggered in rats by perfusing the loop of Henle and early distal tubule with electrolyte-free sera, urine, or peritoneal fluid of patients with ARF and hepatic damage; this effect was not blocked by the addition of furosemide [225].

i. The intraperitoneal administration of dithiothreitol in rats 30 minutes after subcutaneous injection of either UN or $HgCl_2$ prevented or readily ameliorated the heavy metal-induced ARF: only slight alterations were, in fact, observed in GFR (slight fall) and in FE_{Na} (slight increase) in comparison with animals treated with UN or $HgCl_2$ alone; simultaneously both PRA and JGA's renin activity, markedly increased in rats treated with UN or $HgCl_2$ alone, were

completely normalized by dithiothreitol [223].

j. Salt loading, a condition known to cause renin depletion (by a mechanism different from that operating at the macula densa), has been shown to have a protective effect on ARF induced in rats by $HgCl_2$ [226] or by gentamicin [90] despite the persistent occurrence of severe tubular necrosis undistinguishable from that occurring in non-renin-depleted rats.

k. Chronic oral captopril administration, known to lessen endogenous AII formation, has been proven successful in offsetting the impairment in glomerular function induced by gentamicin, with no amelioration of the severe morphologic changes in proximal tubule epithelia [90].

l. The administration of converting-enzyme inhibitor SQ20,881 prior to or shortly after UN injection in dogs has been found to markedly attenuate the fall in GFR [227].

6.3.2 *Observations Arguing Against a Key Role of RAS in the Pathogenesis of ARF* It has been well demonstrated that PRA does not have any effect on the severity of ARF [13, 33, 228]. Any condition, in fact, that can block the effects of circulating renin does not usually protect the experimental animals against nephrotoxic ARF; this is the case with immunization to renin [187], active or passive immunization to AII [229], administration of saralasin, the competitive antagonist of AII [176]. But all these observations left open the possibility that antibodies and pharmacologic inhibitors do not affect the local production of angiotensin [228] because of the intracellular site of this production [230]. It remained possible that the behavior of the renal cortical renin content, as an index of the intrarenal activity of the RAS, could play the key role in the induction of ARF.

Some recent experimental data, however, appear to argue against a primary pathogenetic role for the intrarenal RAS in experimental ARF:

a. Although the TGF is still operative in ARF, the magnitude of the glomerular response to the changes in macula densa signal is clearly reduced in many models of ARF [212] (it is not reduced, however, following 45-minute ischemia) [127].

b. Long-term (five to six weeks) NaC1 loading induced not only a clear suppression of plasma renin but also an intrarenal renin depletion in rats; yet the animals were not protected against UN- or HgC1$_2$-induced ARF in the absence of increased NaC1 intake and/or excretion [228]. Similar observations were reported in rats with ischemic ARF [231].

c. Long-term (three to five weeks) NaC1 loading has been shown to diminish both the renin activity in JGAs and the TGF response to different perfusion rates of the macula densa with Ringer's solution, but did not improve inulin clearance after either 45-minute ischemia or intra-aortic injection of UN [127].

d. Acute ECV expansion by saline infusion partially protected against UN-induced ARF (i.e., it increased inulin clearance) despite an only mild depression of both the renin activity in JGAs and the TGF response to different distal perfusion rates [127].

e. Long-term (five to six weeks) sodium depletion induced a significant increase in renal cortical renin content in rats; yet the animals were protected against UN- or HgCl$_2$-induced ARF by short-term (48 hours) increase in NaC1 intake and/or excretion [228].

f. In two-kidney Goldblatt rats, the ARF due to either arterial occlusion [127] or UN [127], or HgCl$_2$ [232], or glycerol [178] was equal in severity in both kidneys despite different degrees of renal cortical renin content.

g. The increased solute excretion induced in rats by pretreatment with diuretics clearly protected the animals against HgCl$_2$-induced ARF, although no change in renal renin content had occurred [233].

h. Pretreatment with beta-blocking agents prevented the rise in plasma and renal cortical renin activities in HgCl$_2$-injected rats; yet ARF occurred in all animals even though in attenuated form [32].

These observations, therefore, argue against an important role of both intrarenal renin and TGF either in inducing or influencing the severity of ischemic or nephrotoxic ARF: renin suppression confers, in fact, no protection against experimental ARF [127]. NaCl intake and/or excretion may influence the severity of ARF, but this influence seems to occur regardless of the JGA renin activity [127, 228]. In other words, NaCl has an independent effect on renal cortical renin content and on the severity of ARF. The short-term increase in NaCl intake and/or excretion, in fact, reduced the severity, shortened the maintenance phase, and hastened the recovery of HgCl$_2$-induced ARF, whatever the intrarenal renin content [228].

As stated by Thurau et al. [202], however, even if we assume that AII is the mediator of the TGF, local AII concentration cannot be predicted from the activity of renin, which is only one of the enzymes involved in AII production. Thus, for instance, sodium bromide perfusion of macula densa segment did not increase JGA renin activity, yet it induced a feedback response.

Furthermore, some still undefined factors may influence the sensitivity of the TGF. Thus, it has been recently demonstrated that the high interstitial hydrostatic pressure in the kidneys of rats with ECV expansion is associated with a reduced feedback sensitivity, while the low interstitial pressure observed in rats in conditions of dehydration, hypotension, or hypovolemia is associated with an increased feedback sensitivity [234]. These observations may account for the protection of acute salt loading against experimental ARF.

Finally, the RAS should not be regarded as an isolated mechanism; other intrarenal systems (such as prostaglandins, kinins, etc.) may influence renin secretion as well as the TGF [235] in a manner still controversial. Thus, some authors have given evidence that PGI$_2$ decreases the feedback sensitivity (probably through an increase in renal interstitial pressure), while PGE$_2$ does not change feedback characteristics in normal animals but increases to normal level the reduced feedback sensitivity that follows unilateral nephrectomy [234]. However, other authors have shown that blockage of PG synthesis will reduce the feedback response that is restored by intra-aortic infusion of PGI_2 or PGE_2 [195]. Furthermore, it has been demonstrated that inhibition of the PG system by indomethacin increases the severity of gentamicin-induced ARF and that gentamicin decreases plasma and urinary kallikrein [75].

The observations on the protective effects of acute salt loading have, at any rate, very important clinical implications since long-term salt loading appears to be unnecessary in the prevention of ARF; acute ECV expansion or 48-hour increase in NaCl intake is quite sufficient for protective purposes [127, 228]. The failure of expansion in protecting against ARF reported by some authors in ischemic [131, 149] or glycerol models [159] may be attributed to inadequacy of ECV expansion [127]. The mechanism of this protection is still a matter of debate; it is not yet established whether the ECV expansion per se or the resulting solute diuresis is the important factor. The inhibition of proximal tubular reabsorption by ECV expansion may decrease the intraluminal concentration of nephrotoxins, in this way lessening the tubular insult [127]; thus, for instance, salt-loading in rats prior to $HgCl_2$ injection exhibited partial protection against the development of ARF, which was associated with a decrease in renal cortical Hg^{++} levels [236]. On the other hand, the increased diuresis will increase nephrotoxin excretion [127, 174, 228]. Thus urinary excretion of $HgCl_2$ [236] and gentamicin [85] has been found clearly increased in salt-loaded rats undergoing intoxication by $HgCl_2$ and gentamicin, respectively. Finally, increased urine output will minimize obstruction by washing out cellular debris from tubular lumina.

Undoubtedly long- or short-term saline loading may also contribute to some renal function improvement by correcting volume depletion, which may result from the high urine output and salt excretion in early stage of experimental ARF [127].

6.3.3 *The Slow-Acting TGF Mechanism Activated by Prolonged Tubular Blockade* It has been recently suggested that, in addition to the fast-acting, negative TGF mechanism sensitive to

acute increases in distal tubule fluid flow, a slow-acting positive TGF mechanism is also operative in individual nephrons; this mechanism is activated by prolonged tubular blockade [237, 238]. It has been, in fact, demonstrated that 12 to 24 hours following blockade of single tubules in the rat kidney, a clear decrease both in GCP and in glomerular blood flow occurs, suggesting an afferent arteriolar constriction [24, 239], a pattern similar to that observed 24 hours after unilateral ureteral obstruction with a normal contralateral kidney [240]. The JGA is undoubtedly involved in this mechanism, since the glomerular response to chronic tubule blockade does not occur in the Necturus kidney, the JGA of which is poorly developed without a macula densa [241].

It seems that the signal initiating this slow-acting TGF is not given by the increase in diameter and/or in pressure in the loop of Henle (it occurs, in fact, also in case of proximal tubule blockade), nor by the increase in pressure in Bowman's space (it occurs also with a hole in the tubule proximal to the blockade site), but by a decrease in fluid delivery to the macula densa [237].

The extent of afferent arteriolar constriction elicited by prolonged tubular blockade is not severe enough to stop the glomerular filtration rate in the involved nephron. When SNGFR was measured, in fact, in rats 26 hours following tubular blockade while the ITP was maintained normal during fluid collection (it was much higher before collection), a mean value 42% lower than normal was obtained [237]. This observation suggests that SNGFR in undisturbed obstructed nephrons is quite low, but its fall is accounted for both by a feedback mechanism (through an afferent arteriole vasoconstriction) and by the increased ITP (through the decrease in glomerular transcapillary hydraulic pressure difference).

6.3.4 *Role of Angiotensin II (AII) in GFR Regulation* AII is undoubtedly involved in the physiologic regulation of GFR, as shown by the following well-established observations:

a. Renin, AI-converting enzyme, AI, and AII coexist in epithelioid cells of JGA

[242–244], and AII is formed by an intracellular mechanism independent from the extracellular RAS [245].

b. AII has been shown to decrease RBF [246].
c. AII decreases GFR [21].
d. AII has been demonstrated to reduce K_f [21]; even the reduction of K_f observed after PTH, PGE_2, PGI_2, and cAMP seems to be mediated by AII [47].
e. After i.v. injection in rats, tritiated AII has been located by autoradiography in the glomerular mesangial cells [247].
f. Scanning electron microscopy has demonstrated a marked shrinkage of glomerular tufts following AII administration in rats [248] presumably due to the contractile myofilaments contained in glomerular mesangial cells; the resulting decrease of the surface area of the glomerular capillaries may well account for the reduction in K_f. It seems that only AII and arginine vasopressin are capable of stimulating mesangial cell contraction in vitro [249].
g. An AII-mediated vasoreactivity of rat glomeruli has been demonstrated in "in vitro" preparation: the diameter of isolated glomeruli decreased in proportion with the increase in concentration of ^{125}I-AII [250].
h. Specific AII receptors have been demonstrated in isolated rat glomeruli; asparaginyl^1-ileu^5-ileu^8-AII and sarcosine^1-ileu^8-AII (analogs of AII that block the pressor and myotropic activity of AII) appeared effective competitive inhibitors of ^{125}I-AII binding to the isolated glomeruli [250]. AII receptors in glomeruli seem to differ from those in the renal vasculature [251].

Recent studies have demonstrated a dissociation between intrarenal renin and intrarenal AII [7]. Thus, oral sodium loading in rats for three weeks has been shown to suppress PRA and intrarenal renin, as already well known, but to leave unchanged intrarenal AII in comparison with rats on normal sodium intake; in sodium deprived rats, instead, a significant inverse linear relationship was observed between intrarenal AII and urinary sodium concentration [214].

These observations leave open the question concerning the role of AII in the pathogenesis of ARF. It is possible that factors other than renin may lead to angiotensin synthesis; thus AII may be formed directly from renin substrate through an alternative pathway catalized by the beta-converting enzyme "tonin" [252], which is not inhibited by the available converting enzyme blockers [253]. But the demonstration that i.p. injection of the converting-enzyme inhibitor SQ20,881 clearly depresses intrarenal AII one hour after injection (while PRA is elevated and intrarenal renin remains unchanged) appears to support the key role played by the classical "converting enzyme" or by the "AII-forming enzyme" [254] in the production of intrarenal AII [214].

6.4 SYMPATHETIC NERVE ACTIVITY AND CIRCULATING CATECHOLAMINES

The kidney receives a rich sympathetic innervation. Adrenergic nerve fibers enter the kidney with the arterial supply; they are distributed in the cortex along the intrarenal arteries up to afferent and efferent arterioles, reaching both juxtaglomerular cells and tubular structures [255]. Adrenergic innervation has also been demonstrated in the "vasa recta" of the outer medulla, but not in the inner medulla. Chemical measurement of NE in renal tissue has shown a NE distribution well correlated with the histochemical demonstration of nerve fibers [256].

Adrenergic nerve stimulation and exogenous catecholamines are known to induce the following effects:

a. Direct renal vasoconstriction, by a direct effect on afferent arterioles [197]. This effect is so important that an experimental model of ARF has been created by NE infusion, as widely discussed. On the other hand, clinical observations in humans have shown a fall in renal function after i.v. infusion of NE as well as the occurrence of prerenal ARF in those forms of acute myocardial infarction in which increase in catecholamine secretion has been demonstrated [1].
b. Renal renin release [257]. This effect seems to be beta-adrenegically mediated since it is blocked by propranolol. The resulting AII

production will amplify the adrenergic tone both by stimulating catecholamine release from the adrenal glands and by enhancing the NE release from sympathetic nerve terminals [256]. Furthermore, AII will, by itself, potentiate the afferent arteriole vasoconstriction. Beta-blocking agents (mainly propranolol) have been shown to partially protect against experimental ARF [32, 126, 148, 258, 259]. Possibly this protection is the result of suppression of RAS, but it may be due to the inhibition of tubular beta receptors with a consequent decrease in cellular impairment [148, 259]; it has also been proposed that beta blockers inhibit the presynaptic facilitatory beta receptors that increase NE release during nerve stimulation, thus reducing the sympathetic tone [32].

c. Renal PG's synthesis and release [256]. This effect appears to be alpha adrenergically mediated since it is specifically blocked by phenoxybenzamine but not by the beta-adrenergic blocking agent propranolol [256].

It has been demonstrated, at least in unanesthetized rats, that basal renal PGE_2 production is not regulated by basal renal nerve activity, but that adrenergic stimulation and prolonged elevation in plasma NE promote a sustained PGE_2 synthesis by the kidneys [260].

The PGs released by catecholamines will antagonize the vasoconstrictor actions of adrenergic stimulation both by their direct vasodilator activity and by their demonstrated inhibition of NE release induced by adrenergic stimulation (a form of negative feedback) [256].

AII has been shown to be the major ischemic factor in dogs with hemorrhagic hypotension, but renal sympathetic nerve activity is also undoubtedly contributing to the increased renal resistance in this condition [261, 262]. Thus, dogs with hemorrhagic hypotension exhibited reduced RBF and GFR, especially when PGs were inhibited by pretreatment with indomethacin; unilateral intrarenal infusion of a specific AII antagonist could attenuate the impairment of renal perfusion and function, but only when renal denervation was also associated was a

great protection of RBF and GFR observed [261, 262].

The adrenergic system has been shown to be involved in some unknown way in the TGF mechanism in normal rats; TGF response was, in fact, markedly reduced during beta blockade with propranolol (because of a reduction in renin release?) [205]. But no appreciable effect on TGF response was observed during alpha blockade with phenoxybenzamine or phentolamine, nor following chemical renal denervation with 6-hydroxydopamine (which is known to destroy adrenergic nerve terminals), nor following depletion of adrenergic nerve vescicles with reserpine [205]. Thus, nervous transmission does not appear involved in TGF; and this is consistent with the preservation of TGF in completely isolated blood-perfused dog kidneys [263]. It seems, instead, that circulating catecholamines play some role [205]. Thus, TGF response has been found consistently increased in rats following hemorrhagic hypotension: factors other than blood volume, renal perfusion pressure, or RAS had to be considered as responsible for this observation, and circulating catecholamines have been implicated [264].

6.5 PROSTAGLANDINS (PGs)

PGs constitute a heterogeneous group of arachidonate metabolites. The arachidonic acid (an unsaturated fatty acid) is formed from cell membrane phospholipids by the enzyme phospholipase A_2. Under the action of cyclooxygenase, arachidonic acid is transformed into two unstable endoperoxide intermediates, PGG_2 and PGH_2, which are further metabolized to the prostaglandins PGE_2, $PGF_{2\alpha}$, PGI_2 (prostacyclin), PGD_2, and to thromboxane A_2 (TxA_2) [265] (figure 1–1). PGA_2, initially identified as a PG synthesized in the renal medulla, has then been shown to be an artifactual product formed from PGE_2 during the isolation procedure [266, 267]. PGs and their precursor are unbiquitous in the human body. But the kidney is undoubtedly the main site of PG synthesis [268]. This renal biosynthesis was initially believed to be confined to the renal medulla, probably because the amount of PGE_2 synthesized in the medulla is much larger than the total PGs synthesized in the cortex [269].

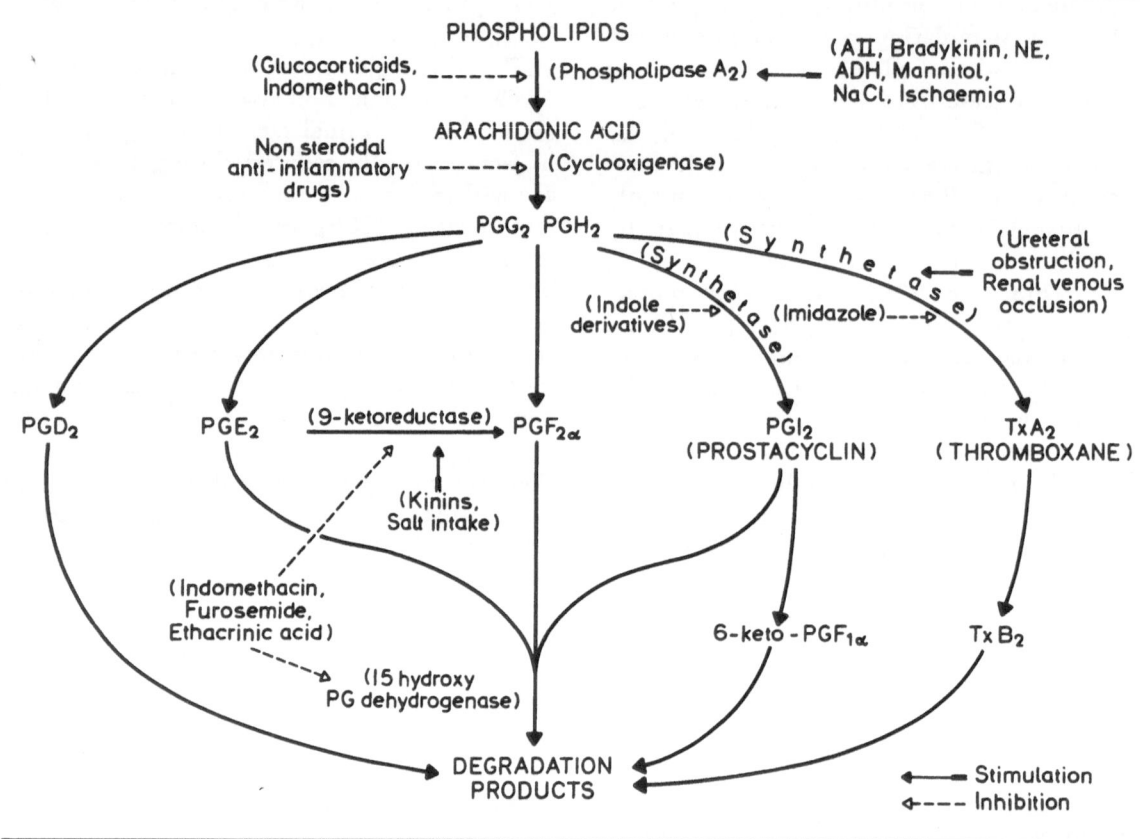

FIGURE 1–1. Synthesis and degradation of prostaglandins.

It is now well established, instead, that PG synthesis, within the kidney, occurs both in the cortex (mainly PGI_2) and in the medulla (mainly PGE_2) [269].

Synthesis of PGs have been located at least in the following sites: (a) glomeruli [270], mainly in epithelial [PGI_2] but also in mesangial cells (PGE_2) [267, 271]; (b) endothelial cells of arteries and afferent arterioles [266]; (c) cortical collecting ducts [267]; (d) medullary collecting ducts [272]; (e) interstitial cells of the medulla [273]; and (f) ascending limb of Henle's loops [274].

PGs are not stored. Their release is due to de novo synthesis, and their effects are exerted close to their sites of synthesis [184]. This accounts for the compartimentation of the synthesis of different PGs. Thus, even though PGI_2, the unstable vasodilator and anti-aggregating compound, would appear as a trivial

PG in a whole kidney preparation, its synthesis on a regional basis is very important considering the functional role played in the renal cortex [269]. While PGE_2 and $PGF_{2\alpha}$ are, in fact, the predominant "classical" PGs synthesized both in the cortex and in the medulla (the more active PGE_2 is transformed into $PGF_{2\alpha}$ by 9-ketoreductase), PGI_2 (prostacyclin) is the PG produced predominantly by cortical arteries and arterioles [266], suggesting its primary role in regulating renal vascular tone in the renal cortex [267].

Renal PGs are mainly matabolized within the kidney, even though stop-flow experiments have demonstrated that unchanged PGE_2 and $PGF_{2\alpha}$ are secreted into the loop of Henle, so that their urinary excretion reflects their synthesis within the kidneys [275]; PGE_2 and $PGF_{2\alpha}$ may also enter the renal venous blood [276] to be almost completely degraded by the lung during one passage through pulmonary circulation. PGI_2, instead, is not metabolized by the lung so that it may function as circulating hormone [267].

Obviously, the renal concentration of PGs is the net result of synthesis and degradation (or excretion). Furthermore, tissue measurements may yield some degradation products with little or no biologic activity, which can be taken, however, as an index of the parent PG biosynthesis; this is the case with 6-keto-$PGF_{1\alpha}$ and TxB_2, the spontaneous degradation products of the chemically unstable PGI_2 and TxA_2, respectively. It was because of this chemical instability of the latter PGs that for many years it was thought that the only PGs were the chemically stable PGE_2 and $PGF_{2\alpha}$ [277].

6.5.1 PG Stimulators and Inhibitors

PG synthesis and degradation may be stimulated or inhibited at various steps of the arachidonate metabolism (figure 1–1). Thus, while AII, NE, bradykinin, arginin vasopressin, mannitol, NaCl, and ischemia appear to stimulate phospholipase A_2 activity, the latter is inhibited by glucocorticoids and indomethacin [267]. Cyclooxygenase activity is inhibited by nonsteroidal anti-inflammatory drugs (indomethacin, aspirin, acetaminophen, phenylbutazone, phenacetin, ibuprofen, naproxen) [267]. Prostacyclin synthetase is inhibited by indole derivatives; thromboxane synthetase is inhibited by imidazole and stimulated by renal venous occlusion [278] and by prolonged (18 to 24 hours) ureteral obstruction [184, 186, 279]. There is some evidence, instead, that acute (up to four to five hours) ureteral obstruction elicits renal vasodilation [240] that is mediated by vasodilator PGs [184, 280]. The enzyme 9-ketoreductase, responsible for the transformation of PGE_2 into $PGF_{2\alpha}$, is stimulated by the high salt intake and by kinins and inhibited by indomethacin, furosemide, and ethacrinic acid [267]. Finally, furosemide, ethacrinic acid, sulphasalazine analogues, and indomethacin inhibit PG breakdown [267].

6.5.2 Effects of Vasodilator PGs on RBF and GFR

It is generally stated that the infusion of PGs (with the exception of TxA_2) into the renal artery causes vasodilation, with a decrease in renal vascular resistance and an increase in RBF. This is not actually correct since species dependency of renal vascular effects of PGs has been reported by many authors. Thus, while PGE_2 and PGD_2 have been shown to be potent renal vasodilators in dogs and rabbits, they appeared to function as vasoconstrictors in rats [281]. $PGF_{2\alpha}$ has either a slight vasodilatory action or no vascular effect at all. PGI_2 (prostacyclin) is the only major PG that unequivocally reduces renal vascular resistance in both dogs and rats [195, 282]. It has been stated, however, that the vasoconstriction often reported with PGE_2 in rats is probably due to the capacity of PG to stimulate renin release, thereby causing AII-induced vasoconstriction. When the latter effect, in fact, is antagonized, the intrarenal infusion of PGE_2 will cause a clear vasodilation [267].

The formation of PGs within the renal cortex suggests that modulations in PG synthesis and degradation should play a local regulatory function either by a direct action or by modulating the response of cortical arterioles to pressure hormones such as AII and catecholamines [195, 266, 267]. The physiologic role of PGs in the regulation of RBF and GFR, however, has not been completely defined as yet. It seems that in normal condition, in which vasoconstrictor influences are minimal, PGs play very little role in determining the resting tone of renal vessels. Thus, in normal subjects and in conscious dogs and baboons, inhibition of PG synthesis does not affect RBF [283, 284]. The role of PGs, instead, becomes really important in conditions of marked renal vasoconstrictor influences, such as after AII infusion [285] or endogenous AII production, following hypotension or renal hypoperfusion [261, 262, 286], and after catecholamine administration or renal nerve stimulation [256, 283]. In these circumstances, in fact, indomethacin will greatly increase renal vascular resistance, significantly reducing RBF and GFR.

The above observations have led to the conclusion that an increased local synthesis of vasodilatory PGs plays a crucial role in counteracting those mechanisms (e.g., AII, NE, alpha-adrenergic neural stimulation), which raise arteriolar resistance and reduce RBF and GFR; the local action of newly synthesized vasodilator PGs will cause, in fact, that reduction in vascular resistance that is required to maintain kidney perfusion and function [195]. Such a fine mechanism appears to work because of the stimulating effect of vasoconstrictors (AII, NE, and sympathetic nervous system) on PG biosynthesis.

Apparently, the control of renal vascular resistance is based mainly on the interaction of PGs and AII [267]; circulating AII exerts, directly, a renal vasoconstriction and may cause, indirectly through its stimulation of PG (PGI_2?) biosynthesis, a renal vasodilation. In basal state the low levels of circulating AII will balance the direct and indirect effects. In conditions of increased circulating levels of AII (e.g., low salt intake or hypotension), the direct vasoconstriction effect of AII is blunted by the concomitant increase in AII-dependent PG synthesis; the blockade of PG synthesis by indomethacin in this condition will cause an increase in renal vascular resistance because of the unopposed direct vasoconstriction of AII [267]. The sympathetic nervous system also plays an important role in this control of renal resistance. AII receptor blockade in dogs pretreated with indomethacin and then made hypotensive by hemorrhage did not totally inhibit the renal vasoconstriction; total inhibition occurred instead when the kidney was also denervated [262].

This mechanism of interaction between vasoconstrictors and renal PGs is very important since renal PGs act locally (without any influence on other vascular beds) and prevent the deleterious effects on renal function of increased renal nerve activity and circulating vasoconstrictors [267]. In this hemodynamic regulation, actually all vasoconstrictors and vasodilators appear deeply involved. Should, for instance, a contraction of ECV occur for any reason, the simultaneous intrarenal activation of the adrenergic system, RAS, PGs, and kallikrein-kinin system would, on one side, allow the extrarenal effects of AII and catecholamines (i.e., peripheral arteriolar vasoconstriction for maintaining systemic blood pressure, release of mineralcorticoids, etc.) and, on the other side, prevent

their intrarenal vasoconstrictive effects (which would impair the renal function) by the activation of vasodilator PGs and kallikrein-kinin system [195].

Perhaps the best evidence of the important role of PGs in preserving renal function is given by the deleterious effects of PG synthetase inhibition in clinical conditions of reduced "effective" blood volume [268]. Thus, ascitic patients with chronic liver disease exhibited an acute renal insufficiency with extreme sodium retention after treatment with indomethacin [287]; and nephrotic patients showed a significant fall in GFR under indomethacin, a condition readily reversed with the withdrawal of the drug [288]. It has been suggested that PGs also play a key role in maintaining RBF during the hemodynamic stresses associated with trauma, surgery, hemorrhage [261, 262, 282].

Recent micropuncture experiments have given some evidence that PGs are very important in the TGF mechanism [195, 289, 290]. An integrity of the PG system, in fact, has appeared necessary for the feedback response to be elicited. Thus, when PG synthesis was inhibited by intravenous or intratubular application of indomethacin, the feedback response was greatly reduced [289, 290] to be then restored with the intra-aortic infusion of PGI_2 and PGE_2 [195, 290]. Hence, the vasoconstrictor response of the afferent arteriole requires a vasodilator PG; this paradoxical effect has still to be explained [195]. It has been suggested that PGs are not directly involved in changing the vascular tone, but are necessary to afferent arterioles for responding to the macula densa signal [195]. In other words, PGs may mediate in some way between the signal sensed by the macula densa and the RAS. This seems supported by the observation that indomethacin did not affect the feedback response in rats on a low salt diet; apparently despite PG inhibition the little amount of PG formed in the juxtaglomerular cells is sufficient to activate the RAS when RAS is stimulated by a low salt diet [289].

The effect of PGs on GFR parallels their effect on RBF with all the mentioned implications of the relationship between RAS and PGs. But in addition to the hemodynamic factor, PGs may affect GFR by modifying K_f.

PGI_2 and PGE_2, in fact, have been shown to regularly decrease K_f [291]; this decrease, however, is abolished by saralasin, suggesting that the effect on K_f is not due to a direct action of PGE_2 and PGI_2, but is the result of PG-stimulated AII production [47, 291].

6.5.3 Effect of Thromboxane on Renal Vascular Resistance Thromboxane (TxA_2) is another unstable arachidonate metabolite, a platelet-aggregating substance with a direct vasoconstrictive effect in many tissues, the kidney included. Possibly, TxA_2 contributes to the basal renal vascular tone in normal kidneys since the intra-aortic infusion of imidazole in rats causes an increase in RBF [267]. Produced particularly in platelets, where the arachidonic acid is mainly converted into TxA_2, this vasoconstrictor arachidonate metabolite is undoubtedly also synthesized in the kidney; and its synthesis is increased by uretheral obstruction [184, 186, 279] and by renal venous occlusion [278].

6.5.4 Effects of Vasodilator PGs on Renin Release Mainly PGI_2, but also PGE_2 and perhaps PGD_2, stimulates renin release "in vivo"; inhibition of PG synthesis by indomethacin, in fact, has been shown to blunt the increase in renin secretion that follows hypotensive hemorrhage [292] or sodium restriction [284]. The influence of PGs on renin release has also been demonstrated "in vitro," in renal cortical slices, and in isolated glomeruli [293, 294]; the only PG effective "in vitro", however, is PGI_2 [294]. These observations suggest that PGs may influence renin release through two mechanisms: (a) an indirect mechanism that is neural, baroreceptor-, or macula densa-mediated and (b) a direct intracellular mechanism, at renal sites common to RAS and PGs, which is independent of external hemodynamics, tubular, neural, or other influences [294]. The latter mechanism involves only PGI_2, which is the typical PG of the vascular endothelium (and this is consistent with a direct interaction between PGI_2 and RAS at the vascular pole of the glomeruli) [294].

The PG system has been recently suggested to be the common mediator of RAS stimulation evoked both by baroreceptor and macula densa mechanisms; only the beta adrenergic mechanism of renin release seems nonmediated by PGs [215].

6.6 THE RENAL KALLIKREIN-KININ SYSTEM
Kallikreins (word derived from the Greek name of pancreas) are a heterogenous group of serum protease, which are found in the plasma (plasma kallikrein) and in glandular tissue (glandular kallikrein) such as the pancreas, kidney, and salivary and sweat glands. They act on alpha-2 globulin substrates—the kininogens—liberating some peptides—the kinins: bradykinin, a nonapeptide generated by plasma kallikreins, and lysyl-bradykinin (kallidin), a decapeptide released by glandular kallikreins [295, 296]. The plasma kallikrein system is well known to play an important role in blood coagulation and fibrinolysis. Much less known is the renal kallikrein-kinin system.

Urinary kallikrein reflects renal synthesis; urinary kinins are generated in the renal cortex, in distal nephrons, where kallikrein has been located in the tubular cells which are juxtaposed to the wall of afferent arterioles, the site of juxtaglomerular cells [297]. An aminopeptidase converts part of lysyl-bradykinin into bradykinin; lysyl-bradykinin, however, remains the major urinary kinin. Intrarenal kininases (kininase I and kininase II) quickly inactivate kinins by converting them into inactive peptides [297]. Hence, the intrarenal activity of the renal kallikrein-kinin system depends on the balance between generation and inactivation of kinins [295, 296].

The kallikrein-kinin system has been shown to be activated by PGs [295, 296]. In turn, kinins do stimulate PG (PGE_2 and PGI_2) synthesis and release [295, 296, 298]. But when PGE synthesis was inhibited by intrarenal infusion of indomethacin, the renal response to the intrarenal administration of bradykinin (i.e., increase in RBF) was not significantly attenuated [299]. Thus, the effects of these vasodilator systems, PGs, and kinins, are additive and independent of each other [298, 299]. They appear to play an important role in renal hemodynamics by reducing the renal vascular reactivity to the pressure hormones, A II, and catecholamines, and by promoting renal vaso-dilation [295, 296] with the consequent increase in RBF. GFR, however, has been shown to remain unchanged during bradykinin infusion in dogs, suggesting a decrease of both afferent and efferent vascular resistance [300].

But the renal kallikrein-kinin system is also linked to the RAS. Thus, the most abundant renal kininase, the kininase II, is identical with the AI-converting enzyme. Kininase II is located in the brush border of proximal tubules; this accounts for the very small contribution of filtered bradykinin to urinary kinins [297]. But kininase II is also located along the luminal surface of endothelial cells; this accounts both for the conversion of AI into AII and for the inactivation of circulating kinins, strongly supporting the contention that renal kinins act locally and are not circulating hormones [301, 302].

The RAS stimulates kallikrein release presumably through an effect of aldosterone [302]. Furthermore, the infusion of AII in the renal artery of dogs increases the urinary excretion of kallikrein; this effect, however, seems mediated by the AII-induced PG synthesis [302].

In turn, the renal kallikrein-kinin system has been shown to stimulate RAS: urinary kallikrein, in fact, (a) correlates with the active renin in plasma, (b) converts prorenin to renin in vitro, and (c) releases active renin from renal cortical slices [302].

Bradykinin has been shown to decrease K_f; since infusion of bradykinin increases renal and glomerular cAMP levels and the effect of cAMP on K_f is mediated by AII, it is possible that the bradykinin effect on K_f is also AII-mediated [47].

It has been recently postulated that the kallikrein-kinin system may be involved in the TGF [205]. The increased tubular flow through the "macula densa" segment may elicit a reduction in the generation of vasodilator bradykinin; a constriction of afferent arteriole may result with the fall in GFR. Since SQ20,881 inhibits not only the AI-converting enzyme activity but also the kininase activity of kininase II-converting enzyme, an excess of bradykinin in the juxtaglomerular cells may account for the observed greater inhibitory effect of

SQ20,881 on TGF compared to that of AII antagonists [205]. There is no direct evidence, however, that bradykinin is formed in the JGA.

6.7 INTRAVASCULAR COAGULATION IN THE PATHOGENESIS OF ARF

The typical form of human ARF that is believed to result from intravascular coagulation is the renal cortical necrosis [303]. It has been suggested however, that this same mechanism may also play an important pathogenetic role in the classical form of ARF (ATN) [304, 305]. In favor of this hypothesis may be the following observations:

a. Shock, sepsis, intravascular hemolysis, as well as severe tissue trauma, may activate intravascular coagulation [305] but also cause ARF [188].

b. Elevated plasma fibrinogen levels have been observed 24 hours after induction of experimental ARF in rats by glycerol or $HgCl_2$ [44].

c. Increase in plasma fibrinogen has been found in various forms of human ARF [304].

d. Fibrin(ogen) degradation products (FDP) have been found clearly increased in the serum and urine of rats developing ARF (but not in those refractory) after glycerol injection [188].

e. FDP levels have been found to be increased in the serum during the anuric phase and in the urine during recovery in humans with various forms of ARF [304].

f. On light microscopic examination of renal biopsies, glomeruli have been found completely normal, but platelets, fibrin, and products of fibrin and fibrinogen degradation have been instead observed in glomerular capillaries by electron microscopy in human ARF [303, 304], suggesting stasis and thrombosis within the capillary lumina.

g. The intravenous infusion of thrombin in rats leads to deposition of fibrin in the kidneys (and in other organs) with a marked fall in GFR; but fibrin will rapidly disappear because of fibrinolysis and GFR will therefore normalize. If i.v. infusion of thrombin is associated with inhibition of fibrinolysis by tranexamic acid injection, the severe fibrin deposition in the glomeruli will lead to ARF [306]. This ARF can be prevented by chronic NaCl loading [306], by beta-adrenergic blockade with propranolol [307], and by saralasin [308]; the protection in all cases is due to a reduction in fibrin deposition in the kidneys [309] with no relation with RBF [310]. AII has been shown to increase, PGE_2 and PGI_2 to decrease fibrin deposition in the glomeruli [309, 310]. Since glomerular deposition of fibrin does not occur in obstructed nephrons (in which filtration does not occur), it has been suggested that glomerular filtration is important for deposition of fibrin in renal glomeruli [310].

It is suggested that either the intravascular clotting may mechanically impair RBF or the vasoactive fibrinopeptides and platelet serotonin released after intravascular coagulation may cause renal vasoconstriction [304, 305, 310]. Recovery of function may be accounted for by fibrinolysis; the high urinary excretion of FDP observed in humans with ARF [304] appears to support such a view.

We should admit, however, that in human ARF fibrin deposition in the glomeruli does not usually appear as frequent as suggested by Clarkson et al. [304].

The pathogenetic role of intravascular coagulation in various forms of ARF is widely discussed in chapter 6.

6.8 VARIATION OF CONTACT BETWEEN TUBULAR AND VASCULAR COMPONENTS OF THE JGA

Three-dimensional studies of the juxtaglomerular apparatus in the rat kidney by Barajas and his coworkers [311–313] using serial semithin sections of plastic-embedded tissue have clearly demonstrated that (a) the distal tubule has a long and constant contact with the efferent arteriole while the extent of contact with afferent arteriole is very small; (b) there are two types of contact between tubular and vascular components of JGA (as observed by electron mi-

croscopy): a permanent contact between distal tubule and efferent arteriole, with a continuous basement membrane between the two structures and a reversible contact between tubular and vascular structures with a simple apposition of their basement membranes. On the basis of these observations, Barajas proposed a model in which variation in the extent of contact between the macula densa and the afferent arteriole (where juxtaglomerular granular cells are mainly located) may control renin secretion under physiological and pathological conditions [313].

6.9 ROLE OF TUBULAR OBSTRUCTION AND BACKLEAK OF FILTRATE IN THE PATHOGENESIS OF ARF

As mentioned above, following the initial plasma membrane damage, heavy metals accumulate within the cells and cause further toxic effects on intracellular structures (as shown by mitochondrial functional impairment) mainly in the "pars recta," where they lead to cell killing [27, 28]. Similarly, a clear impairment of mitochondrial respiratory activity persists long after the ischemic insult; the increase in cytosolic calcium content of tubular cells leads to cell necrosis [129].

Epithelial necrosis is confined to the "pars recta" both in ischemic and nephrotoxic ARF. This occurs, in ischemic ARF, because of the greater susceptibility to ischemia of S_3 cells [113], which are mainly located in the "pars recta," and possibly because of poor reflow into this area in the post-ischemic period [27, 141]. In nephrotoxic ARF, it may occur because of the accumulation of heavy metals in the "pars recta" (active transport); the ischemic effects of the associated alteration in renal hemodynamics (fall and redistribution in RBF) may also contribute to the necrotic lesion.

The late occurrence of progressive tubular cell damage resulting in epithelial necrosis in the "pars recta" may create new conditions within the tubules, which may maintain the reduced GFR by mechanisms other than changes in renal hemodynamics. Thus, the backleak of filtrate through the necrotic tubular wall and the obstruction of tubular lumina by cellular debris may represent two important pathogenetic factors, possibly associated with a reduced glomerular K_f, in the maintenance stage of ARF [33].

That tubular obstruction can markedly reduce GFR is demonstrated by the occurrence of ARF in rats injected i.v. with folic acid at high doses; with tubular fluid reabsorption along the nephron, folic acid precipitates totally obstructing individual tubules [314]. Tubular obstruction may impair filtration both by the slow-acting, positive TGF and by a decrease in glomerular transcapillary hydraulic pressure difference.

Much more difficult is the evaluation of the meaning of studies showing tubular leakage of microinjected inulin. As mentioned by Oken [314], if we consider that the capacity of a normal rat proximal tubule is 1.8 to 3.4 nanolitres, the sudden injection of 4 to 7 nanolitres of inulin solution in a severely damaged proximal tubule, with a reduced absorptive capacity and possibly with obstruction of the lumen, may easily cause artifactual lesions of tubular walls, thus making meaningless any detection of leakage.

6.10 PATHOGENETIC HYPOTHESIS

In my opinion, the occurrence and the maintenance of oligo-anuria in ARF is the result of the contribution of all mentioned factors. As outlined in figure 1–2, in fact, hemorrhagic hypotension or severe salt depletion with contraction of ECV will result in afferent arteriole constriction (prerenal ARF). The persistent reduction in RBF will increase renin secretion in JGA and cause ischemic disfunction of proximal tubules with restriction of active salt reabsorption by proximal tubular cells. A similar effect is caused by the tubular damage due to noxious substances, such as nephrotoxic drugs. The increased tubular fluid delivery to the macula densa will increase the volume of the distal tubule and therefore the contact between mac-

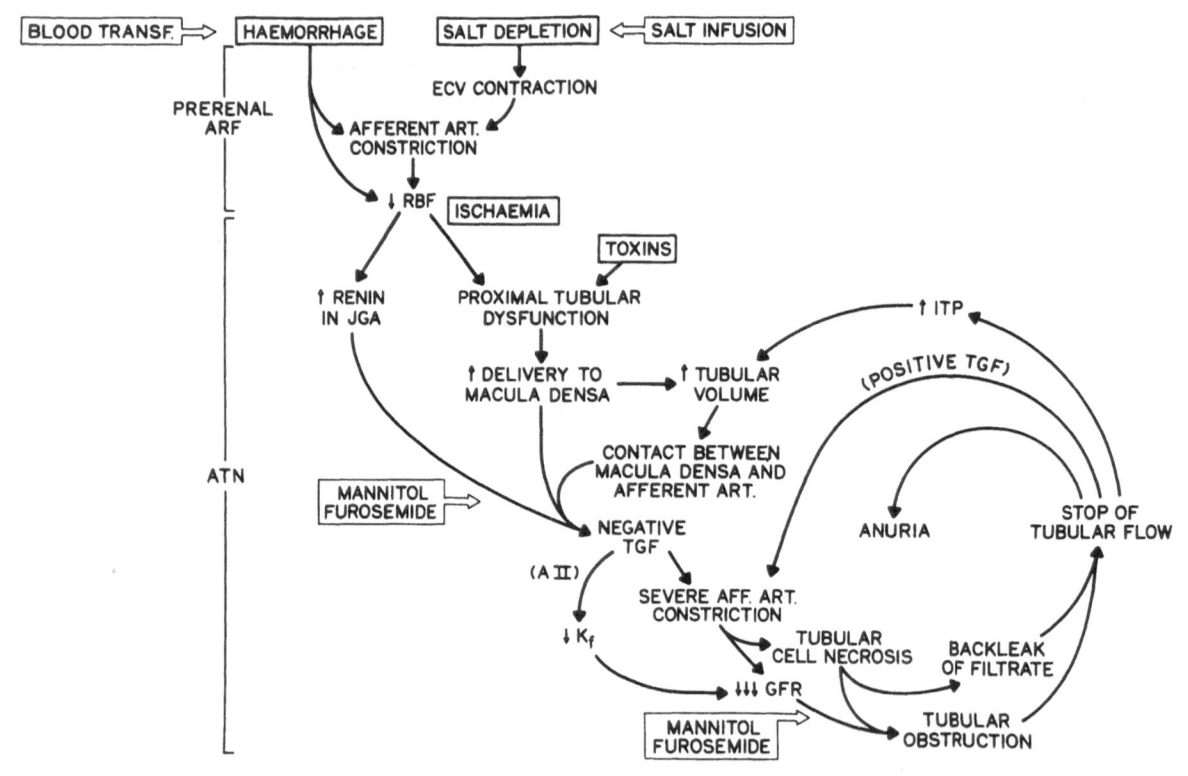

FIGURE 1–2. Pathogenesis of acute renal failure.

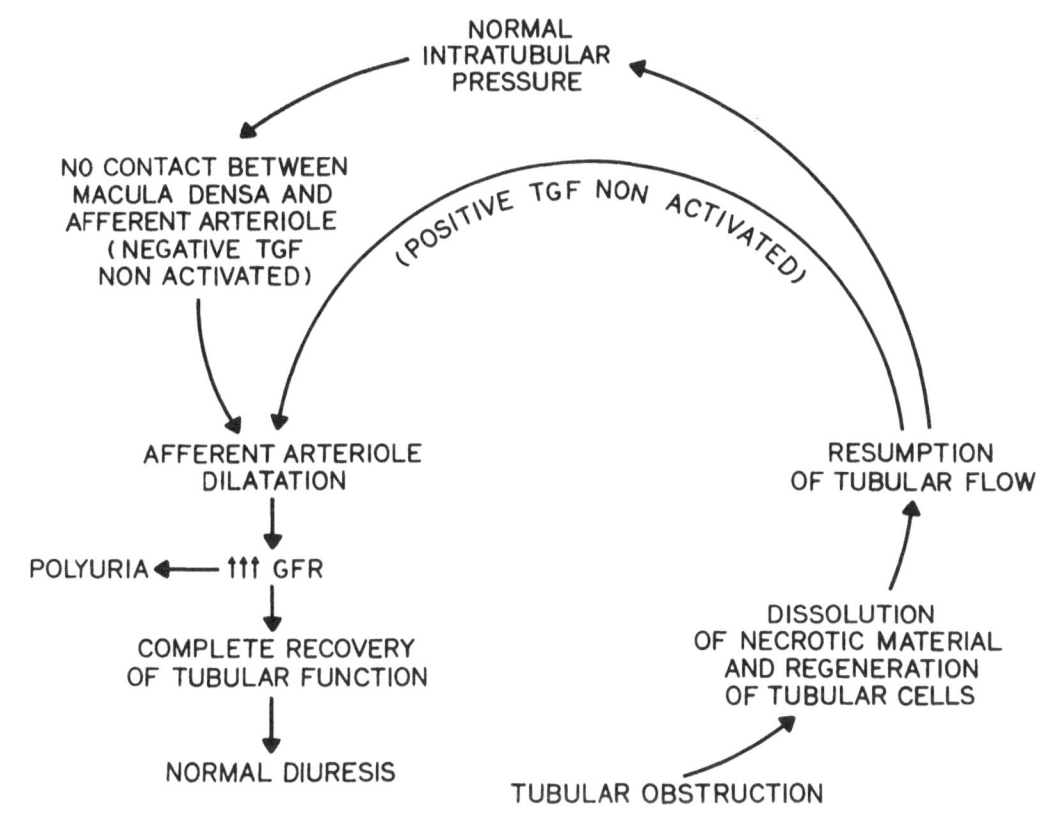

FIGURE 1-3. Recovery from acute renal failure.

ula densa and afferent arteriole. The activation of the negative TGF mechanism will lead to severe constriction of the afferent arteriole and reduction in K_f (by AII), thus responsible for a low GFR. The persisting ischemia with the consequent tubular cell necrosis will cause backleak of filtrate. Cell necrosis and low GFR will lead to tubular obstruction. The result will be the oligo-anuria. But the blockade of the tubular lumen will increase ITP, which will maintain the large contact between macula densa and afferent arteriole and decrease the glomerular transcapillary pressure. On the other hand, the prolonged tubular obstruction will activate the slow-acting, positive TGF mechanism, which will maintain a severe constriction of the afferent arteriole, in this way closing the circle (figure 1-2).

This hypothesis may well account for the following still unsolved phenomena:

a. The disparity between renal function impairment and integrity of renal structures so frequently remarked both in humans and in experimental animals in early stage of ARF.

b. The persistent renal function impairment despite normalization of RBF, late in the course of ARF.

c. The recovery of renal function with time: the dissolution of necrotic debris will, in fact, release the obstruction and the regeneration of epithelial cells will abolish any backleak of filtrate (figure 1-3).

d. The polyuric phase during recovery: the regenerated tubular cells are initially unable to normally reabsorb filtrate. The complete recovery of tubular cell function will ensue a normal diuresis with concentrated urine (figure 1-3).

Note

1. Proximal tubules of rat kidneys have three distinctive cell types, named S_1, S_2, and S_3; S_1 cells occur in the first segments of the proximal convoluted tubules, S_2 cells in the remaining segments of proximal convoluted tubules and in the first part (less than half) of the proximal straight tubules ("pars recta"), and S_3 cells in the remaining part of the "pars recta". S_1 and S_2 cells are therefore located in the cortex; S_3 cells are located in the outer stripe of the medulla and in the medullary rays.

References

1. Andreucci VE, Dal Canton A. Can acute renal failure in humans be prevented? Proc EDTA 17: 123–132, 1980.
2. Thurau K, Boylan JW, Mason J. Pathophysiology of acute renal failure. In Renal Disease, Black D, Jones NF (eds). Oxford: Blackwell Scientific Publ, 1979 (4th ed), pp. 64–92.
3. Siegler RL, Bloomer HA. Acute renal failure with prolonged oliguria. An account of five cases. JAMA 225: 133–137, 1973.
4. Oken DE. Acute renal failure (vasomotor nephropathy): Micropuncture studies of the pathogenetic mechanisms. Ann Rev Med 26: 307–319, 1975.
5. Lameire N, Vanholder R, Vakaet L, Pattyn P, Quatacker J, Ringoir S. Renal hemodynamics in nephrotoxic acute renal failure. Proc NIH Conference on effect of drugs and environmental toxicants on the kidneys, Pinehurst, 1981.
6. Sudo M, Honda N, Hishida A, Nagase M. Renal hemodynamics in uranyl acetate-induced acute renal failure of rabbits. Kidney Int 11: 35–43, 1977.
7. Mendelsohn FAO, Smith EA. Intrarenal renin, angiotensin II and plasma renin in rats with uranyl nitrate-induced and glycerol-induced acute renal failure. Kidney Int 17: 465–472, 1980.
8. Flamenbaum W, McNeil JS, Kotchen TA, Saladino AJ. Experimental acute renal failure induced by uranyl nitrate in the dog. Circ Res 31: 682–698, 1972.
9. Stein JH, Gottschall J, Osgood RW, Ferris TF. Pathophysiology of a nephrotoxic model of acute renal failure. Kidney Int 8: 27–41, 1975.
10. Flamenbaum W, Huddleston ML, McNeil JS, Hamburger RJ. Uranyl nitrate-induced acute renal failure in the rat: Micropuncture and renal hemodynamic studies. Kidney Int 6: 408–418, 1974.
11. Kleinman JG, McNeil JS, Flamenbaum W. Uranyl nitrate acute renal failure in the dog: Early changes in renal function and hemodynamics. Clin Sci 48: 9–16, 1975.
12. Stein JH, Sorkin MI. Pathophysiology of a vasomotor and nephrotoxic model of acute renal failure in the dog. Kidney Int 10 (Suppl 6): 586–593, 1976.
13. Flamenbaum W. Pathophysiology of acute renal failure. Arch Intern Med 131: 911–928, 1973.
14. Mauk RH, Patak RV, Fadem SZ, Litschitz MD, Stein JH. Effects of prostaglandin E administration in a nephrotoxic and a vasoconstrictor model of acute renal failure. Kidney Int 12: 122–130, 1977.
15. Hostetter TH, Wilkes BM, Brenner BM. Mechanisms of impaired glomerular filtration in acute renal failure. In Acute Renal Failure, Brenner BM, Stein JH (eds). New York: Churchill Livingstone, 1980, pp. 52–78.
16. Lindner A, Cutler RE, Goodman WG. Synergism of dopamine plus furosemide in preventing acute renal failure in the dog. Kidney Int 16: 158–166, 1979.
17. Blantz RC. The mechanism of acute renal failure after uranyl nitrate. J Clin Invest 55: 621–635, 1975.
18. Avasthi PS, Evan AP, Hay D. Glomerular endothelial cells in uranyl nitrate-induced acute renal failure in rats. J Clin Invest 65: 121–127, 1980.
19. Cachia R, Savin VJ, Patak RV, Ridge SM. Effect of mercuric chloride and uranyl nitrate on ultrafiltration coefficient in isolated glomeruli. Kidney Int 19: 236, 1981.
20. Mendelsohn FAO. Angiotensin II: Evidence for its role as an intrarenal hormone. Kidney Int 22 (Suppl 12): 578–581, 1982.
21. Blantz RC, Konnen KS, Tucker BJ. Angiotensin II effects upon the glomerular microcirculation and ultrafiltration coefficient of the rat. J Clin Invest 57: 419–434, 1976.
22. Ryan R, McNeil JS, Flamenbaum W, Nagle R. Uranyl nitrate-induced acute renal failure in the rat. Effect of varying doses and saline loading. Proc Soc Exp Biol Med 143: 289–296, 1973.
23. Mason JX, Olbricht CY, Takabatake T, Thurau K. The early phase of experimental acute renal failure. I Intratubular-pressure and obstruction. Pflügers Arch 370: 155–163, 1977.
24. Arendshorst WJ, Finn WF, Gottschalk CW. Nephron stop-flow pressure response to obstruction for 24 hours in the rat kidney. J Clin Invest 53: 1497–1500, 1974.
25. Flamenbaum W, Hamburger RJ, Huddleston ML, Kaufman J, McNeil JS, Schwartz JH, Nagle R. The initiation phase of experimental acute renal failure: An evaluation of uranyl nitrate-induced acute renal failure in the rat. Kidney Int 10 (Suppl 6): S115–S122, 1976.
26. Flamenbaum W, Hamburger R, Kaukman J. Distal tubule [Na$^+$] and juxtaglomerular apparatus renin activity in uranyl nitrate-induced acute renal failure in the rat. Pflügers Archiv 364: 209–215, 1976.
27. Zalme RC, McDowell EM, Nagle RB, McNeil JS, Flamenbaum W, Trump BF. Studies on the pathophysiology of acute renal failure. Virchows Arch B Cell Pathol 22: 197–216, 1976.
28. McDowell EM, Nagle RB, Zalme RC, McNeil JS, Flamenbaum W., Trump BF. Studies on the

pathophysiology of acute renal failure I. Virchows Arch B Cell Path 22: 173–196, 1976.

29. Churchill S, Zarlengo MD, Carvalho JS, Gottlieb MN, Oken DE. Normal renocortical blood flow in experimental acute renal failure. Kidney Int 11: 246–255, 1977.

30. Sherwood T, Lavender JP, Russell SB. Mercury-induced renal vascular shutdown. Observations in experimental acute renal failure. Eur J Clin Invest 4: 1–8, 1974.

31. Conn HL, Wilds L, Helwig J, Ibach P. A study of the renal circulation, tubular function and morphology, and urinary volume and composition in dogs following mercury poisoning and transfusion of human blood. J Clin Invest 35: 732–741, 1954.

32. Gaal K, Siklos J. Effect of beta-receptor antagonists on $HgCl_2$-induced acute renal failure in rats. Renal Physiol 5:245–255, 1982.

33. Stein JH, Lifschitz MD, Barnes LD. Current concepts on the pathophysiology of acute renal failure. Am J Physiol 234: F171–F181, 1978.

34. Sahaphong S, Trump BF. Studies of cellular injury in isolated kidney tubules of the flounder. Am J Pathol 63: 277–298, 1971.

35. Wockel W, Stegner HE, Janisch W. Zum topochemischen Quecksilbermachweis in der Niere bei experimenteller Sublimatvergiftung. Arch Pathol Anat Physiol 334: 503–509, 1961.

36. Hsu CH, Kurtz TW, Rosensweig J, Weller JM. Renal hemodynamics in $HgCl_2$-induced acute renal failure. Nephron 18: 326–332, 1977.

37. Vanholder RC, Praet MM, Pattyn PA, Leusen IR, Lameire NH. Dissociation of glomerular filtration and renal blood flow in $HgCl_2$-induced acute renal failure. Kidney Int 22: 162–170, 1982.

38. Hsu CH, Kurtz TW. Renal hemodynamics in experimental acute renal failure. Nephron 27: 204–208, 1981.

39. Kurtz TW, Hsu CH. Systemic hemodynamics in $HgCl_2$-induced acute renal failure. Nephron 21: 100–106, 1978.

40. Flanigan WJ, Oken DE. Renal micropuncture study of the development of anuria in the rat with mercury-induced acute renal failure. J Clin Invest 44: 449–457, 1965.

41. Baehler RW, Kotchen TA, Burke JH, Galla JH, Bhathena D. Considerations in the pathophysiology of mercuric chloride-induced acute renal failure. J Lab Clin Med 90: 330–340, 1977.

42. Finckh ES: The pathogenesis of uraemia in acute renal failure abnormality of intrarenal vascular tone as possible mechanism. Lancet 2: 330–333, 1962.

43. Andreucci VE. Manual of Renal Micropuncture. Naples: Idelson, 1978.

44. Kurtz TW, Slavicek JM, Hsu CH. Blood viscosity in experimental acute renal failure. Nephron 30: 348–351, 1982.

45. Sraer JD, Baud L, Sraer J, Delarve F, Ardaillou R. Stimulation of PGE_2 synthesis by mercuric chloride in rat glomeruli and glomerular cells in vitro. Kidney Int 21 (Suppl 11): S63–S68, 1982.

46. Baylis C, Deen WM, Myers BD, Brenner BM. Effects of some vasodilator drugs on transcapillary fluid exchange in renal cortex. Am J Physiol 230: 1148–1156, 1976.

47. Brenner BM, Schor N, Ichikawa I. Role of angiotensin II in the physiologic regulation of glomerular filtration. Am J Cardiol 49: 1430–1433, 1982.

48. Biber TUL, Mylle M, Baines AD, Gottschalk CW, Oliver JR, Mac Dowell MC. A study by micropuncture and microdissection of acute renal damage in rats. Am J Med 44: 664–705, 1968.

49. Flamenbaum W, McDonald FD, Di Bona GF, Oken DE. Micropuncture study of renal tubular factors in low-dose mercury poisoning. Nephron 8: 221–234, 1971.

50. Richards AN. Direct observations of change in function of the renal tubule caused by certain poisons. Trans Assoc Am Physicians 44: 64–76, 1929.

51. Barenberg RL, Solomon S, Papper S, Anderson R. Clearance and micropuncture study of renal function in mercuric chloride-treated rats. J Lab Clin Med 72: 473–484, 1968.

52. Steinhausen M, Eisenbach GM, Helmstadter V. Concentration of lissamine green in proximal tubules of antidiuretic and mercury poisoned rats and the permeability of these tubules. Pflügers Arch 311: 1–15, 1969.

53. Olbricht C, Mason J, Takabatake T, Hohlbrugger G, Thurau K. The early phase of experimental acute renal failure. II Tubular leakage and the reliability of glomerular markers. Pflügers Arch 378: 251–258, 1977.

54. Chopra S, Kaufman JS, Jones TW, Hong WK, Gehr MK, Hamburger RJ, Flamenbaum W, Trump BF. Cis-diamminedichlorplatinum-induced acute renal failure in the rat. Kidney Int 21: 54–64, 1982

55. Cvitkovic E, Spaulding J, Bethune V, Martin J, Whitmore WF. Improvement of cis-dichlorodiammineplatinum (NSC 119875): Therapeutic index in an animal model. Cancer 39: 1357–1361, 1977.

56. Choie DD, Longnecker DS, Del Campo AA. Acute and chronic cisplatin nephrotoxicity in rats. Lab Invest 44: 397–402, 1981.

57. Levi J, Jacobs C, Kalman SM, McTigue M, Weiner MW. Mechanism of cis-platinum nephrotoxicity: I Effects of sulphydryl groups in rat kidneys. J Pharmacol Exp Ther 213: 545–550, 1980.

58. Porter GA, Bennett WM. Nephrotoxic acute renal failure due to common drugs. Am J Physiol 241: F1–F8, 1981.

59. Jones TW, Chopra S, McDowell EM, Flamenbaum W, Trump BF. Morphological alterations associated with cis-diamminedichlor-platinum-induced acute renal failure in the rat. In Acute Renal Failure, Eliahou HE (ed). London: John Libbey, 1982, pp. 78–82.

60. Vaamonde CA, Teixeira RB, Morales J, Roth D,

Kelley J, Alpert H, Pardo V. A new model for studying drug-induced acute renal failure: The rat with untreated diabetes mellitus. In Acute Renal Failure, Eliahou HE (ed). London: John Libbey, 1982, pp. 96–101.

61. Madias NE, Harrington JT. Platinum nephrotoxicity. Am J Med 65: 307–314, 1978.

62. Dobyan DC, Levi J, Jacobs C, Kosek J, Weiner MW. Mechanism of cis-platinum nephrotoxicity. II Morphologic observations. J Pharmacol Exp Ther 213: 551–556, 1980.

63. de Rougemont D, Oeschger A, Konrad L, Thiel G, Torhorst J, Wenk M, Wunderlich P, Brunner FP. Gentamicin-induced acute renal failure in the rat. Effect of dehydration, DOCA-saline and furosemide. Nephron 29: 176–184, 1981.

64. Bennett WM. Aminoglycoside nephrotoxicity. Experimental and clinical considerations. Mineral Electrolyte Metab 6: 277–286, 1981.

65. Kaloyanides GJ, Pastoriza-Munoz E. Aminoglycoside nephrotoxicity. Kidney Int 18: 571–582, 1980.

66. Harrison WO, Silverblatt FJ, Turck M. Gentamicin nephrotoxicity: Failure of three cephalosporins to potentiate injury in rats. Antimicrob Agents Chemother 8: 209–215, 1975.

67. Luft FC, Patel V, Yum MN, Kleit SA. Nephrotoxicity of cephalosporin-gentamicin combination in rats. Antimicrob Agents Chemother 9: 831–839, 1976.

68. Dolislager D, Fravert D, Tune B. Interaction of aminoglycosides and cephaloridine in the rabbit kidney. Res Comm Chem Path Pharm 26: 13–23, 1979.

69. Dellinger P, Murphy T, Pinn V, Barza M, Weinstein L. Protective effect of cephalothin against gentamicin-induced nephrotoxicity in rats. Antimicrob Agents Chemother 9: 172–178, 1976.

70. Barza M, Pinn V, Tanguay P, Murray T. Nephrotoxicity of newer cephalosporins and aminoglycosides alone and in combination in a rat model. J Antimicrob Chemother 4 (Suppl A): 59–68, 1978.

71. Bloch R, Luft FC, Rankin LI, Sloan RS, Yum MN, Maxwell DR. Protection from gentamicin nephrotoxicity by cephalothin and carbenicillin. Antimicrob Agents Chemother 15: 46–49, 1979.

72. Barr GA, Mazze RI, Cousins MJ, Kosek JC. An animal model for combined methoxyflurane and gentamicin nephrotoxicity. Brit J Anaesth 45: 306–311, 1973.

73. Bennett WM, Hartnett, MN, Gilbert D, Houghton D, Porter GA. Effect of sodium intake on gentamicin nephrotoxicity in the rat. Proc Soc Exp Biol Med 151: 736–738, 1976.

74. Adelman RD, Spangler WL, Beasom F, Ishizaki G, Conzelman GM. Furosemide enhancement of experimental gentamicin nephrotoxicity. Comparison of functional and morphological changes with activities of urinary enzymes. J Infect Dis 140: 342–352, 1979.

75. Suemitsu-Higa EM, Schor N, Boim M, Ajzen H, Ramos OL. Humoral factors in gentamicin nephrotoxicity: 2-Role of the prostaglandin system. In Acute Renal Failure, Eliahou HE (ed). London: John Libbey, 1982, pp. 88–90.

76. Hsu CH, Kurtz TW, Easterling RE, Weller JM. Potentiation of gentamicin nephrotoxicity by metabolic acidosis. Proc Soc Exp Biol Med 146: 894–897, 1974.

77. Cronin RE. Aminoglycoside nephrotoxicity: Pathogenesis and prevention. Clin Nephrol 11: 251–256, 1979.

78. Luft FC, Kleit SA. Renal parenchymal accumulation of aminoglycoside antibiotics in rats. J Infect Dis 130: 656–659, 1974.

79. Fabre J, Rudhardt M, Blanchard P, Regamey C. Persistence of sisomicin and gentamicin in renal cortex and medulla compared with other organs and serum of rats. Kidney Int 10: 444–449, 1976.

80. Fabre J, Fillastre JP, Morin JP, Rudhardt M. Nephrotoxicity of gentamicin. Contr Nephrol 10: 53–62, 1978.

81. Luft FC, Patel V, Yum MN, Patel V, Kleit SA. Experimental aminoglycoside nephrotoxicity. J Lab Clin Med 86: 213–220, 1975.

82. Schentag JJ, Jusko WJ. Renal clearances and tissue accumulation of gentamicin. Clin Pharmacol Ther 22: 364–370, 1977.

83. Kosek JC, Mazze RI, Cousins MJ: Nephrotoxicity of gentamicin. Lab Invest 30: 48–57, 1974.

84. Pastoriza-Munoz E, Bowman RL, Kaloyanides GJ. Renal tubular transport of gentamicin in the rat. Kidney Int 16: 440–450, 1979.

85. Senekjian HO, Knight TF, Weinman EJ. Micropuncture study of the handling of gentamicin by the rat kidney. Kidney Int 19: 416–423, 1981.

86. Sheth AU, Senekjian HO, Babino H, Knight TF, Weinman EJ. Renal handling of gentamicin by the Munich-Wistar rat. Am J Physiol 241: F645–F648, 1981.

87. Houghton DC, Hartnett M, Campbell-Boswell M, Porter G, Bennett W. A light and electron microscopic analysis of gentamicin nephrotoxicity in rats. Am J Pathol 82: 589–612, 1976.

88. Baylis C, Rennke HR, Brenner BM. Mechanisms of the defect in glomerular ultrafiltration associated with gentamicin administration. Kidney Int 12: 344–353, 1977.

89. Vandewalle A, Farman N, Morin JP, Fillastre JP, Hatt PY, Bonvalet JP. Gentamicin incorporation along the nephron: Autoradiographic study on isolated tubules. Kidney Int 19: 529–539, 1981.

90. Schor N, Ichikawa I, Rennke HG, Troy JL, Brenner BM. Pathophysiology of altered glomerular function in aminoglycoside-treated rats. Kidney Int 19: 288–296, 1981.

91. Morin JP, Viotte G, Vandewalle A, Van Hoof F, Tulkens P, Fillastre JP. Gentamicin-induced nephrotoxicity: A cell biology approach. Kidney Int 18: 583–590, 1980.

92. Teixeira RB, Kelley J, Alpert H, Pardo V, Vaamonde CA. Complete protection from gentamicin-induced acute renal failure in the diabetes mellitus rat. Kidney Int 21: 600–612, 1982. 148–155, 1982.

93. Sastrasinh M, Knauss TC, Weinberg JM, Humes HD. Identification of the gentamicin receptor of renal brush border membranes. Kidney Int 19: 213, 1981.

94. Whelton A, Solez K. Aminoglycoside nephrotoxicity. A tale of two transports. J Lab Clin Med 99: 148–155, 1982.

95. Whelton A, Stout RL, Carter GG, Craig TJ, Bryant HH, Herbst DV, Walker WG. Modulation of renal cortical aminoglycoside uptake by concurrent amino acid administration. In Nephrotoxicité, Ototoxicité Médicamenteuses, Fillastre JP (ed). Rouen: Inserm, 1982, pp. 39–54.

96. Malis CO, Solez K. Whelton A. Nephrotoxicity of a Single Dose of Gentamicin in Lysine-Treated Rats. (In press.)

97. Solez K, Stout R, Bendush B, Silvia CB, Whelton A. Adverse effect of amino acid solutions in aminoglycoside-induced acute renal failure in rabbits and rats. In Acute Renal Failure, Eliahou HE (ed). London; John Libbey, 1982, pp. 241–247.

98. Houghton DC, Plamp CE, De Fehr JM, Bennett WM, Porter G, Gilbert D. Gentamicin and tobramycin nephrotoxicity. Am J Pathol 93: 137–152, 1978.

99. Luft FC, Rankin LI, Sloan RS, Yum MN. Recovery from aminoglycoside nephrotoxicity with continued drug administration. Antimicrob Agents Chemother 14: 284–287, 1978.

100. Gilbert DN, Houghton DC, Bennett WM, Plamp CE, Reger K, Porter GA. Reversibility of gentamicin nephrotoxicity in rats: Recovery during continued drug administration. Proc Soc Exp Biol Med 160: 99–103, 1979.

101. Luft FC, Yum MN, Kleit SA. The effect of concomitant mercuric chloride and gentamicin on kidney structure and function in the rat. J Lab Clin Med 89: 622–631, 1977.

102. Lane AZ, Wright GE, Blair DC. Ototoxicity and nephrotoxicity of amikacin. Am J Med 62: 911–918, 1977.

103. Cowan RH, Jukkola AF, Arant BS Jr. Pathophysiologic evidence of gentamicin nephrotoxicity in neonatal puppies. Pediatr Res 14: 1204–1211, 1980.

104. Avasthi PS, Evan AP, Huser JW, Luft FC. Effect of gentamicin on glomerular ultrastructure. J Lab Clin Med 98: 444–454, 1981.

105. Evan AP, Luft FC. Gentamicin-induced glomerular injury. In Néphrotoxicité. Ototoxicité Médicamenteuses, Fillastre JP (ed). Rouen: Inserm, 1982, pp. 67–78.

106. Myers BD, Deen WM, Brenner BM. Effects of norepinephrine and angiotensin II on the determinants of glomerular ultrafiltration and proximal tubule fluid reabsorptions in the rat. Circ Res 37: 101–110, 1975.

107. Mc Caa RE, Hall JE, Mc Caa CS. The effects of angiotensin I converting-enzyme inhibitors on arterial blood pressure and urinary sodium excretion: Role of the renal renin-angiotensin and kallikrein-kinin system. Circ Res 43: 132–139, 1978.

108. Luft FC, Aronoff GR, Evan AP, Connors BA, Weinberger MH, Kleit SA. Effect of captopril on gentamicin-induced acute renal failure. In Acute Renal Failure, Eliahou HE (ed). London: John Libbey, 1982, pp. 108–111.

109. Soberon L, Bowman RL, Pastoriza-Munoz E, Kaloyanides GJ. Comparative nephrotoxicities of gentamicin, metilmicin and tobramycin in the rat. J Pharmacol Exp Ther 210: 334–343, 1979.

110. Newman RA, Weinstock LB, Gump DW, Hacker MP, Yates JW. Effect of osmotic diuresis on gentamicin-induced nephrotoxicity in rats. Arch Toxicol 45: 213–221, 1980.

111. Taguma Y, Sasaki Y, Kyogoku Y, Arakawa M, Shioji R, Furuyama T, Yoshinaga K. Morphological changes in an early phase of norepinephrine-induced acute renal failure in unilaterally nephrectomized dogs. J Lab Clin Med 96: 616–632, 1980.

112. Mason J, Beck F, Dorge A, Rick R, Thurau K. Intracellular electrolyte composition following renal ischemia. Kidney Int 20: 61–70, 1981.

113. Venkatachalam MA, Bernard DB, Donohoe JF, Levinsky NG. Ischemic damage and repair in the rat proximal tubule: Differences among the S_1, S_2 and S_3 segments. Kidney Int 14: 31–49, 1978.

114. Finn WF, Chevalier RL. Recovery from postischemic acute renal failure in the rat. Kidney Int 16: 113–123, 1979.

115. Cronin RE, Erickson AM, de Torrente A, McDonald KM, Schrier RW. Norepinephrine-induced acute renal failure: A reversible ischemic model of acute renal failure. Kidney Int 14: 187–190, 1978.

116. Cox JW, Baehler RW, Sharma H, O'Dorisio T, Osgood RW, Stein JH, Ferris TF. Studies on the mechanism of oliguria in a model of unilateral acute renal failure. J Clin Invest 53: 1546–1558, 1974.

117. Finn WF. Enhanced recovery from postischemic acute renal failure. Micropuncture studies in the rat. Circ Res 46: 440–448, 1980.

118. Arendshorst WJ, Finn WF, Gottschalck CW. Pathogenesis of acute renal failure following renal ischemia in the rat. Circ Res 37: 558–568, 1975.

119. Burke TJ, Cronin RE, Duchin KL, Peterson LN, Schrier RW. Ischemia and tubule obstruction during acute renal failure in dogs: Mannitol in protection. Am J Physiol 238: F305–F314, 1980.

120. Finn WF. Nephron heterogeneity in polyuric acute renal failure. J Lab Clin Med 98: 21–29, 1981.

121. de Torrente A, Miller PD, Cronin RE, Paulsen PE, Erickson AL, Schrier RW. Effects of furosemide and acetylcholine in norepinephrine-induced acute renal failure. Am J Physiol 235: F131–F136, 1978.

122. Flores J, Di Bona DR, Beck CH, Leaf A. The role of cell swelling in ischemic renal damage and the protective effect of hypertonic solute. J Clin Invest 51: 118–126, 1972.

123. Frega NS, Di Bona DR, Leaf A. Ischemic renal injury. Kidney Int 10 (Suppl 6): S17–S25, 1976.

124. Riley AL, Alexander EA, Migdal S, Levinsky NG. The effect of ischemia on renal blood flow in the dog. Kidney Int 7: 27–34, 1975.

125. Weber PC, Held E, Uhlich E, Eigler J: Reaction constants of renin in juxtaglomerular apparatus and plasma renin activity after renal ischemia and hemorrhage. Kidney Int 7: 331–341, 1975.

126. Iaina A, Solomon S, Eliahou HE. Reduction in severity of acute renal failure in rats by beta-adrenergic blockade. Lancet II: 157–159, 1975.

127. Mason J, Kain H, Shiigai T, Welsch J. The early phase of experimental acute renal failure. V The influence of suppressing the renin-angiotensin system. Pflügers Arch 380: 233–243, 1979.

128. Patak RV, Fadem SZ, Lifschitz MD, Stein JH. Study of factors which modify the development of norepinephrine-induced acute renal failure in the dog. Kidney Int 15: 227–237, 1979.

129. Schrier RW, Arnold PE, Burke TJ. Alterations in mitochondrial respiration and calcium movements in norepinephrine-induced acute renal failure: Modification by mannitol. In Acute Renal Failure, Eliahou HE (ed). London; John Libbey, 1982, pp. 21–22.

130. Jensen PK, Steven K. Influence of intratubular pressure on proximal tubular compliance and capillary diameter in the rat kidney. Pflügers Arch 382: 179, 1979.

131. Tanner GA, Sloan KL, Sophasan S. Effects of renal artery occlusion on kidney function in the rat. Kidney Int 4: 377–389, 1973.

132. Tanner GA, Steinhausen M. Tubular obstruction in ischemia-induced acute renal failure in the rat. Kidney Int 10 (Suppl. 6): S65–S73, 1976.

133. Solez K, Racusen LC, Whelton A. Glomerular epithelial cell changes in early post-ischemic acute renal failure in rabbits and man. Am J Path 103: 163, 1981.

134. Racusen LC, Solez K, Whelton A. Glomerular podocyte changes and increased permeability to protein in early post-ischemic acute renal failure. In Acute Renal Failure, Eliahou HE (ed). London: John Libbey, 1982, pp. 215–218.

135. Savin VJ, Patak RV, Marr G. Glomerular filtration in ischemic renal failure. Kidney Int 16: 776, 1979.

136. Chan L, Thulborn KR, Waterton JC, Ledingham JGG, Ross BD, Radda GK. Prevention of ischemic acidosis: A new approach to acute renal failure. Proc EDTA 17: 681–685, 1980.

137. Chan L, Ledingham JGG, Dixon JA, Thulborn KR, Waterton JC, Radda GK, Ross BD. Acute renal failure: A proposed mechanism based upon ^{31}P nuclear magnetic resonance studies in the rat. In Acute Renal Failure, Eliahou HE (ed). London: John Libbey, 1982, pp. 35–41.

138. Chan L, Ledingham JGG, Clarke J, Ross BD. The importance of pH in acute renal failure. In Acute Renal Failure, Eliahou HE (ed). London: John Libbey, 1982, pp. 58–61.

139. Donohoe JF, Venkatachalam MA, Bernard DB, Levinsky NG. Tubular leakage and obstruction after renal ischemia: Structural-functional correlations. Kidney Int 13: 208–222, 1978.

140. Thurau K, Beck F, Mason J, Rick R, Dörge A. Intracellular electrolytes of proximal and distal tubular cells following renal ischemia. In Acute Renal Failure, Eliahou HE (ed). London: John Libbey, 1982, pp. 10–14.

141. Glaumann B, Trump BF. Studies on the pathogenesis of ischemic cell injury. III Morphological changes of the proximal pars recta tubules (P_3) of the rat kidney made ischemic in vivo. Virchows Arch B Cell Path 19: 303–323, 1975.

142. Reimer KA, Jennings RB. Alterations in renal cortex following ischemic injury: I PAH uptake by slices of cortex after ischemia or autolysis. Lab Invest 25: 176–184, 1971.

143. Reimer KA, Ganote CE, Jennings RB. Alterations in renal cortex following ischemic injury: III Ultrastructure of proximal tubules after ischemia or autolysis. Lab Invest 26: 347–365, 1972.

144. Glaumann B, Glaumann H, Berezesky IK, Trump BF. Studies on cellular recovery from injury. II Ultrastructural studies on the recovery of the pars convoluta of the proximal tubule of the rat kidney from temporary ischemia. Virchows Arch Cell Pathol 24: 1, 1977.

145. Glaumann B, Glaumann H, Trump BF. Studies on cellular recovery from injury. III Ultrastructural studies on the recovery of the pars recta of the proximal tubule (P_3 segment) of the rat kidney from temporary ischemia. Virchows Arch Cell Pathol 25: 281, 1977.

146. Steinhausen M, Thederan H, Nolinski D, Dallenbach FD, Schwaier A. Further evidence of tubular blockage after acute ischemic renal failure in Tupaia balangeri and rats. Virchow Arch 381: 13, 1978.

147. Arendshorst WJ, Finn WF, Gottschalk CW. Micropuncture study of acute renal failure following temporary renal ischemia in the rat. Kidney Int 10 (Suppl 6): S100–S105, 1976.

148. Chevalier RL, Finn WF. Effects of propranolol on postischemic acute renal failure. Nephron 25: 77–81, 1980.

149. Cronin RE, de Torrente A, Miller PD, Bulger RE, Burke TJ, Schrier RW. Pathogenic mechanisms in early norepinephrine-induced acute renal failure: Functional and histological correlates of protection. Kidney Int 14: 115–125, 1978.

150. Myers BD, Chui F, Hilberman M and Michaels AS. Transtubular leakage of glomerular filtrate in

human acute renal failure. Am J Physiol 237: F319–325, 1979.

151. Myers BD, Carrie BJ, Yee RR, Hilberman M, Michaels AS. Pathophysiology of hemodynamically mediated acute renal failure in man, Kidney Int 18: 495–504, 1980.

152. Myers BD, Hilberman M, Carrie BJ, Spencer RJ, Stinson EB, Robertson CR. Dynamics of glomerular ultrafiltration following open-heart surgery. Kidney Int 20: 366–374, 1981.

153. Hanley MJ. Isolated nephron segments in a rabbit model of ischemic acute renal failure. Am J Physiol 239: F17–F23, 1980.

154. Thiel G, Wilson DR, Arce ML, Oken DE. Glycerol induced hemoglobinuric acute renal failure in the rat. II The experimental model, predisposing factors and pathophysiologic factors. Nephron 4:276–297, 1967.

155. Cabili S, Charney AN. Lack of an effect of saline loading on glycerol-induced acute renal failure. Nephron 30: 73–76, 1982.

156. Papanicolau N, Callard P, Bariety J, Milliez P. The effect of indomethacin and prostaglandin (PGE₂) on renal failure due to glycerol in saline-loaded rats. Clin Sci Mol Med 49: 507–510, 1975.

157. Ayer G, Grandchamp A, Wyler T, Truniger B. Intrarenal hemodynamics in glycerol-induced myohemoglobinuric acute renal failure in the rat. Circ Res 29: 128–135, 1971.

158. Oken DE, Arce ML, Wilson DR. Glycerol-induced hemoglobinuric acute renal failure in the rat. I Micropuncture study of the development of oliguria. J Clin Invest 45: 724–735, 1966.

159. Wilson DR, Thiel G, Arce ML, Oken DE. Glycerol-induced hemoglobinuric acute renal failure in the rat: III Micropuncture study of the effects of mannitol and isotonic saline on individual nephron function. Nephron 4: 337–355, 1967.

160. Chedru MF, Baethke R, Oken DE: Renal cortical blood flow and glomerular filtration in myohemoglobinuric acute renal failure. Kidney Int 1: 232–239, 1979.

161. Kurtz TW, Maletz RM, Hsu CH. Renal cortical blood flow in glycerol-induced acute renal failure in the rat. Circ Res 38: 30–35, 1976.

162. Hsu CH, Kurtz TW, Waldinger TP. Cardiac output and renal blood flow in glycerol-induced acute renal failure in the rat. Circ Res 40: 178–182, 1977.

163. Ramos B, Lopez-Novoa JM, Hernando L. Role of hemodynamic alterations in the partial-protection afforded by uninephrectomy against glycerol-induced acute renal failure in rats. Nephron 30: 68–72, 1982.

164. Hofbauer KG, Konrads A, Bauereiss K, Möhring B, Möhring J, Gross F. Vasopressin and renin in glycerol-induced acute renal failure in the rat. Circ Res 41: 424–428, 1977.

165. Hofbauer KG, Forgiarini P, Imbs F, Wood JM.

Effects of a competitive vasopressin antagonist in glycerol-induced acute renal failure in rats. In Acute Renal Failure, Eliahou HE (ed). London: John Libbey, 1982, pp. 194–198.

166. Reineck HJ, O'Connor GJ, Lifschitz MD, Stein JH. Sequential studies on the pathophysiology of glycerol-induced acute renal failure. J Lab Clin Med 96:356–362, 1980.

167. Wilkes BM, Hollenberg NK. Saline and glycerol-induced acute renal failure: "Protection" occurs after insult. Nephron 30: 352–356, 1982.

168. Flamenbaum W, McNeil JS, Kotchen TA, Lowenthal D, Nagel RB. Glycerol-induced acute renal failure after acute plasma renin activity suppression. J Lab Clin Med 82: 587–596, 1973.

169. Konrads A, Hofbauer KG, Bauereiss K, Mohring J, Gross F. Glycerol-induced acute renal failure in Brattleboro rats with hypothalamic diabetes insipidus. Clin Sci 56: 133–138, 1979.

170. Perez-Garcia R, Lopez-Novoa JM, Casado S, Hernando L. Partial protection against acute renal failure in rats with reduced renal mass. Proc EDTA 15: 402–411, 1978.

171. Thiel G, McDonald FD, Oken DE. Micropuncture studies of the basis for protection of renin depleted rats from glycerol-induced acute renal failure. Nephron 7: 67–79, 1970.

172. Di Bona GF, Sawin LL: The renin-angiotensin system in acute renal failure in the rat. Lab Invest 25: 528–532, 1971.

173. Oken DE, Mende CW, Tarabe I, Flamenbaum W. Resistance to acute renal failure by prior renal failure. Examination of the role of renal renin content. Nephron 15:131, 1975.

174. Hsu CH, Kurtz TW, Goldstein JR, Keinath RD, Weller JM. Intrarenal hemodynamics in acute myohemoglobinuric renal failure. Nephron 17: 65–72, 1976.

175. Baranowski RL, O'Connor GJ, Kurtzman NA. The effect of l-sarcosine, 8-leucyl angiotensin II on glycerol-induced acute renal failure. Arch Int Pharmacodyn 217: 322–331, 1975.

176. Ichikawa I, Hollenberg NK. Pharmacologic interruption of the renin-angiotensin system in myohemoglobinuric acute renal failure. Kidney Int 10: S183–S190, 1976.

177. Greven J, Koelling B, Schraufstatter J: Effects of saralasin and indomethacin on glycerol-induced acute renal failure in rats. In Acute Renal Failure, Seybold D, Gessler U (eds). Basel: Karger, 1982, pp. 130–138.

178. Churchill P, Bidani A, Fleischmann L, Becker-McKenna B. Glycerol-induced acute renal failure in the two-kidney Goldblatt rat. Am J Physiol 233: F247–F252, 1977.

179. Mendelsohn FAO. Failure of suppression of intrarenal angiotensin II in the contralateral kidney of one-clip two-kidney hypertensive rats. Clin Exp Pharmacol Physiol 7: 219–223, 1980.

180. Baranowski RL, Westenfelder C, Kurtzman NA. Intrarenal renin and angiotensins in glycerol-induced acute renal failure. Kidney Int 14: 576–584, 1978.

181. Werb R, Clark WF, Lindsay RM, Jones EOP, Turnbull DI, Linton AL. Protective effect of prostaglandin (PGE₂) in glycerol-induced acute renal failure in rats. Clin Sci Mol Med 55: 505–507, 1978.

182. Torres VE, Strong CG, Romero JC, Wilson DM: Indomethacin enhancement of glycerol-induced acute renal failure in rabbits. Kidney Int 7: 170–178, 1975.

183. Benabe JE, Klahr S, Hoffman MK, Morrison AR. Production of thromboxane A₂ by the kidney in glycerol-induced acute renal failure in the rabbit. Prostaglandins 19: 333–347, 1980.

184. Morrison AR, Benabe JE. Prostaglandins and vascular tone in experimental obstructive nephropathy. Kidney Int 19: 786–790, 1981.

185. Papanicolau N. Investigation on the mechanism of prostaglandin release. Experientia 28: 275–276, 1972.

186. Zipser RD, Morrison AR. Prostaglandins and renal disease. Mineral Electrolyte Metab 6: 82–89, 1981.

187. Flamenbaum W, Kotchen TA, Oken DE. Effect of renin immunization on mercuric chloride and glycerol-induced renal failure. Kidney Int 1: 406–412, 1972.

188. Carvalho JS, Carvalho ACA, Vaillancourt RA, Page LB, Colman RW, Landwehr DM, Oken DE. The pathogenetic significance of intravascular coagulation in experimental acute renal failure. Nephron 22: 484–491, 1978.

189. Brenner BM, Badr KM, Schor N, Ichikawa I. Hormonal influences on glomerular filtration. Mineral electrolyte Metab. 4: 49–56, 1980.

190. Suzuki T, Mostofi FK: Electron microscopic studies of acute tubular necrosis: Early changes in the lower tubules of rat kidney after subcutaneous injection of glycerin. Lab Invest 23: 15–28, 1970.

191. Westenfelder C, Arevalo GJ, Crawford PW, Zerwer P, Baranowski RL, Birch FM, Earnest WR, Hamburger RK, Coleman RD, Kurtzman NA. Renal tubular function in glycerol-induced acute renal failure. Kidney Int 18: 432–444, 1980.

192. Oken DE, DiBona GF, McDonald FD. Micropuncture studies of the recovery phase of myohemoglobinuric acute renal failure in the rat. J Clin Invest 49: 730–737, 1970.

193. Tyrakowski T, Knapowski J, Baczyk K. Disturbances in electrolyte transport before the onset of uranyl acetate-induced renal failure. Kidney Int 10 (Suppl 6): S144–S152, 1976.

194. Schwartz JH, Flamenbaum W. Uranyl nitrate and HgCl₂-induced alterations in ion transport. Kidney Int 10 (Suppl 6): S123–S127, 1976.

195. Schnermann J, Briggs JP. Participation of renal cortical prostaglandins in the regulation of glomerular filtration rate. Kidney Int 19: 802–815, 1981.

196. Andreucci VE. Glomerular hemodynamics and autoregulation. Proc EDTA 11: 77–88, 1974.

197. Andreucci VE, Dal Canton A, Corradi A, Stanziale R, Migone L. Role of the efferent arteriole in glomerular hemodynamics of superficial nephrons. Kidney Int 9: 475–480, 1976.

198. Schnermann J, Ploth DW, Hermle M: Activation of tubulo-glomerular feedback by chloride transport. Pflügers Arch 362: 229–240, 1976.

199. Francisco LL, Sawin LL, Di Bona GF. On the signal for activation of tubuloglomerular feedback. J Lab Clin Med 99: 722–730, 1982.

200. Briggs J, Schubert G, Schnermann J. Further evidence for an inverse relationship between macula densa NaCl concentration and filtration rate. Pflügers Archiv 392: 372–378, 1982.

201. Schnermann J, Briggs J. Concentration-dependent sodium chloride transport as the signal in feedback control of glomerular filtration rate. Kidney Int 22 (Suppl 12): S82–S89, 1982.

202. Thurau K, Grüner A, Mason J, Dahlheim H. Tubular signal for the renin activity in the juxtaglomerular apparatus. Kidney Int 22 (Suppl 22): S55–S62, 1982.

203. Bell PD, Navar LG. Relationship between tubuloglomerular feedback responses and perfusate hypotonicity. Kidney Int 22: 234–239, 1982.

204. Bell PD, Navar LG. Macula densa feedback control of glomerular filtration: Role of cytosolic calcium. Mineral Electrolyte Metab 8: 61–77, 1982.

205. Stowe N, Schnermann J, Hermle M. Feedback regulation of nephron filtration rate during pharmacologic interference with the renin-angiotensin and adrenergic systems in rats. Kidney Int 15: 473–486, 1979.

206. Briggs JP, Wright FS. Feedback control of glomerular filtration rate: Site of the effector mechanism. Am J Physiol 236: F40–F47, 1979.

207. Schnermann J, Persson AEG, Agerup B. Tubuloglomerular feedback: Nonlinear relation between glomerular hydrostatic pressure and loop of Henle perfusion rate. J Clin Invest 52: 862–869, 1973.

208. Ichikawa I. Hemodynamic influence of altered distal salt delivery on glomerular microcirculation. Kidney Int 22 (Suppl 12): S109–S113, 1982.

209. Persson AEG, Wright FS. Evidence for feedback mediated reduction of glomerular filtration rate during infusion of acetazolamide. Acta Physiol Scand 114: 1–7, 1982.

210. Tucker BJ, Blantz RC. Studies on the mechanism of reduction in glomerular filtration rate after Benzolanide. Pflügers Arch 388: 211–216, 1980.

211. Thurau K, Vogt C, Dahlheim H. Renin activity in the juxtaglomerular apparatus of the rat kidney during post-ischemic acute renal failure. Kidney Int 10 (Suppl 6): S177–S182, 1976.

212. Mason J. Tubulo-glomerular feedback in the early

stages of experimental acute renal failure. Kidney Int 10 (Suppl 6): S106–S114, 1976.

213. Mason J, Takabatake T, Olbricht C, Thurau K. The early phase of experimental acute renal failure. III Tubuloglomerular feedback. Pflügers Arch 373: 69–76, 1978.

214. Mendelsohn FAO. Evidence for the local occurrence of angiotensin II in rat kidney and its modulation by dietary sodium intake and converting enzyme blockade. Clin Sci 57: 173–179, 1979.

215. Gerber JG, Olson RD, Nies AS. Interrelationship between prostaglandins and renin release. Kidney Int 19: 816–821, 1981.

216. Müller-Suur R, Persson AEG, Ulfendahl HR. Tubuloglomerular feedback in juxtamedullary nephrons. Kidney Int 22 (Suppl 12): S104–S108, 1982.

217. Hollenberg NK, Epstein M, Rosen SM, Basch RI, Oken DE, Merrill JP. Acute oliguric renal failure in man: Evidence for preferential renal cortical ischemia. Medicine 47: 455–474, 1968.

218. Ploth DW, Roy RN: Renal and tubuloglomerular feedback effects of Sar^1, Ala^8 angiotensin II in the rat. Am J Physiol 11: F149–F157, 1982.

219. Ploth DW, Rudulph J, Lagrange R, Navar LG. Tubuloglomerular feedback and single nephron function after converting enzyme inhibition in the rat. J Clin Invest 64: 1325–1335, 1979.

220. Schnermann J, Nagel W, Thurau K. Die frühdistale Natriumkonzentration in Rattennieren nach renaler Ischämie und hämorrhagischer Hypotension. Pflügers Arch 287: 296–310, 1966.

221. Kaufman JS, Hamburger RJ, Flamenbaum W. Renal renin responses to changes in volume status and perfusion pressure. Am J Physiol 238: F488–F490, 1980.

222. Rauh W, Oster P, Dietz R, Gross F. The renin-angiotensin system in acute renal failure of rats. Clin Sci 48: 467–473, 1975.

223. Kleinman JG, McNeil JS, Schwartz JH, Hamburger RJ, Flamenbaum W. Effect of dithiothreitol on mercuric chloride and uranyl nitrate-induced acute renal failure in the rat. Kidney Int 12: 45–121, 1977.

224. Wright FS, Schnermann J: Interference with feedback control of glomerular filtration rate by furosemide, triflocin, and cyanide. J Clin Invest 53: 1695–1708, 1974.

225. Wunderlich PF, Brunner FP, Davis JM, Haberle DA, Tholen H, Thiel G. Feedback activation in rat nephrons by sera from patients with acute renal failure. Kidney Int 17: 497–506, 1980.

226. DiBona GF, McDonald FD, Flamenbaum W, Dammin GJ, Oken DE. Maintenance of renal function in salt-loaded rats despite severe tubular necrosis induced by $HgCl_2$. Nephron 8: 205–220, 1971.

227. Lindner Ā, Cutler RE. Angiotensin blockade and acute renal failure in the dog. In Acute Renal Failure, Eliahou HE (ed). London: John Libbey, 1982, pp. 203–205.

228. Bidani A, Churchill P, Fleischmann L. Sodium-chloride-induced protection in nephrotoxic acute renal failure: Independence from renin. Kidney Int 16: 481–490, 1979.

229. Oken DE, Cotes SC, Flamenbaum W, Powell-Jackson JD, Lever AF. Active and passive immunization to angiotensin in experimental acute renal failure. Kidney Int 7: 12–18, 1975.

230. Semple PF, Brown JJ, Lever AF, Mac Gregoir J, Morton JJ, Powell-Jackson JD, Robertson JIS. Renin, angiotensin II and III in acute renal failure: Notes on the measurement of angiotensin II and III in rat blood. Kidney Int 10 (Suppl 6): S169–S176, 1976.

231. de Rougemont D, Brunner FP, Torhorst J, Thiel G: Superficial nephron function in ischemic renal failure with or without protection. In Acute Renal Failure, Eliahou HE (ed). London: John Libbey, 1982, pp. 65–68.

232. Churchill PC, Bidani A, Fleischmann L, Becker-McKenna B. $HgCl_2$-induced acute renal failure in the Goldblatt rat. J Lab Clin Med 91: 660–665, 1978.

233. Thiel G, Brunner F, Wunderlich P, Huguenin M, Bienko B, Torhorst J, Peters-Haefeli L, Kirchertz EJ, Peters G. Protection of rat kidney against $HgCl_2$-induced acute renal failure by induction of high-urine flow without renin supression. Kidney Int 10 (Suppl 6): S191–S200, 1976.

234. Persson AEG, Boberg U, Hahne B, Müller-Suur R, Norlen BJ, Selen G. Interstitial pressure as a modulator of tubuloglomerular feedback control. Kidney Int 22 (Suppl 12): S122–S128, 1982.

235. Gillies A, Morgan T. Activity of renin in the juxtaglomerular apparatus. Kidney Int 22 (Suppl 12): S67–S72, 1982.

236. Kirschbaum BB, Sprinkle FM, Oken DE. Renal function and mercury level in rats with mercuric nephrotoxicity. Nephron 26: 28–34, 1980.

237. Tanner GA. Nephron obstruction and tubuloglomerular feedback. Kidney Int 22 (Suppl 12): S213–S218, 1982.

238. Tanner GA. Tubuloglomerular feedback after nephron obstruction. In Acute Renal Failure, Eliahou HE (ed). London: John Libbey, 1982, pp. 47–49.

239. Tanner GA. Effects of kidney tubule obstruction on glomerular function in rats. Am J Physiol 237: F379–F385, 1979.

240. Dal Canton A, Andreucci VE. Glomerular hemodynamics in ureteral obstruction. In Renal Pathophysiology, Recent Advances, Leaf A, Giebisch G, Bolis L, Gorini S (eds). New York: Raven Press, 1980, pp. 189–201.

241. Tanner GA, Yum MN. Effects of chronic tubular obstruction in Necturus kidney. Am J Physiol 234: F112–F116, 1978.

242. Celio MR. Angiotensin II immunoreactivity coex-

isting with renin in the human juxtaglomerular epithelioid cells. Kidney Int 22 (Suppl 12): S30–S32, 1982.

243. Rightsel WA, Okamura T, Inagami T, Pitcock JA, Takii Y, Brooks B, Brown P, Muirhead EE. Juxtaglomerular cells grown as monolayer cell culture contain renin, angiotensin I-converting enzyme and angiotensin I and II/III. Circ Res 50: 822–829, 1982.

244. Taugner R, Hackenthal E, Rix E, Nobiling R, Poulsen K. Immunocytochemistry of the renin-angiotensin system: Renin, angiotensinogen, angiotensin I, angiotensin II, and converting enzyme in the kidney of mice, rats and three shrews. Kidney Int 22 (Suppl 12): S33–S43, 1982.

245. Naruse K, Inagami T, Celio MR, Workman RJ, Takii Y. Immunohistochemical evidence that angiotensin I and II are formed by intracellular mechanism in juxtaglomerular cells. Hypertension 4 (Suppl II): II70–II74, 1982.

246. Regoli D, Gauthier R. Site of action of angiotensin and other vasoconstrictors on the kidney. Can J Physiol Pharmacol 49: 608–612, 1971.

247. Osborne M, Meyer P, Droz B, Morel F. Localisation intraénale de l'angiotensive tritiée dans les cellules mésangiales par radioautographie. C R Acad Sci (Paris) 276: 2457–2460, 1973.

248. Hornich H, Beaufils M, Richet G: The effect of exogenous angiotensin on superficial and deep glomeruli in the rat kidney. Kidney Int 2: 336–342, 1972.

249. Ausiello DA, Kreisberg JI, Roy C, Karnovsky MJ. Contraction of cultured rat glomerular cells of apparent mesangial origin after stimulation with angiotensin II and arginin vasopressin. J Clin Invest 65: 754–760, 1980.

250. Sraer JD, Sraer J, Ardaillou R, Mimoune O. Evidence for renal glomerular receptors for angiotensin II. Kidney Int 6: 241–246, 1974.

251. Caldicott WJH, Taub KJ, Margulies SS, Hollenberg NK. Angiotensin receptors in glomeruli differ from those in renal arterioles. Kidney Int 19: 687–693, 1981.

252. Boucher R, Asselin J, Genest J. A new enzyme leading to the direct formation of angiotensin II. Circ Res 34 & 35 (Suppl 1): 1203–1209, 1974.

253. Boucher R, Demassieux S, Garcia R, Genest J. Tonin, angiotensin II system. A review. Circ Res 41 (Suppl 2): 26–29, 1977.

254. Burghardt W, Schweisfurth H, Dahlheim H. Juxtaglomerular angiotensin II formation. Kidney Int 22 (Suppl 12): S49–S54, 1982.

255. Barajas L, Muller J. The innervation of the juxtaglomerular apparatus and surrounding tubules: A quantitative analysis by serial section electron microscopy. J Ultrastruct Res 43: 107–132, 1973.

256. Needleman P, Douglas JR, Jakschik B, Stoecklein PB, Johnson EM. Release of renal prostaglandins by catecholamines. Relationship renal endocrine function. Pharmacol Exp Ther 188: 453–460, 1974.

257. Davis JO, Freeman RH. Mechanisms regulating renin release. Physiol Rev 56: 1–56, 1976.

258. Eliahou HE, Iaina A, Solomon S, Gavendo S. Alleviation of anoxic experimental acute renal failure in rats by beta-adrenergic blockade. Nephron 19: 158–166, 1977.

259. Gaal K. Effect of beta-receptor antagonists on $HgCl_2$-induced acute renal failure in rats; functional and morphological investigations. In Acute Renal Failure, Seybold D, Gessler U (eds). Basel: Karger, 1982, pp. 162–177.

260. Diz DI, Baer PG, Nasjletti A. Effect of norepinephrine and renal denervation on renal PGE_2 and kallikrein in rats. Am J Physiol 241: F477–F481, 1981.

261. Henrich WL, Anderson RJ, Berns AS, McDonald KM, Paulsen PJ, Berl T, Schrier RW. Role of renal nerves and prostaglandins in control of renal hemodynamics and plasma renin activity during hypotensive hemorrhage in the dog. J Clin Invest 61: 744–750, 1978.

262. Henrich WL, Berl T, McDonald KM, Anderson RJ, Schrier RW. Angiotensin II, renal nerves, and prostaglandins in renal hemodynamics during hemorrhage. Am J Physiol 235: F46–F51, 1978.

263. Schnermann J, Stowe N, Yarimizu S, Magnussen M, Tingwald G. Feedback control of glomerular filtration rate in isolated, blood-perfused dog kidneys. Am J Physiol 233: F217–F224, 1977.

264. Kaufman JS, Hamburger RJ, Flamenbaum W. Tubuloglomerular feedback response after hypotensive hemorrhage. Renal Physiol 5: 173–181, 1982.

265. Lands WEM. The biosynthesis and metabolism of prostaglandins. Ann Rev Physiol 41: 633–653, 1979.

266. Anggard E, Oliw E. Formation and metabolism of prostaglandins in the kidney. Kidney Int 19: 771–780, 1981.

267. Levenson DJ, Simmons CE, Brenner BM. Arachidonic acid metabolism, prostaglandins and the kidney. Am J Med 72: 354–374, 1982.

268. Epstein M, Lifschitz MD. Volume status as a determinant of the influence of renal PGE on renal function. Nephron 25: 157–159, 1980.

269. Whorton AR, Smigel M, Oates JA, Frölich JC. Regional differences in prostacyclin formation by the kidney. Prostacyclin is a major prostaglandin of renal cortex. Biochim Biophys Acta 529: 176–180, 1978.

270. Schlondorff D, Roczniak S, Satriano JA, Folkert VW. Prostaglandin synthesis by isolated rat glomeruli: Effect of angiotensin II. Am J Physiol 8: F486–F495, 1980.

271. Kreisberg JI, Karnovsky MJ, Levine L. Prostaglandin production by homogeneous cultures of rat glomerular epithelial and mesangial cells. Kidney Int 22: 355–359, 1982.

272. Bohman SO: Demonstration of prostaglandin syn-

thesis in collecting duct cells and other cell types of the rabbit renal medulla. Prostaglandins 14: 729–744, 1977.

273. Muirhead EE, German GS, Leach BE, Brooks B, Stephenson P. Renomedullary interstitial cells (RIC): Prostaglandins (PG) and the antihypertensive function of the kidney. Prostaglandins 3: 581–594, 1973.

274. Smith WL, Bell TG. Increased renal tubular synthesis of prostaglandins in the rabbit kidney in response to ureteral obstruction. Prostaglandins 18: 269–277, 1979.

275. Williams WM, Frolich JC, Nies AS, Oates JA. Urinary prostaglandins: Site of entry into renal tubular fluid. Kidney Int 11: 256–260, 1977.

276. Zambraski EJ, Dunn MJ. Renal prostaglandin E_2 secretion and excretion in conscious dogs. Am J Physiol 236: F552–F556, 1979.

277. Moncada S, Vane JR. Prostacyclin: Homeostatic regulator or biological curiosity? Clin Sci 61: 369–372, 1981.

278. Zipser R, Myers S, Needleman P. Exaggerated prostaglandin and thromboxane synthesis in the renal vein constricted rabbit. Cir Res 47: 231–237, 1980.

279. Whinnery MA, Shaw JO, Beck N. Thromboxane B_2 and prostaglandin E_2 in the rat kidney with unilateral ureteral obstruction. Am J Physiol 242: F220–F225, 1982.

280. Schramm LP, Carlson DE. Inhibition of renal vasoconstriction by elevated ureteral pressure. Am J Physiol 228: 1126–1133, 1975.

281. Gerber JG, Nies S. The hemodynamic effects of prostaglandins in the rat: Evidence for important species varications in renovascular responses. Circ Res 44: 406–410, 1979.

282. Gerber JG, Nies AS. The role of prostaglandins in the control of renal hemodynamics. Mineral Electrolyte Metab 6: 27–34, 1981.

283. Swain JA, Hendrix GR, Boettcher DH, Vatner SF. Prostaglandin control of renal circulation in the unanesthetized dog and baboon. Am J Physiol 229: 826–830, 1975.

284. Donker AJM, Arisz L, Brentjens JRH, Van Der Hem GK, Hollemans HJC. The effect of indomethacin on kidney function and plasma renin activity in man. Nephron 17: 288–296, 1976.

285. Baylis C, Brenner BM. Modulation by prostaglandin synthesis inhibitors of the action of exogenous angiotensin II on glomerular ultrafiltration in the rat. Circ Res 43: 889–898, 1978.

286. Oliver JA, Sciacca RR, Pinto J. Participation of the prostaglandins in the control of renal blood flow during acute reduction of cardiac output in the dog. J Clin Invest 67: 229–239, 1981.

287. Zipser RD, Hoefs JC, Speckart PF, Zca PK, Horton R. Prostaglandins. Modulators of renal function and pressor resistance in chronic liver disease. J Clin Endocr Metab 48: 895–900, 1979.

288. Arisz L, Donker AJ, Brentjens JR, Vanderhem

GK. The effect of indomethacin on proteinuria and kidney function in the nephrotic syndrome. Acta Med Scand 199: 121–125, 1976.

289. Schnermann J, Schubert G, Hermle M, Herbst R, Stowe NT, Yarimizu S, Weber PC. The effect of inhibition of prostaglandin synthesis on tubuloglomerular feedback in the rat kidney. Pflügers Arch 379: 269–279, 1979.

290. Schnermann J, Weber PC. Reversal of indomethacin-induced inhibition of tubuloglomerular feedback by prostaglandin infusion. Prostaglandins 24: 351–361, 1982.

291. Schor N, Ichikawa I, Brenner BM. Mechanisms of action of various hormones and vasoactive substances on glomerular ultrafiltration in the rat. Kidney Int 20: 442–451, 1981.

292. Romero JC, Dunlap CL, Strong CG. The effect of indomethacin and other anti-inflammatory drugs on the renin-angiotensin system. J Clin Invest 58: 282–288, 1976.

293. Whorton AR, Misono K, Hollifield J, Frölich JC, Inagami T, Oates JA. Prostaglandins and renin release: I Stimulation of renin release from rabbit renal cortical slices by PGI_2. Prostaglandins 14: 1095–1104, 1977.

294. Beierwaltes WH, Schryver S, Sanders E, Strand J, Romero JC. Renin release selectively stimulated by prostaglandin I_2 in isolated rat glomeruli. Am J Physiol 243: F276–F283, 1982.

295. Nesjletti A, Malik KU. Renal kinin-prostaglandin relationship: Implications for renal function. Kidney Int 19: 860–868, 1981.

296. Nasjletti A, Malik KU. The renal kallikrein-kinin and prostaglandin system interaction. Annu Rev Physiol 43: 597–609, 1981.

297. Nasjletti A, Colina-Chourio J, McGiff JC. Disappearance of bradykinin in the renal circulation of dogs: Effects of kininase inhibition. Circ Res 37: 59–65, 1975.

298. Flamenbaum W, Gagnon J, Ramwell P. Bradykinin-induced renal hemodynamic alterations: Renin and prostaglandin relationship. Am J Physiol 237: F433–F440, 1980.

299. Strand JC, Gilmore JP. Prostaglandins do not mediate the renal effects of bradykinin. Renal Physiol 5: 286–296, 1982.

300. Thomas CE, Bell PD, Navar LG. Influence of bradykinin and papaverine on renal and glomerular hemodynamics in dogs. Renal Physiol 5: 197–205, 1982.

301. Carretero OA, Scicli AG. The renal kallikrein-kinin system. Am J Physiol 238: F247–F255, 1980.

302. Smith MC, Dunn MJ. Renal kallikrein, kinins and prostaglandins in hypertension. In Hypertension, Brenner BM, Stein JH (eds). New York: Churchill Livingstone, 1981, pp. 168–202.

303. Koffler D, Paronetto F. Fibrinogen deposition in acute renal failure. Am J Path 49: 383–395, 1966.

304. Clarkson AR, MacDonald MK, Fuster V, Cash

JD, Robson JS. Glomerular coagulation in acute ischemic renal failure. Quart J Med 39: 585–599, 1970.

305. Wardle EN: Intravascular coagulation in experimental acute renal failure. Thromb Diath Haemorrh 29: 579–591, 1973.

306. Rammer L, Gerdin B. Protection against the impairment of renal function after intravascular coagulation in the rat kidney by increased ingestion of sodium chloride. Nephron 14: 433–441, 1975.

307. Rammer L, Stahl E. Effect of beta-adrenergic blockade by propranolol upon intravascular coagulation in the rat kidney. Nephron 24: 246–249, 1979.

308. Stahl E, Gerdin B, Rammer L. Protective effect of angiotensin II inhibition on acute renal failure after intravascular coagulation in the rat. Nephron 29: 250–257, 1981.

309. Rammer L, Stahl E. Acute renal failure due to intravascular coagulation in the rat. In Acute Renal Failure, Eliahou HE (ed). London: John Libbey, 1982, pp. 58–61.

310. Stahl E, Karlberg BE, Rammer L. Fibrin deposition in the kidney and renal blood flow during intravascular coagulation in the rat: Influence of the renin-angiotensin system. Clin Sci 62: 35–41, 1982.

311. Barajas L, Latta H. A three-dimensional study of the juxtaglomerular apparatus in the rat. Light and electron microscopy observations. Lab Invest 12: 257–269, 1963.

312. Barajas L, Latta H. Structure of the juxtaglomerular apparatus. Circ Res 21–22 (Suppl II): 15–28, 1967.

313. Barajas L. Anatomy of the juxtaglomerular apparatus. Am J Physiol 237: F333–F343, 1979.

314. Oken DE, Landwehr DM, Kirschbaum BB. On the pathogenesis of murine experimental acute renal failure. In Acute Renal Failure, Seybold D, Gessler U (eds). Basel: Karger, 1982, pp. 1–8.

2. DIFFERENT FORMS OF ISCHEMIC/ TOXIC ACUTE RENAL FAILURE IN HUMANS

Vittorio E. Andreucci

1 Introduction

We may define acute renal failure (ARF) as a rapid deterioration of renal function associated with retention of nitrogenous wastes in the body [1]. On the basis of this definition, ARF may occur as result of many different causes, as summarized in table 2–1. In this chapter, only ischemic and toxic forms of ARF in humans are reviewed.

Initially defined as "lower nephron nephrosis," ARF resulting from ischemic and/or toxic conditions was then called acute tubular necrosis (ATN) [2] to focus attention on tubular necrosis as the essential renal lesion. Although a frank necrosis is not constant or, at least, not readily apparent, the term ATN has been maintained and has become popular for defining the renal shutdown that cannot be reversed by adequate fluid replacement. I have, therefore, decided to maintain this popular term (ATN).

As fully discussed in chapter 1, both in man and in experimental animals, ATN may be ei-

TABLE 2–1. Causes of acute renal failure (ARF)

Ischemic disorders (prerenal ARF, ATN)
Nephrotoxins (ATN, drug-induced acute interstitial
    nephritis)
Diseases of the renal interstitium
Primary glomerular diseases
Vascular nephropathies
Obstruction of the urinary tract (postrenal ARF)

V.E. Andreucci (ed.). ACUTE RENAL FAILURE.
All rights reserved. Copyright © 1984.
Martinus Nijhoff Publishing, Boston/The Hague/
Dordrecht/Lancaster.

ther the result of a direct toxic effect on renal tubules or the secondary consequence of an ischemic insult. Under the latter condition, however, with only a few exceptions (e.g., the ATN following the temporary interruption of blood flow during renal transplantation), ATN is usually preceded by a functional ARF, better known as prerenal ARF. We may define the prerenal ARF as that abrupt impairment of renal function that occurs in conditions of renal hypoperfusion that may be reversed by adequate fluid replacement (in the form of blood, plasma, and/or saline solutions). Should prerenal ARF remain uncorrected for a prolonged time, ATN will result.

2. Hypovolemic ARF

The normal kidney is able to withstand wide variations in renal perfusion pressure, maintaining practically unchanged RBF and GFR; this phenomenon is called renal autoregulation [3]. When renal perfusion pressure falls below the lower limit of autoregulatory range (i.e., below a blood pressure of 80 mm Hg), RBF and/or glomerular capillary pressure are reduced, thus leading to a decrease in GFR. On the other hand, the diminution of blood volume may stimulate the adrenergic nervous system and release vasoconstrictor factors; both phenomena will cause renal vasoconstriction, which leads to more severe renal hypoperfusion and/or greater fall in glomerular capillary pressure. The immediate consequence is a reduction in GFR, which is mirrored by the rise in serum creatinine. However, the hypoperfusion of renal parenchyma secondary to ECV depletion causes tubular overreabsorption, occurring mainly, but not exclusively, in proximal tubules, with the aim of normalizing the blood volume and consequently the renal perfusion. A reduced volume of highly concentrated urine, with very low sodium concentration (sodium is reabsorbed more avidly than water), will be produced with normal urinalysis. This is typically a functional, prerenal ARF.

Severe hypovolemia (i.e., diminution of total intravascular volume) may result from external or internal fluid losses. External fluid losses include hemorrhage and renal and extrarenal losses. Internal fluid losses include internal hemorrhage, intestinal sequestration of fluid, peritonitis, and acute pancreatitis.

2.1 HEMORRHAGE

Severe hypovolemia may obviously result from external acute blood loss following trauma or from gastrointestinal bleeding. The latter may not be immediately apparent; nasogastric suction, inspection of the stool, or even gastric or rectal endoscopy may help in the diagnosis. Gross hematuria in uremic patients with polycystic renal disease may sometimes cause hypovolemia and acute worsening of renal function. Trauma on the kidney (as from a heavy abdominal blow) may cause perirenal hematoma and/or gross hematuria, with severe hypovolemia and hypotension.

Internal hemorrhage (hematomas, hemoperitoneum, hemothorax) should be suspected any time hypovolemia occurs without evident blood loss or salt depletion.

Severe hemorrhage causes a fall in blood pressure and requires immediate blood transfusion. The faster the replacement of the lost blood, the less the risk of ATN.

2.2 RENAL FLUID LOSS

Much salt and water may be lost by the kidney itself. Thus, some uremic patients may lose great amounts of sodium with the consequent contraction in ECV, fall in blood pressure, and worsening of renal function [4]. This represents the so-called "salt-losing nephritis," usually secondary to chronic urinary obstruction, poly-

cystic kidney disease, phenacetin nephropathy, and chronic pyelonephritis with urinary infection [5]. A classical cause of prerenal ARF in chronic uremic patients, this condition is readily reversed by salt replacement (figure 2–1).

Severe diabetic acidosis represents another condition characterized by renal loss of salt and water that may cause ARF (figure 2–2). As blood sugar rises in untreated (or inadequately treated) patients, the filtered load of sugar increases, exceeding the maximal capacity of the proximal tubule to reabsorb glucose ($Tm_{glucose}$). In this condition glucose behaves as a nonreabsorbable solute, preventing the reabsorption of water and salt and leading to a greater urine output (osmotic diuresis). This osmotic diuresis will be the major cause of water, sodium, and chloride losses in diabetic patients, causing ECV contraction, renal hypoperfusion, and prerenal ARF [6]. In this form of ARF, the associated hyponatremia is due to a continuous diffusion of water from the intracellular compartment to the extracellular fluids because of the increase in effective osmotic pressure due to high glucose levels; if hypernatremia is present despite hyperglycemia, it indicates a great degree of water loss from the body, which is markedly in excess of sodium [6]. Taken together these data clearly demonstrate that patients with severe diabetic acidosis have to be treated with parenteral administration of large volumes of water and salt (water in excess of salt). In patients with marked ECV depletion and severe hypotension or hypovolemic shock, isotonic saline should be given first and in adequate volume (e.g., two to three liters i.v.) [6] (see chapter 21). Should these patients remain untreated too long, prerenal ARF will be converted into ATN.

Diuretics may cause ECV contraction or, more frequently, may worsen pre-existent salt depletion. Too frequently, in fact, patients who become oliguric following vomiting, diarrhea, severe sweating, or other conditions of extrarenal fluid losses are mistakenly treated with high doses of loop diuretics (usually furosemide). The resulting functional ARF is difficult to evaluate by urinary tests because of the high urinary sodium concentration and FE_{Na};

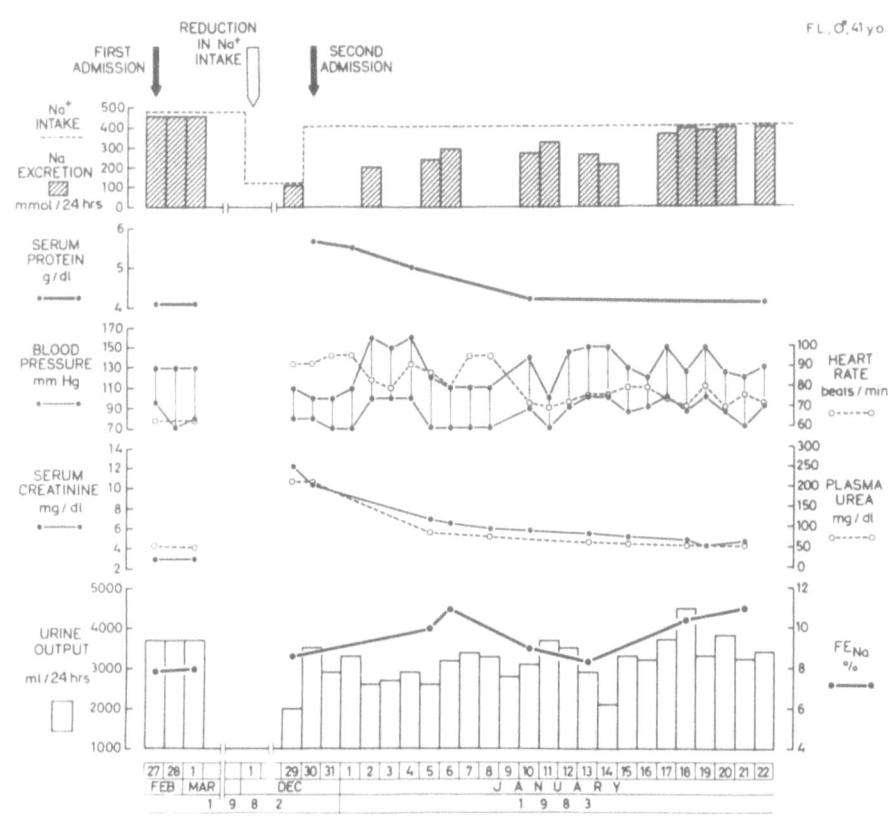

FIGURE 2–1. Salt-losing nephritis. A 41-year-old male patient with paraplegia and permanent catheter for bladder drainage was first admitted to our unit in February 1982. A sodium intake of 480 mmol/24 hours was necessary to balance urinary sodium excretion. Under such circumstances blood pressure was 130/75 mm Hg, urine output 3,800 ml/24 hours, serum creatinine 248 μmol/l (2.8 mg/dl), plasma urea 10.82 mmol/l (65 mg/dl), and serum protein 4.1 g/dl (the patient had marked proteinuria due to renal amyloidosis). The patient was discharged on 1 March 1982 with sodium intake of 480 mmol/24 hours. Many months later, the patient decided to reduce sodium intake. On 29 December, he was admitted again to our unit. Blood pressure was 110/70 mm Hg, urine output 2,000 ml/24 hours, urinary sodium excretion 100 mmol/24 hours, serum creatinine 1,087 μmol/l (12.3 mg/dl), plasma urea 35.13 mmol/l (211 mg/dl), serum protein 5.8 g/dl. This prerenal ARF was readily reversed by adequate salt replacement.

the diagnosis should be based on the history (revealing extrarenal fluid losses and diuretic therapy) and physical examination (revealing signs of severe dehydration) (see chapter 7).

2.3 EXTRARENAL FLUID LOSS

2.3.1 Vomiting and Nasogastric Suction
Vomiting, even without food expulsion (the patient frequently denies vomiting because of lack of food expulsion), is responsible for loss

of fluid with hydrochloric acid, sodium, and potassium, leading to ECV depletion, hypokalemia, and alkalosis. The extent of these losses is variable depending on the extreme variation in the composition of the gastric content; the latter may vary according to the basal or stimulated gastric juice secretion, the swallowed saliva, and the degree of fluid refluxing from the duodenum [7]. Obviously, the metabolic consequences of nasogastric suction or spontaneous gastric fistula are similar to those

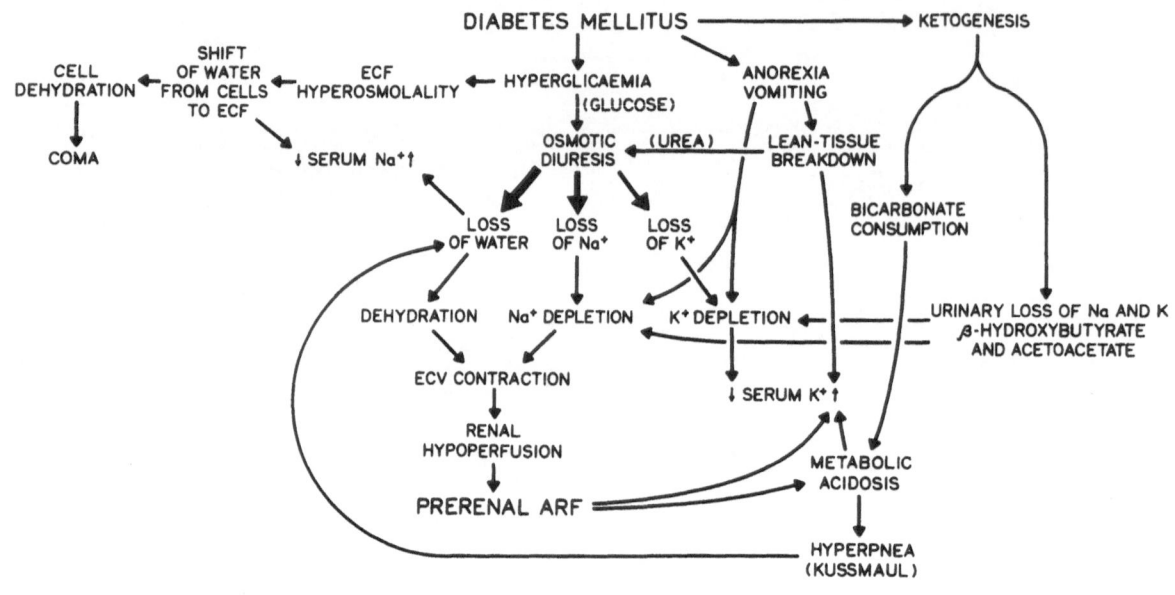

FIGURE 2–2. Metabolic consequences of untreated diabetic acidosis.

of vomiting. It should be stressed that the occurrence of metabolic alkalosis and potassium depletion under such circumstances is due not only to the gastrointestinal losses of water, acid, sodium, and potassium, but also to the increased renal tubular secretion of hydrogen and potassium [7–9] (see chapter 7).

2.3.2 Diarrhea and Intestinal Drainage or Fistula

Severe diarrhea may cause a daily loss of 5 to 10 liters of fluid containing sodium, potassium, and bicarbonate, leading to ECV depletion, hypokalemia, and acidosis. The metabolic consequences of spontaneous intestinal fistulae or post-surgical intestinal drainage are similar to those of diarrhea with some variations on cation and anion losses, depending on the site of the fistula or drainage (see chapter 7).

2.3.3 Excessive Sweating

Excessive sweating may lead to ECV depletion because of loss of water and salt (concentration of sodium in sweat ranges from 18 to 97 mmol/l with a mean of 45 mmol/l) [10] and potassium depletion (concentration of potassium in sweat ranges from 1 to 15 mmol/l, with a mean of 4.5 mmol/l) [10].

Losses of water and sodium from sweating are too frequently disregarded even though they may become life threatening. Excessive sweating usually occurs in subjects living in hot climates, but it may be observed in ill patients with hyperpyrexia. Severe water depletion is unusual in healthy sweating subjects since the sensation of thirst will induce the individual to drink. But sodium losses may be substantial and will not be replaced by simple water-drinking unless salt supplements are given. A sick patient, sweating because of increased body temperature and allowed to drink but not to eat (as may occur in the first days following myocardial infarction), may develop severe salt depletion and consequently prerenal ARF (figure 2–3).

2.3.4 Burns

ECV depletion with a significant reduction of effective arterial blood volume may occur following extensive and severe burns. The thermal injury of the skin, when involving epidermis and dermis either in part (second-degree burns or partial-thickness burns) or totally (third-degree burns or full-thickness burns) will be associated initially with local edema and subsequently with severe

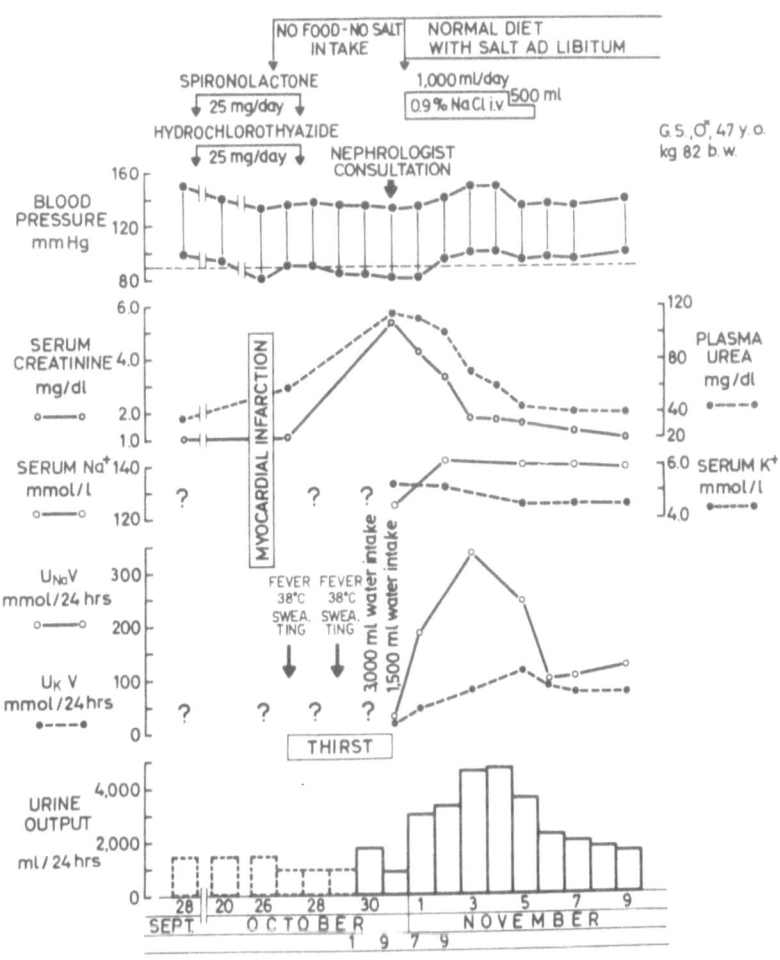

FIGURE 2–3. Salt depletion and prerenal ARF after myocardial infarction. The use of diuretics and the occurrence of fever with profuse sweating (with no food or salt intake for several days) were followed by a fall in urine output and rise in serum creatinine. The patient was in excellent condition. The i.v. infusion of 154 mmol/l (0.9 g/dl) NaCl normalized urine output and renal function. (Reprinted with permission from Andreucci VE and Dal Canton A, Proc, EDTA 17: 123–132, 1980.)

evaporation of water from the wound surface and, sometimes, with diffuse edema [11]. Burn edema is due to a rapid leak of fluid from the vascular bed into the wound and occurs mainly in the first six to eight hours (but may continue up to 48 hours) after injury; it is caused by dilatation and increased permeability of the damaged capillaries so that the edema

fluid has the same composition of plasma with a protein content of 40 to 50 g/l [11].

In the days following, when full-thickness burns involve more than 30% of body surface, diffuse edema may occur in undamaged areas quite far from the site of thermal injury; this edema has been attributed to a fall of oncotic pressure resulting from the massive loss of plasma protein into the wound [11]. Finally, after the initial thermal injury, a long-lasting and serious fluid loss from the burn surface occurs because of water vaporization; this loss may vary with the temperature and humidity of the room (it may be decreased by heating the room and saturating the air with water vapor) and with the extension of the thermally damaged skin. Thus, water loss, in full-thickness burns, may reach 300 ml/hour/square meter of burned skin between the fifth and the tenth postburn days [11]. This water loss will continue, even though at a much lower rate, with burn eschar and terminates only when the wound has been completely covered by epithelium.

Thermal trauma may cause local thrombosis and may damage circulating erythrocytes traversing the wound area during burning; this may lead to immediate and delayed hemolysis and to RBC agglutination, with loss of erythrocyte mass.

Loss of plasma into the burn wound, evaporation of water from the wound surface, and hemolysis causes a severe decrease of blood volume with renal hypoperfusion and prerenal ARF. Furthermore, direct thermal injury and secondary tissue hypoxia may cause potassium release from tissue cells, metabolic acidosis, and superimposed bacterial infection.

When prerenal ARF in burned patients is not adequately treated or when adequate protein, salt and fluid replacement are given too late after thermal injury, ATN (frequently a nonoliguric form) may result, which usually requires early and intensive dialysis therapy and high-calorie feeding because of severe hypercatabolism [12].

2.4 INTERNAL SEQUESTRATION OF FLUID

Severe plasma volume depletion may also occur during the course of intestinal obstruction or ileus, because of intestinal sequestration of several liters of fluid. Mechanical obstruction of the gut, in fact, results in decreased absorption from distended bowel and then in intraluminal secretion of sodium and water; the damage of the intestinal mucosa leads to protein loss from blood to the intestinal lumen, with bacteria and their toxins moving in the opposite direction; resulting peritonitis causes further loss of fluid into the peritoneal cavity, which will greatly contribute, with associated vomiting, to severe hypovolemia [7].

Similar effects may follow adynamic or spastic ileus (functional obstruction of the bowel), which is commonly observed in association with peritonitis [7]. Under such circumstances both severe hypovolemia and endotoxemia may

account for the shock condition leading to ARF and frequently to death.

Internal sequestration of fluid, with hypovolemic ARF may occur following acute pancreatitis. Under such circumstances, hypovolemia with hemoconcentration and severe hypotension are accounted for by a tremendous subcapsular and peripancreatic edema, accumulation of bloody peritoneal exudate (chemical peritonitis) and intestinal sequestration of fluid (paralytic ileus) and may be worsened by associated vomiting. Hypotension may be aggravated by pancreatic release of kallikrein and the consequent production of vasodilator bradykinin. In acute hemorrhagic pancreatitis, blood loss from circulation may greatly contribute to refractory hypotension and shock and requires immediate blood transfusion.

As mentioned elsewhere in this chapter, however, ARF may also occur in acute pancreatitis without hypovolemia and/or hypotension.

Peritonitis, whether due to bacterial or chemical injury, causes fluid loss into the peritoneal cavity. The peritoneum, with its large surface area, normally allows fast transport of water and electrolytes from the peritoneal cavity to the circulating blood. In peritonitis this transport system is impaired and fluid is sequestered into the peritoneal cavity; this sequestration is further increased by the concomitant exudation of plasma protein [7]. Hypovolemia, hypotension, and ARF may follow and may be initially reversed by adequate protein and fluid replacement.

2.5 POSTSURGICAL ARF

ARF is undoubtedly frequent after surgical procedures. In a review of 104 cases of ARF, 82 patients had undergone surgery [13]. Many factors favor post-surgical ARF. As mentioned elsewhere in this chapter, anesthesia may play an important role. But, undoubtedly, hypovolemia is usually predominant and may result from (a) preoperative fluid restriction, (b) surgical fluid loss, (c) surgical blood loss, or (d) gastric and/or enteric drainage of fluids [14]. The resulting hypovolemic ARF may be aggravated by prophylactic use of nephrotoxic antibiotics. Under such circumstances, the toxic injury is added to the ischemic damage on tubular epithelium.

3 Endotoxin-Induced ARF in Septic Shock Patients

Invasion of the blood stream by bacteria may follow urinary tract infection, biliary or intraperitoneal sepsis, or sepsis following abortion, pelvic surgery or severe trauma with exposed wounds. Sometimes the portal of entry is not evident. Bacteremia is usually characterized by a sudden fever, with chills, dyspnea, mental confusion, and, frequently, unexplained hypotension. Prolonged hypotension characterizes the shock syndrome and consequent ARF.

In recent years, great importance has been attributed to the role played by endotoxemia in septic shock not only for the "shock lung" (acute respiratory distress syndrome) but also for the "shock kidney" [15].

Endotoxin is the lipopolysaccharide component of the cell wall of gram-negative bacteria. The real toxin is the lipid-A, which is concealed within the bacterial cell; when lipid-A is liberated, its fatty acids insert into the phospolipids of the cell membranes, causing those cellular reactions that are typical of endotoxin shock [16].

3.1 EFFECTS OF ENDOTOXEMIA IN SEPTIC PATIENTS

As pointed out by Wardle, in septic patients endotoxemia may cause many effects, either directly or indirectly (figure 2–4): (a) decrease in effective arterial blood volume due to enhanced capillary permeability (with the consequent escape of protein-rich fluid), pooling of blood in the splanchnic area, opening of arteriovenous shunts; (b) decrease in venous return and cardiac output; (c) arteriolar vasoconstriction (due to sympathetic nervous activation and increase in catecholamine release); (d) endothelial cell damage with release of tissue thromboplastin

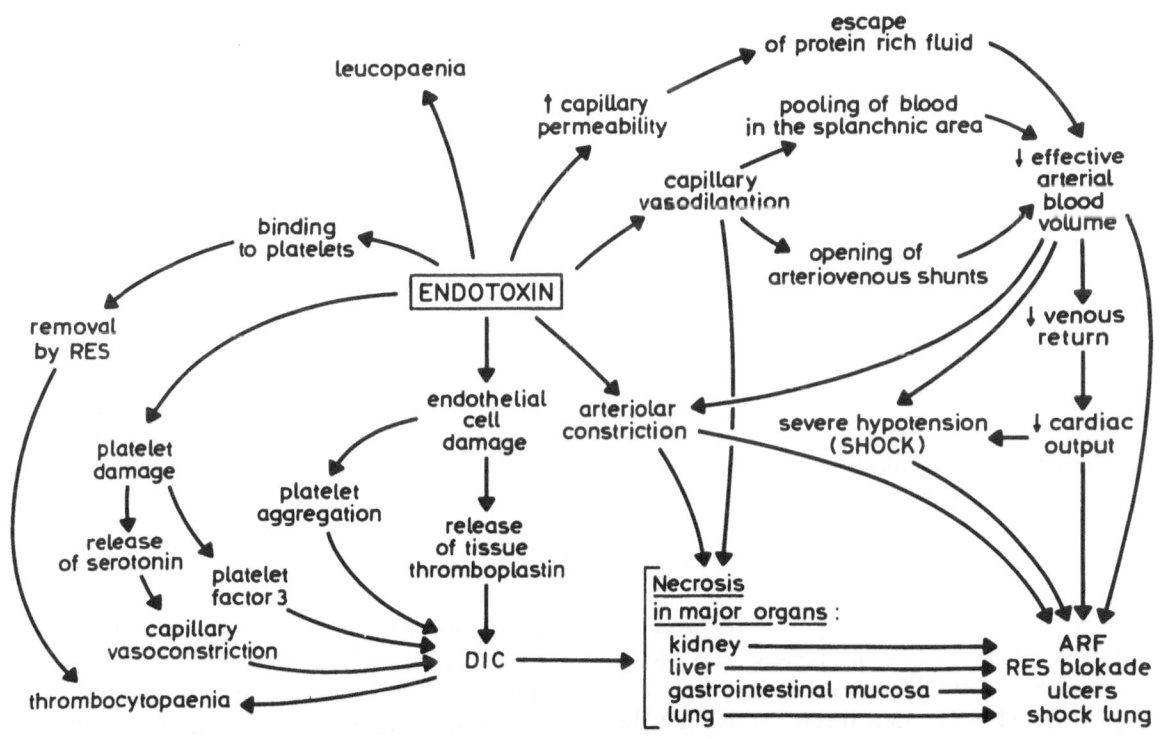

FIGURE 2–4. Endotoxin effects in septic patients. (RES = reticuloendothelial system; DIC = disseminated intravascular coagulation).

leading to microthrombi formation and disseminated intravascular coagulation (DIC); (e) platelet damage with release of serotonin and exposure of lipoprotein platelet factor 3 (activating coagulation); (f) thrombocytopenia, due to removal from circulating blood of entotoxin-carrying platelets by the reticuloendothelial system (RES) and to DIC; (g) leukopenia; (h) complement activation (by triggering both classical and alternate pathways); (i) hyperglycaemia with increase in plasma insulin levels and, then, lactic-acidemia with hypoglycemia; (j) increased lipolysis with high blood levels of free fatty acids and, then, hyperlipidemia; (k) hyponatremia, hypocalcemia, hypophosphatemia [17].

The consequences of a combined number of these direct or indirect endotoxin effects will be (a) hypovolemic shock with reduced cardiac output and severe hypotension; (b) DIC; (c) tissue necrosis in gastrointestinal mucosa (ulcers), liver (RES blockade), lung (shock lung), and kidneys [17].

3.2 ENDOTOXIN EFFECTS ON RENAL FUNCTION

At the renal level, ARF due to endotoxemia may result from the following endotoxin effects: (a) the renal hemodynamic consequences of severe hypovolemia and low cardiac output; (b) the severe renal arteriolar constriction, induced both directly and indirectly through the activation of the sympathetic nervous system and the release of catecholamines; (c) the activation of the renin-angiotensin system; (d) the intravascular coagulation (DIC) resulting from direct damage to white cells, platelets, and endothelial cells and from activation of both complement and coagulation cascades [15, 17, 18]. With mild endotoxemia, the production of kinins and prostaglandins partially protects against renal vasoconstriction, while adequate protection against DIC is given by the fibrinolytic activity of blood and the removal of thromboplastins, fibrin complexes, and endotoxins by RES cells (Kuppfer cells in particular) [17]. Prerenal ARF may result, which can be reversed by improving renal perfusion. More severe endotoxemia causes severe vasoconstriction with hemostasis, local acidosis, and co-

agulation, while endothelial damage prevents prostacyclin release and its protective effect as vasodilator and inhibitor of platelet aggregation; meanwhile the toxic effect on Kuppfer cells and vasoconstriction within the liver impairs the protective role normally played by RES [16]. ATN results, greatly worsening the prognosis of these severely ill patients. Conditions of defective fibrinolysis (such as during pregnancy or following trauma) or poisoning of Kuppfer cells by alcohol or general anesthetics greatly decrease the natural defenses against DIC and may be fatal [17].

There is direct experimental evidence that endotoxemia may cause ARF. Thus, when Escherichia coli endotoxin was injected i.v. in rats, an immediate fall in urine output and in PAH and inulin clearances occurred, secondary to endotoxin-induced increase in renal arteriolar resistances, which was followed by tubular necrosis [19–21]. This observation is very important when we recall that there is great species difference in the degree of endotoxin resistance and that while rats are usually resistant, man is particularly sensitive [16]. Unfortunately, normal humans do not have protective antiendotoxin (antilipid-A) antibodies unless they have chronic pyelonephritis or inflammatory bowel disease or have suffered previous gram-negative infections [17, 22, 23].

3.3 PREVENTION AND TREATMENT OF ENDOTOXIN SHOCK

When nephrotoxic bactericidal antibiotics are used in patients with sepsis for gram-negative bacteremia, it is frequently difficult to decide whether the ARF is due to the antibiotic or to the secondary endotoxemia or to both [16]. Even though only a few studies have been performed to detect endotoxin at the onset of ARF [24], it has been suggested that patients should not be loaded with bactericidal antibiotics alone (for fear of a massive release of endotoxin) but should receive them in combination with short-term steroids in massive doses [16].

Promising preliminary experimental results have been obtained with prostacyclin (PGI_2), which appeared to protect against lethal endotoxemia [25] and against the onset of ARF [26]. PGI_2, in addition to its potent renal va-

sodilatation and inhibition of platelet aggregation (see chapter 1) minimizes cell damage by
raising intracellular cyclic AMP, particularly in
platelets and white cells [16].

Hemoperfusion through charcoal or resin
seems to be particularly useful for removing
endotoxin from circulating blood [27].

4 ARF Secondary to Acute Myocardial Infarction

Prerenal ARF (less commonly ATN) is widely
known to follow acute myocardial infarction.
This occurrence is usually believed, however,
to be only in association with massive myocardial infarction, severe hypotension, and cardiogenic shock. It has been stated, in fact, that
"when failure of the cardiac pump is so severe
as to lead to ARF," the poor prognosis is determined by the pump failure [28].

However, ARF may occur a few days after
mild myocardial infarction, when the patient
appears in excellent clinical condition (although renal function is severely impaired),
and the ARF may fail to be diagnosed for some
time, unless reduction in urine output attracts
the attention of the physician [14] (figure 2-3).

In a recent report, a significant fall in GFR
has been observed, on the third postinfarction
day, in as many as 11 out of 40 patients with
acute myocardial infarction (an incidence,
therefore, of 27.5%) [29].

4.1 THE PATHOGENETIC ROLE OF THE LOW CARDIAC OUTPUT

In terms of left ventricular function, acute
myocardial infarction cannot be regarded as a
single disease, but should be considered as a
series of different hemodynamic conditions that
include (a) hyperdynamic ventricular function,
a rare condition (4% incidence) with high
stroke work (SW) and reduced left ventricular
filling pressure (LVFP); (b) normal left ventricular function (11% incidence) with SW and
LVFP, which are both normal; (c) left ventricular failure (53% incidence) with low SW and
elevated LVFP; (d) cardiogenic shock (28% incidence) with very low SW and elevated LVFP;
(e) hypovolemic condition (4% incidence) with
SW and LVFP both reduced [30]. The cause of

these conditions is usually impairment of left
ventricular performance. This causes either left
ventricular failure (with pulmonary congestion
and dyspnea), which is a predominant "backward failure" of the left ventricle, or cardiogenic shock (with reduced left ventricular output), which is a predominant "forward failure"
[31]. Less frequently, left ventricle function is
either normal or even hyperdynamic (presumably because of circulating catecholamines) or
associated with hypovolemia [30].

Thus, cardiac output is frequently reduced
even in patients without clinical shock [31];
this reduction may by itself cause renal hypoperfusion and prerenal ARF. A proportional
fall in cardiac output and in RBF (with a RBF-
cardiac output ratio maintained around the
normal value of 0.20) has been reported in hypotensive patients with myocardial infarction,
but without shock [32].

The hypoperfusion of renal parenchyma secondary to low cardiac output is "sensed" by the
kidneys as a real ECV depletion even though
only the effective blood volume is reduced. The
renal response will be a markedly increased tubular reabsorption, occurring mainly, but not
exclusively, in proximal tubules with the aim
of normalizing renal perfusion. A reduced volume of highly concentrated urine, with very
low sodium concentration (sodium is reabsorbed more avidly than water), is produced,
but urinalysis is normal. This retention of salt
and water is an appropriate compensating
mechanism when the kidney is hypoperfused
due to volume depletion, but is not appropriate in conditions of low cardiac output without
hypovolemia [33].

4.2 ACUTE MYOCARDIAL INFARCTION AND HYPOVOLEMIA

While ARF appears secondary to reduced cardiac output in most cases of myocardial infarction, on some occasions hypovolemia may contribute to the renal shutdown (figure 2-3).

Hypovolemia may result from increased external loss of extracellular fluid through vomiting and/or sweating, especially in conjunction with reduced food (and salt) intake [14].
Internal shift of intravascular fluid (sequestration of plasma in low-flow areas and/or extra-

vasation of fluid out of the vascular bed because of the increase in capillary hydrostatic pressure) [31] may also contribute greatly to the fall in effective blood volume. This is due to activation of the sympathetic nervous system, which has been demonstrated in the acute phase of myocardial infarction [34, 35]. Sympathetic nervous stimulation and circulating catecholamines, on the other hand, will also cause direct renal vasoconstriction, particularly in patients with shock. Thus, a reduced renal fraction of cardiac output (i.e., a RBF-cardiac output ratio much less than 0.20) has been observed in patients with myocardial infarction a few hours after shock developed [36]. Under such circumstances, part of the original renal blood flow is made available to other vascular areas with greater needs for blood perfusion [31].

Obviously, when myocardial infarction is associated with hypovolemia, the salt and water retention of prerenal ARF works to the patient's advantage, and diuretics are contraindicated; their use, in fact, will aggravate hypovolemia and lead to ATN. The right therapeutic strategy relies on controlled volume loading (figure 2–3).

4.3 CLINICAL EVALUATION OF PATIENTS WITH MYOCARDIAL INFARCTION

LVFP should be measured in patients with acute myocardial infarction by continuously monitoring pulmonary capillary wedge pressure. Should the latter be too high (more than 18 to 20 mm Hg, "backward failure"), pulmonary congestion or even acute pulmonary edema (values greater than 30 mm Hg) would ensue. Under such circumstances, diuretic therapy is necessary with the aim of lowering pulmonary wedge pressure below those levels that cause pulmonary congestion (i.e., below 18 mm Hg) but not so much as to reduce cardiac output (i.e., not below 15 mm Hg) [30]. Should pulmonary capillary wedge pressure be too low (i.e., below 15 mm Hg) as occurs in hypovolemia, stroke volume may be reduced and may be improved with volume loading until a pulmonary capillary wedge pressure of 15 mm Hg is achieved; further increase in pulmonary capillary wedge pressure should be avoided since it does not increase stroke volume but may cause pulmonary congestion [30].

5 ARF Following Open-Heart Surgery

The occurrence of ARF in the first few days following open-heart surgery is not uncommon. An overall incidence as high as 30% has been reported [37, 38]. The occurrence of non-oliguric ARF is more frequent (25%) than that of oliguric ARF (3 to 5%) [37, 38].

Presumably, this ARF is hemodynamically mediated [39]. It may occur as prerenal ARF, with a transient reduction of renal function that is readily reversed with the improvement of cardiac performance [37–40], or as ATN, which may be so protracted as to require dialysis therapy [41].

During cardiopulmonary bypass, the kidneys are underperfused (200 to 500 ml/min) and GFR is markedly reduced [39]. At the end of surgery, however, GFR returns to normal in most patients, provided cardiac output is satisfactory.

5.1 PRERENAL ARF

The prerenal ARF observed in some patients usually results from a cardiac functional impairment lasting for a few days following surgery. Myers et al. [39] have recently demonstrated, in patients with prerenal ARF observed one to four days after open-heart surgery, that the fall in GFR was associated with a reduction (a) in left ventricular function (low left ventricular stroke work and low cardiac output), (b) in systemic blood pressure, and (c) in renal blood flow (RBF). This occurred despite an ECV expansion (15% body weight gain) induced by i.v. infusion of lactate Ringer's solution, with added mannitol, prior to surgery and maintained throughout cardiopulmonary bypass and in the early postoperative period. The fall in GFR in these patients, however, was disproportionate to the decrease in RBF. A reduction in transcapillary glomerular pressure and in glomerular ultrafiltration coefficient K_f (see chapter 1) (which was ingeniously calculated by the authors) accounted for this severe fall in filtration fraction and were attributed to severe hypotension and decrease of cardiac output [39]. It has therefore been suggested that serum creatinine should be monitored in these patients when using vasodilator drugs (such as sodium nitroprusside, given to reduce systemic vascular resistance) since a fall in blood pressure below the autoregulatory range may greatly reduce GFR [39].

5.2 ATN

Following open-heart surgery, however, ATN may occur, probably as a result of more severe and prolonged impairment in renal hemodynamics. Under such circumstances a backleak of filtered inulin has been demonstrated by clearance techniques [41, 42]. Thus, when clearances of inulin (molecules with radius of 13.5 Å) and of larger dextran molecules (radius of 22 to 28 Å) were simultaneously performed in patients with ATN following open-heart surgery, the clearance of dextran exceeded that of inulin, although limitation of filtration was predicted for the large dextran molecules but not for inulin. This observation suggested that the leak of filtered inulin through necrotic tubular epithelium exceeded that of dextran [41–43]. Since the damaged tubular epithelium is permeable to inulin, it must be permeable also to other constituents of tubular fluid. Thus, a transtubular backleak of glomerular filtrate is peculiar to this human form of ATN and has been even suggested as a test to differentiate prerenal ARF (no backleak) from ATN [43].

Myers et al. [41] have also observed that there was no delay in the urinary appearance of the inulin infused intravenously. Therefore, should tubular obstruction occur in these patients, it cannot be homogeneous, but a subpopulation of tubules must remain widely patent [41].

6 ARF Secondary to Nonsteroidal Anti-Inflammatory Drugs (NSAID)

Many reports have demonstrated that aspirin, indomethacin, and other new nonsteroidal anti-inflammatory drugs (NSAID), such as ibuprofen, naproxen, and fenoprofen, may clearly decrease RBF and/or GFR in patients with pre-existent renal disease. Since these drugs, which are structurally dissimilar, are well known inhibitors of prostaglandin (PG) synthesis and PGs play a very important role in regulating renal hemodynamics (see chapter 1), it has been suggested that such inhibition of PG synthesis is responsible for the renal functional impairment by NSAID.

When given to normal subjects, indomethacin may cause a slight reduction of renal function; but when previously volume depleted, these subjects exhibit a significant fall in GFR with indomethacin [44, 45] or aspirin [46]. This observation is consistent with the major role played by vasodilator PGs in preserving renal function when vasoconstrictor stimuli are challenging the kidneys; under such circumstances, in fact, PG synthesis is clearly enhanced [47–50].

Vasoconstrictor stimuli (angiotensin, catecholamines) are potentiated in all conditions of effective blood volume depletion. These include, therefore, ECV depletion, cirrhosis with ascites, nephrotic syndrome, low-output heart failure (when the kidneys perceive a salt depletion state) [51, 52]. Should indomethacin or aspirin or other NSAID be given under such circumstances, ARF might either occur or be potentiated [44, 45, 51–53]; vasoconstrictor stimuli, in fact, will no longer be balanced or attenuated by PGs, the synthesis of which has been inhibited (see chapter 1). The resulting enhanced vasoconstriction may cause a functional ARF (prerenal ARF), which is readily reversed with drug withdrawal (44, 45, 51, 54–56). When the resulting ischemic insult is more severe, however, ATN may result. This was the case, for instance, with the patient with lupus nephritis reported by Kimberly et al. [57] who was treated with aspirin and ibuprofen; renal biopsy revealed patchy ultrastructural ischemic changes in proximal tubular epithelium. Similarly, in two other patients reported by Fong and Cohen [58], ibuprofen (800 mg three times daily) significantly increased serum creatinine in a few days of therapy (in one patient dialysis was necessary); renal biopsies revealed proximal tubular lesions by light and electron microscopy: disruption of brush border, fragmentation of cytoplasm, and even disintegration of cells with debris accumulation in the tubular lumina.

On the basis of the above clinical experience, aspirin, indomethacin, and all NSAID must be used with caution in conditions of renal hypoperfusion (including salt depletion, heart failure, cirrhosis, nephrotic syndrome) and in patients with underlying renal disease [54, 59], particularly lupus nephritis [55, 57, 60]. According to Kimberly et al. [60], patients with systemic lupus erythematosus have high levels of urinary PG excretion. Caution is also necessary in the use of NSAID in association with triamterene, since prerenal ARF has been observed in healthy subjects receiving combined triamterene and indomethacin [56]. Serum creatinine should be monitored during treatment and the drug withdrawn immediately if any impairment of renal function is observed.

As mentioned elsewhere in this chapter, NSAID may also cause acute interstitial nephritis.

7 Aminoglycoside-Induced ARF in Humans

Aminoglycosides are very important antibiotics used extensively in the treatment of infections caused by gram-negative bacteria. It has been stated that as many as 4 million people are treated yearly with these drugs [61, 62]. Unfortunately, all of these drugs are nephrotoxic, hence, any structural modification in newer aminoglycosides with the purpose of increasing their antibacterial activity is also accompanied by an increase in nephrotoxicity [63].

Neomycin is no longer available for parenteral use because of its toxicity; for the same reason, treatment with kanamycin is usually avoided.

7.1 INCIDENCE

Among the most widely used aminoglycosides, nephrotoxicity is similar for gentamicin and amikacin [64–67] while tobramycin is somewhat less toxic [68–71]. The last observation is still a matter of debate. Thus, in a prospective

randomized clinical trial, Fong et al. [72] observed that nephrotoxicity occurred in 10% of patients treated with gentamicin and in 8% of those treated with tobramycin, but the difference was not statistically significant. According to the authors, however, it is possible that longer duration of treatment and larger doses may result in minor toxicity of tobramycin. In randomized studies, Smith et al. [70, 71] have observed, in fact, an incidence of nephrotoxicity of 10 to 12% with tobramycin, and 21 to 26% with gentamicin, and Kumin [61] an incidence of 15% and 55.2%, respectively, using similar doses (3.33 mg/kg/day with a mean cumulative dose of 2.2 g/patient for tobramycin, and 3.37 mg/kg/day with a mean cumulative dose of 2.1 g/patient for gentamicin).

Sisomicin has nephrotoxicity as great as or even greater than that of gentamicin [63].

Netilmicin, a new semisynthetic derivative of sisomicin, seems to be less nephrotoxic and ototoxic than other aminoglycosides. Thus, in only 8 out of 890 courses of netilmicin, in doses ranging from 3 to 8 mg/kg b.w./day i.m. or i.v., a significant impairment of renal function was observed, with an incidence of 0.9%; the incidences of ototoxicity and vestibular dysfunction were 0.4% and 0.6% respectively [73]. In a review of prospective studies on the effect of netilmicin on renal function, however, the incidence of "probable" nephrotoxicity appeared to range from 0 to 11.5% (mean of 4%) and that of "probable but in several cases doubtful" nephrotoxicity appeared to range from 0 to 30% (mean of 12.6%) [74].

Streptomycin is the least nephrotoxic aminoglycoside in experimental animals [63], and no cases of ARF have been reported after this drug.

It has been stated that a better knowledge of aminoglycoside nephrotoxicity has decreased the incidence of renal functional impairment, especially in patients with pre-existing renal disease [75]; thus Hewitt [76] observed that the 7.7% incidence of gentamicin nephrotoxicity in the years 1965 and 1966 fell to 2.9% in the years 1970 to 1973. However greater incidences in recent years have been reported by others (as mentioned above).

7.2 AMINOGLYCOSIDE NEPHROTOXICITY AND PATIENT AGE

Nephrotoxicity of aminoglycosides in newborn infants is rarely described. The relative tolerance of neonates to aminoglycosides has been attributed to a preferential distribution of RBF to the juxtamedullary cortex at birth; this will prevent the accumulation of the drug in the outer cortex where the more numerous superficial nephrons are located [77]. The centrifugal redistribution of RBF with increasing age increases the delivery of aminoglycosides to superficial nephrons which will no longer be protected.

In advanced age the susceptibility to aminoglycoside nephrotoxicity is greatly increased [78].

7.3 PATHOGENESIS AND RENAL PATHOLOGY

In chapter 1 we extensively discussed the pathogenesis of gentamicin-induced ARF. The pathogenetic mechanism is presumably not dissimilar for other aminoglycosides. In human renal biopsies, aminoglycoside nephrotoxicity has shown pathologic changes in the proximal tubule varying from ultrastructural, subcellular damage (increase in lysosomes, presence of numerous myeloid bodies in lysosomes, etc.) to overt cell necrosis [79–84] in a fashion quite similar to that of experimental gentamicin-induced ARF (chapter 1). It is interesting to note that in at least one case, gentamicin has induced acute interstitial nephritis (AIN, biopsy diagnosis), which was reversed by high-dose methylprednisolone [85].

7.4 CLINICAL FEATURES

Aminoglycosides also cause nonoliguric ARF in humans, with an increase in urine volume, which usually precedes the fall in GFR [86]. Sometimes, however, oliguric ARF occurs [14, 87]. But it is undoubtedly very difficult to figure out the single pathogenetic contribution of so many coexisting factors. These factors include, in addition to aminoglycosides, other nephrotoxic drugs (such as cephalosporin, loop diuretics, etc.)—the primary disease for which these drugs (including aminoglycosides) have been prescribed—any pre-existing renal dysfunction, advanced age [78], ECV depletion

[86], and metabolic acidosis [88]. Thus, although it has been demonstrated that nephrotoxicity is dose-dependent, and despite the statement that excessive levels of the drug precede the rise in serum creatinine [63], it is today well established that renal damage may occur despite serum drug concentrations maintained within the accepted therapeutic range [64, 71, 72, 89–91]. On the other hand, high serum levels of aminoglycosides in treated patients may represent only the consequence rather than the cause of the fall in GFR since these drugs are excreted almost entirely by glomerular filtration [90, 92, 93]. That is why, in my opinion, determination of serum concentrations of the drugs is unpractical and unnecessary.

After discontinuation of treatment, aminoglycosides are excreted in the urine for many days, being continuously released from tissue stores [94]. This urinary excretion may last more than 10 days after tobramycin and even a month after the last dose of gentamicin [61]; it has been stated that gentamicin can be detected in the urine of humans as long as six months after the end of the therapy [62]. Thus, especially with gentamicin, renal injury may continue and ARF may occur and frequently persist several days and even several weeks after treatment ends [95, 96], when the cause-and-effect relationship is no longer so evident.

ARF secondary to aminoglycoside nephrotoxicity is usually reversible after discontinuation of the drug, but it may require dialysis and may even lead to uremic death [63]. Sometimes the return of renal function to normal may be very slow [63, 97]. We have recently observed a 57-year-old male patient who was dialyzed for two months (thrice weekly) for gentamicin-induced ARF; his renal function returned to complete normality only after a year.

7.5 ASSOCIATION OF AMINOGLYCOSIDES WITH OTHER NEPHROTOXIC AGENTS

As mentioned in chapter 1, in contrast with experimental animals in which cephalosporins may even protect against aminoglycoside nephrotoxicity, the administration of an aminoglycoside combined with a cephalosporin (not only cephaloridine, but also cephalothin) in humans will greatly increase the incidence and severity of renal injury [14, 87, 89, 94, 98–104]. Thus, in the series of Klastersky et al. [101], the incidence of renal functional impairment in patients treated with the association cephalothin + tobramycin was 21% against an incidence of 6% with the association tircacillin + tobramycin and 2% with the association tircacillin + cephalothin. Similarly, in a prospective, randomized, double-blind trial, Wade et al. [89] found a significant rise in serum creatinine in 30.4% of the patients treated with cephalothin + gentamicin, in 20.8% of those treated with cephalothin + tobramycin, against an average incidence of 7% in patients treated with combined methicillin + aminoglycoside (gentamicin or tobramycin). Finally, in a large trial by the EORTC (International Antimicrobial Therapy Project Group) [105], nephrotoxicity was observed in 16% of patients receiving combined gentamicin + cephalothin against 6% and 3% incidences in patients treated with carbenicillin + cephalothin and carbenicillin + gentamicin, respectively.

All of these studies appear, undoubtedly, to be strong evidence for the potentiation of aminoglycoside nephrotoxicity by cephalothin, which has to be taken into account when prescribing antibiotic therapy [104].

Similarly, other medications, which are frequently administered in conjunction with aminoglycosides to critically ill patients, may enhance their nephrotoxicity. Among these medications we should mention furosemide [106, 107], methoxyflurane [108], cis-platinum [109], amphotericin B [110], and clindamycin [111].

Finally, there are clinical conditions that have been shown to potentiate aminoglycoside nephrotoxicity: dehydration [112], sodium depletion [86, 107, 113], potassium depletion [114], metabolic acidosis [88], and pre-existing renal dysfunction.

Aminoglycosides should never be given to salt-depleted patients. Furthermore, serum creatinine should be monitored during treatment of severely ill patients. In patients with CRF, drug dosage should be adjusted to the degree of renal function impairment (see chapter 3).

8   ARF Secondary to Cephalosporins

It is demonstrated that cephaloridine may cause proximal tubular necrosis at therapeutic dosage [115]. This observation has raised some concern about the clinical use of all cephalosporins, especially the widespread practice of using them in combination with aminoglycosides [102]. The association of cephalosporins and aminoglycosides has shown an additive toxicity in humans [14, 89, 100, 101, 116] but not in rats [102, 117–120] nor in rabbits [121]. This discrepancy between humans and animals is not surprising since a great difference in sensitivity to antibiotic nephrotoxicity has been observed between species [122]. Thus, while rats are resistant to cephalosporins [115, 123, 124], rabbits, guinea pigs, monkeys, and humans are not [14, 115, 116, 124].

There is increasing evidence that furosemide, even at moderate doses, will increase the nephrotoxicity of cephalosporins [125–127].

8.1   CEPHALORIDINE

Undoubtedly, cephaloridine is cytotoxic to proximal tubular cells [115, 128, 129]; this cytotoxicity is prevented by probenecid [128, 130, 131]. Its excretion, however, is accomplished by glomerular filtration without any net tubular secretion [122]. There is evidence that the drug is actively transported into proximal tubular cells at the antiluminal membrane by an organic anion secretory carrier (probably the same involved in PAH secretion) [132, 133] but without any further movement from the cell to the tubular fluid [122, 133, 134]. Thus, the high concentration in the renal cortex, observed after cephaloridine administration, is mainly due to the intracellular fraction; probenecid, in fact, will greatly reduce the cortical concentration of cephaloridine without affecting its urinary excretion [122].

One to five hours after cephaloridine injection, proximal tubular cells exhibit focal losses of brush border, an increase in apical vacuoles and in membranous structures, loss of basolateral interdigitations, and rounded shape of mitochondria [122, 129]; these changes then progress to widespread tubular necrosis [115]. Although the mechanism of cellular toxicity is not known, there is evidence that it is at least in part mediated by alterations in mitochondrial respiration [122].

The nephrotoxicity of cephaloridine is exacerbated (a) by high dosage of the drug [135, 136], (b) by pre-existent renal insufficiency, and (c) by furosemide [126, 137, 138]. Presumably, the potentiating effect of furosemide is due to its capability of increasing the serum half-life of the antibiotic by a mechanism not yet identified [127].

Clinically, the patient becomes oliguric, and established ARF frequently requires dialysis. Recovery of renal function usually occurs, but the patient may die because of complications.

8.2 CEFAZOLIN

Cefazolin has been shown to cause proximal tubular necrosis in rabbits, rats, and guinea pigs when used in very large doses [124, 139, 140]. It is filtered by glomeruli and secreted by proximal tubules like PAH [122]; its renal cortical concentration is usually lower than that of the more toxic cephaloridine, but greater than that of the less toxic cephalothin [118]. Cefazolin toxicity is prevented by probenecid [122, 140].

It has been stated that cefazolin is not toxic in humans [141, 142]. Although no cases of ATN have been reported up to now, two cases of AIN following cefazolin have been recently described [143].

8.3 CEPHALOTHIN

Cephalothin is one of the least nephrotoxic antibiotics of the cephalosporin group [124, 144, 145]. Its renal excretion, only partly due to glomerular filtration is mainly due to secretion by the proximal tubules [122].

Massive administration of cephalothin has been shown to cause ARF in rabbits and rats [124] and in humans [102, 146] with clinical and laboratory changes consistent with ATN. It seems that nephrotoxicity similar to that in-

duced by cephaloridine is induced by cephalothin when high intracellular concentration of the drug is achieved [140]. This nephrotoxicity is potentiated by furosemide [126, 138]. In some patients, however, reversible renal failure has occurred, associated with eosinophilia and rash, with typical renal biopsy appearances, of cephalothin-induced AIN [102, 147–149]. Furthermore, cephalothin may aggravate AIN due to methicillin or nafcillin [150, 151].

It has been stated that prophylactic treatment with cephalothin may impair renal function of transplanted kidneys, but this conclusion is still a matter of debate [63].

As already mentioned, in humans (but not in experimental animals) cephalothin will increase the incidence and the severity of renal injury due to aminoglycosides [14, 87, 98–101, 105, 152].

8.4 CEPHALEXIN

Reversible nonliguric ARF has also been reported sporadically after therapy with oral cephalexin [153–155]. AIN with fever, rash, arthralgia, and oliguric ARF has been observed during therapy with cephalexin [138].

8.5 OTHER CEPHALOSPORINS

Cephapirin, cephacetrile, cephradine [136, 138], cefadroxil [156], cefoxitin [63, 157], and cefotaxime [158, 159] have all been reported as free of nephrotoxicity, at least when given in moderate therapeutic doses.

A recent interesting observation concerning cefoxitin points out that serum creatinine may appear falsely elevated with most assay systems when determined soon after cefoxitin administration [160].

Lentnek et al. [161] have recently reported one case of cefamandole-induced ARF with acute tubular necrosis on renal biopsy: a 52-year-old patient with Hemophilus parainfluenzae endocarditis was cured after 20 days of cefamandole therapy; for 12 days cefamandole was given at high-doses (4 grams every 4 hours); he became oliguric and was dialyzed for three weeks; renal function then returned to normal. Since no report of significant nephrotoxicity of cefamandole exists up to now when

66

the drug is used at a therapeutic dosage (i.e., 0.5 to 1 g every 4 to 8 hours with a maximal dose of 2 g every 4 hours), it may be concluded that for this semisynthetic cephalosporin, there is a considerable margin between therapeutic and nephrotoxic doses [161].

9 Cisplatinum-Induced ARF

Among the antineoplastic agents effective against solid tumors, the heavy metal compound cis-diamine dichloroplatinum (cisplatinum), because of its property of interfering with DNA synthesis [162], plays an important role, especially in disseminated testicular cancer, but also in ovarian and urinary bladder carcinomas and tumors of the neck and head. Cisplatinum is the only platinum compound available for clinical use. Its major adverse effects include nausea and vomiting (almost invariable), hematologic depression, high-frequency hearing loss, renal magnesium wasting, increased urinary loss of calcium and amino-acids, and, more important, impairment of renal function [109, 163–172].

Nephrotoxicity of cisplatinum has been shown to be dose-related in experimental animals in which an experimental model of ARF has been produced (see chapter 1). Since nephrotoxicity is also dose-related in humans, the adverse effect of cisplatinum on renal function represents a dose-limiting factor in its clinical use.

9.1 RENAL DAMAGE BY CISPLATINUM
The tubular lesions caused by cisplatinum in experimental animals have been fully described in chapter 1. Those in humans have been located mainly in distal convoluted tubules and in collecting ducts [163, 165], but also in the S_3 segment ("pars recta") of proximal tubules; they consist of epithelial necrosis, tubular dilation, and cast formation in the tubular lumen [163, 165, 167, 169, 173].

9.2 INCIDENCE AND SEVERITY OF RENAL FUNCTION IMPAIRMENT
Renal function impairment by cisplatinum, when given alone, occurs in as many as 50 to 75% of treated patients [171]. In combination

with other nephrotoxic drugs (such as aminoglycosides or cephalosporins), both the incidence and the severity of renal damage is increased [109, 165].

ARF is usually of nonoliguric type but may on occasion be oliguric [163]. It has been considered a reversible ARF, but many patients never regain their pretreatment level of renal function [109, 166].

Urinary magnesium wasting is another common adverse effect of cisplatinum even in patients without renal function impairment; hypomagnesemia, hypocalcemia, and hypokalemia may result from magnesium deficiency [171, 172, 174, 175]. It may be potentiated by the association of aminoglycoside antibiotics [176].

9.3 PROTECTIVE EFFECTS OF CHLORIDE-CONTAINING VEHICLES
Experimental studies in animals have indicated that the administration of cisplatinum in chloride-containing vehicles (such as 0.9% saline solution) rather than in chloride-free solutions may reduce the nephrotoxicity of the drug. Apparently, when dissolved in water, cisplatinum undergoes an aquation reaction and consequent transformation into the monochloro-monoaquo-diammine-platinum or diaquo-diammine-platinum; these aquation products are involved both in the antineoplastic and nephrotoxic effects of the drug [171]. But the aquation reaction does not occur in chloride-containing solutions (e.g., 0.9% saline solution); since the intracellular chloride concentration is very low (i.e., 10 to 15% of that in extracellular fluid), aquation of cisplatinum can occur intracellularly [171]. On the basis of these observations, it may be postulated that the use of chloride-containing vehicles will prevent the aquation reaction until cisplatinum has reached the intracellular compartment. In favor of this theory are experimental studies in rats that have demonstrated that the administration of cisplatinum (9 mg/Kg b.w.) in distilled water was followed by death of 100% of the treated rats; this percentage was reduced to 66% and 0% when the vehicle for cisplatinum was either 0.9% saline or 4.5% saline, respectively [171]. No protective effect was observed

when hypertonic saline was infused simultaneously [but at a different site] with cisplatinum dissolved in distilled water [171]. Apparently, the solvent vehicle does not affect the antineoplastic efficacy of cisplatinum [171].

9.4 PROTECTIVE EFFECT OF HYDRATION AND SALINE INFUSIONS

As mentioned, tubular lesions due to cisplatinum are mainly located in distal tubules and collecting ducts, i.e., in that part of the nephron where urine becomes highly concentrated. The massive administration of water in patients treated with cisplatinum, therefore, by greatly reducing tubular water reabsorption in the distal nephron, will decrease cisplatinum concentration in the tubular fluid, thereby decreasing its toxic effects. Thus, when intensive i.v. hydration was performed before, during, and after cisplatinum administration, the incidence of renal function impairment was greatly reduced [177].

However, cell damage also occurs in the proximal tubules. ECV expansion by i.v. infusion of isotonic saline is the best way to dilute cisplatinum in proximal tubular fluid by inhibiting proximal tubular reabsorption. The dilutional effect will simultaneously protect proximal and distal tubular cells. The i.v. infusion of saline has been shown to decrease the renal tissue content of platinum and to increase its urinary excretion [171, 177].

9.5 TREATMENT AND PREVENTION

Once established, cisplatinum-induced ARF should be treated as any other form of ischemic/toxic ARF (see chapters 21 and 22), including, when necessary, hemodialysis (see chapter 23) or peritoneal dialysis (see chapter 24). It is, however, much more important to prevent cisplatinum-induced ARF, through reduction in dosage of the drug, adequate hydration, saline infusion, and use of mannitol or loop diuretics (see chapter 3).

10 Radiocontrast-Induced ARF

Half a century ago, clinicians and radiologists were really concerned about the possible nephrotoxicity of radiographic contrast materials

that had been introduced to clinical practice. Thus, intravenous pyelography (IVP) was considered as contraindicated in renal disease or at least in renal failure. In 1963, however, Schwartz et al. [178] suggested the routine use of IVP with high doses of diatrizoate (Hypaque®) (approximately twice the usual dose) in patients with chronic renal failure (CRF); the authors demonstrated its diagnostic utility and safety. Schencker [179] introduced the drip infusion pyelography (DIP) technique for CRF patients. The essential feature of DIP was the slow administration of the large dose of contrast agent (2.2 ml/Kg b.w. of Hypaque 50%) diluted with an equal volume of 278 mmol/l (5g/dl) glucose solution. Since then high-dose IVP and DIP have been widely used as diagnostic procedures in chronic uremia. It was later demonstrated that the same urinary concentration of contrast agent is obtained if the same amount is given by i.v. injection or by drip infusion, so that DIP remained a convenient technique for delivering large volumes of contrast agents [180].

In recent years many reports of contrast nephropathy have appeared in the literature.

Contrast nephropathy or radiocontrast-induced ARF may be defined as an acute deterioration of renal function (usually an increment of at least 88.4 μmol/l [1mg/dl] in serum creatinine) associated with the use of radiocontrast agents, when no other etiologic factor appears responsible for the renal damage. In other words, it is an iatrogenic ARF that usually follows (a) the use of diatrizoate, iothalamate, or metrizoate for IVP, angiography, and even computerized tomography (CT); (b) the use of sodium bunamiodyl or iopanoic acid for cholecystography; or (c) the use of iodipamide for cholangiography.

The increasing incidence of deterioration of renal function following contrast media in recent years (mainly in the last 10 years) is in part due to the increased use of contrast agents, in part to the increase in their dosage [181]; but it is also partly due to the careful evaluation of renal function in the days following the radiographic procedures. Thus, changes in serum creatinine, which would have not been recognized because of lack of clinical symptoms and their usual reversibility, are to-day recorded and taken into consideration.

This ARF may range from a subclinical, transient, slight impairment of renal function (in most cases) to an abrupt oliguric ARF.

It should also be mentioned that in surveys on acute reactions to contrast media conducted by radiologists, nephrotoxicity might have been omitted because contrast-induced ARF usually occurs hours to days after the radiographic procedure, when the patient is no longer under the observation of the radiologist [181].

It has been stated that radiocontrast-induced ARF accounts for 2 to 9% of all cases of ARF [170].

10.1 RADIOCONTRAST MEDIA

Radiocontrast media are radiopaque compounds used in diagnostic radiology and are also commonly called contrast agents or materials or dyes or drugs; the term *contrast drugs* seems quite appropriate since they behave as drugs even though their pharmacologic activity is very weak [181]. And as for other drugs, contrast media exhibit untoward side reactions, such as renal toxicity in the form of ARF.

All contrast agents used in clinical practice are tri-iodinated derivatives of benzoic acid, which may be chemically distinguished from each other by the substitution on the carbon atoms of the benzene ring and by the composition of the side chains [182]. Thus, oral cholecystographic agents, namely sodium bunamiodyl (Orabilex®) and iopanoic acid (Telepaque®, Cistobil®), have no substitution on the carbon atom at position 5 of the benzene ring. The cholangiographic agent iodipamide (Cholografin®, Biligrafin®, Endocistobil®) is a two-ring compound also with incomplete substitution. Contrast agents commonly used for IVP, angiography, and CT—namely sodium or meglumine diatrizoate (Urografin®, Angiografin®, Selectografin®, Hypaque®, Renografin®) iothalamate (Conray®), and metrizoate (Isopaque®)—have, instead, a fully substituted benzene ring [182]. The contrast agents with a completely substituted benzene ring are not consistently bound to plasma proteins and are highly water soluble and lipid insoluble; thus they distribute in the extracellular space, are freely filtered by the glomeruli, and are not reabsorbed by the tubules (they are not secreted, at least in man), being readily excreted in the urine [181]; this allows a ready visualization of kidneys and urinary tract.

Incompletely substituted compounds are strongly bound to albumin so they cannot be freely filtered by glomeruli but undergo hepatic excretion [182]. Thus, they can be used for oral cholecystography and cholangiography. Iopanoic acid (Telepaque®, Cistobil®) is a lipid-soluble compound and is conjugated by the liver to form a water-soluble compound subsequently undergoing hydrolysis in the gallbladder; iodipamide (Cholografin®, Biligrafin®, Endocistobil®), instead, is excreted by the liver without conjugation [182]. These compounds, therefore, allow the visualization of the biliary tract.

The contrast media used for IVP, angiography, and CT are usually given intravenously or intra-arterially as hyperosmotic solutions. Their plasma concentration is a function of the dose, the speed of the injection, and the body size [182]. After a fast i.v. injection, a peak value is obtained almost immediately; the plasma decay curve exhibits an initial steep slope due to mixing of the contrast medium throughout the blood pool, which is followed by a less steep slope due to urinary excretion with a t½ of approximately 2 hours in normal man [181–183]. In conditions of reduced GFR, the decline in plasma concentration of the contrast medium is reduced.

The slow i.v. infusion of a contrast medium for IVP does not give the initial peak but a lower sustained plasma concentration [182].

10.2 ARF DUE TO UROGRAPHIC AND ANGIOGRAPHIC CONTRAST AGENTS

10.2.1 Predisposing factors Contrast-induced ARF is undoubtedly favored by one or more of the following predisposing factors.

10.2.1.1 PRE-EXISTING IMPAIRMENT OF RENAL FUNCTION. This appears the most frequent risk factor: 90% of the reported cases of contrast-induced ARF occurred in patients with impaired renal function [184]. No correlation has been observed between the occurrence of contrast nephropathy and the type of pre-existing renal disease [185].

In a survey of IVP in 377 hospitalized patients, the incidence of contrast-induced ARF [abrupt increase of serum creatinine by more than 88.4 μmol/l, 1mg/dl even without oliguria] was 4.8%; but the percentage fell to 0.6% when the study was limited to 169 patients with no evidence of renal disease [186]. In a careful retrospective study by Cattell's group, only 3 out of 40 patients with CRF exhibited a transient, slight rise in serum creatinine without oliguria following high-dose IVP [600mg I/Kg b.w. of sodium diatrizoate-Hypaque 45®] [187]. Retrospective studies, however, are not accurate and may not include all patients undergoing the radiologic procedures.

In a prospective study on the effect of IVP on renal function in 124 patients, transient deterioration of renal function, without oliguria, was observed in 27 cases (21.8%); the incidence fell to 15.3% when only 85 patients with normal renal function were considered, and increased to 55% in the 20 patients with CRF [188]. In another prospective study in 378 hospitalized patients undergoing nonrenal angiography, the incidence of contrast-induced ARF (usually subclinical ARF) was 2% in subjects with normal renal function and 33% in patients with CRF [189].

ARF has been observed following CT procedures since CT is usually performed with the aid of contrast enhancement (see chapter 9). Thus, ARF has been reported in patients following head or body scan using sodium or meglumine iothalamate with iodine doses ranging from 0.59 to 2.11g/Kg [190,191]; most of these patients had pre-existing renal insufficiency [191].

It seems that the greater the degree of pre-existing renal failure, the greater the risk of nephrotoxicity by contrast media [186]. Thus, as many as 40% of patients with serum creatinine greater than 398 μmol/l (4.5 mg/dl) had acute decrement of their renal function [186].

10.2.1.2 DIABETES MELLITUS Diabetes mellitus is considered another important risk factor of contrast-induced ARF. More than 50% of the reported cases of contrast nephropathy were, in fact, diabetics, but almost all of them also had CRF [184]. Taken together, the observations reported in the recent literature suggest the following three conclusions. First, diabetic patients (especially with juvenile onset or type-I diabetes) [192] with CRF are at prohibitively high risk of exacerbation of their renal failure, a condition that may frequently require permanent hemodialysis [184, 186, 192, 193]. It has been shown that the higher the pre-existing serum creatinine in diabetic patients, the greater the risk of permanent exacerbation of renal failure by contrast media [192]. Blood hyperviscosity, reduced deformability of erythrocytes, increased platelet aggregation, and, more important, the severe vascular lesions particularly in the afferent and efferent glomerular arterioles—all are typical changes of diabetes mellitus, represent important predisposing factors; the abnormal rheology and the basal impairment of renal perfusion may, in fact, be aggravated by contrast media [194]. Obviously, the association of other predisposing factors, such as dehydration, salt and water depletion, severe hypertension, or high dosage of contrast dye may potentiate the risk of renal function impairment [194]. The second conclusion is that at similar degrees of CRF, the risk is greater in diabetic patients than in nondiabetic ones [186]. The third and final conclusion is that diabetes mellitus associated with normal renal function does not seem to represent a risk factor [184, 186, 189]. Thus, only 3 out of 49 type-2 diabetic patients with serum creatinine less than 177 μmol/l (2mg/dl) developed reversible impairment of renal function [194], while none of 19 diabetics with serum creatinine less than 133 μmol/l (1.5 mg/dl) exhibited any renal function deterioration [186]. It has therefore been stated that IVP can be safely performed in type-2 diabetic patients with creatinine clearance greater than 35 ml/min provided that proteinuria is not greater than 2 g/24 hours and other disposing factors are not associated [194]. It should be mentioned, however, that irreversible deterioration of renal function has occasionally been reported in diabetics with creatinine clearance of 50 ml/min (serum creatinine of 133 μmol/l, 1.5 mg/dl) and proteinuria much less than 2 g/24 hours [195].

10.2.1.3 VASCULAR DISEASES INVOLVING THE KID-NEYS. Vascular diseases involving the kidneys, such as nephrosclerosis, diabetic nephropathy, or polyarteritis nodosa, may predispose to contrast nephropathy. Thus, ARF has been observed after angiography in a case of polyarteritis nodosa with impairment of renal function that was largely irreversible [196].

Hypertension has been reported to increase the incidence of contrast-induced ARF in patients with and without pre-existing renal insufficiency [188].

10.2.1.4 DEHYDRATION. In the early days of IVP, fluid restriction was advised before the radiographic procedure in order to visualize better the urinary tract. Undoubtedly, since modern radiocontrast media are filtered by glomeruli and neither reabsorbed nor secreted by tubules, their intratubular concentration progressively increases along the tubule reaching the maximum in the collecting duct. Thus, fluid restriction, by increasing ADH secretion and consequently water reabsorption in the distal nephron, may raise the concentration of contrast media in tubular fluid; this occurs, however, only in the collecting tubules, thereby limiting the contribution of dehydration to predisposing to contrast nephrotoxicity. On the other hand, ARF by contrast agents has also been observed in well-hydrated patients [184, 193].

However, even though there is no clear evidence that the incidence of contrast nephropathy is reduced by hydration, it is commonly accepted that adequate hydration will prevent oliguria and permanent renal damage, especially in high-risk patients [184].

10.2.1.5 SALT AND WATER DEPLETION. Perhaps too much attention has been given to dehydration as a predisposing factor, and too little attention to the role of salt and water depletion [182]. Undoubtedly, the proximal tubule is the site of maximal salt and water reabsorption (isosmotic reabsorption) and, therefore, the site of maximal concentration of unreabsorbable solutes (such as contrast media) in tubular fluid. In salt and water depletion, proximal tubular reab-sorption is markedly enhanced; the same occurs in any other condition of renal underperfusion, such as congestive heart failure. This will prolong the transit time of the contrast medium through the nephron and increase its intratubular concentration, both effects leading to a greater nephrotoxicity. On the other hand, the osmotic activity of the contrast agent within the tubular lumen will initially limit water reabsorption and subsequently (through a decrease of sodium concentration in the tubular fluid) sodium reabsorption, leading to salt and water diuresis (osmotic diuresis); this diuretic effect is less marked when effective blood volume is reduced [182].

It is therefore advisable to avoid the use of diuretics and preparation of patients by cleansing enemas and to correct any volume depletion prior to radiographic procedures.

10.2.1.6 MULTIPLE MYELOMA. It is commonly known that multiple myeloma represents a predisposing factor to ARF following radiographic procedures. The pathogenetic mechanism of this ARF, however, seems to be different than that usually observed in contrast nephropathy. The impairment of renal function is, in fact, due to tubular obstruction by protein casts that are formed by precipitation of abnormal proteins by the contrast agent. It is therefore predictable that dehydration or salt and water depletion will facilitate this mechanism.

With the use of diatrizoate and its isomers, the incidence of ARF following radiocontrast procedures in patients with multiple myeloma has greatly decreased; this is probably due to a decreased protein binding of these contrast media compared to the older ones [184]. Thus, in a review of 508 patients with multiple myeloma exposed to contrast media, only five patients exhibited ARF [181] and at least two of them had pre-existing impairment of renal function [197]. It seems, therefore, that the coexistence of CRF, multiple myeloma, and salt and water depletion or dehydration will increase the risk of ARF [184, 197].

10.2.1.7 MARKED PROTEINURIA. Apparently, marked proteinuria is not, by itself, a predisposing factor, but it may become so when associated with other predisposing conditions.

Thus, in patients with CRF who developed radiocontrast nephrotoxicity, proteinuria was greater than in those who did not exhibit ARF following IVP [198, 199]. On the other hand, it has been shown that both serum albumin and urographic contrast agents decrease the solubility of Tamm-Horsfall mucoprotein in the urine (see below); it is conceivable that their effects are cumulative.

10.2.1.8 ADVANCED AGE. Nephrotoxicity of contrast media has been stated to be greater in advanced age. It has been shown, in fact, that most of the cases of contrast-induced ARF reported in the literature occurred in patients between 50 and 80 years of age; this relationship to age, however, seems to reflect the incidence of radiographic procedures [181]. On the other hand, in the older population, underlying vascular disease and reduction in renal mass may predispose to renal damage by radiocontrast media [200].

10.2.1.9 DOSAGE OF THE CONTRAST AGENT. Nephrotoxicity seems to be favored by large and repeated doses of contrast agents [185, 193], even though (a) some authors have not observed any correlation between dosage and incidence or severity of contrast nephropathy [200, 201]; (b) the dosage of the contrast agent used for performing angiography in patients who then developed ARF ranged from 30 to 146 g iodine (i.e., 12 to 42 g iodine/hour) [202]; and (c) in a recent review of the literature, ARF has been observed to occur frequently after doses of media in common use [181].

It has been therefore suggested that the lowest possible dose should be used in high-risk patients and that frequent exposure to contrast procedures over a short period of time should be avoided in order to prevent cumulative effects [184, 185].

It must be mentioned, however, that dosage apart, site (e.g., peripheral vein or renal artery) and rate of injection (e.g., bolus or continuous infusion) may vary the dilution of contrast media in the blood perfusing the kidney [181]. Thus, should a rapid achievement of very high plasma concentration of contrast media be the crucial point for nephrotoxicity, ARF would be expected to occur more frequently following arteriography than after IVP [181]. From the clinical data, however, this does not seem to be the case. Thus, in a recent prospective study of 378 hospitalized patients undergoing nonrenal angiography (cases of renal angiography were excluded to avoid the influence of underlying renal disease), no influence of the site of injection was observed on the incidence of ARF [189].

It seems that no difference in toxicity exists between diatrizoate, iothalamate, metrizoate, and ioxithalamate and between sodium and meglumine salts [181].

10.2.2 *Renal histopathology* With the exception of the form occurring in multiple myeloma (in which tubular casts have been observed), very little is known concerning the renal histopathology of contrast-induced ARF. In a retrospective study in which renal biopsy was performed in 211 patients wtihin 10 days of IVP or renal arteriography employing diatrizoate, iothalamate, or ioxithalamate, tubular lesions of "osmotic nephrosis" (vacuolization of cytoplasm in tubular epithelium), limited to the proximal convoluted tubules, were observed in 47 renal specimens (incidence of 22%) [203]. "Osmotic nephrosis" was more frequent in patients with impaired renal functions, with a positive correlation between the amount of injected iodine, the severity of renal failure, and the extent of epithelial "osmotic" lesion [203]. Even six anuric ARF patients exhibited diffuse or focal "osmotic nephrosis." Most of the cases with this lesion have been biopsied less than four days after contrast injection, while "osmotic nephrosis" was never observed in 514 patients who underwent renal biopsy more than 10 days after the radiographic procedure [203]. In 27 out of 47 renal specimens, partial and/or focal tubular necrosis or atrophy was observed [203].

It is difficult to understand the possible consequences of this "osmotic" lesion. Osmotic swelling of cytoplasm of the tubular cells in proximal convoluted tubules cannot cause anuria through mechanical tubular obstruction since "osmotic nephrosis" was also observed in patients whose renal function was preserved intact [203]. On the other hand in another study in which renal biopsy was performed, in two patients with contrast-induced ARF, one and 14 days after IVP, structural changes of ATN were reported [186].

Thus, the morphologic basis of contrast-induced ARF is still not known [181].

10.2.3   Clinical Features and Outcome

10.2.3.1 OLIGURIC ARF.   In a recent review of the literature on the reports of ARF secondary to contrast media, the most common clinical feature of nephrotoxicity was an oligo-anuric ARF (200 cases), with a severe fall in urine output occurring usually within 24 hours after the radiographic procedure without significant associated symptoms [181]. The decrease of GFR was mirrored by the rise in serum creatinine, which reached a peak most frequently on the third day (but in some cases even on the seventh to eighth day) after the administration of contrast media [181]. The outcome of these cases of oliguric ARF was (a) complete recovery of renal function (with serum creatinine not more than 44 μmol/1, 0.5 mg/dl, greater than control), 66% of the 200 cases; (b) recovery but with partial permanent impairment of renal function (serum creatinine more than 44 μmol/l, 0.5 mg/dl, greater then control), 13%; and (c) death or RDT or transplantation, 21% [181]. There appeared to be the same degree of renal impairment with nonrenal angiography as with IVP [181].

Complete or partial recovery of renal function usually occurs within one to two weeks [185, 186].

10.2.3.2 NONOLIGURIC ARF.   Nonoliguric ARF has also been reported, even though less frequently than the oliguric form (with a relation of 1 to 6) [181]. The outcome of this nonoliguric form was similar to that observed in the oliguric ARF, with incidence of 67%, 10%, and 23%, respectively, for complete recovery; partial recovery; and permanent dialysis or transplantation, or death [181].

10.2.3.3 HYPERSENSITIVITY REACTION TO CONTRAST MEDIA.   An anaphylactic reaction is the most severe and unpredictable complication of the use of radiocontrast agents. It may occur with and without severe hypotension, and it may cause ARF by itself or as the consequence of the severe fall in blood pressure and in renal perfusion [181].

The sensitivity reaction may vary in type and severity, extending from nausea, vomiting, "hot flush," maculopapular rash with eosinophilia [204–206], to severe respiratory, neurologic, and cardiovascular disturbances that may be fatal [206]. Symptoms usually begin one to three minutes after the start of injection and are complete within the first ten minutes. Among the severe reactions, grand mal epileptic seizures, angioneurotic edema, asthma, and laryngeal edema have been reported [205, 206]. The most frequent reactions, however, are cardiovascular: hypotension with erythematous rash, bradycardia, or arrhythmia; the patient may be in shock, unconscious, with relaxation of tongue, and laryngeal muscles; this may cause airway obstruction, anoxia, and cardiac arrest [206].

Fortunately, these severe reactions are rare (from 1/1,100 to 1/14,000 in different statistical studies). Mortality from IVP is exceptional (from 1/40,000 to 1/116,000 in different statistical surveys) [205, 206].

Occasionally, serum antibodies against the contrast medium (iothalamate) [207] and reversible nephrotic syndrome with proliferative glomerulonephritis on renal biopsy, maculopapular rash, and eosinophilia [204, 208] have been reported.

When ARF occurs, it is usually reversible even though proteinuria may last for a long time. Transient or even massive proteinuria may sometimes be observed following IVP or renal angiography; it should be noted, however, that urinary acidification may cause visible precipitation, which may give false positive results for any test for urinary protein that requires acidification [181].

A higher incidence of reactions to radiocontrast agents has been observed in patients with a history of clinical hypersensitivity (e.g., asthma, allergic conditions, etc.) [206]. It is interesting to note, however, that patients who have experienced a reaction to a contrast agent do not necessarily exhibit clinically important reactions on reinjection of the same agent for re-examination [206]. It is advisable whenever re-examination becomes necessary, however, to pretreat with corticosteroids and antihistamines those patients who have a history of severe reactions [206].

Unfortunately, sensitivity tests to identify those patients who may exhibit reactions to contrast agents have completely failed; hence intradermal, subcutaneous, ocular, sublingual, or intravenous tests are completely useless [205, 206].

10.2.3.4 ALLOGRAFT REJECTION. There is some evidence that following renal transplantation radiocontrast media may increase the incidence of allograft rejection [209].

10.2.4 *Diagnosis* Contrast-induced ARF is frequently asymptomatic and may go unrecognized, especially in its nonoliguric form, unless renal function is carefully evaluated following radiographic procedures. Thus, in patients at risk, especially in those with pre-existing renal insufficiency, it is advisable to measure serum creatinine 24 and 48 hours after contrast infusion [189] and to examine a radiographic abdominal flat plate, in order to detect persistence of nephrographic contrast material 24 hours after the radiographic procedure. It has been demonstrated, in fact, that a dense, late (24-hour) nephrogram (following an early normal excretory pyelogram) is the most sensitive index of contrast nephropathy [189, 210]. It is undoubtedly an inaccurate test by itself since the false-positive rate is high (76%); but false negatives have not been observed [189].

BUN also increases, in contrast-induced ARF, although its increment (2.86 mmol/l, 8 mg/dl, per 88.4 μmol/l, 1mg/dl, of creatinine) is less than usual [181].

Careful examination of urine sediment may help in recognizing contrast nephropathy, especially when a rise in serum creatinine is present, but less than 88.4 μmol/l (1 mg/dl, the increment commonly used to recognize a significant impairment of renal function). A point system for an ARF index based on urinary sediment has been recently defined [189]: detection of white blood cells in urine sediment represent 1 point; isolated renal tubular cells or hyaline casts or granular casts, 2 points; casts

of renal tubular cells, 3 points; and dark, coarsely granular casts, 4 points. This ARF index is positive when, after the exposure to radiocontrast media, an increment of at least five points is observed above the baseline (obtained prior to the radiographic test); it is borderline with increments of 3 to 4 points [189].

In the oliguric form, oliguria occurs within 24 to 48 hours persisting, usually for two to three days [186] (sometimes up to five days) despite treatment with loop diuretics or volume expansion, so that dialysis may be required (in about 25% of the cases).

Urinary concentration of sodium (U_{Na}) has been reported usually to be low, with values less than 30 mmol/l [186, 196, 211]. In a recent report on 12 consecutive patients with oliguric radiocontrast-induced ARF, U_{Na} values ranged from 1 to 17 mmol/l, with a mean of 7.5 mmol/l [212].

The fractional excretion of sodium (FE_{Na}) is also low, consistently less than 1%; it ranged from 0.03 to 0.9% in the above report on 12 cases of oliguric contrast-induced ARF [212]; FE_{Na} remains low throughout the oliguric phase of ARF [212]. In patients with CRF who were hydrated with i.v. saline solution in the 12 to 16 hours preceding the IVP, FE_{Na} was high (greater than 1%) prior to the radiographic procedure and increased significantly only in those patients exhibiting ARF [199, 201].

Urinary osmolality has been reported to range from 350 to 400 mOsm/Kg water, with a mean value of 350 mOsm/Kg water (n = 12 patients) [212].

The urine-to-plasma–creatinine ratio (U/P Cr) has been reported to range from 6 to 42 [212]. When hydration with i.v. saline was performed in patients with CRF prior to IVP, U/P Cr decreased only in those cases exhibiting ARF [199].

10.2.5 *Pathogenesis* The following mechanisms have been suggested as responsible for contrast-induced ARF.

10.2.5.1 DECREASE IN RBF. Contrast-induced ARF may be due to reduction in renal perfusion with consequent ischemic damage. Experimental studies in dogs have shown a biphasic response to the administration of contrast media into the renal artery: an initial transient renal vasodilation with a rise in RBF is followed by a prolonged renal vasoconstriction with decrease in RBF [200, 213, 214]. This vasoconstriction appears to occur only in the kidney [200] and has been attributed to ECV depletion resulting from diuresis and natriuresis secondary to osmotic load and, possibly, to a direct depressive effect of contrast media on active sodium transport [200, 215]. Thus, while some authors have observed similar transient changes in RBF and GFR following i.v. injection of either diatrizoate or osmotically similar mannitol-containing solution [214], others have demonstrated that the natriuretic effect of contrast media is greater than that of equiosmolar loads of mannitol [216] and that diuresis by contrast agents occurs within three minutes of their i.v. injection [217].

When ECV depletion was prevented by replacement of urine volume, vasoconstriction did not occur [92].

Renal vasoconstriction may be enhanced by salt depletion and the resulting renal ischemia may be prolonged and intensified in patients with pre-existent renal impairment.

Newer contrast media, such as iopamidolo (Iopamiro®) with an osmolality (400–800 mOsm/Kg water) much lower than that of commonly used agents (approximately 1500 mOsm/Kg water) are expected to cause less hemodynamic changes [200].

It should be noted, however, that other factors, such as erythrocyte aggregation and increase in blood viscosity, induced by contrast media, may contribute to the fall in RBF.

In favor of the "prerenal" nature (i.e., reduced renal perfusion) of radiocontrast-induced ARF appear the low values of both urinary concentration of sodium and FE_{Na}.

Two observations, however, argue against an ischemic mechanism: (a) the early excretory pyelogram is normal, and the initial normal opacification of pelvis, ureter, and bladder suggests that glomerular filtration is initially preserved; and (b) acute, severe hypotension during radiographic procedures utilizing contrast agents was, in many occasions, not followed by ARF [181].

10.2.5.2 TUBULAR OBSTRUCTION. If the decrease in RBF represents the initiating factor, tubular obstruction may account for the maintenance phase of contrast-induced ARF.

Tubular obstruction may result from (a) precipitation of contrast agents, (b) precipitation of other urinary solutes, or (c) interaction between contrast media and some components of the urine [181].

Precipitation of contrast media. Since modern contrast media (i.e., the salts of triiodinated derivatives of benzoic acid) are extremely soluble, it is unlikely for their solubility limits to be exceeded even after severe dehydration or salt depletion [181].

Precipitation of other urinary solutes. Tubular obstruction may be due to uric acid crystals. Radiocontrast media, in fact, have been shown to have a uricosuric effect. This effect, particularly evident also with cholecystographic agents [218, 219] results from an enhanced tubular secretion of uric acid. The increased uric acid excretion coupled with the maximal urine concentration (resulting from volume depletion secondary to osmotic diuresis) will greatly increase intratubular concentration of uric acid and cause precipitation of uric acid crystals in collecting ducts [219]. If this mechanism is operative, hyperuricemia is expected to favor contrast-induced ARF and to worsen its prognosis. Renal biopsy findings consistent with acute urate nephropathy have been reported in a patient with CRF and hyperuricemia following IVP [184]. But when plasma uric acid before the radiographic procedure was evaluated in relation to the urine output and the outcome of ARF due to contrast agents, no correlation was observed [181]. Intraluminal precipitation of oxalate has also been implicated as a possible cause of tubular obstruction in patients with pre-existing renal insufficiency undergoing angiographic procedures; urinary excretion of oxalate, in fact, was found clearly increased after angiography with diatrizoate in 14 patients [220]. The increase in oxalate excretion (from 29 to 44 mg/24 hours) was, however, too low to represent the sole cause of ARF [184].

Interaction between contrast media and some components of the urine. It has been stated that interaction between contrast media and Tamm-

Horsfall mucoprotein may cause tubular obstruction [181]. Tamm-Horsfall protein is a normal component of the urine and a major constituent of urinary casts; synthesized and secreted by the cells of the ascending limb of the loop of Henle and early distal tubule, this mucoprotein may be normally detected within these tubular cells as well as in the lumen of the tubule; its excretion is increased following acute renal lesions when the protein may be detected also in the renal interstitium [181]. Tamm-Horsfall mucoprotein becomes less soluble in the presence of urine with low pH, or high salt concentration, or serum albumin, or Bence-Jones protein. Its solubility is also decreased by urographic contrast agents [181, 221]. Since an increased urinary excretion of Tamm-Horsfall protein has been reported during the recovery phase of contrast-induced ARF [210], it has been suggested that urographic contrast agents cause precipitation of Tamm-Horsfall protein, formation of luminal casts, and, consequently, tubular obstruction [210, 221]. It is interesting to note that, in recent prospective studies on the incidence of contrast-induced ARF in patients with CRF, proteinuria was greater in those patients who developed ARF compared to patients "protected" by mannitol or diuretics [198, 199]. It is possible that serum albumin and urographic contrast agents have cumulative effects in decreasing the solubility of Tamm-Horsfall mucoprotein in the urine.

10.2.5.3 DIRECT TOXICITY OF CONTRAST MEDIA ON TUBULAR EPITHELIAL CELLS. The occurrence of enzymuria following the use of radiocontrast agents [222] has suggested a direct toxic effect on tubular epithelium. But the tubular damage responsible for the enzymuria may result from the hypertonicity of contrast media. Enzymuria was, in fact, observed not only after iodinated agents, but also following i.v. infusion of noniodinated hypertonic solutions [223]. On the other hand, as already mentioned, renal biopsies in human subjects, performed within 10 days of radiocontrast procedures, have frequently exhibited a vacuolization of proximal tubular cell cytoplasm [203]. Furthermore, when diatrizoate and iothalamate salts and equiosmolar control solutions were tested "in vitro," in isolated toad bladders, a depression of sodium transport was detected with all hypertonic solutions [215].

A direct toxic effect due to triiodinated contrast molecules and unrelated to hypertonicity has also been suggested as contributing to epithelial damage [200].

10.2.6 Treatment There is no effective therapy for contrast-induced ARF. Neither hypertonic mannitol nor furosemide, in fact, have demonstrated any effect in helping recovery when ARF occurred in patients with CRF after IVP [199]. Clinical management of patients with contrast nephropathy is similar to that of any "organic" ARF.

10.3 ARF FOLLOWING BILATERAL RETROGRADE PYELOGRAPHY
ARF has also been reported after bilateral retrograde pyelography [224, 225]. The resulting anuria may be due either to ureteral edema causing obstructive uropathy [225] (in this case ureteral recatheterization will restore urine flow) or to intrarenal obstructive nephropathy [224]. The latter condition has been accounted for by a pyelorenal backflow of contrast medium for which there has been clear radiological evidence; in this case the reinsertion of urethral catheters did not result in the return of urine flow [224].

10.4 ARF DUE TO CHOLECYSTOGRAPHIC AND CHOLANGIOGRAPHIC AGENTS
ARF has been reported in several occasions following a single dose [226], but, more frequently, multiple doses of oral cholecystographic agents, namely, sodium bunamiodyl (Orabilex®) [227–231] and, more recently, iopanoic acid (Telepaque®, Cistobil®) [232, 233]. ARF has also been associated with the use of meglumine iodipamide (Cholografin®) for intravenous cholangiography [233]. The patients who developed this type of ARF usually had clinical and/or laboratory evidence of biliary tract or hepatocellular disease. Some of them also had renal impairment [232], but in others renal function was normal [231, 233].

The triiodinated aromatic nucleus of oral cholecystographic media has been considered responsible for renal toxicity; since aromatic compounds are usually excreted by hepatic conjugation, reduced clearance due to liver disease may expose the kidneys to a large load of these nephrotoxic media [233].

The uricosuric effect of iopanoic acid (Telepaque®, Cistobil®) (which is the most potent uricosuric agent, comparable in magnitude to that of probenecid) [226] and meglumine iodipamide (Cholografin®) has suggested the possibility of acute urate nephropathy [218, 219], which may be favored by hyperuricemia and dehydration [233]. Urinalysis with massive amounts of amorphous urates that dissolved immediately upon alkalinization of the urine have been reported in some cases [226]. The uricosuric effect of cholecystographic agents, however, has been shown to increase the ratio of urinary uric acid/creatinine concentration, but this ratio never exceeded 0.90 [218]. Since in acute urate nephropathy this ratio is greater than 1 [234], ARF following radiocontrast procedures cannot be regarded as acute urate nephropathy [200].

Tubular obstruction by calcium oxalate-containing crystals has also been suggested as a possible pathogenetic mechanism of ARF due to oral cholecystographic agents [227, 229].

11 Acute Renal Failure Following Anesthesia

The first observation that anesthesia may damage the kidneys goes back to the beginning of this century, when Dublin surgeons observed that ether anesthesia was followed by a fall in urine volume and a decrease in urinary excretion of nitrogenous metabolites [235]. Since then other anesthetics have been used, and nephrotoxicity has been demonstrated particularly for methoxyflurane.

Nephrotoxicity due to anesthetic agents is difficult to investigate. Unless anesthetics are tested in normal volunteers, in fact, it is not easy to separate the effects of anesthesia itself from those of surgery, other drugs given simultaneously or subsequently, and other conditions, such as hypotension, hypovolemia, and disturbances of pulmonary gas exchange [235].

Furthermore, the evaluation of renal blood flow by clearance technique is not adequate since it has been well demonstrated that tubular transport of PAH is depressed by inhalational agents; this makes PAH clearance meaningless unless the renal extraction of PAH is also measured [235].

General anesthesia is based on the sequential administration of premedicants and induction and inhalational agents; all of these agents may impair renal function.

11.1 PREMEDICANTS
Morphine is the most commonly used narcotic analgesic drug. It may cause, in clinical dosage, reduction in urine output and in solute excretion, increase in urine concentration, presumably through enhanced ADH release, and a reversible fall in GFR and RBF [235]. The latter is apparently a hemodynamic effect secondary to the increased secretion of catecholamines that follows morphine administration [236].

Phenothiazines, at least in small doses, and atropine do not affect RBF and GFR in man, while there are no studies on the effect of benzodiazepines on renal function [235].

11.2 INDUCTION AGENTS
Urine volume, RBF, and GFR usually show a transient fall after barbiturate induction of anesthesia as a result of the hemodynamic effects of barbiturates (impairment of myocardial contractility, reduction in cardiac output, hypotension). Similar minor and transient disturbances of renal function are expected after althesin and propanidid and have been demonstrated after neuroleptanesthesia (e.g., with fentanyl + droperidol, 50:1 [235].

11.3 INHALATIONAL ANESTHETIC AGENTS
Today, anesthesia is usually maintained by fluorinated inhalational anesthetic agents. These agents (methoxyflurane, in particular) have been implicated as responsible for many cases of ARF following surgery.

11.3.1 Methoxyflurane In 1964, Paddock et al. [237] reported three cases of reversible ARF secondary to methoxyflurane anesthesia. In 1966, Crandell et al. [238] described a toxic nephropathy in 16 out of 94 patients who received methoxyflurane during its first year of use. Many other retrospective reports then followed attributing postoperative impairment of renal function to this fluorinated anesthetic agent.

The first prospective study was that of Mazze et al. [239], who compared the renal function of 12 patients anesthetized with methoxyflurane with that of 10 patients receiving halothane. Methoxyflurane caused an increase in serum concentration of creatinine, blood urea nitrogen, and uric acid; polyuria; and prolonged reduction in renal concentrating ability unresponsive to vasopressin injection.

The ARF due to methoxyflurane is usually of nonoliguric type. It was polyuric in 74 out of 104 cases reviewed by Churchill et al. [240], while in six cases the urine output was normal; only in 10 cases ARF was oliguric; in the remaining 14 it was uncertain.

The degree of renal dysfunction has been correlated to the dose of anesthetic administered [241, 242] and to the serum level of inorganic fluoride reached after methoxyflurane anesthesia [243].

In most cases ARF was reversible, but some patients failed to recover normal renal function [238, 240, 244].

11.3.1.1 PATHOPHYSIOLOGY OF METHOXYFLURANE-INDUCED ARF. Methoxyflurane is metabolized to inorganic fluoride and oxalic acid [245, 246]. Both metabolites have been implicated in the nephrotoxicity of methoxyflurane [240, 241, 247].

Both serum concentration and urinary excretion of inorganic fluoride have been reported to be significantly increased after methoxyflurane anesthesia [241, 245, 246]. The vasopressin-resistant concentrating defect observed in man following methoxyflurane has been attributed to its fluoride metabolite [240, 241], since inorganic fluoride has been demonstrated to cause vasopressin-resistant polyuria [248], presumably through inhibition of the adenyl cyclase enzyme [246]. But being an inhibitor of anerobic metabolism, fluoride may also impair the concentration mechanism of urine by inhibiting sodium chloride reabsorption in the ascending limb of the loop of Henle [240, 249]. It seems that renal toxicity by methoxyflurane (in

the form of polyuria unresponsive to vasopressin and an increase in serum uric acid) occurs when peak serum inorganic fluoride levels exceed 50 μmol/liter [240, 242, 243, 250]. Severe clinical toxicity usually occurs with more than 5 MAC-h exposure (serum fluoride above 90 μmol/liter) (see note 1 on page 104) [235, 242].

Urinary excretion of oxalate is also significantly increased following anesthesia with methoxyflurane, especially in those cases exhibiting nephrotoxicity [246]. The high urinary excretion of oxalate and the extensive deposition of oxalate crystals in the renal tissue in cases of methoxyflurane-induced ARF have focused attention on oxalic acid as the nephrotoxic metabolite of methoxyflurane [240], although it is quite possible that it represents a secondary phenomenon since oxalate nephropathy is usually associated with oliguria and not with polyuria [251]. Oxalate crystals, in fact, may be observed occasionally in the kidney in any form of ARF with prolonged oliguria [252]; the number of these crystals, however, is much greater after methoxyflurane anesthesia [253] when deposition of oxalate crystals has also been observed in lungs and meninges [244]. This may be due to an increased oxalate load following methoxyflurane. The chronic interstitial fibrosis observed as a long-term result of methoxyflurane-induced ARF has been attributed to a reaction to the oxalate crystals [240, 244] although it has also been observed after long-term fluoride ingestion [240].

The controversy as to whether inorganic fluoride or oxalate was the nephrotoxic metabolite of methoxyflurane seemed to be solved by Cousins et al. [247]. These authors observed that rats receiving fluoride to such an extent as to reach a serum concentration similar to that obtained with methoxyflurane exhibited polyuric nephrotoxicity, while rats receiving oxalic acid did not show any renal damage.

11.3.1.2 PATHOLOGY OF METHOXYFLURANE-INDUCED ARF. The renal lesions in methoxyflurane-induced ARF, as observed by light and electron microscopy, include [240, 241] tubular epithelial cell degeneration, ranging from swelling to frank necrosis mainly in the proximal tubules [241]; deposition of birefringent crystals of calcium oxalate in the tubular lumina (mainly in the cortical tubules), and also, occasionally, within the epithelial cells and in the interstitium [240, 244, 253]; tubular dilatation; and interstitial edema [240]. Glomeruli are normal.

11.3.1.3 PREDISPOSING FACTORS TO METHOXYFLURANE-INDUCED ARF.

a. A large total dose of the anesthetic, dependent on the depth and duration of anesthesia, will undoubtedly favor ARF [240]. Mild nephrotoxicity has been observed with the MAC-hour value exceeding 2.5, more severe toxicity with 5.0 MAC-hours.

b. Methoxyflurane nephrotoxicity seemed to be potentiated by some antibiotics such as tetracycline [238, 254–256], penicillins [253], and gentamicin [108, 240, 257] given either preoperatively or postoperatively. It should be borne in mind that gentamicin interferes with urinary excretion of inorganic fluoride [257] and that methoxyflurane may persist in fat deposits for as long as one week [108]. Thus, the additive nephrotoxic effects of methoxyflurane and gentamicin may occur several days after the anesthesia, especially in obese patients (see below).

c. Obesity is undoubtedly a predisposing factor, the adipose tissue functioning as a reservoir of methoxyflurane. This is, in fact, a highly lipid-soluble anesthetic agent with very high oil-water solubility, which is around 970 (i.e., the agent is 970 times as soluble in oil as in water); this lipid solubility makes methoxyflurane the most potent inhalational agent [235, 255]. But its high water-gas solubility (13 at 37°C) is responsible for slow induction and recovery from anesthesia [235].

d. Long-term treatment with barbiturate or tolbutamide has been suggested predisposing to methoxyflurane nephrotoxicity [240]. There is experimental evidence that long-term phenobarbital treatment significantly enhances defluorination of methoxyflurane [258].

e. Methoxyflurane nephrotoxicity seems to be intensified by hydropenia, presumably through a reduction in inorganic fluoride renal clearance [235].

11.3.2 *Enflurane* Enflurane is a fluorinated methylethyl ether, chemically more stable than methoxyflurane [259]; furthermore, because its fat solubility is lower, the substrate pool for post-anesthetic metabolism is smaller [250]. Thus, although enflurane is also metabolized to inorganic fluoride, nephrotoxic serum levels of this metabolite are not usually reached [260].

Mazze et al. [261] have observed a peak serum level of 33.6 μmol/liter of inorganic fluoride in healthy volunteers after prolonged enflurane anesthesia (9.6 MAC-h). Järnberg et al. [262] found a mean maximal plasma fluoride level of 17.4 μmol/liter two hours after the end of enflurane anesthesia in seven women undergoing histerectomy. Only occasionally were high peak values of fluoride observed following enflurane: 52 μmol/liter in one obese patient and 106 μmol/liter in another patient receiving multiple medication [263]. It is, however, a common observation that ARF does not occur in patients with normal renal function following enflurane anesthesia [243, 264] although slight decreases in RBF, GFR, and urine flow and fractional excretion of sodium were observed during anesthesia [243, 265] as described also for halothane and isoflurane [266]. Even prolonged (eight hours) and repeated (twice at seven-day intervals), anesthesia with enflurane has not caused renal damage in dogs as observed by light and electron microscopy [250].

There are three reports of ARF following enflurane anesthesia, but all the patients had pre-existing renal disease. Thus, Eichhorn et al. [267] reported a case of anuric ARF occurring two days after six-hour enflurane anesthesia in a 66-year-old man; peak value of serum inorganic fluoride was 93 μmol/liter on the second postanesthetic day (the true peak might have been even higher soon after the anesthesia). Loehning et al. [268] have also reported a polyuric form of ARF following enflurane in a patient with a failing transplanted kidney with acute damage of proximal tubules on renal biopsy (in addition to the typical changes of chronic allograft rejection). Finally, Hartnett et al. [269] described a case of transient polyuria with renal function impairment, although serum fluoride was not measured.

It is possible that a diseased kidney may have a lower urinary excretion of inorganic fluoride allowing the occurrence of high, toxic serum levels of fluoride that do not occur in normal subjects. It has also been postulated that the threshold for fluoride-induced nephrotoxicity is lower in the diseased kidney so that ARF occurs even with normal serum levels of inorganic fluoride [268].

Fluoride kinetic studies in man have shown that fractional fluoride excretion is decreased during enflurane anesthesia and that, in the postanesthetic period, tubular reabsorption of fluoride is inversely related to tubular fluid pH; it has been therefore suggested that alkalinization of urine may increase fluoride excretion and protect from enflurane nephrotoxicity [265]. According to Schiffl and Binswanger [270], on the other hand, fractional excretion of fluoride positively correlates with water excretion while urine pH has no effect.

Since enflurane like methoxyflurane, is metabolized to oxalic acid and inorganic fluoride [243], deposition of oxalate crystals in the kidneys has been predicted after enflurane anesthesia. Wickstrom and Stefansson [250], however, did not observe any increase in urinary oxalate excretion, nor deposition of oxalic acid crystals in renal tissues of dogs after prolonged enflurane anesthesia; thus the authors have suggested that enflurane is not completely defluorinated to oxalic acid [250].

It may be concluded that enflurane is a safe anesthetic. Care must be taken during long anesthesia, especially in obese patients, in those receiving multiple medication, and in patients with pre-existing renal disease [235].

11.3.3 Isoflurane

Apparently, isoflurane is better than enflurane [271]. It has been recently released for general use in the United States and in Canada.

Isoflurane is the structural isomer of enflurane, therefore belonging to the fluorinated methyl-ethyl ethers. Its original synthesis occurred in 1965, but it was not used for many years because of suspected carcinogenic potential; this was then completely excluded.

Isoflurane is similar to enflurane, but with lower solubility in blood and tissues and lower susceptibility to biodegradation; thus, uptake, distribution, and elimination are fast and the onset and recovery from anesthesia very rapid [271].

Following 3 MAC-h isoflurane anesthesia, serum fluoride levels never exceeded 5.5 μmol/liter, being comparable to those following halothane, much less than those found after methoxyflurane, and even enflurane anesthesia [266].

Mazze et al. [266] have reported a mean peak of serum inorganic fluoride of 4.4 μmol/liter six hours after isoflurane anesthesia in nine surgical patients. Intra-anesthetic fall of RBF, GFR, and urine flow was similar during isoflurane (nine patients) and during halothane anesthesia (in six control surgical patients); but in both groups postanesthetic renal function, including the response to vasopressin, was completely normal [266].

11.3.4 Halothane

Halothane is the most widely used volatile anesthetic agent. There are no reports on renal damage after prolonged halothane anesthesia.

Furthermore, halothane is a lipid-soluble agent, but its oil-water partition coefficient is 330, i.e., much less than that of methoxyflurane. Halothane is not metabolized to inorganic fluoride to such an extent as to reach toxic serum levels of this metabolite [247, 272]; the maximal mean concentration achieved in man following halothane anesthesia is around 20 μmol/liter [263, 265].

Prolonged (eight hours) and repeated (twice at seven-day intervals) anesthesia with halothane has not caused any renal damage in dogs even on electron microscopic study [250]. The intra-anesthetic slight fall of RBF, GFR, and urine flow are followed by complete normalization of renal function, including response to vasopressin, in the postanesthetic period [266].

11.3.5 Effect of Ventilation on Renal Function

Very frequently, patients treated by intermittent positive pressure ventilation retain sodium and water by a mechanism still not elucidated. Hemodynamic changes, presumably related to the decreased venous return with a consequent reduction in cardiac output, seem to account for this phenomenon, which may cause pulmonary edema.

Hypocapnia may contribute to the salt and water retention in hyperventilated patients, while hypoxia may result in renal vasoconstriction (secondary to sympathetic stimulation) and fall in GFR [235].

12 ARF Secondary to Ethylene Glycol Intoxication

Acute ethylene glycol intoxication is an unfrequent but quite severe condition that may cause ARF. The ingestion of the poison may occur by error or by humans attempting suicide.

Ethylene glycol is an odorless, colorless liquid commonly used in many commercial products, including, for instance, radiator antifreeze.

12.1 CLINICAL OUTCOME OF ETHYLENE GLYCOL INTOXICATION

When ingested in large amounts (more than 1.4 ml/kg b.w.), it will cause a severe acute poisoning due to its rapid conversion, in the liver and in the kidneys, to toxic metabolites: aldehydes (which inhibit glycolysis and Kreb's cycle), lactic acid (which causes severe metabolic acidosis), and oxalate (which causes calcium oxalate crystallization in many organs) [273].

The clinical outcome of this poisoning has been divided into three stages [274]. The stage 1 or neurologic stage, occurs 30 minutes to 12 hours after the ingestion and is characterized by neurologic symptoms: the patient is inebriated (but without alcohol odor on breath); ophthalmoplegia, nystagmus, papilledema, seizures, and depressed reflexes may all occur and may be followed by coma. If the patient survives, a stage 2 or cardiopulmonary stage, will follow, with tachicardia, tachypnea, cyanosis, and pulmonary congestion. Should the patient survive this severe cardiopulmonary derangement, he enters the stage 3 or renal stage, in which flank pain and oliguric ARF may occur.

12.2 RENAL INJURY BY ETHYLENE GLYCOL

Calcium oxalate crystallization occurs in many organs, but mainly in the kidneys [275, 276] so that the observation of oxalate crystals in the urinary sediment is of great diagnostic value.

ARF may result from intratubular precipitation of calcium oxalate or from toxic tubular damage by metabolites such as glycolic acid, glyoxylic acid, and glycoaldehyde; renal lesions include dilation of proximal tubules, degeneration of tubular epithelium, and deposition of oxalate crystals in the cells and in tubular lumina [273, 274].

12.3 CLINICAL DIAGNOSIS OF ETHYLENE GLYCOL POISONING

In acute ethylene glycol poisoning, a marked anion gap (sodium glycolate replacing sodium bicarbonate) metabolic acidosis occurs, associated with a clear increase in delta osmolality. Delta osmolality is the difference between the measured and the calculated plasma osmolality (calculated as $P_{Osm} = 2 ([Na^+] + [K^+]) +$ BUN (mg/dl)/2.8 + blood glucose (mg/dl)/18), which does not usually exceed 5 mOsm/kg water [277]. When plasma delta osmolality is greater than 5 mOsm/kg water, a solute other than urea, glucose, sodium, and potassium and their anions is present in the circulating plasma; in ethylene glycol poisoning this solute is either ethylene glycol itself or its metabolic products. The association of a wide plasma anion gap and a high plasma delta osmolality is typical of either methanol or ethylene glycol intoxication, but it is combined with calcium oxalate crystals in the urine only in the latter [274]. Hypocalcemia, requiring calcium therapy intravenously, and leukocytosis may also occur.

12.4 TREATMENT OF ETHYLENE GLYCOL POISONING

Since ethylene glycol is oxidized to toxic derivatives by alcohol dehydrogenase, ethyl alcohol is a competitive inhibitor of this oxidation [278, 279]. Hence, treatment of ethylene glycol intoxication is based (after gastric lavage, which is, however, of limited benefit since the poison is rapidly absorbed) on immediate oral (via nasogastric tube) load of 0.6 g of 50% ethanol/kg b.w., with an oral maintenance dose of 109 of 20% ethanol/kg b.w./hour (237 mg/kg b.w./hour during hemodialysis) [280] in order to maintain a blood level of 100–200 mg/dl of ethyl alcohol [274]. Ethyl alcohol, however, enhances the formation of lactic acid from pyruvate, making the metabolic acidosis more marked. Hence an immediate i.v. infusion of bicarbonate is also necessary (i.v. calcium infusion will prevent tetany) before and in addition to dialysis therapy.

Dialysis should be instituted promptly not only because the large amounts of sodium bicarbonate required to treat metabolic acidosis will represent a large sodium load that cannot be excreted by the patient, but also in order to prevent rather than treat ARF [281]. Hemodialysis, possibly with bicarbonate-containing dialysate [274] is more effective than peritoneal dialysis in removing ethylene glycol, oxalate, and their toxins from the body [274, 280–282]. Large doses of thiamine and pyridoxine may be useful, since these vitamins are essential in promoting the degradation of ethylene glycol to less toxic derivatives [283]. When plasma oxalate has reached very high levels, it becames almost impossible to lower it even by dialysis therapy [282]. Survival after ingestion of large amounts of ethylene glycol has been obtained when therapy was started within two hours of poison ingestion [273].

13. Acute Uric Acid Nephropathy (UAN)

Hyperuricemia and hyperuricosuria may cause renal injury by three different mechanisms: (a) deposition of sodium urate crystals in the renal interstitium thereby causing chronic urate nephropathy and leading to progressive CRF; (b) precipitation of uric acid in the urinary tract, resulting in uric acid nephrolithiasis—but the enhanced uric acid excretion will also promote calcium oxalate stone formation; and (c) deposition of uric acid in collecting ducts [284, 285] causing an intrarenal obstructive nephropathy known as acute uric acid nephropathy (UAN) [234, 286].

Impairment in renal function may "per se" cause hyperuricemia. Renal failure is, in fact, characterized by retention of waste products of nitrogen metabolism. These include uric acid, the serum concentration of which is increased with the fall of renal function, even though this hyperuricemia is blunted by the increase in uric acid clearance per residual nephron (uric acid clearance to creatinine clearance is, in

fact, increased) (see below). It is not surprising, therefore, that hyperuricemia is observed in both CRF and in ARF. There are conditions, however, in which serum uric acid is increased out or proportion of the degree of renal failure. This is quite frequent, although not constant [234] in UAN, in which hyperuricemia is regarded as the cause rather than the consequence of renal shutdown.

13.1 URIC ACID METABOLISM

Uric acid is the end-product of purine metabolism [287, 288]. The purines adenine and guanine are present in the body mainly as components of nucleic acids, ribonucleic acid (RNA), and deoxyribonucleic acid (DNA). The major source of uric acid production is the hydrolysis of endogenous nucleic acids, while less than 20% of uric acid production derives from hydrolysis of ingested nucleic acids. The enzymatic oxidation of adenine and guanine leads to inosinic acid, hypoxanthine, xanthine, and uric acid. The enzyme xanthine oxidase catalyzes the oxidation of hypoxanthine to xanthine and then of xanthine to uric acid. Xanthine oxidase is inhibited by a structural analogue of hypoxanthine, allopurinol, which reduces, therefore, the formation of uric acid.

Of the 700 mg of uric acid produced daily in man, about 500 mg (normally never more than 600 mg/24 hours) are excreted by the kidney involving glomerular filtration, tubular secretion (in proximal tubules), and tubular reabsorption (in proximal and/or distal tubules); the remainder is eliminated by intestinal uricolysis [288].

Uric acid is an organic acid with a pK of 5.75. Since urine pH may be frequently below 5.75, the solubility of uric acid in urine is low; it has been demonstrated, in fact, that it falls from 12 mmol/l (200 mg/dl) to 1.27 mmol/l (15 mg/dl) as urine pH is decreased from 7.4 to 5.0 [289]. An increase in serum levels of uric acid increases its renal excretion by raising both the filtered load and the tubular secretion. Hence hyperuricemia leads to hyperuricosuria. But hyperuricosuria may occur in the absence of hyperuricemia. Thus, ECV expansion (e.g., by saline i.v. infusion) will increase the uric acid clearance by decreasing tubular reabsorption. Conversely, hyperuricemia may result from a reduced tubular secretion or increased tubular reabsorption of uric acid. The reduced tubular secretion may occur in conditions of either retention or increased production of other organic acids that compete with uric acid for the secretory site in the kidney; this may be the case during ketoacidosis of diabetes or lactic acidosis of exercise, alcohol ingestion, or toxemia of pregnancy. Even low doses of aspirin or i.v. infusion of sodium lactate may cause hyperuricemia by inhibiting uric acid secretion [288]. An increase in tubular reabsorption of uric acid may occur in congestive heart failure, in cirrhosis, in prerenal ARF, and, typically, in long-term treatment with diuretics, particularly thiazides; in the latter condition, however, interference of diuretics with organic acid secretory mechanism has also been suggested as a contributory factor [288].

13.2 RENAL INJURY FOLLOWING HYPERURICEMIA

Hyperuricemic ARF usually occurs in patients with malignancies (in particular leukemias, lymphomas, and, less frequently, multiple myeloma and large solid tumors), that is, in conditions of massive destruction of tumor cells, being the rule during chemotherapy or radiation therapy. Thus, it may occur prior to cytolytic therapy in patients with rapidly growing solid tumors, but, more frequently, during aggressive treatment of the neoplastic disorders.

The release of great amounts of nucleoproteins and their metabolites because of cell destruction and the consequent formation of unusual amounts of uric acid causes severe hyperuricemia (values greater than 5.35 mmol/l, 90 mg/dl, have been reported), which may lead to ARF [290].

Severe hyperuricemia (which may lead to ARF) may occur in other disorders associated with increased production of uric acid (because of accelerated breakdown of tissue nucleotides) and, consequently, enhanced uric acid excretion. This is the case in primary gout (20% to 25% of gouty patients have a primary increase in uric acid production) [289], in hypercatabolic states, and in conditions of severe tissue hypoxia (such as acute myocardial infarction,

cardiomyopathy, cardiogenic or hemorrhagic shock, rhabdomyolysis) [291]. The underlying disorder responsible for the hyperuricemia, however, is not always apparent (figure 2–5).

Oliguric ARF of UAN has been attributed to massive intratubular crystallization of uric acid that has been demonstrated in the collecting ducts [284] where tubular fluid becomes very concentrated and uric acid solubility is decreased because of the acidic pH [286]. This widespread tubular obstruction by uric acid crystals results in an increase in intratubular pressure in proximal and distal tubules, dilatation of these tubular segments, and fall in GFR [284]. A decline in RBF has also been observed [286] and attributed to obstruction of the distal renal vasculature either due to urate deposits in deep cortical and medullary vessels or to compression of these vessels secondary to the increases in tubular and interstitial pressure or both [284]. But tubular obstruction undoubtedly plays the primary pathogenetic role, and dehydration, by markedly concentrating the urine, result in an oversaturated state that favors uric acid precipitation in the collecting ducts [290]. From these observations it appears evident that it is the hyperuricosuria (rather than the hyperuricemia) with the high urinary concentration of uric acid that is of primary importance in UAN; this disorder will never occur in patients with hyperuricemia due to reduced urinary excretion (such as that due to CRF or prolonged use of diuretics) [289]. As mentioned elsewhere in this chapter, the hyperuricosuria (due to enhanced tubular secretion of uric acid) that follows the use of urographic or cholecystographic agents has been invoked as playing a pathogenetic role in radiocontrast-induced ARF [218, 219].

More rarely, ARF is of postrenal type due to obstruction of the ureter by uric acid stones. In these cases, symptoms of acute obstructive uropathy may occur, such as colicky pain or back pain. It has been stated that acute obstructive uropathy occurs predominantly in those cases exhibiting gradual onset of hyperuricemia, while intrarenal obstructive nephropathy is typical of a sharp rise in serum uric acid [290]. The obstructive uropathy may be demonstrated by ultrasonography, high-dose IVP, or gamma

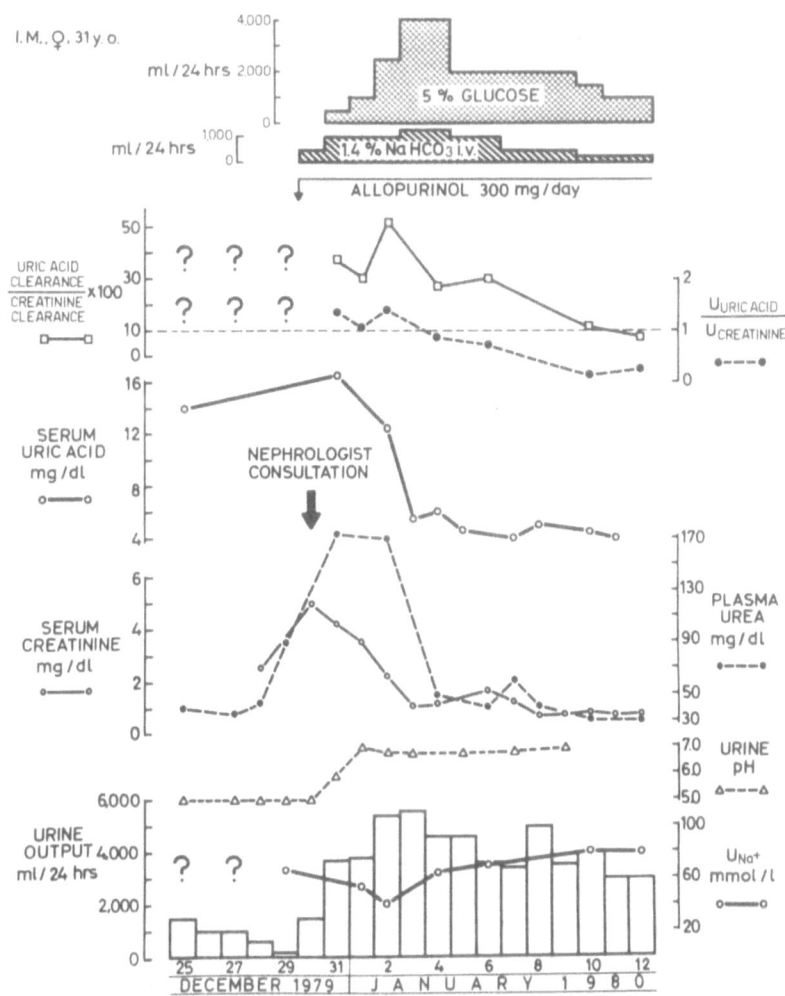

FIGURE 2-5. Acute uric acid nephropathy. A pregnant woman (28th week of gestation) with a history of stones in the right kidney, was admitted to the hospital because of lumbar pain. Oligo-anuria occurred with acidic urine (Ph = 5). Ultrasonography of both kidneys was negative for renal stones or pyelocalyceal dilation. Adequate hydration, alkalinization by NaHCO₃ infusion, and allopurinol normalized urine output and renal function. Two months later, a healthy girl was born. After delivery, IVP did not show renal stones. (Reprinted with permission from Andreucci VE and Dal Canton A, Proc EDTA 17: 123–132, 1980.)

camera renography (see chapter 19). It is, however, possible for the two conditions (obstructive nephropathy and uropathy) to coexist in the same patient, both contributing to renal shutdown.

In some patients with malignancies, the severe hyperuricemia that follows antineoplastic treatment is associated with an extremely high serum concentration of phosphorus that is out of proportion to the degree of renal failure [290]. This hyperphosphatemia has been attributed to a release of intracellular phosphorus because of the extensive cell destruction. The practical consequence is the danger of metastatic calcification, which may be prevented by aluminum hydroxide administration prior to the onset of chemotherapy [290]. As mentioned in this chapter, in some patients with acute lymphoblastic leukemia whose serum uric acid was kept normal by pretreatment with allopurinol, ARF that followed cytolytic therapy was attributed to acute nephrocalcinosis due to the massive phosphate release [292, 293].

13.3 CLINICAL COURSE OF UAN

Usually, the patient experiences an abrupt onset of oliguria or even anuria without any symptom or, on occasion, just a flank pain that may be due to associated ureteral obstruction. Many patients with nephrolithiasis, however, may have no symptoms at all. Serum creatinine and BUN increase, but frequently there is a disproportional increase in serum uric acid that usually exceeds 0.89 mmol/l (15 mg/dl), up to 5.35 mmol/l (90 mg/dl) or even more (whereas in uncomplicated renal failure it is usually less than 0.70 mmol/l, 12 mg/dl) [289] (figure 2–5).

The extensive tissue breakdown is frequently associated with release of intracellular ions; hyperkalemia and hyperphosphatemia may result, which require adequate treatment; hypocalcemia may follow the hyperphosphatemia because of precipitation of calcium phosphate [289].

13.4 DIAGNOSIS OF UAN

Since UAN is readily and completely reversible with appropriate early treatment, an early diagnosis is absolutely necessary.

The use of serum-uric-acid-to-BUN ratio [294] has been proven to be inadequate to identify all patients with UAN [234].

It has been stated that urine sediment of UAN patients will show many uric acid crystals or amorphous urates [295]. This is not always true and may be limited to early phases since in several reported cases of proven UAN no crystals have been found in the urine and urinalysis was normal [234, 296]. Occasionally, microscopic or gross hematuria may occur [295].

Urinary excretion of uric acid may increase earlier and to a greater extent than serum uric acid in patients who will then develop UAN; thus, patients with mild hyperuricemia and urinary uric acid excretion greater than 5.95 mmol/24 hours (1,000 mg/24 hours) should be considered at risk for UAN [289].

It has been demonstrated that the urinary excretion of uric acid is reduced with the decrease in GFR, but less than expected from the impairment in renal function; thus, the uric-acid-clearance-to-creatinine-clearance ratio (C_{UA}/C_{Cr}) usually rises as GFR falls, reflecting the relative preservation of uric acid secretion [297]. This behavior is similar in gouty and nongouty individuals at comparable levels of serum uric acid [297]. For GFR values between 170 and 190 ml/min, C_{UA}/C_{Cr} averaged 0.06, while it averaged 0.26 with GFR between 3.7 and 20 ml/min [297]. In UAN uric acid clearance may easily exceed 26% (figure 2–5), reflecting a striking hyperuricosuria. Consequently, the ratio urinary uric acid/creatinine concentration (normal values 0.30-0.90) has been suggested as a useful test for differentiating UAN (ratio greater than 1) from ARF due to other causes (ratio less than 1) [234]. Thus, while in five patients with UAN, the ratio averaged 1.68 ± 0.63 SD (the lowest value being 1.0), in 27 patients with ARF from other causes this ratio averaged 0.43 ± 0.19 SD (the highest value being 0.9) [234]. More recently, it has been stated that the ratio should be measured in 24-hour urine specimens rather than in spot urine samples [298].

When these tests are associated with a history of neoplastic disease and the institution of cytolytic therapy, the diagnosis is very easy.

It may be useful to mention that two other disorders are associated with ARF and hyperuricemia: (a) prerenal ARF and (b) ATN secondary to trauma or hypotension. In prerenal ARF, proximal tubular reabsorption is increased in the attempt to correct ECV depletion; hence, not only sodium but also uric acid is retained with a consequent rise in serum uric acid out of proportion to the degree of renal failure. The laboratory findings typical of prerenal ARF (see chapter 7) and a urinary uric acid/creatinine ratio less than 1 will exclude UAN [289]. The same ratio will differentiate UAN from ATN secondary to trauma or hypotension in which the severe tissue breakdown may mimic UAN [289].

Intravenous pyelography is of no help in UAN since obstruction of collecting ducts does not allow an adequate pyelocalyceal visualization; retrograde pyelography may only visualize associated uric acid stones (when present) in the urinary tract [289]. Uric acid stones are radiolucent and cannot be seen on plain films of the abdomen.

13.5 TREATMENT OF UAN

As mentioned, this oliguric ARF secondary to severe hyperuricemia with hyperuricosuria may be reversed if adequately treated (figure 2–5). The following procedures are suggested:

a. A high urinary flow rate should be produced as early as possible in order to flush out obstructing uric acid crystals. This may be achieved either by the use of loop diuretics (e.g., high-dose furosemide) or by i.v. infusion of saline and/or glucose solutions or both. The use of mannitol has also been suggested. Both solute and water diuresis may prevent further uric acid deposition within the collecting ducts by diluting uric acid in the urine, thereby enhancing its solubility. In volume-expanded patients, saline infusion may be hazardous and loop diuretics may be used alone.

b. Alkalinization should be performed by a constant i.v. drip infusion of sodium bicarbonate (lactate is contraindicated since it inhibits tubular secretion of uric acid) in order to increase the solubility of urinary uric acid. Alternatively, sodium bicarbonate may be given per os in frequent divided doses in order to obtain a urine pH between 6.5 and 7 (greater values may increase the hazard of crystallization of calcium salts and monosodium urate) [295, 299].

c. Sometimes acetazolamide should be combined with sodium bicarbonate administration in order to reduce tubular reabsorption of bicarbonate and to alkalinize the urine (particularly during the night) [234, 299]. In volume-expanded patients, bicarbonate infusion may be hazardous; in these patients acetazolamide may replace sodium bicarbonate administration [288, 290]. Since acetazolamide inhibits hydrogen ion secretion leading to metabolic acidosis, it is contraindicated in lactic acidosis (which may complicate leukemia) [288].

d. Allopurinol, the specific competitive inhibitor to xanthine oxidase has to be given at high dosage (300 to 900 mg daily) particularly in patients with extremely high levels of serum uric acid [290]. Particular care should be used in patients treated with 6-mercaptopurine, azathioprine, or cyclophosphamide, since allopurinol potentiates their action and toxicity; hence, the dosage of these drugs should be appropriately reduced [295, 300]. As mentioned in this chapter, allopurinol may cause, in some patients, AIN [301, 302], which may account for the occurrence of refractoriness in recovery from UAN. Thus, it is worthwhile to perform a renal biopsy in refractory ARF.

e. Patients with hyperphosphatemia should be given aluminum hydroxide in large amounts in order to prevent metastatic calcification [290] and acute nephrocalcinosis.

f. Severe hyperkalemia should be treated immediately, even before starting dialysis (see chapter 21).

g. If hemodialysis becomes necessary in patients with hyperuricemic ARF secondary to antineoplastic chemotherapy and hyperphosphatemia, dialysate calcium should be decreased in order not to elevate serum calcium too rapidly (which may cause metastatic calcification) [290]. Hemodialysis is 10 to 20 times more efficient than peritoneal dialysis in removing uric acid [290]. But even peritoneal dialysis may be of great help (see chapter 24).

h. If the patient responds to conservative management (alone or combined with dialysis) with a dramatic increase in urine output, hydration, alkalinization, and allopurinol administration has to be pursued until a complete recovery of renal function and the return of serum uric acid to normal values.

13.6 PROPHYLAXIS IN PATIENTS WITH MALIGNANCIES

Experimental studies in rats have clearly demonstrated that high tubular fluid flow rate, whether induced by solute diuresis (high-dose furosemide) or water diuresis (Brattleboro rats with pituitary diabetes insipidus) plays a primary role in protection against UAN [285]. Hence, a high urinary flow rate must be the crucial aim for preventing UAN in patients with rapidly growing solid tumors and in patients with any neoplastic disease who have to be submitted to aggressive chemotherapy or radiation therapy. Urine output should possibly exceed three liters daily [289]. This may be obtained by i.v. saline infusion alone or associated with loop diuretics (solute diuresis) and/or i.v. infusion of glucose solution (water diuresis).

Adequate hydration (urine output should probably exceed three liters daily) [289], alkalinization, administration of allopurinol, and, eventually, aluminum hydroxide should be started several days before institution of chemotherapy [290] and continued throughout the treatment, adjusting the doses according to urine output and pH and according to the serum levels of uric acid and phosphorus (see chapter 3).

14   ARF Secondary to Multiple Myeloma

Renal failure is very frequent in multiple myeloma, occurring in more than 50% of patients [303, 304]. It is the second most common cause of death in this disease after infection [305]. ARF, on the other hand, is not so frequent, occurring in only 7.5% of patients [306].

Many factors may cause ARF in multiple myeloma, the most important being the urinary excretion of immunoglobulin light chains.

14.1 ROLE OF IMMUNOGLOBULIN LIGHT CHAINS IN CAUSING ARF ("MYELOMA KIDNEY")

In multiple myeloma, abnormal plasma cells produce monoclonal globulins (containing heavy and light chains) and free light chains. The latter are filtered by the glomeruli and then mostly reabsorbed (and catabolized) by proximal tubules; thus, urinary excretion of light chains is low, usually less than 30 mg/24 hours. In about 50% of patients with myeloma, however, light chain production is massive so that the reabsorptive capacity of proximal tubules is exceeded; a great amount of light chains (or Bence Jones proteins) will

therefore appear in the urine, ranging from 100 mg to more than 20 g/24 hours [289]. Although a good correlation has been found between the occurrence of Bence Jones proteinuria and ARF, high urinary excretion of Bence Jones protein is not always followed by ARF [303].

The mechanism by which light chains may impair renal function is not known. The most widely accepted theory is that GFR is reduced because of tubular obstruction by casts containing light chains and other proteins. Consistent with this hypothesis is the frequent observation, in renal biopsy specimens, of intratubular casts, with tubular atrophy and degeneration, mainly located in distal tubules and collecting ducts [303, 307, 308]. If this theory is correct, the occurrence of ARF in patients with heavy Bence Jones proteinuria may be greatly influenced by predisposing factors (such as dehydration and acidosis) that favor intraluminal precipitation of casts. Dehydration, particularly when associated with acidosis, favors interaction between Bence Jones protein and Tamm-Horsfall mucoprotein [306]; the solubility of Tamm-Horsfall mucoprotein in urine has been demonstrated to be reduced by low pH, high salt concentration or the presence of Bence Jones protein. Urographic contrast agents may further reduce Tamm-Horsfall protein solubility, thereby accounting for the greater incidence of radiocontrast-induced ARF in myeloma, particularly in dehydrated or salt-depleted patients (see section 10 of this chapter). It is therefore advisable to avoid dehydration or salt depletion in all patients with multiple myeloma and to hydrate them before radiocontrast procedures.

Another theory postulates a direct toxic effect of light chains on the epithelium of both proximal and distal tubules [309]. Light chains may even reach tubular cells from peritubular capillaries. Consistent with this hypothesis is the biopsy observation that some patients with severe impairment of renal function have only a mild degree of tubular casts but diffuse tubular necrosis [303, 308, 309]. The occurrence of heavy Bence Jones proteinuria without ARF may be accounted for by difference in the nephrotoxicity of light chains (which are chemically different from patient to patient) [289].

Whatever the mechanism, both kappa and lambda light chains may impair renal function and cause ARF. This may therefore be reversed by those therapeutic measures that decrease serum concentration of light chains. Treatment of primary tumor by melphalan (or other alkylating agent) and prednisone will reduce light chain production and improve renal function. Peritoneal dialysis has been proven to remove moderate amounts of light chains [305, 308]. But, undoubtedly, plasmapheresis is the best therapeutic measure for rapidly decreasing serum levels of light chains and frequently reversing ARF [308, 310, 311].

14.2 HYPERVISCOSITY SYNDROME AND ARF
Because of the important contribution of plasma proteins to blood viscosity, the hyperviscosity syndrome may occur in multiple myeloma (in 5 to 15% of patients) as a result of production of abnormal gamma globulins. Hyperviscosity is more frequent in myeloma of IgG and IgA type and when there is a high serum concentration of monoclonal protein. The syndrome often causes hemorrhagic diathesis, central nervous system dysfunction, ocular disturbances, and Ménière's syndrome. Sometimes ARF occurs as a result of alterations in renal microcirculation [305, 310]. Rapid reduction in serum viscosity has been obtained in such patients by plasmapheresis [310]. A single plasmapheresis, exchanging two to three liters of plasma, has been shown to decrease serum immunoglobulin and light chain levels by 50% [308]. Peritoneal dialysis may also be useful [305]. Obviously, chemotherapy and/or irradiation therapy should be given in combination.

14.3 ACUTE URIC ACID NEPHROPATHY IN MULTIPLE MYELOMA
Hyperuricemia is frequent in multiple myeloma, and UAN may occur in some patients either spontaneously or, more frequently, as a consequence of chemotherapy [305] (see section 13 of this chapter). Prevention and treatment in such circumstances will be those of UAN.

14.4 ACUTE HYPERCALCEMIC NEPHROPATHY IN MULTIPLE MYELOMA
Hypercalcemia is frequent in multiple myeloma, its incidence varying from 40% to more than 60% [304, 307, 312]. Hypercalcemia may result either from direct bone destruction by the neoplasia of plasma cells (which are normal constituents of bone marrow) or from the action on bone of an osteoclast-activating factor that is produced by myeloma cells [313]. Immobilization may further increase calcium release from bone. Acute hypercalcemic nephropathy may result in some cases, causing ARF. Under such circumstances, the treatment will be that of acute hypercalcemic nephropathy (see section 15 of this chapter).

14.5 TREATMENT OF ARF SECONDARY TO MULTIPLE MYELOMA
As mentioned above, ARF secondary to myeloma will frequently exhibit a beneficial effect from treatment of primary tumor with melphalan alone or in the form of triple alkylating regimen (melphalan, cyclophosphamide, and carmustine) in combination with prednisone, under careful monitoring of leukocyte and platelet counts. In some patients high doses of furosemide and/or saline infusion may be useful presumably by flushing out obstructing protein casts. Plasmapheresis is undoubtedly the best procedure for lowering serum light chains and reversing ARF. Hemodialysis or peritoneal dialysis may be particularly useful in patients with hypercalcemia or hyperuricemia. Hyperuricemic patients should also be given allopurinol and sodium bicarbonate.

Myeloma patients are susceptible to infections, which require antibiotic therapy. Apparently, the nephrotoxicity of nephrotoxic antibiotics is increased in myeloma. These antibiotics should possibly be avoided or at least used with caution.

15   Acute Hypercalcemic Nephropathy
ARF may also be caused by severe hypercalcemia, in the so-called acute hypercalcemic nephropathy.

Hypercalcemia is usually due to an increase

in bone resorption, which is commonly secondary to malignancies (such as solid tumors, lymphomas, multiple myeloma) through direct bone invasion or osteolytic metastases, or to primary hyperparathyroidism through a release of parathyroid hormone. Less frequently, hypercalcemia may result from increased intestinal absorption of calcium, such as in hypervitaminosis D, sarcoidosis, and the milk-alkali syndrome.

15.1 PATHOGENESIS AND RENAL PATHOLOGY

The mechanisms by which hypercalcemia may cause ARF include (a) a decrease in renal blood flow (RBF), (b) reduction in glomerular capillary ultrafiltration coefficient (K_f), and (c) tubular obstruction.

15.1.1 Decrease in RBF

The fall in GFR observed after acute hypercalcemia has been attributed to a reduction in RBF [314, 315]. Actually, hypercalcemia may increase the intracellular calcium concentration. An increase in the calcium content of smooth muscle cells of afferent arterioles may cause vasoconstriction and consequently a marked fall in RBF [315]; this phenomenon has also been postulated as the initiating mechanism of ischemic ARF [316, 317]. Consistent with this cellular effect of calcium is the observation that verapamil, a blocker of calcium influx into cells, protected the dogs against the ischemic experimental model of ARF. A similar effect has been observed with mannitol. In both circumstances, the calcium content of mitochondria from the renal cortex has been found to be clearly reduced [316, 317].

15.1.2 Reduction of K_f

Experimental studies have clearly demonstrated that the significant decline in GFR observed in rats with acute hypercalcemia is due primarily to a reduction in glomerular capillary ultrafiltration coefficient (K_f) [318, 319]. Since this effect on GFR and K_f was not observed in thyroparathyroidectomized rats but was reproduced by the combined infusion of calcium chloride (to induce acute hypercalcemia) and PTH, the reduction in K_f (and the consequent decline in GFR) after acute hypercalcemia must depend on the presence of PTH [319]. Thus, even though circulating PTH is expected to be reduced in patients with acute hypercalcemia, at least some of the hormone must be present to elicit the fall in K_f. On the other hand, it has been demonstrated that PTH itself causes reduction in K_f and GFR [320].

15.1.3 Tubular Obstruction

The increased filtered load of calcium and its increased transit across the proximal tubular epithelium may damage tubular cells. In their attempt to maintain a normal intracellular concentration of calcium, mithocondria swell, increase their calcium content, and disintegrate; necrosis of tubular epithelial cells results [315]. Calcified cellular debris will form, obstructing casts within the tubular lumen [321]; tubular obstruction in turn will cause a fall in GFR.

Calcium phosphate deposition within the kidney (which is the histological lesion typical of hypercalcemia) and consequent ARF may also occur in conditions of acute and marked hyperphosphatemia [289]. Thus, severe hyperphosphatemia (with hypocalcemia) has been reported to cause ARF in patients with acute lymphoblastic leukemia following cytolytic therapy [292, 293]. In these cases, hyperuricemia had been prevented by allopurinol administration, and the ARF was therefore attributed to acute nephrocalcinosis secondary to the massive phosphate release following the rapid cell lysis; the serum calcium-phosphorus product was in fact extremely high [292, 293].

15.2 CLINICAL OUTCOME

Hypercalcemia may be discovered incidentally since it is usually asymptomatic when less than 3 mmol/l (12 mg/dl). On some occasions, symptoms may include asthenia, anorexia, nausea, vomiting, dry mouth and metallic taste, polydipsia and polyuria, abdominal pain, constipation, impaired memory, lack of concentration, headache, confusion, and lethargy. Hypertension is frequently observed, probably due to the vascular effects of calcium or to increased renin secretion [289]. Band keratopathy (calcium deposition along the margins of the cornea) may be seen on slit-lamp examination.

Anorexia, vomiting, and polyuria (due to impaired renal-concentrating ability resistant to ADH) may cause dehydration, volume depletion, and hypokalemia. An increase in the urinary excretion of phosphate may lead to hypophosphatemia. When ARF is established, however, hyperphosphatemia and hyperkalemia will occur.

In all cases of acute hypercalcemic nephropathy, a plain film of the abdomen with nephrotomography becomes necessary to rule out nephrocalcinosis and nephrolithiasis.

15.3 TREATMENT OF ACUTE HYPERCALCEMIC NEPHROPATHY

First of all, hypercalcemic patients should receive an i.v. infusion of isotonic saline to correct the hypovolemia that frequently coexists. Second, attempts should be made to decrease the serum calcium level since normalization of serum calcium may reverse ARF or at least improve renal function.

Furosemide is effective in reducing serum calcium by inhibiting sodium and calcium reabsorption at the ascending limb of the loop of Henle, thereby enhancing urinary excretion of sodium, calcium, and potassium; obviously, the diuretic response to furosemide will require adequate replacement of the urinary losses of sodium and potassium. I.V. infusion of isotonic saline is also very effective in increasing urinary excretion of calcium; the resulting ECV expansion, in fact, will reduce sodium and calcium reabsorption, especially in the proximal tubule. The combined use of furosemide and isotonic saline will potentiate their calciuric effects, thus speeding up the normalization of serum calcium. The high tubular flow rate obtained with furosemide and with isotonic saline will also flush out intratubular casts (if they are present), re-establishing the patency of renal tubules.

It should be stressed that i.v. infusion of 278 mmol/l (5 g/dl) dextrose (or similar salt-free solutions) is completely ineffective in reducing serum calcium since water diuresis does not increase urinary excretion of calcium.

Immobilization of the patient should possibly be avoided since it may increase calcium release from bones. Thiazide diuretics must be avoided because they increase tubular reabsorption of calcium.

Corticosteroids (e.g., 40 mg/kg b.w./day of prednisone) are effective in lymphomas and multiple myeloma by antagonizing bone resorption, and in sarcoidosis, hypervitaminosis D and milk-alkali syndrome by blocking the action of vitamin D on intestinal calcium absorption. Steroids are ineffective in primary hyperparathyroidism and in some tumors [289].

Calcitonin may be used at doses of 100 to 200 MRC (Medical Research Council) units to reduce bone resorption and works better when combined with corticosteroids.

Hemodialysis and peritoneal dialysis may be necessary to correct severe hypercalcemia.

16 Drug-Induced Acute Interstitial Nephritis (AIN)

The other major mechanism accounting for drug-mediated nephrotoxicity involves the activation of immunological responses. Acute interstitial nephritis (AIN) may result, the diagnosis of which may be suspected clinically but can be confirmed only by renal biopsy. The latter will show interstitial infiltrates of inflammatory cells (usually mononuclears, lymphocytes, and plasma cells), disrupted tubules, and spared glomeruli.

Actually, an immunological mediated drug-induced ARF may occur in man in the form of acute glomerulonephritis (by penicillin G or sulfonamides) [322, 323], acute angiitis (by penicillin G, sulfonamides, thiazides, allopurinol) [322–325] and AIN. In this section the discussion will be limited to AIN.

16.1 DRUGS RESPONSIBLE FOR AIN IN MAN

First described during treatment with methicillin [151, 326–333], drug-induced AIN has since been reported after the therapeutic administration of many different drugs: penicillin [322, 327, 334–339]; ampicillin [334, 340–344]; rifampicin [345–349]; sulfonamides [344, 350, 351], and co-trimoxazole in particular [85, 352–355]; the anticoagulant phenindione [356–361]; the analgesic drugs glafenin [362–370] and antrafenin [371]; diphenylhydantoin [372, 373]; and, less frequently, cephalothin [102, 148, 149, 374, 375]; cephalexin [155, 344]; cefazolin [143]; cephradine [376]; nafcillin [63]; oxacillin [147]; amoxicillin [377]; carbenicillin [378, 379]; tetracycline and in particular minocycline [380]; gentamicin [85]; polymixins [381]; piromidic acid [382]; diuretics and in particular furosemide [383–385] and hydrochlorothiazide [344, 383, 385, 386]; allopurinol [301, 302]; nonsteroidal anti-inflammatory agents, such as naproxen [387], ibuprofen [344], fenoprofen [388–392], indomethacin [393], aspirin [394], pyrazolon derivatives such as phenazone (antipyrine) [395], and phenylbutazone [396–398]; the histamine H_2-receptor antagonist cimetidine [399–401]; the uricosuric agent sulfinpyrazone [344]; phenobarbital [402]; azathioprine [403]; para-aminosalicylic acid [404]; gold and bismuth salts [405]; the angiotensin-converting-enzyme inhibitor captopril [406].

Undoubtedly, the incidence of this type of ARF is increasing with the increasing practice of performing renal biopsy in those cases of ARF in which the cause is obscure. Thus, among 218 out of 976 patients with ARF in whom renal biopsy was performed, Richet et al. [407] observed AIN in 29 cases; this represents an incidence of 14% of biopsied patients (3% of all cases of ARF). An incidence of 10% was similarly reported by Wilson et al. [408] in 84 biopsied patients with unexplained ARF.

It should be borne in mind, however, that an acute inflammatory lesion of renal interstitium, which is also AIN, may occur in various infections, as we will mention later in this chapter. Furthermore, even in ATN a cellular interstitial reaction may be observed, which may make the differential diagnosis by renal biopsy very difficult with the AIN [409–410], especially if we consider that many drugs (such as gentamicin, cephalothin, and cephalexin) may cause either ATN or AIN. For this reason, some authors have sometimes defined the adverse renal reaction to drugs as "acute tubulo-interstitial nephropathy" in order to indicate an "intermediate phase" between ATN and AIN [410].

Things are even more difficult if we consider

that in other diseases, such as irradiation nephritis, medullary cystic disease, and even some types of glomerulonephritis (membranous, membranoproliferative, SLE) [411], the interstitium may present a moderate to severe infiltrate in the form of a "chronic" inflammatory pattern [344, 409] so that drug nephrotoxicity in these conditions may create problems for diagnosis by renal biopsy.

Drug-induced AIN may occur in patients with glomerulonephritis and may appear clinically simply as progressive degradation of renal function. This situation was experienced by Lyons et al. [383]. These authors decided to repeat the renal biopsy in a patient with nephrotic syndrome and membranous glomerulonephritis treated by diuretics, just because of the observation of persistently normal kidney size despite a slow (in terms of months) but progressive deterioration of renal function. A diagnosis of superimposed diuretic-induced AIN was made, and the deterioration of renal function was interrupted by withdrawing diuretic therapy [383].

Thus, the only way to recognize the causative role of a drug dissociated from the underlying disease is the observation of the reversibility of the renal damage when the drug is withdrawn [151, 344]. Sometimes a second and even a third episode of ARF has occurred in the same patient after assumption of the same drug even at very low dosage [395]. Things are more difficult when several drugs are given simultaneously, as usually occurs in severely ill patients.

Recurrent episodes of AIN due to different drugs (co-trimoxazole and gentamicin) have also occurred in the same patient and were reversed by drug withdrawal and by a short course of high-dose steroid therapy (1 gram methyl prednisolone i.v. for a few days) [85]. On the other hand, cross-reactivity between methicillin and ampicillin was earlier reported by Gilbert et al. [334]: ampicillin, inadvertently given to a patient sensitive to methicillin, reproduced a typical picture of AIN.

16.2 PATHOGENESIS OF AIN
The activation of immunological responses in drug-induced AIN is suggested by its frequent

(but not constant) occurrence with symptoms such as fever, cutaneous rash, and arthralgia, sometimes associated with (a) an increase in numbers of eosinophils in blood, urine, and renal tissue; (b) increase in serum IgE levels [328, 344]; and (c) detection of hemagglutinating antibodies to the responsible drug (e.g., ampicillin or methicillin) [340].

16.2.1 Experimental AIN

As recently reviewed by van Ypersele [410], AIN may be induced experimentally by three immunologic mechanisms: (a) formation of immune complexes; (b) formation of antitubular basement membrane (anti-TBM) antibodies; and (c) induction of delayed hypersensitivity.

16.2.1.1 FORMATION OF IMMUNE COMPLEXES. Repeated injection of either homologous cytoplasmic tubular antigens or heterologous bovine albumin in rabbits causes AIN; in the former case the immune complexes (cytoplasmic tubular antigens diffusing from tubular cells plus circulating antibodies arriving from blood flow) are formed "in situ"; in the latter case immune complexes (bovine albumins plus anti-bovine albumin antibodies) are brought to the kidney through the circulation.

16.2.1.2 FORMATION OF ANTI-TBM ANTIBODIES. Injection of rabbit tubular membranes into guinea pigs induces the formation of circulating anti-TBM antibodies, complement activation, and induction of AIN with linear deposits of IgG and C3 along the tubular basement membrane.

16.2.1.3 INDUCTION OF DELAYED HYPERSENSITIVITY. This experimental model is based on the injection of bovine gamma globulins into guinea pigs or rats; if the aggregated bovine gamma globulins are then injected into the kidneys (subcortical injection), AIN is induced.

16.2.2 AIN in Man

So far as clinical AIN is concerned, if we limit the discussion to the forms unaccompanied by glomerular lesions, we may distinguish, as suggested by Richet (a) an AIN with interstitial infiltration of polymorphonuclear cells and (b) an AIN with interstitial infiltration of mononuclear cells.

16.2.2.1 AIN WITH INTERSTITIAL INFILTRATION OF POLYMORPHONUCLEAR CELLS (ACUTE BILATERAL PYELONEPHRITIS). This type is usually secondary to septicaemic states with or without bacterial endocarditis; interstitial infiltrates may form microabscesses in both kidneys; there is pyuria, and renal failure is progressive and only partially reversible if adequately and promptly treated [412]. This is obviously a form distinct from acute pyelonephritis secondary to urinary tract infection.

The incidence of this type of AIN was 6% in the Richet series of 218 biopsied patients with unexplained ARF [407].

16.2.2.2 AIN WITH INTERSTITIAL INFILTRATION OF MONONUCLEAR CELLS This type of AIN may be induced both by infections and by drugs and is termed "acute" because of the acute clinical presentation, despite the infiltration of mononuclear cells (mainly lymphocytes) [409].

Among the infections that may cause AIN, the following have been reported: diphtheria, scarlet fever, brucellosis, syphilis, leptospirosis, toxoplasmosis, measles, mononucleosis, and Mycoplasma pneumoniae infection [323, 410, 413]. However, AIN may also be caused by many different drugs when given at their normal dosage, or even at dosages much lower than normal.

It has been postulated that the etiological factor (bacterial or viral antigen in infection-induced AIN, and the responsible drug in drug-induced AIN) reaches the renal interstitium either with blood flowing within the peritubular capillaries or from the tubular lumen through the damaged tubular wall. Once in the renal interstitium, it causes either local formation of antibodies by plasmocytes or the arrival of delayed hypersensitivity lymphocytes, which will create an inflammatory reaction [410].

Undoubtedly, in some patients with drug-induced AIN, an immunological reaction of antibody-mediated type is suggested by the detection of circulating anti-TBM antibodies or antibodies to the responsible drug (e.g., ampicillin, methicillin) [340] and by linear deposits of IgG, C3, and, on occasion, even drug (methicillin) antigen along the TBM [327, 328, 332, 351]. The responsible drug may alter the antigenicity of the TBM; anti-TBM antibodies will be formed that will react with TBM, thus stimulating an interstitial inflammatory reaction.

In many patients, however, there is no evidence of anti-TBM antibodies. Thus, cell-mediated immunity may be postulated as responsible for the AIN; the interstitial infiltration of mononuclear cells, particularly lymphocytes, is suggesting a delayed hypersensitivity reaction [327, 344, 355, 394, 414, 415].

In favor of a cell-mediated type of immune response are the following tests reported as positive in a number of patients: intradermal skin test to the responsible drug [327, 328], lymphocyte blast transformation test [373, 394], leukocyte migration inhibition test and basophil degranulation test [416].

It is possible, however, that, in some cases of drug-induced AIN, both antibody-mediated and cell-mediated types of immune response occur in the same patient [416, 417].

16.3 HYPERSENSITIVITY REACTION TO RIFAMPICIN

The oliguric ARF that has been reported in patients who have taken rifampicin intermittently deserves special mention. It is a hypersensitivity reaction to rifampicin that may appear in two different forms, AIN and ATN (347).

16.3.1 The Rifampicin-Induced AIN This is a rare condition, with interstitial edema and infiltration with mononuclear cells typical of drug-induced AIN; it occurs days after the onset of treatment, sometimes with no clinical symptoms at all [351, 418].

16.3.2 The Rifampicin-Induced ATN This condition is a more frequent one that starts clinically a few hours after the ingestion of a single low dose of the drug, with an anaphylactic reaction, followed by oliguric ARF.

Symptoms may include fever, chills, dizziness, skin rash, lumbar and/or abdominal pain, nausea, vomiting, diarrhea, oliguria, and, more rarely, hemolysis and thrombocytopenia. These clinical manifestations occur on assumption of a dose of the drug days or even months after the preceding treatment with the same drug. Sometimes linear deposits of C3 or even IgG on tubular membrane have been observed [347, 351]. Antirifampicin antibodies have been detected in the serum of some patients with this peculiar form of rifampicin-dependent ARF [345, 346, 416, 419–423], and symptoms have been attributed to the interaction of circulating antibodies with the reintroduced antigen [424, 425]. An interesting observation has been reported by Decroix et al.[346]: serum antirifampicin antibodies were detected in their patients during the reaction to rifampicin and, five months later, when they were no longer detected, the administration of 300 mg of rifampicin did not elicit any reaction.

Lymphocyte transformation test and leukocyte migration test have been reported positive in some patients [416, 426, 427].

In some cases, however, general symptoms of intolerance have occurred after the first dose of rifampicin [425].

It should be mentioned that while ATN has been usually observed on renal biopsy [347, 428], on some occasions renal biopsy showed essentially normal glomeruli and tubules with little or no change in the interstitium [425].

It has been proposed that a vasomotor substance is produced from a reaction between antigen and antibody (local activation of renin-angiotensin system?) that may cause renal ischemia [345, 429]. However, this type of ARF is reversible with return of renal function in days or weeks [425, 430]. Permanent renal damage has, however, been reported [429].

16.4 CLINICAL DIAGNOSIS OF AIN

As described above symptoms of fever, skin rash, and/or arthralgia associated with ARF in patients under treatment with any drug should suggest drug-induced AIN.

Laboratory findings usually include mild to moderate proteinuria, microscopic hematuria, and leucocyturia, which represent nonspecific signs of renal damage.

Macroscopic hematuria has been reported especially with the first observations of methicillin-induced AIN [151].

Heavy proteinuria (16 to 17 g/24 hours) with nephrotic syndrome has been described in some patients with drug-induced AIN [330, 388, 392, 431]; when a renal biopsy was performed, a typical pattern of AIN with a number of eosinophils was observed, which was associated with a fusion of epithelial foot processes as the only glomerular lesion, typical of the minimal change nephrotic syndrome. The observation of high serum IgE and eosinophilia in some cases and the recovery upon withdrawal of the incriminated drug clearly demonstrated that an adverse drug reaction was the cause of the AIN with nephrotic syndrome.

While the observation of leukocyturia is not specific and does not help in the diagnosis of AIN, it is helpful to demonstrate numerous eosinophils in the urine sediment by Wright's stain [344]. Eosinophils may represent more than 33% of all urinary leukocytes [355], but this finding is not constant and is helpful only if positive.

More frequent (60 to 100% of reported cases) is the increase in eosinophil count (greater than $0.7 \times 10^9/1$); but for this test too, a normal count does not exclude AIN [344].

Increased serum levels of IgE (greater than 80 μg/dl) have been found in about 50% of cases of AIN in which the diagnosis was confirmed by renal biopsy [330, 344, 432].

Other immunologic tests may represent useful support for the diagnosis of drug-induced AIN: the detection of serum anti-TBM antibodies, Coombs reaction, inhibition of lymphocyte migration, lymphoblastic transformation, intradermal skin test to the responsible drug [410].

Urine-to-plasma osmolality ratio does not show a constant behavior (1 to 1.4 values have been reported) [344].

Recently, evidence has been presented that abdominal scanning after intravenous injection of gallium citrate (^{67}Ga) shows an intense and uniform renal uptake of ^{67}Ga in AIN, but not in ATN [344, 433]. Gallium citrate scanning may therefore represent a useful test for separating patients with AIN from those with ATN [344]. Some patchy and less intense ^{67}Ga uptake may be observed in other conditions, such as glomerulonephritis and pyelonephritis; intense and diffuse uptake similar to that of AIN has been reported in patients with minimal change nephrotic syndrome, and attributed either to the increased glomerular permeability or to a functional alteration of glomerular mesangial cells [344].

16.5 CLINICAL COURSE OF AIN

16.5.1 Acute Bilateral Pyelonephritis Secondary to Septicemia As mentioned above, this condition occurs in patients with septicemic states, especially those due to group A streptococci or coagulase-positive staphylococci [409]. There may be a bacterial endocarditis.

There is no way to differentiate clinically this type of ARF from that due to ATN in the course of septicemia. It may be suspected in septic patients without shock, with clear pyuria, with no evidence of drug toxicity and with no signs of glomerular disease. In the forms due to group A streptococci, however, acute glomerulonephritis may occur in association with acute pyelonephritis [409].

16.5.2 Drug-Induced AIN In the typical case, drug-induced AIN is characterized by the association of acute renal impairment and acute allergic reaction with the triad of fever, skin rash, and arthralgias [151, 344, 434]. But these clinical manifestations are by no means constant since it is becoming more and more evident that quite frequently one or more of these symptoms are missing. Thus, although the diagnosis may be sometimes suspected on clinical grounds, it should be considered in all cases of unexplained ARF [344].

Fever is the most frequent but not specific symptom with an incidence of 60 to 100% [151, 355, 416, 434]. The skin rash is frequent too, with an incidence of 45% [344]; it is erythematous, maculopapular, and transient [151, 344, 355]. Arthralgia is less frequent and is rarely prominent. Severe lumbar pain has been reported in several cases, presumably related to capsular distention because of kidney enlargement due to interstitial edema; it is usually bilateral but in a few occasions it was unilateral [410].

The delay between the exposure to the drug and the onset of ARF may vary from a few hours (presumably in presensitized patients) to 45 days [416]. It may be, for instance, quite short (a few hours) with rifampicin, clearly longer (12 to 56 days) with phenindione.

Renal function deteriorates suddenly; but sometimes renal failure develops insidiously. The resulting ARF is nonoliguric in 30 to 40% of cases [330, 355]. Sometimes dialysis is necessary for a certain period of time.

Renal specimens obtained by renal biopsy (sometimes at autopsy) reveal infiltrates of mononuclear cells, usually lymphocytes, but also plasma cells and eosinophils, in the renal interstitium and, in some patients, epithelioid cell granulomata with giant cells [416]. Tubules are often disrupted, but glomeruli are spared.

It has been suggested recently that (bilateral) renal papillary necrosis may complicate drug-induced allergic AIN [344].

16.6   TREATMENT OF DRUG-INDUCED AIN

ARF due to drug-induced AIN is a reversible condition provided that the responsible drug is withdrawn. Readministration of the same drug will reproduce ARF [383]. If the condition is not recognized and the drug administration continued, it may even lead to death [327]. Recovery of ARF is usually followed by normalization of renal function; but permanent residual impairment of renal function has been reported on some occasions [329, 355, 360, 416, 435–437]. There are reports of patients who could never stop dialysis following drug-induced AIN [394].

Follow-up renal biopsies carried out by Pasternack et al. [438] have shown that chronic interstitial changes are frequent.

Recovery seems to be favored by steroid therapy [85, 344, 355, 377, 383, 385, 434, 439–441]. Thus, Galpin et al. [355] have reported recovery of renal function in an average of 9.6 days in patients with methicillin-induced AIN treated with 60 mg daily of prednisone while 54 days were necessary for recovery of untreated patients. Linton et al. [344] have observed a clear improvement of renal function within two days of therapy with prednisone (60 mg/day) in seven patients with drug-induced AIN who were not showing re-

covery of renal function. Frommer et al. [441] have reported a patient on regular dialysis treatment for three months; when a renal biopsy was finally performed and AIN observed, steroid treatment was instituted and shortly followed by significant recovery of renal function. Saltissi et al. [85] succeeded on three occasions in reversing ARF due to drug-induced AIN by giving high-dose steriod therapy.

17   Other Toxic Forms of ARF

17.1   PARACETAMOL/(ACETAMINOPHEN)-INDUCED ARF

Paracetamol (acetaminophen) is an analgesic compound that is usually without adverse side effects when used in therapeutic doses. However, overdosage may cause fulminant hepatic failure that may be fatal.

ARF has been reported to occur after paracetamol poisoning, usually in association with massive hepatic necrosis with hepatic failure dominating the clinical setting [442–444].

In recent years, however, several reports have emphasized that ARF may occur after paracetamol overdosage even without fulminant liver failure [445–447]. It usually took the form of oliguric ARF, with high values of both urinary sodium concentration and FE_{Na} [447, 448], in the absence of hepatic failure, hypotension, and/or volume depletion. Liver function in these cases was only mildly impaired, the clinical picture being dominated by ARF, with associated nausea, vomiting, and abdominal pain.

17.1.1   *Pathophysiology*   The toxic effect of paracetamol has been attributed to its metabolic deactivation to an arylating metabolite by the microsomal cytochrome P-450 oxygenase system that controls most drug oxidations in the liver, kidney, and other tissues. Since this enzyme system is more concentrated in renal cortex and in liver, these are the sites of toxic injury by paracetamol [445]. Apparently, glutathione is capable of binding the reactive metabolite, thereby protecting against its toxic effect. The greater concentration of glutathione in renal cortex than in liver may account for the usually greater resistance of the kidney against paracetamol toxicity [170]. When the availability of glutathione is reduced, paracetamol exerts a greater toxic effect [170]. Thus, depletion of glutathione by diethylmaleate in rats has been shown to increase paracetamol nephrotoxicity, whereas the administration of cysteine, a precursor of glutathione, reduces it [445]. This is why acetylcysteine has been suggested for the treatment of paracetamol poisoning [449].

The occurrence of severe renal damage without major hepatic injury has been attributed to a gradual (over a period of many hours) ingestion of high doses of the drug rather than to a single large ingestion. In the latter condition, a high serum peak of the drug is rapidly achieved, particularly in the portal vein, explaining the severe hepatic damage; in the former condition, peak serum levels will be less high but more protracted, allowing renal injury [448]. However, the picture of dominant ARF has been observed after a single large (16 grams) ingestion of paracetamol [446].

17.1.2 Renal Pathology In one case of paracetamol-induced ARF in which the renal damage dominated the clinical picture, a pathological study was carried out on a renal biopsy obtained in the oliguric phase. Light and electron microscopy sections showed severe epithelial necrosis, particularly in the proximal tubules, with the tubular lumina filled with shed cells and necrotic debris; frequent breaks in integrity of tubular basement membrane were also observed [446].

17.1.3 Clinical Course The possibility of an ARF after paracetamol overdosage without clinical signs of severe hepatic failure should warn physicians to inquire about the recent use of analgesic preparations containing paracetamol when taking the history of patients with ARF of unknown origin. Too frequently, patients do not spontaneously mention the consumption of analgesic drugs; they consider these drugs to be safe since no prescription is needed [448].

The clinical course is that of oliguric ARF secondary to a renal toxic insult, worsened by

a concomitant more or less severe hepatic failure.

Prognosis is undoubtedly grave, particularly when hepatic failure dominates. ARF, however, is reversible, and complete return of renal function may be observed [446].

17.1.4 Prevention of Hepatic and Renal Failure after Paracetamol Overdosage Early treatment of paracetamol poisoning with intravenous N-acetylcysteine has been found very successful in preventing hepatic and renal failure. Thus, Prescott et al. [449] have demonstrated complete protection against liver damage in 40 patients who received acetylcysteine within eight hours after ingestion of the poison; the efficacy decreased progressively with increases in the interval between ingestion and treatment, to become completely ineffective after 15 hours. When patients given supportive treatment only were compared with patients given acetylcysteine, the incidence of severe liver damage fell from 58% (33 out of 57 patients) to a little more than 1% (1 out of 62 patients) [449]. Important protection was also observed against renal damage; thus, when acetylcysteine was given within 10 hours after paracetamol ingestion no patients exhibited a rise in serum creatinine over 300 μmol/l (3.4 mg/dl), whereas in untreated patients with paracetamol poisoning, ARF occurred in 11% of the cases (in 6 out of 57 patients) [449].

The following management protocol has been suggested [449]:

a. Gastric aspiration and lavage should be performed in all patients who are admitted within four hours after paracetamol ingestion or in those in coma.

b. Acetylcysteine should be given i.v. (oral administration has been proven unsuccessful) at an initial dose of 150 mg/Kg b.w. in 200 ml of 278 mmol/l (5g/dl) dextrose, in 15 minutes.

c. Then 50 mg/Kg b.w. of acetylcysteine in 500 ml of 278 mmol/l dextrose should be infused i.v. over a four-hour period, followed by 100 mg/Kg in 1.000 ml of 278 mmol/l dextrose over the next 16 hours. Overall treatment, therefore, will be 300 mg/Kg b.w. of acetylcysteine over 20 hours [449].

d. This treatment should start within 15 hours (better within 8 hours) after paracetamol ingestion.

e. Since treatment with acetylcysteine is not harmful and has no side effects, it may be instituted even if the interval between ingestion and treatment is 15 to 24 hours [449].

17.2 GLAPHENIN-INDUCED ARF

Glaphenin is an analgesic compound widely used in France where it represents one of the most common causes of toxic ARF [450]. The first case of glaphenin-induced ARF was reported in 1972 [362]. In some patients, an immunoallergic acute interstitial nephritis (AIN) has been postulated [369, 370], while in others hypersensitivity phenomena have been absent despite histopathological findings compatible with AIN on renal biopsy specimens [362, 363, 451] (see section 16 of this chapter).

In most patients, ARF occurs following the ingestion of extremely high doses (up to 10 grams) of glaphenin, frequently in a suicide attempt [450], or when the usual therapeutic dose (maximum 1.2 g daily) is ingested in a single dose rather than in divided doses [369].

Recent experimental studies in rats have produced clear evidence that tubular obstruction plays a predominant role in the pathogenesis of this nonoliguric form of ARF, in a fashion quite similar to that due to folic acid or uric acid [450]. A marked increase in intratubular hydrostatic pressure (three times higher than normal) was recorded by micropuncture techniques in proximal convoluted tubules 90 minutes after glaphenin administration and remained significantly elevated throughout the following days. Intratubular deposits of a glaphenin metabolite (hydroxyglaphenin acid) were observed, on the other hand, in renal histopathological preparations, taken 90 minutes after the oral administration of glaphenin, mainly in the medullary collecting ducts, but also in the distal tubules; these deposits increased with time up to 24 hours later [450, 452].

While inhibition of the renin-angiotensin system by SQ 14, 225 (captopril) did not prevent glaphenin-induced ARF, increase in urine output by saline infusion and/or furosemide administration had a clear protective effect, presumably through an increase in tubular fluid flow rate with the consequent wash-out of intratubular precipitates. However, nonsaline-loaded Brattleboro rats (with congenital diabetes insipidus), were not protected, presumably because water diuresis raises the tubular fluid flow rate only in the terminal portion of the collecting duct while intratubular deposits in glaphenin-induced ARF occur in the proximal segments [450]. An increase in nephrotoxin clearance and in medullary blood flow, by reducing the nephrotoxin accumulation in the papillary region, may also contribute to protection following saline loading and/or furosemide [450]. It does not seem that the inhibition of prostaglandin (PGE_2) synthesis by glaphenin has an important pathogenetic role in glaphenin-induced ARF, since salt-loaded rats were protected from ARF despite low PGE_2 synthesis (as mirrored by the reduced urine excretion of PGE_2) [450].

17.3 ARF SECONDARY TO HERBICIDE POISONING (PARAQUAT, DIQUAT)

Paraquat and diquat are two bipyridilium compounds used as weed killers. Their activity and toxicity in mammalians are due to liberation of hydrogen peroxide; this leads to tissue destruction [453].

Both paraquat and diquat are commercially available either as liquid concentrate or as granular preparations, the former being used in farming and forestry work, the latter in domestic gardening. Poisoning may occur from accidental ingestion or as a suicide attempt. Inhalation of paraquat spray droplets has been also reported as a possible way of poisoning in agricultural workers [454, 455].

Large quantities of paraquat or diquat lead to death in several hours to a few days by pulmonary edema or hemorrhage and necrosis of heart, liver, and kidney. Smaller quantities may cause delayed symptoms; vomiting, abdominal cramps, diarrhea, and erosion of oral, esophageal, and gastrointestinal mucosa occur more slowly and may be followed by an asymptomatic period of 24 to 48 hours [453, 456, 457]. This period of lack of serious symptoms is misleading and may give a false sense of security; symptoms of poisoning, in fact, will reappear, and the patient may die from pulmonary fibrosis and progressive respiratory failure after paraquat poisoning or from gastrointestinal or cerebral haemorrhage after diquat poisoning [453]. Sometimes, intestinal paralysis with gastrointestinal fluid sequestration and hypovolemic shock may occur following diquat ingestion [453].

ARF after diquat or paraquat poisoning may result from hemodynamic alterations (hypovolemia, decrease in cardiac output, shock). But in some cases ARF occurred in the context of preserved hemodynamic status, suggesting a direct toxic effect on tubular epithelium [453]. Renal pathology was that of diffuse necrosis in proximal tubules [453–455, 458, 459].

Therapeutic measures include gastric and intestinal lavage, administration of absorbents (e.g., Fuller's earth) [460] and purgatives; when the poison is in the circulation, repeated sessions of hemoperfusion or, less efficiently, hemodialysis become necessary [457]. Large quantities of fluid (isotonic saline) infused i.v. to force diuresis may protect the kidney from damage, provided that ATN has not occurred as yet.

It should be stressed that a symptom-free interval after poison ingestion should not delay therapeutic measures. Furthermore, after diquat ingestion, (a) gastric and intestinal lavage requires special care because of the risk of gastric or intestinal perforation; (b) intestinal sequestration of fluid requires adequate hydration; and (c) the risk of cerebral hemorrhage should suggest special caution (reduced dosage) with heparin for dialysis [453].

17.4 AMPHOTERICIN B NEPHROPATHY
This antifungal agent (Fungizone), which is so important for treating life-threatening fungal infections, when given at high dosage may cause ARF sometimes preceded by renal tubular acidosis of the distal type, hypokalemia (due to enhanced urinary loss of potassium), and impaired concentrating ability [461].

Renal biopsy usually shows tubular necrosis and nephrocalcinosis. The renal damage has been attributed to renal vasoconstriction [461] and/or a direct toxic effect on tubular epithelium [170]. Alkalinization of urine and administration of mannitol have been reported to reduce the nephrotoxicity of amphotericin in experimental animals but not in patients [170].

17.5 COLISTIN (COLOMYCIN)-INDUCED ARF
Colistimethate or colistin (colomycin) is a very toxic antibiotic. Its toxicity includes neurological reactions and renal impairment in the form of ATN. Renal function may continue to deteriorate for about a week after the end of therapy, as happens with aminoglycosides [462]. In combination with a cephalosporin, it seems to enhance its nephrotoxicity. Pre-existent chronic renal failure represents a predisposing factor and requires reduction in dosage (see chapter 3).

17.6 MUSHROOM POISONING AND ARF
The ingestion of as little as 50 grams of *Amanita phalloides* mushroom is sufficient to kill an adult. Death usually occurs from hepatic coma. Amanitine is the main toxin (10 to 20 times more toxic than phallotoxins), which causes cell death by impairing RNA synthesis [463]. The first symptoms occur 8 to 12 hours after ingestion and include acute abdominal pain, nausea, vomiting, and watery or bloody diarrhea, with consequent severe volume depletion (with extreme thirst), shock, and ARF [464]; 36 to 40 hours after ingestion, hepatic disease will start dominating the clinical course leading to hepatic coma; death from acute yellow atrophy of the liver usually occurs within four days of ingestion. Adequate replacement of fluid and electrolyte losses (due to vomiting and diarrhea) may prevent ARF [463]. Amanitatoxins, however, must be removed from circulation to improve survival, and this should be done within 36 hours after ingestion. Forced diuresis (by saline infusion and/or mannitol), hemodialysis, hemoperfusion, and plasmapheresis have all been suggested for this purpose [170, 463]. However, mortality remains high.

17.7 ARF SECONDARY TO INFECTION BY RICKETTSIA RICKETTSII

ARF has been observed as a common complication of severe cases of Rocky Mountain spotted fever, an infection by Rickettsia rickettsii. Despite the observation of focal perivascular interstitial nephritis on histologic sections of the kidney, and the demonstration of Rickettsia rickettsii by immunofluorescence in renal tissue, the pathogenesis of ARF seems to be related to hypovolemia and hypotension; volume depletion may, in fact, result from the severe increase in capillary permeability due to the rickettsial-induced diffuse vasculitis [465].

17.8 ARF FOLLOWING SNAKEBITE

Snakebite may cause ARF by one or more of the following mechanisms: intravascular hemolysis, disseminated intravascular coagulation, shock or severe hypotension, or direct nephrotoxic effect of the snake venom [466]. Renal histopathology may vary from acute proliferative glomerulonephritis (on a hypersensitivity basis) [467] to ATN [468] and patchy to diffuse bilateral renal cortical necrosis [468, 469]. ARF frequently required dialysis and was usually reversible; in some cases, however, the patients had irreversible renal failure [468, 469].

17.9 ARF SECONDARY TO ACUTE PANCREATITIS

It has been reported that ARF occurs in as many as 78% of patients with acute pancreatitis [470]. As already mentioned, acute pancreatitis may cause hypovolemic ARF, through blood, plasma, and fluid losses, hypotension and shock. If this functional ARF remains inadequately treated (by blood transfusion and/or i.v. infusion of plasma, human albumin, and electrolyte solutions), ATN ensues, greatly worsening the prognosis of the disease.

ARF, however, has also been reported by Goldstein et al. [471] in patients with mild forms of acute pancreatitis (serum amylase ranging from 290 to 1,450 units/dl and urine amylase from 960 to 4,000 units/dl) who did not develop shock, hypotensive episodes, or ECV depletion. It was an oliguric ARF (requiring peritoneal dialysis in one case), with high

urinary sodium concentration (greater than 53 mmol/l), low urinary osmolality (less than 435 mOsm/kg H_2O), normal urinalysis, and no urinary uric acid crystals. ARF occurred early (within 24 hours) after the onset of symptoms of pancreatitis and was constantly associated with severe hyperuricemia (serum uric acid ranging from 0.89 to 1.43 mmol/l, 15 to 24 mg/dl). This marked increase in serum uric acid was attributed to the enhanced tissue breakdown secondary to the pancreatic release of proteolytic enzymes; but acute uric acid nephropathy was ruled out as responsible for the renal impairment since the hyperuricemia did not adversely affect but actually decreased, with recovery of renal function and without specific treatment [471]. It has been postulated that toxic products of pancreatic autodigestion, pancreatic release of proteolytic enzymes, intravascular coagulation, and/or pancreatic release of vasoactive factors (activation of kallikrein-kinin system) may contribute to renal dysfunction/damage in these mild forms of acute pancreatitis [470–472].

17.10 ARF WITHOUT HISTOLOGICAL LESIONS ON RENAL BIOPSY

The types of different compounds reported to be responsible for renal shutdown are tremendously numerous. ARF has even been reported following oral consumption of an herbal medicine "impila" (Callilepsis laureola), prescribed by a witch-doctor among a Bantu population for the treatment of impotence [473]. The list of nephrotoxic substances will undoubtedly increase with time. Renal biopsy has clarified in recent years the underlying renal lesion in many instances. For many compounds, however, the histological pattern of the failing kidney is not known, since renal biopsy is still frequently avoided in patients with ARF, usually because of possible postbiopsy complications.

Finally there are reports of ARF in which no renal damage has been observed on renal biopsy. Jones et al. [474], for instance, have reported a patient with meningococcal purulent pericarditis due to Neisseria meningitidis who developed a reversible form of ARF; renal biopsy did not show any significant abnormality on light microscopy, immunofluorescence, and electron microscopy.

Desferrioxamine, used as a nonchelating agent in the parenteral (subcutaneous or intravenous) treatment of secondary hemosiderosis, has been reported to cause ARF without any evidence of significant glomerular, tubular, or interstitial damage in the kidney when studied by light and electron microscopy [475].

A tranquilizing drug, chlorprothixene, usually nontoxic at therapeutic dosage (400 mg/day) has been reported to cause ARF in a case of overdosage (3,000 mg as a single dose in a suicide attempt); renal biopsy did not show any lesion by light microscopy or by immunofluorescence [476].

17.10.1 Cyclosporin A (CyA) Cyclosporin A (CyA), the metabolite from the fungi *Cylindrocarpon lucidum* and *Trichoderma polysporum,* recently introduced in the treatment of transplanted patients for its immunosuppressive properties, has been shown to impair renal function in a reversible fashion [477, 478] without glomerular, tubular, or interstitial lesions on light or electron microscopy [479–481]. It has been suggested that adequate hydration and mannitol infusion performed before starting CyA therapy may protect the kidney [478, 479]. Calne et al. [479] have delayed the administration of CyA until it was clear that the transplanted kidney was making urine six hours after transplantation; if there was no diuresis, the use of CyA was avoided. Klintmalm et al. [477], on the other hand, suggest a preoperative initiation of CyA therapy; since the toxic effect of CyA on the kidney is relatively late (it occurs within a week of starting therapy), early anuria would indicate acute rejection or ATN rather than CyA nephrotoxicity.

It has been stated that nontoxic CyA dosage ranges from 7.4 to 14 mg/kg b.w./day (mean 9.2 mg/kg b.w./day) in liver recipients with normal renal function; in renal recipients, instead, nephrotoxicity occurred in doses as low as 5.2 mg/kg b.w./day [477], suggesting that normal renal function reduces CyA nephrotoxicity. For this reason, it appears advisable to delay CyA therapy until adequate renal function is obtained from transplanted kidneys.

While it has been demonstrated that early CyA nephrotoxicity is reversed on CyA withdrawal, it has recently been reported that long-term treatment with CyA will permanently impair renal function even though such impairment does not seem to be progressive [481]. Histological studies of renal biopsy specimen obtained from transplant recipients treated long term with CyA have shown that fibrosis, tubular atrophy, and interstitial inflammation, is a nonspecific feature, possibly reflecting chronic low-grade rejection [481].

17.10.2 Captopril-induced ARF Captopril is the first inhibitor of angiotensin-converting enzyme-kininase II, which is effective, when given orally, as an antihypertensive agent. Its administration is followed by increase in plasma renin activity, presumably because there is no longer the negative feedback normally exerted by angiotensin II (AII) on renin release [482]. Since the converting enzyme-kininase II is responsible both for converting AI to AII and for inactivating bradykinin (which is a prostaglandin stimulator) [483], its inhibition by captopril is expected to decrease vasoconstrictors such as AII and increase vasodilators such as bradykinin and prostaglandins (PGs), thereby leading to the observed hypotensive effect.

These effects of captopril on kinin and PG levels have been recently demonstrated [484, 485]. Significant increments in plasma concentrations of kinins and PGE_2-M (a metabolite of PGE_2) have been observed by Swartz et al. [484] even after doses as low as 12.5 mg of captopril. The increments of PGE_2-M (but not those of kinins) were dose related and were significantly correlated with the fall in diastolic blood pressure. Although bradykinin has been demonstrated to release PGs from several tissues, only slight increments of kinins have been found after captopril in acute studies [484, 485] and no change at all after long-term treatment [486], making it unreasonable that the increase in PGE_2 production is kinin mediated. Since the hypotensive effect of captopril was blunted by inhibition of PG synthetase by indomethacin, it may be concluded that PGs contribute to captopril's antihypertensive effect and that nonsteroidal anti-inflammatory drugs (aspirin, indomethacin, etc.) should be avoided in order to maximize the hypotensive effect of captopril [485].

Captopril is excreted mainly in the urine, so that its dosage must be reduced in chronic renal failure. Adverse effects of the drug include proteinuria (greater than 1g/day) in 1.2% of the patients, sometimes with nephrotic syndrome and the histological picture of membranous glomerulopathy [482]. Reversible ARF has recently been reported in a number of cases on treatment with captopril [487–492]. This ARF was initially attributed to a direct toxic effect on the kidney [487], to a sudden fall in systemic blood pressure and, consequently, in renal perfusion [489], and to a drug reaction in the form of acute interstitial nephritis [488]. More recently it has been observed that ARF occurs when therapy with captopril is performed in patients with either bilateral renal artery stenosis [491] or renal artery stenosis in a solitary kidney [490, 491], such as in a transplanted kidney [487, 489, 492]. Under such circumstances, ARF is promptly resolved by discontinuation of the drug, suggesting a functional form of ARF (prerenal ARF). It has even been proposed to use this reversible impairment of renal function by captopril as a diagnostic tool for stenosis of the transplanted renal artery in the allograft recipient [492].

Reduction in renal perfusion secondary to a drug-induced decrease in systemic blood pressure has been ruled out as the pathogenetic mechanism; ARF, in fact, also occurred when blood pressure was not reduced by captopril, but did not occur when a decrease in systemic blood pressure was obtained by other antihypertensive agents after discontinuation of captopril [491, 492].

That the causal role was played by the inhibition of a converting enzyme is demonstrated by one of the cases reported by Hricik et al. [491]. A 65-year-old hypertensive (230/100 mm Hg) woman with a bilateral marked (greater than 95%) renal artery stenosis was treated first with captopril; blood pressure fell to 175/85 mm Hg but serum creatinine increased from 160 μmol/l (1.8 mg/dl) to 420 μmol/l (4.8 mg/dl). Upon discontinuation of

captopril, serum creatinine fell immediately and stabilized at 210 μmol/l (2.4 mg/dl). When another converting enzyme inhibitor (MK 421) was given, serum creatinine rose again to 690 μmol/l (7.8 mg/dl) and fell to 220 μmol/l (2.5 mg/dl) upon discontinuation of MK 421 [491].

From these observations, it appears evident that the transient ARF secondary to the administration of converting-enzyme inhibitors is a functional impairment in the autoregulation of GFR induced by these drugs in conditions of marked reduction in renal perfusion pressure.

It has been postulated that when renal perfusion pressure is markedly reduced, the mechanism by which GFR is maintained (through an increase in glomerular capillary pressure, GCP) is an AII-dependent efferent arteriolar constriction [493, 494]. Should this hypothesis be correct, converting enzyme inhibitors would impair this protective mechanism, and the resultant decrease in GCP would cause a fall in GFR [491, 492]. According to Hricik et al. [491], the above sequence of events after captopril would not occur in the absence of renal artery stenosis, because renal perfusion pressure remains within the range in which GFR autoregulation does not rely on an intact renin-angiotensin system (RAS).

I do not agree with this hypothesis. Against a critical role of efferent arteriolar constriction in renal autoregulation are anatomical and experimental studies. Anatomical studies have demonstrated that efferent arterioles have a very thin wall, with very few muscle cells [495, 496]. They are therefore predicted to have a feeble muscular activity and to be practically unable to constrict in response to neural and humoral stimuli. Support for this concept stems from the micropuncture studies in experimental animals. Andreucci et al. [497] have demonstrated in rats that in several experimental conditions in which hemodynamic pressure in glomerular capillaries of superficial nephrons was varied widely, the percentage of pressure dissipated across the efferent arterioles remained constant. This observation appeared to provide evidence against an active role for efferent arterioles in regulating filtration fraction. On the other hand, micropuncture studies in dogs by Navar et al. [498] could not support the contention that blockade of RAS by a converting-enzyme inhibitor (SQ 20,881) results in a preferential reduction in efferent arteriolar resistance.

In my opinion, in the underperfused kidney the impairment of renal function following treatment with captopril is due to ECV depletion, which will further reduce the already impaired renal perfusion. Since captopril has been shown to stimulate PG release [484, 485] and PGs are known to reduce tubular sodium reabsorption thereby increasing urinary sodium excretion [498], I hypothesize that long-term treatment with captopril in high dosage will cause ECV depletion through a sustained PG-mediated increase in urinary sodium excretion. Brenner et al. [499] have demonstrated that a filtration pressure equilibrium is achieved at the efferent end of glomerular network when glomerular plasma flow (GPF) is low; under such circumstances GFR is GPF dependent. Since a kidney with severe renal artery stenosis has reduced perfusion, its GFR will be GPF dependent; under such circumstances even a modest contraction of ECV (as may occur with high doses of captopril), which would not have any effect in a normal (without renal artery stenosis) kidney, will significantly reduce GFR.

Support for this hypothesis stems from the following observations:

a. While the effect of captopril on arterial blood pressure is very rapid, clearly demonstrating the rapid hormonal response to the drug, the rise in serum creatinine requires days of therapy. This delayed effect on renal function fits with progressive salt depletion but not with RAS inhibition.
b. Unlike most antihypertensive drugs (with the exception of diuretics), which reduce urinary sodium excretion with the fall in blood pressure, captopril has been shown to increase sodium excretion and urine output [498, 500].
c. Significant and marked increments of PGE_2 production have been demonstrated to follow captopril administration in hypertensive patients on high- or low-sodium intake [484].

d. In transplanted kidneys with renal artery stenosis, the rise in serum creatinine following captopril administration was associated with a fall in renal plasma flow [492]. This reduction in renal perfusion may be accounted for by volume depletion, but not by release of the postulated efferent arteriole constriction.
e. In all reported cases of captopril-induced ARF, the drug was given in high doses and/or associated with diuretics. Under such conditions a significant urinary loss of sodium may have occurred, resulting in ECV depletion.
f. In a boy with a transplanted kidney and renal artery stenosis who was studied in my unit, serum creatinine rose significantly when captopril was given either in high doses or combined with a diuretic agent; under such circumstances urinary sodium excretion and urine output increased and body weight fell. Serum creatinine, on the other hand, remained at basal levels when captopril was given at low dosage (12.5 mg daily) and without diuretics; under such circumstances urine output and urinary sodium excretion were relatively low (figure 2–6).
g. In two cases with transplant renal artery stenosis, renal biopsy did not show ATN or any other organic damage to the kidney [487, 489].

Should my hypothesis be correct, prerenal ARF after captopril, in underperfused kidneys, would be prevented by ensuring adequate replacement of urinary salt losses.

18 ARF Secondary to Incompatible Blood Transfusion

Transfusion of mismatched blood (usually a nursing error) may cause a hemolytic reaction with ARF and an hemorrhagic diathesis that may be life-threatening.

A functional, readily reversible ARF occurs following the transfusion of small amounts of incompatible blood; after transfusion of 200–500 ml, ATN results; however, unreversible bilateral acute cortical necrosis is rare [501].

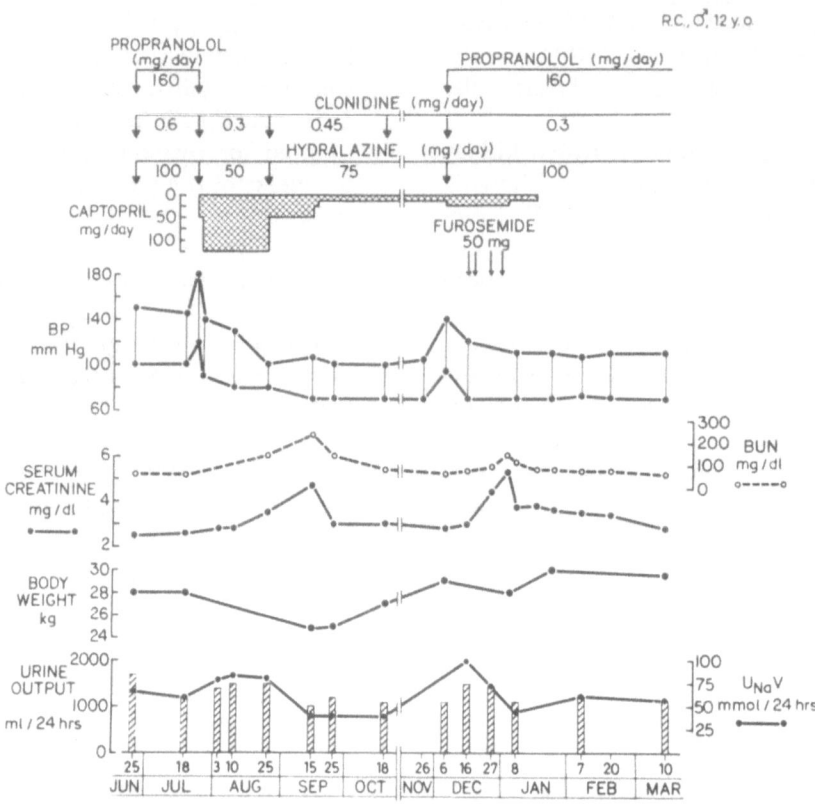

FIGURE 2–6. Effect of different doses of captopril and combined captopril-furosemide on blood pressure, urine output, sodium excretion, and renal function in a 12-year-old boy with renal artery stenosis of a transplanted kidney.

The hemorrhagic diathesis has been attributed to disseminated intravascular coagulation (DIC) (see chapter 6) initiated by intravascular hemolysis.

18.1 PATHOGENESIS

It has been stated for a long time that hemoglobin had a direct toxic effect on tubular epithelium, even though such toxicity had not been clearly proven. Convincing experimental evidence against the nephrotoxicity of hemoglobin has been given in dogs and monkeys: the i.v. infusion of large quantities of stroma-free hemoglobin in these animals was, in fact, followed by massive hemoglobinuria without any impairment of renal function [502, 503]. Conversely, when hemoglobin-free incompatible erythrocyte stroma was infused i.v. in two patients, both subjects developed ARF [504]. The latter study clearly demonstrates that hemoglobinemia and hemoglobinuria are not nec-

essary for the induction of ARF that follows incompatible transfusion; however, incompatible erythrocyte stroma is the single factor responsible for renal shutdown [501]. Thus, it has been postulated that a specific antigen-antibody reaction is the cause of ARF that follows incompatible blood transfusion [501, 504]. This ARF will result from the combined effects of intrarenal vasomotor alterations and DIC both triggered by the antigen-antibody reaction and leading to renal ischemia [501]. Incompatible red blood cells, as soon as infused intravenously, react with preformed antibodies (figure 2–7): the antigen-antibody complexes (a) activate the Hageman factor and, through this, the kinin system; (b) act on platelets caus-

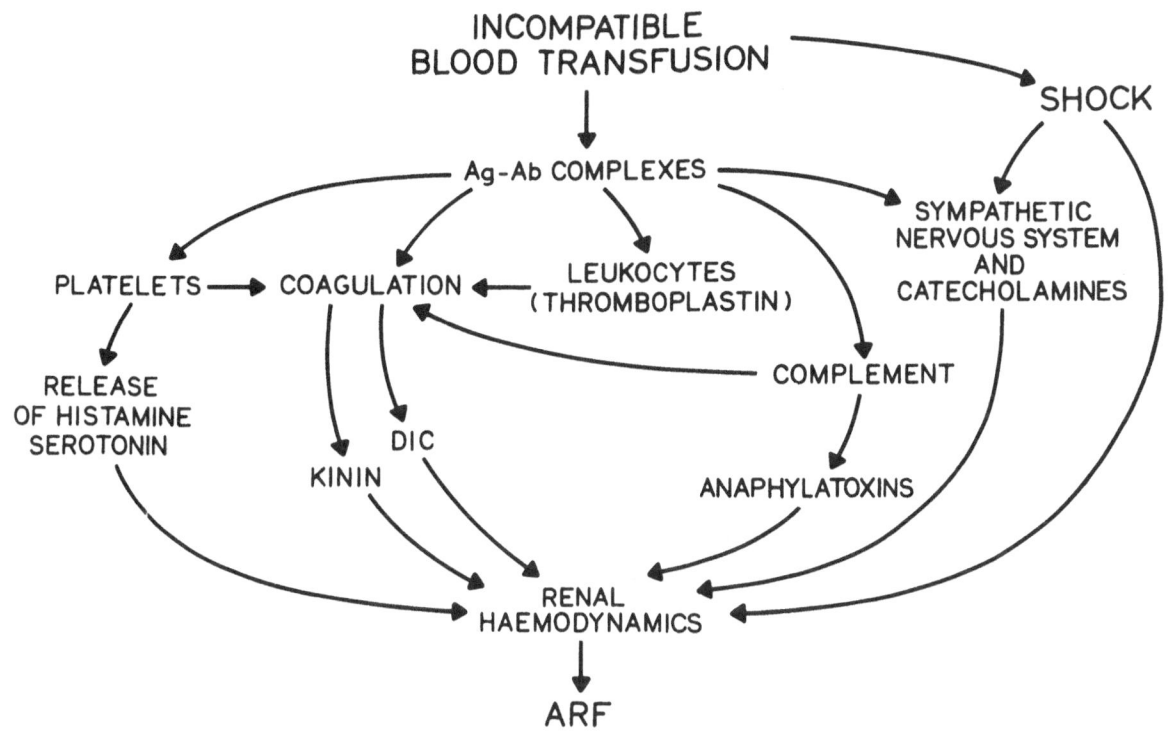

FIGURE 2–7. Renal effects of incompatible blood transfusion.

ing the release of histamine, serotonin, and platelet factor 3; (c) activate the complement system with release of anaphylatoxins, histamine, and serotonin and the activation of coagulation; (d) act on leukocytes causing the release of thromboplastin; (e) activate the sympathetic nervous system and release catecolamines, both directly and indirectly through the shock that usually follows the hemolytic reaction. The resulting alterations in renal hemodynamics lead to ARF (figure 2–7).

18.2 CLINICAL OUTCOME OF MISMATCHED BLOOD TRANSFUSION
Symptoms suggestive of acute hemolytic reaction include fever; shivering; pain in the back, chest, or elsewhere; dyspnea; hypotension; and shock. Some or all of these symptoms may occur within hours or even during the blood transfusion. In the latter case, transfusion must be stopped immediately. A specimen of pa-

tient's blood should be immediately taken and centrifuged, and the plasma examined by naked eye. If the plasma is not pink, hemolysis has not occurred and symptoms are due to other causes (other proteins contained in the blood may have caused reaction, blood may have been infected); under such circumstances, blood transfusion may be continued using a fresh bottle of blood [5]. If the plasma is pink, hemoglobin is present (at least 25 mg/dl), indicating that hemolysis has occurred; no further blood can be given, and the patient should be immediately treated to prevent ARF. It should be stressed however, that severe complications are rare after transfusion of less than 200 ml of red blood cells [501].

18.3 TREATMENT OF ACUTE HEMOLYTIC REACTION TO INCOMPATIBLE BLOOD
Once the diagnosis of acute hemolytic reaction has been supported by the pink color of the patient's blood, renal vasoconstriction secondary to hypovolemia, hypotension, and shock should be overcome by intensive intravenous

infusion of fluids. The i.v. infusion of large amounts (1 to 2 liters) of plasma expanders (such as low-molecular-weight dextran) has been suggested, associated with oxygen administration to increase the plasma-oxygen tension and compensate the resulting anemia [5]. Alternatively, isotonic saline solution should be given in great amounts in order to expand ECV and maintain high urine output.

Loop diuretics (e.g., furosemide 20 to 80 mg i.v.) have also been suggested in addition to saline infusion [501]. If diuretics are used, however, the resulting increase in urine output should be compensated with adequate salt and water replacement.

In case of severe reaction, it has also been suggested that heparin should be started immediately in order to prevent DIC [501]. When haemorrhagic diathesis occurs, in fact, it is an expression of a severe degree of DIC; at this point it is too late to begin anticoagulation [505]. Heparin may be given as 5,000 units loading dose to be followed by continuous i.v. infusion of 1,500 units per hour, for 6 to 24 hours (until the danger of DIC has passed), unless serious complications exclude anticoagulation [501].

Immediate exchange transfusion has been claimed to prevent ARF following mismatched transfusion by removing hemoglobin and circulating immune complexes [5].

Note

1. The MAC of an anesthetic agent is the minimal alveolar concentration of the anesthetic necessary to prevent movement in response to surgical incision in 50% of the patients. MAC-hour is one hour of anesthesia at a concentration of 1 MAC; thus two hours of anesthesia with 0.5 MAC will correspond to 1 MAC-hour.

References

1. Schrier RW, Conger JD. Acute renal failure: Pathogenesis, diagnosis and management. In Renal and Electrolyte Disorders, Schrier RW (ed). Boston: Little Brown and Co, 1980 (2nd ed), pp. 375–408.
2. Bull GM, Joekes AM, Lowe KG. Renal function studies in acute tubular necrosis. Clin Sci 9: 379–404, 1950.
3. Andreucci VE. Glomerular hemodynamics and autoregulation. Proc EDTA 11: 77–88, 1974.
4. Andreucci VE. Chronic renal failure. In The Treatment of Renal Failure, Castro JE (ed). Lancaster: MTP Press Limited, 1982, pp. 33–167.
5. de Wardener HE. The Kidney. An Outline of Normal and Abnormal Structure and Function. Edinburgh: Churchill Livingstone, 1973.
6. Kleeman CR, Narins RG. Diabetic acidosis and coma. In Clinical Disorders of Fluid and Electrolyte Metabolism, Maxwell MH, Kleeman CR (eds). New York: McGraw-Hill Book Co, 1980 (3rd ed), pp. 1339–1377.
7. Phillips SF. Water and electrolytes in gastrointestinal disease. In Clinical Disorders of Fluid and Electrolyte Metabolism, Maxwell MH, Kleeman CR (eds). New York: McGraw-Hill Book Co, 1980, pp. 1267–1290.
8. Seldin DW, Rector FC Jr. The generation and maintenance of metabolic alkalosis. Kidney Int 1: 305–321, 1972.
9. Narins RG, Jones ER, Stom MC, Rudnick MR, Bastl CP. Diagnostic strategies in disorders of fluid, electrolyte, and acid-base homeostasis. Am J Med 72: 496–520, 1982.
10. Arieff AI. Principles of parenteral therapy. In Clinical Disorders of Fluid and Electrolyte Metabolism, Maxwell MH, Kleeman CR (eds). New York: McGraw-Hill Book Co, 1972, pp. 567–589.
11. Orloff MJ, Chandler JG. Fluid and electrolyte disorders in burns. In Clinical Disorders of Fluid and Electrolyte Metabolism, Maxwell MH, Kleeman CR (eds). New York: McGraw-Hill Book Co, 1972, pp. 1043–1062.
12. Davies DM, Pusey CD, Rainford DJ, Brown JM, Bennett JP. Acute renal failure in burns. Scand J Plast Reconstr Surg 13: 189–192, 1979.
13. Minuth AN, Terrell JB Jr, Suki WN. Acute renal failure: A study of the course and prognosis of 104 patients and of the role of furosemide. Am J Med Sci 271: 317–324, 1976.
14. Andreucci VE, Dal Canton A. Can acute renal failure in humans be prevented? Proc EDTA 17: 123–132, 1980.
15. Wardle EN. Endotoxin and acute renal failure: A review. Nephron 14: 321–332, 1975.
16. Wardle N. Acute renal failure in the 1980s: The importance of septic shock and of endotoxemia. Nephron 30: 193–200, 1982.
17. Wardle N. Endotoxin shock. In Contraversies in Surgical Sepsis. New York: Praeger Publishing Co, 1980, pp. 199–206.
18. Wardle EN. Bacteremic and endotoxic shock. Br J Hosp Med 21: 223–231, 1979.
19. Jacob AI, Bistritz J, Spolter D, Bourgoignie JJ. Endotoxemic acute renal failure. Kidney Int 16: 774, 1979 (Abstract).
20. Conger JD, Schrier RW. Renal hemodynamics in acute renal failure. Annual Rev Physiol 42: 603–614, 1980.
21. Conger JD, Falk SA, Gugenheim SJ. Glomerular dynamics and morphological changes of the gener-

alized Shwartzman reaction. J Clin Invest 67: 1334–1346, 1981.

22. Simon G, Reindke S, Marget W. Lipoid-A-Antikörpertiter bei Pyelonephritis und anderen Infektionen mit gram-negativen Bakterien. Infection 2: 178–184, 1974.

23. Blake D, Hamlyn AN, Proctor S, Wardle EN. Anti-endotoxin (anti-Lipid-A) antibodies. Experientia 36: 254–255, 1980.

24. Wardle EN. Endotoxemia and the pathogenesis of acute renal failure. Q J Med 44: 389–395, 1975.

25. Krausz MM, Utsunomiya T, Feverstein G, Wolfe JHN, Shepro D, Hechtman HV. Prostacyclin reversal of lethal endotoxemia in dogs. J Clin Invest 67: 1118–1125, 1981.

26. Oliver JA. Participation of the prostaglandins in the control of renal blood flow during acute reduction of cardiac output in the dog. J Clin Invest 67: 229–237, 1981.

27. Pegues AS, Sofer SS, Mc Callum RE, Hinshaw LB. Removal of 14C-labeled endotoxin by activated charcoal. Int J Art Intern Organs 2: 153–158, 1979.

28. Braunwald E. Heart Disease. Philadelphia: WB Saunders Co, 1980.

29. Moseley MJ, Sawminathan R, Morgan B. Raised plasma urea levels after myocardial infarction. Arch Intern Med 141: 438–440, 1981.

30. Forrester JS, Chatterjee K, Jobin G. A new conceptual approach to the therapy of acute myocardial infarction. Adv Cardiol 15: 111–123, 1975.

31. Cohn JN, Franciosa JA. Pathophysiology of shock in acute myocardial infarction. In Progress in Cardiology, You PN, Goodwin JF (eds). Philadelphia: Lea & Febiger, 1973, pp. 207–234.

32. Hutton I, Pack AI, Lindsay RM, Lawrie TDV. Clinical significance of renal hemodynamics in acute myocardial infarction. Lancet 2:123–125, 1970.

33. Bastl CP, Rudnick MR, Narins RG. Diagnostic approaches to acute renal failure. In Acute Renal Failure, Brenner BM, Stein JH (eds). New York: Churchill Livingstone, 1980, pp. 17–51.

34. Valori C, Thomas M, Shillingford J. Free noradrenaline and adrenaline excretion in relation to clinical syndromes following myocardial infarction. Am J Cardiol 20: 605–617, 1967.

35. Lukomsky PE, Organov RG. Blood plasma catecholamines and their urinary excretion in patients with acute myocardial infarction. Am Heart J 83: 182, 1972.

36. Tristani FE, Cohn JN. Studies in clinical shock and hypotension. VII Renal hemodynamics before and during treatment. Circulation 42:839, 1970.

37. Yeboah ED, Petrie A, Pead JL. Acute renal failure and open-heart surgery. Brit Med J 1: 415, 1972.

38. Bhat JG, Gluck MC, Lowenstein J, Baldwin DS. Renal failure after open-heart surgery. Ann Intern Med 84: 677–682, 1976.

39. Myers BD, Hilberman M, Carrie BJ, Spencer RJ, Stinson EB, Robertson CR. Dynamics of glomerular ultrafiltration following open-heart surgery. Kidney Int 20: 366–374, 1981.

40. Abel R, Buckley J, Austen W, Barnett G, Beck G, Fischer J. Etiology, incidence and prognosis of renal failure following cardiac operations. J Thorac Cardiovasc Surg, 71: 323–333, 1976.

41. Myers BD, Carrie BJ, Yee RR, Hilberman M, Michaels AS. Pathophysiology of hemodynamically mediated acute renal failure in man. Kidney Int 18: 495–504, 1980.

42. Myers BD, Chui F, Hilberman M, Michaels AS. Transtubular leakage of glomerular filtrate in human acute renal failure. Am J Physiol 23: F319–F325, 1979.

43. Myers BD, Hilberman M, Spencer RJ, Jamison RL. Glomerular and tubular function in non-oliguric acute renal failure. Am J Med 72: 642–649, 1982.

44. Donker AJM, Arisz L, Brentjens JRH, Van Der Hem GK, Hollemans HJC. The effect of indomethacin on kidney function and plasma renin activity in man. Nephron 17: 288–296, 1976.

45. Arisz L, Donker AJ, Brentjens JR, Vanderhem GK. The effect of indomethacin on proteinuria and kidney function in the nephrotic syndrome. Acta Med Scand 199:121–125, 1976.

46. Muther RS, Potter DM, Bennett WM. Aspirin-induced depression of glomerular filtration rate in normal humans: Role of sodium balance. Ann Intern Med 94: 317–321, 1981.

47. McGiff JC, Crowshaw K, Terragno NA, Malik KU, Lonigro AJ. Differential effect of noradrenaline and renal nerve stimulation of vascular resistance in the dog kidney and the release of a prostaglandin E-like substance. Clin Sci 42: 223–233, 1972.

48. Gagnon DJ, Gauthclr R, Rejoli D: Release of prostaglandins from the rabbit perfused kidney: Effects of vaso-constrictors. Brit J Pharmacol 50:553–558, 1974.

49. Schnermann J, Briggs JP. Participation of renal cortical prostaglandins in the regulation of glomerular filtration rate. Kidney Int 19: 802–815, 1981.

50. Levenson DJ, Simmons CE, Brenner BM. Arachidonic acid metabolism, prostaglandins and the kidney. Am J Med 72: 354–374, 1982.

51. Walshe JJ, Venuto RC. Acute oliguric renal failure induced by indomethacin: Possible mechanism. Ann Intern Med 91: 47–49, 1979.

52. Zipser RD, Hoefs JC, Speckart PF, Zla PK, Horton R. Prostaglandins: Modulators of renal function and pressor resistance in chronic liver disease. J Clin Endocr Metab 48: 895–900, 1979.

53. Prescott LF. Analgesic nephropathy: A reassessment of the role of phenacetin and other analgesics. Drugs 23: 75–149, 1982.

54. Kimberly RP, Plotz PH. Aspirin-induced depression of renal function. N Engl J Med 296: 418–424, 1977.

55. Kimberly RP, Bowden RE, Keiser HR, Plotz PH.

Reduction of renal function by newer nonsteroidal anti-inflammatory drugs. Am J Med 64: 804–807, 1978.

56. Favre L, Glasson P, Vallotton MB. Reversible acute renal failure from combined triamterene and indomethacin: A study in healthy subjects. Ann Intern Med 96: 317–320, 1982.

57. Kimberly RP, Sherman RL, Mouradian J, Lockshin MD. Apparent acute renal failure associated with therapeutic aspirin and ibuprofen administration. Arthritis Rheum 22: 281–285, 1979.

58. Fong HJ, Cohen AH. Ibuprofen-induced acute renal failure with acute tubular necrosis. Am J Nephrol 2: 28–31, 1982.

59. Tan SY, Shapiro R, Kish MA. Reversible acute renal failure induced by indomethacin. JAMA 241: 2732–2733, 1979.

60. Kimberly RP, Gill JR, Bowden RE, Keiser HR, Plotz PH. Elevated urinary prostaglandins and the effects of aspirin on renal function in lupus erythematosus. Ann Intern Med 89: 336–341, 1978.

61. Kumin GD. Clinical nephrotoxicity of tobramycin and gentamicin. JAMA 244: 1808–1810, 1980.

62. Whelton A, Solez, K. Aminoglycoside nephrotoxicity. A tale of two transports. J Lab Clin Med 99: 148–155, 1982.

63. Appel GB, Neu HC. The nephrotoxicity of antimicrobial agents. N Engl J Med 296: 663–670, 722–728 and 784–787, 1977.

64. Smith CR, Baughman KL, Edwards CQ, Rogers JF, Leitman PS. Controlled comparison of amikacin and gentamicin. N Engl J Med 296: 349–353, 1977.

65. Lau WK, Young LS, Black RE, Winston DJ, Linne SR, Weinstein RJ, Hewitt WL. Comparative efficacy and toxicity of amikacin/carbenicillin versus gentamicin/carbenicillin in leukopenic patients: A randomized prospective trial. Am J Med 62: 959, 1977.

66. Keating MJ, Bodey GP, Valdivieso M, Rodriguez V. A randomized comparative trial of three aminoglycosides: Comparison of continuous infusion of gentamicin, amikacin and sisomycin combined with carbenicillin in the treatment of infections in neutropenic patients with malignancies. Medicine 58: 159, 1979.

67. French MA, Cerra FB, Plaut ME, Schentag JJ. Amikacin and gentamicin accumulation pharmacokinetics and nephrotoxicity in critically ill patients. Antimicrob Agents Chemother 19: 147, 1981.

68. Schor N, Ichikawa I, Rennke HG, Brenner BM. Comparative effects of tobramycin and gentamicin on glomerular function in the Munich-Wistar rat. Kidney Int 16: 776, 1979.

69. Schor N, Ichikawa I, Rennke HG, Troy JL, Brenner BM. Pathophysiology of altered glomerular function in aminoglycoside-treated rats. Kidney Int 19: 288–296, 1981.

70. Smith CR, Lipsky JJ, Laskin OL. Tobramycin is less nephrotoxic than gentamicin. Results of a double-blind clinical trial. 11th Int Congress of Chemotherapy and XIXth Interscience Conference on Antimicrobial Agents and Chemotherapy, 1–5 October 1979, Boston, Mass (Abstract).

71. Smith CR, Lipsky JJ, Laskin OL, Hellmann DB, Mellits ED, Longstreth J, Lietman PS. Double-blind comparison of the nephrotoxicity and auditory toxicity of gentamicin and tobramycin. N Engl J Med 302: 1106–1109, 1980.

72. Fong IW, Fenton RS, Bird R. Comparative toxicity of gentamicin versus tobramycin: A randomized prospective study. J Antimicrob Chemother 7: 81–88, 1981.

73. Herting RL, Lane AZ, Lorber RR, Wright JJ. Netilmicin: Chemical development and overview of clinical research. Scand J Infect Dis 23 (Suppl): 20–29, 1980.

74. Dahlager JI. The effect of netilmicin and other aminoglycosides on renal function. Scand J Infect Dis Suppl 23: 96–102, 1980.

75. Fabre J, Fillastre JP, Morin JP, Rudhardt M. Nephrotoxicity of gentamicin. Contr Nephrol 10: 53–62, 1978.

76. Hewitt WL. Gentamicin: Toxicity in perspective. Postgrad Med 50 (Suppl 7): 55–59, 1974.

77. Cowan RH, Jukkola AF, Arant BS Jr. Pathophysiologic evidence of gentamicin nephrotoxicity in neonatal puppies. Pediatr Res 14: 1204–1211, 1980.

78. Lane AZ, Wright GE, Blair DC. Ototoxicity and nephrotoxicity of amikacin. Am J Med 62: 911–918, 1977.

79. Kosek JC, Mazze RI, Cousins MJ. Nephrotoxicity of gentamicin. Lab Invest 30: 48–57, 1974.

80. Milman N. Renal failure associated with gentamicin therapy. Acta Med Scand 196: 87–91, 1974.

81. Olsen S. Renal histopathology in various forms of acute anuria in man. Kidney Int (Suppl) 10: S–2, 1976.

82. Wellwood JM, Lovell D, Thompson AE, Tighe JR. Renal damage caused by gentamicin. A study of the effects on renal morphology and urinary enzyme excretion. J Path 118: 171–182, 1976.

83. Bennett WM, Gilbert DN, Houghton DC, Porter GA. Gentamicin nephrotoxicity: Morphologic and pharmacologic features. West J Med 126: 65–68, 1977.

84. Solez K, Stout R, Bendush B, Silvia CB, Whelton A. Adverse effect of amino acid solutions in aminoglycoside-induced acute renal failure in rabbits and rats. In Acute Renal Failure, Eliahou HE (ed). London: John Libbey, 1982, pp. 241–247.

85. Saltissi D, Pusey CD, Rainford DJ. Recurrent acute renal failure due to antibiotic-induced interstitial nephritis. Brit Med J 1: 1182–1183, 1979.

86. Bennett WM. Aminoglycoside nephrotoxicity. Experimental and clinical considerations. Mineral Electrolyte Metab 6: 277–286, 1981.

87. Plager JE. Association of renal injury with com-

bined cephalothin-gentamicin therapy among patients severely ill with malignant disease. Cancer 37: 1937–1943, 1976.

88. Hsu CH, Kurtz TW, Easterling RE, Weller JM. Potentiation of gentamicin nephrotoxicity by metabolic acidosis. Proc Soc Exp Biol Med 146: 894–897, 1974.

89. Wade JC, Smith CR, Petty BG, Lipsky JJ, Conrad G, Ellner J, Lietmann PS. Cephalothin plus an aminoglycoside is more nephrotoxic than methicillin plus an aminoglycoside. Lancet II: 604–606, 1978.

90. Cronin RE. Aminoglycoside nephrotoxicity: Pathogenesis and prevention. Clin Nephrol 11: 251–256, 1979.

91. Trollfors B, Alestig K, Krantz I, Norrby R. Quantitative nephrotoxicity of gentamicin in nontoxic doses. J Infect Dis 141: 306–309, 1980.

92. Bennett WM, Luft F, Porter GA. Pathogenesis of renal failure due to aminoglycosides and contrast media used in roentgenography. Am J Med 69: 767–774, 1980.

93. Porter GA, Bennett WM. Nephrotoxic acute renal failure due to common drugs. Am J Physiol 241: F1–F8, 1981.

94. Kaloyanides GJ, Pastoriza-Munoz E. Aminoglycoside nephrotoxicity. Kidney Int 18: 571–582, 1980.

95. Rose BD. Acute renal failure. In Pathophysiology of Renal Disease, Rose BD (ed). New York: McGraw-Hill Book Co, 1981, pp. 55–95.

96. Sethi K, Diamond LH. Aminoglycoside nephrotoxicity and its predictability. Nephron 27: 265–270, 1981.

97. Gary NE, Buzzco L, Salaki J. Gentamicin-associated acute renal failure. Arch Intern Med 136: 1101–1104, 1976.

98. Bobrow SN, Jaffe E, Young RC. Anuria and acute tubular necrosis associated with gentamicin and cephalothin. JAMA 222: 1546–1547, 1972.

99. Kleinknecht D, Ganeval D, Droz D. Acute renal failure after high doses of gentamicin and cephalothin. Lancet 1: 1129, 1973.

100. Fillastre JP, Laumonier R, Humbert G, Dubois D, Metayer J, Delpech A, Leroy J, Robert M. Acute renal failure associated with combined gentamicin and cephalothin therapy. Brit Med J 2: 396–397, 1973.

101. Klastersky J, Hansgens C, Debusscher L. Empiric therapy for cancer patients: Comparative study of ticarcillin-tobramycin, ticarcillin-cephalothin, and cephalothin-tobramycin. Antimicrob Agents Chemother 7: 640–645, 1975.

102. Barza M. The nephrotoxicity of cephalosporins: An overview. J Infect Dis 137: S60–S73, 1978.

103. Leitman PS: Néphrotoxicité de la gentamicine et de la tobramycine associées á la méthicilline ou á la céfazoline. Nouv Presse Med 42: 3833–3834, 1978.

104. Green WH. Cephalosporin and aminoglycoside

nephrotoxic interaction. Ann Int Med 90: 435–436, 1979.

105. EORTC International Antimicrobial Therapy Project Group: Three antibiotic regimens in the treatment of infection in febrile granulocytopenic patients with cancer. J Infect Dis 137: 14–29, 1978.

106. Noel P, Levy VG. Toxicité rénale de l'association gentamicin-furosemide. Nouv Presse Med 7: 351–353, 1978.

107. Adelman RD, Spangler WL, Beasom F, Ishizaki G, Conzelman GM. Furosemide enhancement of experimental gentamicin nephrotoxicity. Comparison of function and morphological changes with activities of urinary enzymes. J Infect Dis 140: 342–352, 1979.

108. Mazze RI, Cousins M. Combined nephrotoxicity of gentamicin and methoxyflurane anesthesia in man. Brit J Anaesth 45: 394–397, 1973.

109. Dentino ME, Luft RC, Yum MN, Einhorn LH. Long-term effect of cis-diamminedichloride platinum on renal function and structure in man. Cancer 41: 1274–1281, 1978.

110. Churchill DN, Seely J. Nephrotoxicity associated with combined gentamicin-amphotericin B therapy. Nephron 19: 176–181, 1977.

111. Butkus DE, De Torrente A, Terman DS. Renal failure following gentamicin in combination with clindamycin. Nephron 17: 307–313, 1976.

112. Chiu PJS, Long JF. Effect of hydration on gentamicin excretion and renal accumulation in furosemide-treated rats. Antimicrob Agents Chemother 14: 214–217, 1978.

113. Bennett WM, Hartnett MN, Gilbert D, Houghton D, Porter GA. Effect of sodium intake on gentamicin nephrotoxicity in the rat. Proc Soc Exp Biol Med 151: 736–738, 1976.

114. Brinker K, Cronin R, Bulger R, Southern P, Henrich W. Potassium depletion risk factor for and consequence of gentamicin nephrotoxicity. Kidney Int 16: 849, 1979.

115. Atkinson RM, Currie JP, Davis B, Pratt DAH, Sharpe HM, Tomich EG. Acute toxicity of cephaloridine, an antibiotic derived from cephalosporin C. Toxicol Appl Pharmacol 8: 398–406, 1966.

116. Foord RD. Cephaloridine, cephalothin and the kidney. J Antimicrob Chemother 1: 119–133, 1975.

117. Harrison WO, Silverblatt FJ, Turck M. Gentamicin nephrotoxicity failure to three cephalosporins to potentiate injury in rats. Antimicrob Agents Chemother 8: 209–215, 1975.

118. Luft FC, Patel V, Yum MN, Kleit SA. Nephrotoxicity of cephalosporin-gentamicin combination in rats. Antimicrob Agents Chemother 9: 831–839, 1976.

119. Dellinger P, Murphy T, Barza M, Pinn V, Weinstein L. Effect of cephalothin on renal cortical concentration of gentamicin in rats. Antimicrob Agents Chemother 9: 587–588, 1976.

120. Bloch R, Luft FC, Rankin LI, Sloan RS, Yum MN, Maxwell DR. Protection from gentamicin

nephrotoxicity by cephalothin and carbenicillin. Antimicrob Agents Chemother 15: 46–49, 1979.

121. Dolislager D, Fravert D, Tune B. Interaction of aminoglycosides and cephaloridine in the rabbit kidney. Res Comm Chem Path Pharm 26: 13–23, 1979.

122. Tune BM, Fravert D. Mechanisms of cephalosporin nephrotoxicity: A comparison of cephaloridine and cephaloglycin. Kidney Int 18: 591–600, 1980.

123. Welles JS, Gibson WR, Harris PN, Small RM, Anderson RC. Toxicity distribution, and excretion of cephaloridine in laboratory animals. Antimicrob Agents Chemother 1965: 863–869, 1966.

124. Silverblatt F, Harrison WO, Turck M. Nephrotoxicity of cephalosporin antibiotics in experimental animals. J Infect Dis 128: S367–S372, 1973.

125. Lawson DH, Macadam RF, Singh H, Gavras H, Linton AL. The nephrotoxicity of cephaloridine. Postgrad Med J (Suppl) 46: 36–38, 1970.

126. Lawson DH, Macadam RF, Singh H, Gavras H, Hartz S, Turnbull D, Linton AL. Effect of furosemide on antibiotic-induced renal damage in rats. J Infect Dis 126: 593–600, 1972.

127. Norrby R, Stenquist K, Elgefors B. Interaction between cephaloridine and furosemide in man. Scand J Infect Dis 8: 209–212, 1976.

128. Child KJ, Dodds MG. Nephron transport and renal tubular effects of cephaloridine in animals. Br J Pharmacol Chemother 30: 354–370, 1967.

129. Silverblatt F, Turck M, Bulger R. Nephrotoxicity due to cephaloridine: A light- and electron-microscopic study in rabbits. J Infect Dis 122: 33–44, 1970.

130. Tune BM. Effect of organic acid transport inhibitors on renal cortical uptake and proximal tubular toxicity of cephaloridine. J Pharmacol Exp Ther 181: 250–256, 1972.

131. Tune BM, Wu KY, Kempson RL. Inhibition of transport and prevention of toxicity of cephaloridine in the kidney: Dose-responsiveness of the rabbit and the guinea pig to probenecid. J Pharmacol Exp Ther 202: 466–471, 1977.

132. Tune BM, Fernholt M. Relationship between cephaloridine and p-aminohippurate transport in the kidney. Am J Physiol 225: 1114–1117, 1973.

133. Tune BM, Fernholt M, Schwartz A. Mechanism of cephaloridine transport in the kidney. J Pharmacol Exp Ther 191: 311–317, 1974.

134. Tune BM, Wu KY, Longerbeam D, Holtzman D. Renal transport and toxicity of cephalosporins, including effects on tubular and mitochondrial respiration. Proc VIIth Int Congress of Nephrology, Basel, S Karger, 1978, pp. 279–287.

135. Kleinknecht D, Jungers P, Fillastre JP. Nephrotoxicity of cephaloridine. Ann Intern Med 80: 421–422, 1974.

136. Mandell GL. Cephaloridine. Ann Intern Med 79: 561–565, 1973.

137. Dodds MG, Foord RD. Enhancement by potent di-uretics of renal tubular necrosis induced by cephaloridine. Brit J Pharmacol 40: 227–236, 1970.

138. Linton AL, Bailey RR, Turnbull DI. Relative nephrotoxicity of cephalosporin antibiotics in an animal model. Can Med Ass J 107: 414–416, 1972.

139. Birkhead HA, Briggs GB, Saunders LZ. Toxicity of cefazolin in animals. J Infect Dis 128: S379–S381, 1973.

140. Tune BM. Relationship between the transport and toxicity of cephalosporins in the kidney. J Infect Dis 132: 189–194, 1975.

141. Turck M, Clark RA, Beaty HN: Cefazolin in the treatment of bacterial pneumonia. J Infect Dis 128: S382–S385, 1973.

142. Reinarz JA, Kier CM, Guckian JC. Evaluation of cefazolin in the treatment of bacterial endocarditis and bacteremias. J Infect Dis 128: S392–S395, 1973.

143. Rossi E, Savazzi GM, Ferrari C, Migone L. Insufficienza renale acuta secondaria a somministrazione di cefazolina. Min Nefrol 28: 493–496, 1981.

144. Perkins RL, Apicella MA, Lee IS, Cuppage FE, Saslaw S. Cephaloridine and cephalothin: Comparative studies of potential nephrotoxicity. J Lab Clin Med 71: 75–84, 1968.

145. Tune BM, Kempson RL. Nephrotoxic drugs. Brit Med J 3: 635, 1973.

146. Carling PC, Idelson BA, Casano AA, Alexander EA, McCabe WR. Nephrotoxicity associated with cephalothin administration. Arch Intern Med 135: 797–801, 1975.

147. Burton JR, Lichtenstein NS, Colvin RB, Hyslop NE Jr. Acute interstitial nephritis from oxacillin. Johns Hopkins Med J 134: 58–61, 1974.

148. Pasternak DR, Stephens BG. Reversible nephrotoxicity associated with cephalothin therapy. Arch Intern Med 135: 599–602, 1975.

149. Engle JE, Drago J, Carlin B, Schoolwerth AC. Reversible acute renal failure after cephalothin. Ann Intern Med 83: 232–233, 1975.

150. Cohen SN, Conte JE Jr. Drug-induced nephropathy. JAMA 227: 325, 1974.

151. Sanjad SA, Haddad GG, Nassar VH. Nephropathy, an underestimated complication of methicillin therapy. J Pediatr 84: 873–877, 1974.

152. Tobias JS, Whitehouse JM, Wrigley PFM. Severe renal dysfunction after tobramycin/cephalothin therapy. Lancet 1: 425, 1976.

153. Kunin CM, Furkleberg Z. Oral cephalexin and ampicillin: Antimicrobial activity, recovery in urine, and persistence in blood of uremic patients. Ann Intern Med 72: 349–356, 1970.

154. Fung-Herrera CG, Mulvaney WP. Cephalexin nephrotoxicity: Reversible nonoliguric acute renal failure and hepatotoxicity associated with cephalexin therapy. JAMA 229: 318–319, 1974.

155. Verma S, Kieff E. Cephalexin-related nephropathy. JAMA 234: 618–619, 1975.

156. Cutler RE, Blair AD, Kelly MR. Cefadroxil kinet-

ics in patients with renal insufficiency. Clin Pharmacol Ther 25: 514–521, 1979.

157. Trollfors B, Norrby R, Kristianson K. Effects on renal function of treatment with cefoxitin sodium alone or in combination with furosemide. J Antimicr Chem 4 (Suppl B): 85–89, 1978.

158. Clumeck N, Vanhoof R, Vanlaethem Y, Butzler JP. Cefotaxime and nephrotoxicity. Lancet 1: 835, 1979.

159. Ninane G. Cefotaxime and nephrotoxicity. Lancet 1: 332, 1979.

160. Saah AJ, Koch TR, Drusano GL. Cefoxitin falsely elevates creatinine levels. JAMA 247: 205–206, 1982.

161. Lentnek AL, Rosenworcel E, Kidd L. Acute tubular necrosis following high-dose cefamandole therapy for hemophilus-para-influenzae endocarditis. Am J Med Sci 281: 164–168, 1981.

162. Rozencweig M, Vanhoff DF, Slavik M, Muggia FM. Cis-diammine dichloroplatinum (II). Ann Intern Med 86: 803–812, 1977.

163. Rossof AH, Slayton RE, Perlia CP. Preliminary clinical experience with cis-diamminedichloroplatinum (II) (NSC 119875, CACP). Cancer 30: 1451–1456, 1972.

164. Lippman AJ, Helson C, Helson L, Krakoff IH. Clinical trials of cis-diamminedichloroplatinum (NSC 119875). Cancer Chemother Rep 57: 191–200, 1973.

165. Gonzales-Vitale JC, Hayes DM, Cvitkovic E, Sternberg SS. The renal pathology in clinical trials of cisplatinum (11) diamminedichloride. Cancer 39: 1362–1371, 1977.

166. Hayes DM, Cvitkovic E, Golbey RB, Scheiner E, Helson L, Krakoff IH. High-dose cis-platinum diamminedichloride. Cancer 39: 1372–1381, 1977.

167. Madias NE, Harrington JT. Platinum nephrotoxicity. Am J Med 65: 307–314, 1978.

168. Krakoff IH. Nephrotoxicity of cis-dichlorodiammineplatinum. Cancer Treat Rep 63: 1523–1525, 1979.

169. Dobyan DC, Levi J, Jacobs C, Kosek J, Weiner MW. Mechanism of cis-platinum nephrotoxicity. II Morphologic observations. J Pharmacol Exp Ther 213: 551–556, 1980.

170. Porter GA, Bennett WM. Nephrotoxin-induced acute renal failure. In Acute Renal Failure, Brenner BM, Stein JH (eds). New York: Churchill Livingstone, 1980, pp. 123–162.

171. Blackley JD, Hill JB. Renal and electrolyte disturbances associated with cisplatin. Ann Intern Med 95: 628–632, 1981.

172. Bitran JD, Desser RK, Billings AA, Kozloff MF, Shapiro CM. Acute nephrotoxicity following cis-dichlorodiammine-platinum. Cancer 49: 1784–1788, 1982.

173. Chopra S, Kaufman JS, Jones TW, Hong WK, Gehr MK, Hamburger RJ, Flammenbaum W, Trump BF. Cis-diamminedichlorplatinum-induced

acute renal failure in the rat. Kidney Int 21: 54–64, 1982.

174. Anderson T, Javadpour N, Schilsky R, Barlock A, Young RC. Chemotherapy for testicular cancer: Current status of the National Cancer Institute Combined Modality Trial. Cancer Treat Rep 63: 1687–1695, 1979.

175. Schilsky RL, Anderson T. Hypomagnesemia and renal magnesium wasting in patients receiving cisplatin. Ann Intern Med 90: 929–931, 1979.

176. Bar RS, Wilson HE, Mazzaferri EI. Hypomagnesemic hypocalcemia, secondary to renal magnesium wasting: A possible consequence of high-dose gentamicin therapy. Ann Intern Med 82: 646–649, 1975.

177. Cvitkovic E, Spaulding J, Bethune V, Martin J, Whitmore WF. Improvement of cis-dichlorodiammineplatinum (NSC 119875): Therapeutic index in an animal model. Cancer 39: 1357–1361, 1977.

178. Schwartz WB, Hurwit A, Ettinger A. Intravenous urography in the patient with renal insufficiency. N Engl J Med 269: 277–283, 1963.

179. Schencker B. Drip infusion pyelography: Indications and applications in urologic roentgen diagnosis. Radiology 83: 12–21, 1964.

180. Fry IK, Cattell WR. Radiology in the diagnosis of renal failure. Brit Med Bull 27: 148–152, 1971.

181. Mudge GH. Nephrotoxicity of urographic radiocontrast drugs. Kidney Int 18: 540–552, 1980.

182. Cattell WR. Excretory pathways for contrast media. Ivest Radiol 5: 473–486, 1970.

183. Newhouse JH, Pfister RC. The nephrogram. Radiol Clin North Am 17: 213–226, 1979.

184. Harkonen S, Kjellstrand C. Contrast nephropathy. Am J Nephrol 1: 69–77, 1981.

185. Milman N, Gottlieb P. Renal function after high-dose urography in patients with chronic renal insufficiency. Clin Nephrol 6:250–254, 1977.

186. Van Zee BE, Hoy WE, Talley TE, Jaenike JR. Renal injury associated with intravenous pyelography in nondiabetic and diabetic patients. Ann Intern Med 89: 51–54, 1978.

187. Webb JAW, Reznek RH, Cattell WR, Fry IK. Renal function after high-dose urography in patients with renal failure. Brit J Radiol 54: 479–483, 1981.

188. Teruel JL, Marcen R, Onaindla JM, Serrano A, Quereda C, Ortuno J. Renal function impairment caused by intravenous urography. A prospective study. Arch. Intern Med 141: 1271–1274, 1981.

189. D'Elia JA, Gleason RE, Alday M, Malarick C, Godley K, Warram J, Kaldany A, Weinrauch LA. Nephrotoxicity from angiographic contrast material. A prospective study. Am J Med 72: 719–725, 1982.

190. Hanaway J, Black J. Renal failure following contrast injection for computerized tomography. JAMA 238: 2056, 1977.

191. Byrd LH, Sherman RL, Stenzel KH, Rubin AL.

Computerized tomography-induced acute renal failure. Arch Intern Med 139: 491, 1979.

192. Harkonen S, Kjellstrand CM. Exacerbation of diabetic renal failure following intravenous pyelography. Am J Med 63: 939–946, 1977.

193. Weinrauch LA, Healy RW, Leland OS Jr, Goldstein HH, Kassissieh SD, Libertino JA, Takacs FJ, D'Elia JA. Coronary angiography and acute renal failure in diabetic azotemic nephropathy. Ann Intern Med 86: 56–59, 1977.

194. Shieh SD, Hirsch SR, Boshell BR, Pino JA, Alexander LJ, Witten DM, Friedman EA. Low risk of contrast media-induced acute renal failure in nonazotemic type 2 diabetes mellitus. Kidney Int 21: 739–743, 1982.

195. Vesely DL, Mintz DH. Acute renal failure in insulin-dependent diabetics. Episodes secondary to intravenous pyelography. Arch Intern Med 138: 1858–1859, 1978.

196. Kaur JS, Goldberg JP, Schrier RW. Acute renal failure following arteriography in a patient with polyarteritis nodosa. JAMA 247: 833–834, 1982.

197. Myers GH, Witten DM. Acute renal failure after excretory-urography in multiple myeloma. Am J Roentgenol 133: 583–588, 1971.

198. Anto HR, Chou SY, Porush JG, Shapiro WB. Infusion intravenous pyelography and renal function. Effects of hypertonic mannitol in patients with chronic renal insufficiency. Arch Intern Med 141: 1652–1656, 1981.

199. Porush JG, Chou SY, Anto HR, Oguagha C, Shapiro WB, Faubert PF. Infusion intravenous pyelography and renal function: Effects of hypertonic mannitol and furosemide in patients with chronic renal insufficiency. In Acute Renal Failure, Eliahou HE (ed). London: John Libbey, 1982, pp. 161–167.

200. Byrd L, Sherman RL. Radiocontrast-induced acute renal failure: A clinical and pathophysiologic review. Medicine 58: 270–279, 1979.

201. Shafi T, Chou SY, Porush JG, Shapiro WB. Infusion intravenous pyelography and renal function: Effects in patients with chronic renal insufficiency. Arch Intern Med 138: 1218–1221, 1978.

202. Swartz RD, Rubin JE, Leeming BW, Silva P. Renal failure following major angiography. Am J Med 65: 31–37, 1978.

203. Moreau JF, Droz D, Sabto J, Jungers P, Kleinknecht D, Hinglais N, Michel JR. Osmotic nephrosis induced by water-soluble triiodinated contrast media in man. Radiology 115: 329–336, 1975.

204. Borra S, Hawkins D, Deguid W, Kaye M. Acute renal failure and nephrotic syndrome after angiocardiography with meglumine diatrizoate. N Engl J Med 284: 592–593, 1971.

205. Davies P, Roberts MB, Roylance J. Acute reactions to urographic contrast media. Brit Med J 2: 434–437, 1975.

206. Witten DM. Reactions to urographic contrast media. JAMA 231: 974–977, 1975.

207. Kleinknecht D, Deloux J, Homberg JC. Acute renal failure after intravenous urography: Detection of antibodies against contrast media. Clin Nephrol 2: 116–119, 1974.

208. Minetti L, Barbiano Di Belgioioso G, Civati G, Durante A, Ratti F, Rovati C. Nefriti da ipersensibilità ai farmaci. Min Nefrol 21: 197–212, 1974.

209. Heideman M, Claes G, Nilson AE. The risk of renal allograft rejection following angiography. Transpl 21: 289–293, 1976.

210. Berdon WE, Schwartz RH, Becker J, Baker DH. Tamm-Horsfall proteinuria: Its relationship to prolonged nephrogram in infants and children and to renal failure following intravenous urography in adults with multiple myeloma. Radiology 92: 714–722, 1969.

211. Carvallo A, Rakowski TA, Argy WP Jr, Schreiner GE. Acute renal failure following drip infusion pyelography. Am J Med 65: 38–45, 1978.

212. Fang LST, Sirota RA, Ebert TH, Lichtenstein NS. Low fractional excretion of sodium with contrast media-induced acute renal failure. Arch Intern Med 140: 531–533, 1980.

213. Norby LH, Dibona GF. The renal vascular effects of meglumine diatrizoate. J Pharmacol Exp Ther 193: 932–940, 1975.

214. Forrest JB, Howards SS, Gillenwater JY. Osmotic effects of intravenous contrast agents on renal function. J Urol 125: 147–150, 1981.

215. Ziegler TW, Ludens JH, Fanestil DD, Talner LB. Inhibition of active sodium transport by radiographic contrast media. Kidney Int 7: 68–76, 1975.

216. Porter GA, Kloster FE, Bristow JD. Sequential effect of angiographic contrast agent on canine renal and systemic hemodynamics. Am Heart J 81: 80–92, 1972.

217. Cunningham JJ, Friedland GW, Thurber B. Immediate diuretic effects of intravenous sodium diatrizoate injections. Radiology 111: 85–88, 1974.

218. Mudge GH. Uricosuric action of cholecystographic agents. N Engl J Med 284: 929–933, 1971.

219. Postlethwaite AE, Kelley WN. Uricosuric effect of radiocontrast agents: A study in man of four commonly used preparations. Ann Intern Med 74: 845–852, 1971.

220. Gelman ML, Rowe JW, Coggins CH, Athanasoulis C. Effects of an angiographic contrast agent on renal function. Cardiov Med. 4: 313–320, 1979.

221. Schwartz RH, Berdon WE, Wagner J, Becker J, Baker DH. Tamm-Horsfall urinary mucoprotein precipitation by urographic contrast agents: In vitro studies. Am J Roentgenol 108: 698–701, 1970.

222. Goldstein EJ, Feinfeld DA, Fleischner GM, Elkin M. Enzymatic evidence of renal tubular damage following renal angiography. Radiology 121: 617–619, 1976.

223. Talner LB, Rushmer HN, Coel MN: The effect of renal artery injection of contrast material on urinary enzyme excretion. Invest Radiol 7: 311–322, 1972.

224. Alfrey AC, Rottschafer OW, Hutt MP. Acute parenchymal dysfunction with acute anuria induced by retrograde pyelography. Arch Intern Med 119: 214–217, 1967.

225. Hurley RM: Acute renal failure secondary to bilateral retrograde pyelography. Clin Pediat 18:754–756, 1979.

226. Krumlovsky FA, Simon N, Santhanam S, Del Greco F, Roxe D, Pomaranc MM. Acute renal failure. Association with administration of radiographic contrast material. JAMA 239: 125–127, 1978.

227. Wennberg JE, Okum R, Hinman EJ, Northcutt RC, Griep RJ, Walker WG. Renal toxicity of oral cholecystographic media. Bunamiodyl sodium and iopanoic acid. JAMA 186: 461–467, 1963.

228. Malt RA, Olken HG, Goade WJ. Renal tubular necrosis after oral cholecystography. Arch Surg 87: 743–746, 1963.

229. Setter JG, Maher JF, Schreiner GE. Acute renal failure following cholecystography. JAMA 184: 102–110, 1963.

230. Borges GF, Asplen CH, Wood C. Acute renal failure after oral cholecystography. Lancet 2: 340–342, 1964.

231. Duggan FJ, Rohner TJ. Acute renal insufficiency following oral cholecystography. J Urol 109: 156–159, 1972.

232. Canales CO, Smith GH, Robinson GD, Remmers AR, Sarles HE. Acute renal failure after the administration of iopanoic acid as an oral cholecystographic agent. N Engl J Med 281: 89–91, 1969.

233. Ansary Z, Baldwin DS. Acute renal failure due to radio-contrast agents. Nephron 17: 28–40, 1976.

234. Kelton J, Kelley WN, Holmes EW. A rapid method for the diagnosis of acute uric acid nephropathy. Arch Intern Med 138: 612–615, 1978.

235. Bevan DR. Renal Function in anesthesia and Surgery. London: Academic Press, 1979.

236. Bailey DR, Miller ED, Kaplan JA, Rogers PW. The renin-angiotensin-aldosterone system during cardiac surgery with morphine-nitrous oxide anesthesia. Anesthesiology 42: 538, 1975.

237. Paddock RB, Parker JW, Guadagni NP. The effects of methoxyflurane on renal function. Anesthesiology 25: 707–708, 1964.

238. Crandell WB, Pappas SG, MacDonald A. Nephrotoxicity associated with methoxyflurane anesthesia. Anesthesiology 27: 591–607, 1966.

239. Mazze RI, Shue GL, Jackson SH. Renal dysfunction associated with methoxyflurane anesthesia. A randomized prospective clinical evaluation. JAMA 216: 278–288, 1971.

240. Churchill D, Knaack J, Chirito E, Barre P, Cole C, Muehrcke R, Gault MH. Persisting renal insuf-

241. Mazze RI, Cousins MJ, Kosek JC. Dose-related methoxyflurane nephrotoxicity in rats: A biochemical and pathologic correlation. Anesthesiology 36: 571–587, 1972.

242. Cousins MJ, Mazze RI. Methoxyflurane Nephrotoxicity. A study of dose response in man. JAMA 225: 1611–1616, 1973.

243. Cousins MJ, Mazze RI. Biotransformation of enflurane (ethrane) and isoflurane (forane). Int Anesth Clin 12: 111, 1974.

244. Frascino JA, Vanamee P, Rosen PP. Renal oxalosis and azotemia after methoxyflurane anesthesia. N Engl J Med 283: 676, 1970.

245. Holaday DA, Rudofsky S, Treuhaft PS. The metabolic degradation of methoxyflurane in man. Anesthesiology 33: 579–593, 1970.

246. Mazze RI, Trudell JR, Cousins MJ. Methoxyflurane metabolism and renal dysfunction: Clinical correlation in man. Anesthesiology 35: 247–252, 1971.

247. Cousins MJ, Mazze RI, Kosek JC, Hitt BA, Love FV. The etiology of methoxyflurane nephrotoxocity. J Pharmacol Exp Ther 190: 530–541, 1974.

248. Frascino JA. Effect of inorganic fluoride on the renal concentrating mechanism. Possible nephrotoxocity in man. J Lab Clin Med 79: 192, 1972.

249. Roman RJ, Carter JR, North WC, Kauker ML. Renal tubular site of action of fluoride in Fischer 344 rats. Anesthesiology 46: 260–264, 1977.

250. Wickstrom I, Stefansson T. Effects of prolonged anesthesia with enflurane or halothane on renal function in dogs. Acta Anaesth Scand 25: 228–234, 1981.

251. Taves Dr, Gillies AJ, Freeman RB, Fry BW. Toxicity following methoxyflurane anesthesia. JAMA 214: 91–97, 1970.

252. Zucker S, Lautsch EV. Methoxyflurane anesthesia and renal function. N Engl J Med 283: 1226, 1970.

253. Aufderheide AC. Renal tubular calcium oxalate crystal deposition. Its possible relation to methoxyflurane anesthesia. Arch Path 92: 162–166, 1971.

254. Kuzucu EY. Methoxyflurane, tetracycline, and renal failure. JAMA 211: 1162–1164, 1970.

255. Panner BJ, Freeman RB, Roth-Moyo LA, Markowitch W Jr. Toxicity following methoxyflurane anesthesia. I Clinical and pathological observations in two fatal cases. JAMA 214: 86–90, 1970.

256. Proctor EA, Barton FL. Polyuric acute renal failure after methoxyflurane and tetracycline. Brit Med J 4: 661, 1971.

257. Barr GA, Mazze RI, Cousins MJ, Kosek JC. An animal model for combined methoxyflurane and gentamicin nephrotoxocity. Brit J Anaesth 45: 306–311, 1973.

258. Baden JM, Rice SA, Mazze RI. Deuterated me-

thoxyflurane anesthesia and renal function in Fischer 344 rats. Anesthesiology 56: 203–206, 1982.

259. Chase RE, Holaday DA, Fiserova-Bergerova V, Saidman LJ, Mack FE. The biotransformation of ethrane in man. Anesthesiology 35: 262–267, 1971.

260. Maduska AL. Serum inorganic fluoride levels in patients receiving enflurane anesthesia. Anesth Analg 53: 351–353, 1974.

261. Mazze RI, Calverley RK, Smith NT. Inorganic fluoride nephrotoxicity: Prolonged enflurane and halothane anesthesia in volunteers. Anesthesiology 46: 265–271, 1977.

262. Järnberg PO, Ekstrand J, Irestedt L, Santesson J. Renal fluoride excretion during and after enflurane anaesthesia: Dependency on spontaneous urinary pH-variations. Acta Anaesth Scand 24: 129–134, 1980.

263. Cousins MJ, Greenstein LR, Hitt BA, Mazze RI. Metabolism and renal effects of enflurane in man. Anesthesiology 44: 44–53, 1976.

264. Graves CL, Downs NH. Cardiovascular and renal effects of enflurane in surgical patients. Anesth Analg 53: 898–903, 1974.

265. Järnberg PO, Ekstrand J, Irestedt L, Santesson J. Fluoride kinetics and renal function during enflurane anesthesia. Acta Anaesth Scand (Suppl 71): 20–23, 1979.

266. Mazze RI, Cousins MJ, Barr GA. Renal effects and metabolism of isoflurane in man. Anesthesiology 40: 536–542, 1974.

267. Eichhorn JH, Hedley-Whyte J, Steinman TI, Kaufmann JM, Laasberg LH. Renal failure following enflurane anesthesia. Anesthesiology 45: 557–560, 1976.

268. Loehning RW, Mazze RI. Possible nephrotoxicity from enflurane in a patient with severe disease. Anesthesiology 40: 203–205, 1974.

269. Hartnett MN Lane W, Bennett WN. Nonoliguric renal failure and enflurane. Ann Intern Med 81: 560, 1974.

270. Schiffl H, Binswanger U. Renal handling of fluoride in healthy man. Renal Physiol 5: 192–196, 1982.

271. Prys-Roberts C. Isoflurane (Editorial). Brit J Anaesth 53: 1243–1245, 1981.

272. Cohen EN, Trudell JR, Edmunds HN, Watson E. Urinary metabolites of halothane in man. Anesthesiology 43: 392–401, 1975.

273. Gordon HL, Hunter JM. Ethylene glycol poisoning. A case report. Anaesthesia 37: 332–338, 1982.

274. Frommer JP, Ayus JC. Acute ethylene glycol intoxication. Am J Nephrol 2: 1–5, 1982.

275. Pons CA, Custer RP. Acute ethylene glycol poisoning. A clinicopathologic report of 18 fatal cases. Am J Med Sci 211: 544–552, 1946.

276. Hagemann PO, Chiffelle TR. Ethylene glycol poisoning. A clinical and pathologic study of three cases. J Lab Clin Med 33: 573–584, 1948.

277. Glasser L, Sternglanz PD, Combie J, Robinson A. Serum osmolality and its applicability to drug overdose. Am J Clin Path 60: 695–699, 1973.

278. Vonwartburg JP, Bethune JL, Vallee BL. Human-liver alcohol dehydrogenase. Kinetic and physicochemical properties. Biochemistry 3: 1775–1782, 1964.

279. Wacker WE, Haynes H, Druyan R, Fisher W, Coleman JE. Treatment of ethylene glycol poisoning with ethyl alcohol. JAMA 194: 173–175, 1965.

280. Peterson CD, Collins AJ, Himes JM, Bullock ML, Keane WF. Ethylene glycol poisoning. Pharmacokinetics during therapy with ethanol and hemodialysis. N Engl J Med 304: 21–23, 1981.

281. Underwood F, Bennett WM. Ethylene glycol intoxication: Prevention of renal failure by aggressive management. JAMA 226: 1453–1454, 1973.

282. Stokes JB, Averon F. Prevention of organ damage in massive ethylene glycol ingestion. JAMA 243: 2065–2066, 1980.

283. Parry MF, Wallach R. Ethylene glycol poisoning. Am J Med 57: 143, 1974.

284. Conger JD, Falk SA, Guggenheim SJ, Burke TJ. A micropuncture study of the early phase of acute urate nephropathy. J Clin Invest 58: 681–689, 1976.

285. Conger JD, Falk SA. Intrarenal dynamics in the pathogenesis and prevention of acute urate nephropathy. J Clin Invest 59: 786–793, 1977.

286. Rieselbach RE, Benzel CJ, Cotlove E, Frei E, Freireich EJ. Uric acid excretion and renal function in the acute hyperuricemia of leukemia. Am J Med 37: 872–884, 1964.

287. Sorensen LB, Levinson DJ. Origin and extrarenal elimination of uric acid in man. Nephron 14: 7–20, 1975.

288. Weinman EJ. Uric acid and the kidney. In The Kidney in Systemic Disease, Suki WN, Eknoyan G (eds). New York: John Wiley, 1976, pp. 141–158.

289. Rose BD. Tubulointerstitial diseases. In Pathophysiology of Renal Disease, Rose BD (ed). New York: McGraw-Hill, 1981, pp. 295–345.

290. Kjellstrand CM, Campbell DCII, von Hartitzsch B, Buselmeier TJ. Hyperuricemic acute renal failure. Arch Intern Med 133: 349–359, 1974.

291. Woolliscroft JO, Colfer H, Fox IH. Hyperuricemia in acute illness: A poor prognostic sign. Am J Med 72: 58–62, 1982.

292. Vanhille, P, Raviart B, Tacquet A, Jovet JP, Huart JJ, Bauters F, Goudemand M. Insuffisance rénale aigüe par hyperphosphatémie majèure an cours de leucémies aiguës lymphoblastiques. Nouv Presse Med 8: 3977–3979, 1979.

293. Kaplan BS, Herbert D, Morrell RE. Acute renal failure induced by hyperphosphatemia in acute lymphoblastic leukemia. Can Med Ass J 124: 429–431, 1981.

294. Warren DJ, Leitch AG, Leggett RF. Hyperuri-

cemic acute renal failure after epileptic seizures. Lancet 2: 385–387, 1975.

295. Klinenberg JR, Kippen L, Bluestone R. Hyperuricemia nephropathy. Pathological features and factors influencing urate deposition. Nephron 14: 88–98, 1975.

296. Crittenden DR, Ackerman GL. Hyperuricemic acute renal failure in disseminated carcinoma. Arch Intern Med 137: 97–99, 1977.

297. Yu TF, Berger L. The Kidney in Gout and Hyperuricemia. Mount Kisco, NY: Futura Publishing, 1982.

298. Wortmann RL, Fox IH. Limited value of uric acid to creatinine ratios in estimating uric acid excretion. Ann Intern Med 93: 822–825, 1980.

299. Lassiter WE. Uric acid and the kidney. In Strauss and Welt's Diseases of the Kidney, third edition, Earley LE, Gottschalk CW (eds). Boston: Little, Brown and Co, 1979, pp. 1217–1228.

300. Andreucci VE. Le Glomerulonefriti. Naples: Idelson, 1977.

301. Gelbart DR, Weinstein AB, Fajardo LF. Allopurinol-induced interstitial nephritis. Ann Intern Med 86: 196–198, 1977.

302. Grussendorf M, Andrassy K, Waldherr R, Ritz E. Systemic hypersensitivity to allopurinol with acute interstitial nephritis. Am J Nephrol 1: 105–109, 1981.

303. DeFronzo RA, Cooke CR, Wright JR, Humphrey RL. Renal function in patients with multiple myeloma. Medicine 57: 151–166, 1978.

304. Bernstein SP, Humes HD. Reversible renal insufficiency in multiple myeloma. Arch Intern Med 142: 2083–2086, 1982.

305. Martinez-Maldonado M. The kidney in sickle cell disease and multiple myeloma. In The Kidney in Systemic Disease, Suki WN, Eknoyan G (eds). New York: John Wiley, 1976, pp. 77–93.

306. Ng RCK, Suki WN. Treatment of acute renal failure. In Acute Renal Failure, Brenner BM, Stein JH (eds). New York: Churchill Livingstone, 1980, pp. 229–273.

307. De Fronzo RA, Humphrey RL, Wright JR, Cooke CR. Acute renal failure in multiple myeloma. Medicine 54: 209–223, 1975.

308. Misiani R, Remuzzi G, Bertani T, Licini R, Levoni P, Crippa A, Mecca G. Plasmapheresis in the treatment of acute renal failure in multiple myeloma. Am J Med 66: 684–688, 1979.

309. Beaufils M, Morel-Maroger L. Pathogenesis of renal disease in monoclonal gammopathies. Current concepts. Nephron 20: 125–131, 1978.

310. Wolf RE, Alperin JB, Ritzmann SE, Levin WC. IgG-K-Multiple myeloma with hyperviscosity syndrome. Response to plasmapheresis. Arch Intern Med 129: 114–117, 1972.

311. Feest TG, Burge PS, Cohen SL. Successful treatment of myeloma kidney by diuresis and plasmapheresis. Brit Med J 1: 503–504, 1976.

312. Kyle RA, Elveback LR. Management and prognosis of multiple myeloma. Mayo Clin Proc 51: 751–760, 1976.

313. Mundy GR, Raisz LG, Cooper RA, Schechter GP, Salmon SE. Evidence for the secretion of an osteoclast stimulating factor in myeloma N Engl J Med 291: 1041–1046, 1974.

314. Epstein FH. Calcium and the kidney. Am J Med 45: 700–714, 1968.

315. Duffy JL, Suzuki Y, Churg J. Acute calcium nephropathy: Early proximal tubular changes in the rat kidney. Arch Pathol 91: 340–350, 1971.

316. Schrier RW, Arnold PE, Burke TJ. Alterations in mitochondrial respiration and calcium movements in norepinephrine-induced acute renal failure: Modification by mannitol. In Acute Renal Failure, Eliahou HE (ed). London: John Libbey, 1982, pp. 21–22.

317. Schrier RW. Acute renal failure. JAMA 247: 2518–2525, 1982.

318. Benabe JE, Martinez-Maldonado M. Hypercalcemic nephropathy. Arch Intern Med 138: 777–779, 1978.

319. Humes HD, Ichikawa I, Troy JL, Brenner BM. Evidence for a parathyroid hormone-dependent influence of calcium on the glomerular ultrafiltration coefficient. J Clin Invest 61: 32–40, 1978.

320. Ichikawa I, Humes HD, Dousa TP, Brenner BM. Influence of parathyroid hormone on glomerular ultrafiltration in the rat. Am J Physiol 234: F393–F401, 1978.

321. Parfitt AM. Hypercalcemic nephropathy. Med J Aust 2: 127–134, 1964.

322. Schrier RW, Bulger RJ, Van Arsdel PP Jr. Nephropathy associated with penicillin and homologues. Ann Intern Med 64: 116–127, 1966.

323. Maher JF. Toxic nephropathy. In The Kidney, Brenner B, Rector FC Jr (eds). Philadelphia: Saunders, 1976, vol 2, pp. 1355–1395.

324. Kjellbo H, Stakeberg H, Mellgren J. Possibly thiazide-induced renal necrotising vasculitis. Lancet 1: 1034–1035, 1965.

325. Mills RM Jr. Severe hypersensitivity reactions associated with allopurinol. JAMA 216: 799–802, 1971.

326. Hewitt WL, Finegold SM, Monzon OT. Untoward side effects associated with methicillin therapy. Antimicrob Agents Chemother 1: 765–772, 1961.

327. Baldwin DS, Levine BB, McCluskey RT, Gallo GR. Renal failure and interstitial nephritis due to penicillin and methicillin. N Engl J Med 279: 1245–1252, 1968.

328. Border WA, Lehman DH, Egan JD, Sass HJ, Glode JE, Wilson CB. Antitubular basement membrane antibodies in methicillin-associated interstitial nephritis. N Engl J Med 291: 381–384, 1974.

329. Mayaud C, Kourilsky O, Kanfer A, Sraer JD. Interstitial nephritis after methicillin. N Engl J Med 292: 1132–1133, 1975.

330. Ooi BS, Wellington J, First MR, Mancilla R, Pollak VE. Acute interstitial nephritis: A clinical and

pathologic study based on renal biopsies. Am J Med 59: 614–629, 1975.

331. Olsen S, Asklund M. Interstitial nephritis with acute renal failure following cardiac surgery and treatment with methicillin. Acta Med Scand 199: 305–310, 1976.

332. Hansen ES, Tauris P. Methicillin-induced nephropathy. Acta Path Microbiol Scand Sect A 84: 440–442, 1976.

333. Mery JPh, Morel-Maroger L. Les néphrites interstitielles aiguës par hypersensibilité médicamenteuse. Ann Med Interne (Paris) 127: 590–595, 1977.

334. Gilbert DN, Gourley R, D'Agostino A, Goodnight SH Jr, Worthen H. Interstitial nephritis due to methicillin, penicillin and ampicillin. Ann Allergy 28: 378–385, 1970.

335. Mery JPh: Les néphropathies interstitielles aiguës provoquées par les pénicillines. Ann Méd Interne (Paris) 121: 811–816, 1970.

336. Kovnat P, Labovits E, Levison SP. Antibiotics and the kidney. Med Clin North Am 57: 1045–1063, 1973.

337. Colvin RB, Burton JR, Hyslop ME Jr, Spitz L, Lichtenstein NS. Penicillin-associated interstitial nephritis. Ann Intern Med 81: 404–405, 1974.

338. Orchard RT, Rooker G. Penicillin-hypersensitivity nephritis. Lancet 1: 689, 1974.

339. Geller M, Kriz RJ, Zimmerman SW, Flaherty DK, Dickie HA. Penicillin-associated pulmonary hypersensitivity reaction and interstitial nephritis. Ann Allergy 37: 183–190, 1976.

340. Tannenberg AM, Wicher KJ, Rose NR. Ampicillin nephropathy. JAMA 218: 449, 1971.

341. Maxwell D, Szwed JJ, Wahle W, Kleit SA. Ampicillin nephropathy JAMA 230: 586–587, 1974.

342. Ruley EJ, Lisi LM. Interstitial nephritis and renal failure due to ampicillin. J Pediat 84: 878–881, 1974.

343. Woodroffe AJ, Weldon M, Meadows R, Lawrence JR. Acute interstitial nephritis following ampicillin hypersensitivity. Med J Aust 1: 65–68, 1975.

344. Linton AL, Clark WF, Driedger AA, Turnbull DI, Lindsay RM. Acute interstitial nephritis due to drugs. Review of the literature with a report of nine cases. Ann Intern Med 93: 735–741, 1980.

345. Kleinknecht D, Homberg JC, Decroix G. Acute renal failure after rifampicin. Lancet 1: 1238–1239, 1972.

346. Decroix G, Pujet JC, Homberg JC, Feldman A, Kleinknecht D. Insuffisance rénal aiguë due à la rifampicine. Nouv Presse Med 2: 2093–2095, 1973.

347. Minetti L, Barbiano Di Belgioioso G, Civati G, Durante A, Scatizzi A, Surian M. Acute renal failure due to rifampicin. Proc EDTA 12: 210–217, 1975.

348. Nessi R, Bonoldi GL, Redaelli B, Di Filippo G. Acute renal failure after rifampicin: A case report and survey of the literature. Nephron 16: 148–159, 1976.

349. Alarcon Zurita A, Dalmau M, Piza C, Morey A, Ull M, Casellas G, De La Calle F. Fracaso renal agudo por rifampicina. Rev Clin Española 150: 209–210, 1978.

350. Robson M, Levi J, Dolberg L, Rosenfeld JB. Acute tubulointerstitial nephritis following sulfadiazine therapy. Isr J Med Sci 6: 561–566, 1970.

351. Minetti L, Barbiano Di Belgioioso G, Busnach G. Immunohistological diagnosis of drug-induced hypersensitivity nephritis. Contr Nephrol 10: 15–29, 1978.

352. Kalowski S, Nanra RS, Mathew TH, Kincaid-Smith P. Deterioration in renal function in association with cotrimoxazole therapy. Lancet 1: 394–397, 1973.

353. Dry J, Leynadier F, Herman D, Pradalier A. L'association sulfa-méthoxazole-triméthoprine (cotrimoxazole). Réaction immunoallergique inhabituelle. Nouv Presse Méd 4: 36, 1975.

354. Bailey RR, Little PJ. Deterioration in renal function in association with cotrimoxazole therapy. Med J Austr 1: 914–916, 1976.

355. Galpin JE, Shinaberger JH, Stanley TM, Blumenkrantz MJ, Bayer AS, Friedman GS, Montgomerie JZ, Guze LB, Coburn JW, Glassock RJ. Acute interstitial nephritis due to methicillin. Am J Med 65: 756–765, 1978.

356. Baker SB de C, Williams RT. Acute interstitial nephritis due to drug sensitivity. Brit Med J 1: 1655–1658, 1963.

357. Galea EG, Young LN, Bell JR. Fatal nephropathy due to phenindione sensitivity. Lancet 1: 920–922, 1963.

358. Hollman A, Wong HO. Phenindione sensitivity. Brit Med J 2: 730, 1964.

359. Smith K. Acute renal failure in phenindione sensitivity. Brit Med J 2: 24–26, 1965.

360. Sraer JD, Beaufils PH, Morel-Maroger L, Richet G. Néphrite interstitielle chronique due à la phènylindanedione faisant suite à une insuffisance rénale aiguë. Nouv Presse Méd 1: 193–196, 1972.

361. Chevet D, Garre M, Thomas R, Ramée MP, Goasguen J, Alquier P. Nephropathies induites par la phényl-indanedione. Intérêt du test d'inhibition de migration des leucocytes. Nouv Presse Med 5: 588, 1976.

362. Gaultier M, Bismuth C, Efthymiou ML, Morel-Maroger L, Romion A. Nephropathie tubulo-interstitielle aiguë au cours d'une introxication par la glafénine. Nouv Presse Med 1: 3125–3128, 1972.

363. Gaultier M, Bismuth C, Morel-Maroger M, Dauchy F. Néphropathie tubulo interstitielle aiguë au cours d'intoxications par la glafénine. Thérapie 29: 579–585, 1974.

364. Chevet D, Ramee MP, Garre M, Thomas R, Cartier F. Néphropathie aigue tubulo interstitelle anurique due à une intoxication par la glafénine. Therapie 29: 575–578, 1974.

365. Duplay H, Mattei M, Barillon D, Bauza R, Gaillot M, Kermarec J. Nephrite Tubulo-interstitielle aiguë par intoxication à la glafenine. Therapie 29: 593–597, 1974.

366. Chivrac D, Marti R, Fournier A, Faille N, Mes-

serschmitt J, Lorriaux A. Hémolyse immuno-aller-gique compliquée d'insuffisance rénale aiguë après ingestion de glafenine. Nouv Presse Med 3: 2578, 1974.

367. Rénier JC, Boasson M, Pitois M, Alquier Ph. In-suffisance rénale aiguë récidivante après ingestion de la glafénine à dose thérapeutique. Nouv Presse Méd 4: 670–671, 1975.

368. Andrieu J, Audebrand C, Chassaigne M, Renier E. Anémie Hémolytique et insuffisance rénale imputa-bles à la glafénine. Nouv Presse Méd 5: 2394–2395, 1976.

369. Rozen J, Homberg JC, Offenstadt G, Hericord Ph, Damecour C, Duron F. Insuffisance rénale aiguë à la glafénine. Nouv Presse Méd 7: 3255–3256, 1978.

370. Lery N, Descotes J, Loupi E, Evreux JC. Les effets indésirables de la glafénine. Lyon Med 240: 37–39, 1978.

371. Lobel A, Vanhille Ph, Dequiedt Ph, Raviart B, Tacquet A: Insuffisance rénale aiguë après ingestion d'antrafénine: Possibilité d'un mécanisme immuno-allergique. Nouv Presse Méd 8: n.13, 1979.

372. Agarwal BN, Cabebe FG, Hoffman BI. Biphenyl-hidantoin-induced acute renal failure. Nephron 18: 249–251, 1977.

373. Hyman LR, Ballow M, Knieser MR. Diphenylhy-dantoin interstitial nephritis. Roles of cellular and humoral immunologic injury. J Pediatr 92: 915–920, 1978.

374. Burton JR, Lichtenstein NS, Colvin RB, Hyslop NE Jr. Acute renal failure during cephalothin ther-apy. JAMA 229: 679–682, 1974.

375. Harrington JT, McCluskey RT. Fever, rash and renal failure after upper-respiratory-tract infection. N Engl J Med 293: 1308–1316, 1975.

376. Wiles CM, Assem ESK, Cohen SL, Fisher C. Ce-phadrine-induced interstitial nephritis. Clin Exp Immunol 36: 342–346, 1979.

377. Appel GB, Garvey G, Silva F, Francke E, Neu HC, Weissman J. Acute interstitial nephritis due to amoxicillin therapy. Nephron 27: 313–315, 1981.

378. Appel GB, Woda BA, Neu HC. Acute interstitial nephritis associated with carbenicillin therapy. Arch Intern Med 138: 1265–1267, 1978.

379. Roselle GA, Clyne DH, Kauffman CA. Carbenicil-lin nephrotoxicity. South Med J 71: 84–86, 1978.

380. Walker RG, Thomson NM, Dowling JP, Ogg CS. Minocycline-induced acute iterstitial nephritis. Brit Med J 1: 524, 1979.

381. Beirne GJ, Hansing CE, Octaviano GN, Burns RO. Acute renal failure caused by hypersensitivity to polymyxin B sulfate. JAMA 202: 62, 1967.

382. Rossi E, Silvestri MG, Manari A, Savazzi G, Mi-gone L. Acute renal failure and piromidic acid. Nephron 32: 80–82, 1982.

383. Lyons H, Pinn VW, Cortell S, Cohen JJ, Har-rington JT. Allergic interstitial nephritis causing reversible renal failure in four patients with idio-pathic nephrotic syndrome. N Engl J Med 288: 124–128, 1973.

384. Fialk MA, Romankiewicz J, Perrone F, Sherman RL. Allergic interstitial nephritis with diuretics. Ann Intern Med 81: 403–404, 1974.

385. Fuller TJ, Barcenas CG, White MG. Diuretic-in-duced interstitial nephritis. Occurrence in a patient with membranous glomerulonephritis. JAMA 235: 1998–1999, 1976.

386. Magil AB, Ballon HS, Cameron EC, Rae A. Acute interstitial nephritis associated with thiazide diuret-ics. Am J Med 69: 939–943, 1980.

387. Cartwright KC, Trotter TL, Cohen ML. Naproxen nephrotoxicity. Ariz Med 36: 124–126, 1979.

388. Brezin JH, Katz SM, Schwartz AB, Chinitz JL. Reversible renal failure and nephrotic syndrome as-sociated with nonsteroidal anti-inflammatory drugs. N Engl J Med 301: 1271–1273, 1979.

389. Handa SP. Renal effects of fenoprofen. Ann Intern Med 93: 508, 1980.

390. Lorch J, Lefavour G, Davidson H, Cortell S. Renal effects of fenoprofen. Ann Intern Med 93: 509, 1980.

391. Wendland ML, Wagoner RD, Holley KE. Renal failure associated with fenoprofen. Mayo Clin Proc 55: 103–107, 1980.

392. Curt GA, Kaldany A, Whitley LG, Crosson AW, Rolla A, Merino MJ, D'Elia JA. Reversible rapidly progressive renal failure with nephrotic syndrome due to fenoprofen calcium. Ann Intern Med 92: 72–73, 1980.

393. Gary NE, Dodelson R, Eisinger RP. Indometha-cin-associated acute renal failure. Am J Med 69: 135–136, 1980.

394. McLeish KR, Senitzer D, Gohara AF. Acute inter-stitial nephritis in a patient with aspirin hypersen-sitivity. Clin Immun Immunopathol 14: 64–69, 1979.

395. Ortuno J, Botella J. Recurrent acute renal failure induced by phenazone hypersensitivity. Lancet II: 1473–1476, 1973.

396. Richardson JH, Alderfer HH. Acute renal failure caused by phenylbutazone. N Engl J Med 268: 809, 1963.

397. Kuhlmann U, Fontana A, Briner J, Steinemann U, Seigenthaler W. Acute interstitielle Nephritis mit oligurischem Nierenversagen nach Phenylbut-tazon- Medikation. Schweiz Med Woch 108: 494–499, 1978.

398. Russel GI, Bing RF, Walls J, Pettigrew NM. In-terstitial nephritis in a case of phenylbutazone hy-persensitivity. Brit Med J 1: 1322, 1978.

399. McGowan WR, Vermillion SE. Acute interstitial nephritis related to cimetidine therapy. Gastroen-terology 79: 746–749, 1980.

400. Richman AV, Narayan JL, Hirschfield JS. Acute interstitial nephritis and acute renal failure associ-ated with cimetidine therapy. Am J Med 70: 1272–1274, 1981.

401. Rudnick MR, Bastl CP, Elfenbein IB, Sirota RA, Yudis M, Narins RG. Cimetidine-induced acute renal failure. Ann Intern Med 96: 180–182, 1982.

402. Faarup P, Christensen E. IgE-containing plasma

cells in acute tubulo-interstitial nephropathy. Lancet 2: 718, 1974.

403. Sloth K, Thomsen AC. Acute renal insufficiency during treatment with azathioprine. Acta Med Scand 189: 145–148, 1971.

404. Owen D. Renal failure due to para-amino salicylic acid. Brit Med J 2: 483, 1958.

405. Fillastre JP, Morel-Maroger L, Mignon F, Mery JPh. Les néphropathies aiguës médicamenteuses. Actualités Nephrol Hôp Necker. Paris: Flammarion, 1969, pp. 155–193.

406. Luderer JR, Schoolwerth AC, Sinicrope RA, Ballard JO, Lookingbill DP, Hayes AH Jr. Acute renal failure, hemolytic anemia and skin rash associated with captopril therapy. Am J Med 71: 493–496, 1981.

407. Richet G, Sraer JD, Kourilsky O, Kanfer A, Mignon F, Whitworth J, Morel-Maroger L. La ponction biopsies rénale dans les insuffisance rénales aiguës. Ann Méd Interne (Paris) 129: 335–337, 1978.

408. Wilson DM, Turner DR, Cameron JS, Ogg CS, Brown CB, Chantler C. Value of renal biopsy in acute intrinsic renal failure. Brit Med J 2: 459–461, 1976.

409. Heptinstall RH. Interstitial nephritis: A brief review. Am J Pathol 83: 214–236, 1976.

410. van Ypersele de Strihou C. Acute oliguric interstitial nephritis. Kidney Int 16: 751–765, 1979.

411. Olsen S, Hansen ES, Jepsen FL. The prevalence of focal tubulointerstitial lesions in various renal diseases. Acta Path Microbiol Scand Sect A 89: 137–145, 1981.

412. Richet G, Mayaud C. The course of acute renal failure in pyelonephritis and other types of interstitial nephritis. Nephron 22: 124–127, 1978.

413. Pasternack A, Helin H, Vanttinen T, Jarventie G, Vesikari T. Acute tubulointerstitial nephritis in a patient with mycoplasma pneumoniae infection. Scand J Infect Dis 11: 85, 1979.

414. Andres GA, McCluskey RT. Tubular and interstitial renal disease due to immunologic mechanisms. Kidney Int 7: 271–289, 1975.

415. Van Zwieten MJ, Leber PD, Bhan AK, McCluskey RT. Experimental cell-mediated interstitial nephritis induced with exogenous antigens. J Immunol 118: 589–593, 1977.

416. Kleinknecht D, Kanfer A, Morel-Maroger L, Mery JPh. Immunologically mediated drug-induced acute renal failure. Contrib Nephrol 10: 42–52, 1978.

417. Mery JP, Morel-Maroger L. Acute interstitial nephritis. A hypersensitivity reaction to drugs. Proc 6th Int Congress of Nephrology (Florence, June 8–12, 1975) S Karger Publ, Basel, 1976, pp. 524–529.

418. Gabow PA, Lacher JW, Nelf TA. Tubulointerstitial and glomerular nephritis associated with rifampicin. JAMA 235: 2517–2518, 1976.

419. Poole G, Stradling P, Worlledge S. Potentially serious side effects of high-dose twice weekly rifampicin. Brit Med J 3: 343–347, 1971.

420. Lakshminarayan S, Sahn SA, Hudson LD. Massive hemolysis caused by rifampicin. Brit Med J 2: 282–283, 1973.

421. Stradling P. Side Effects observed during intermittent rifampicin therapy. Scand J Resp Dis 84: S129–S131, 1973.

422. Möhring K, Asbach HW, Schubothe H, Weber S. Hämolytische Krise mit akutem Nierenversagen unter Rifampicin-Behandlung. Dt med Wschr 99: 1458–1462, 1974.

423. Germann HJ, Hoppe-Seyler GF, Boesken WH. Akutes Nierenversagen nach Rifampicin. Dt med Wschr 99: 1454–1457, 1974.

424. Poole G, Stradling P, Worlledge S. Postgrad Med J 47: 742, 1971.

425. Flynn CT, Rainford DJ, Hope E. Acute renal failure and rifampicin: Danger of unsuspected intermittent dosage. Brit Med J 1: 482, 1974.

426. Tacquet A, Devulder B, Lelievre G, Duchatelle P, Capier P, Cuvelier D, Wambergue F. Pharmacocinétique et tolérance renale de la rifampicin. Lille Méd 17: 1366–1377, 1972.

427. Devulder B, Lelievre G, Capier P, Tacquet A. Insuffisance rénale aigué due à la rifampicine. Nouv Presse Méd 2: 2691, 1973.

428. Campese UM, Marzullo F, Schena FP, Coratelli P. Acute renal failure during intermittent rifampicin therapy. Nephron 10: 256–261, 1973.

429. Kleinknecht D, Adhemar JP. Les insuffisances rénales aiguës dues à la rifampicine. Méd Mal Infect 7: 117–121, 1977.

430. Rothwell DL, Richmond DE. Hepatorenal failure with self-initiated intermittent rifampicin therapy. Brit Med J 2: 481–482, 1974.

431. Rennke HG, Roos PC, Wall SG. Drug-induced interstitial nephritis with heavy glomerular proteinuria. N Engl J Med 302: 691–692, 1980.

432. Ooi BS, First MR, Pesce AJ, Pollak VE, Bernstein IL, Jao W. IgE levels in interstitial nephritis. Lancet 1: 1254–1256, 1974.

433. Wood BC, Sharma JN, Germann DR, Wood WG, Crouch TT. Gallium citrate Ga 67 imaging in noninfectious interstitial nephritis. Arch Intern Med 138: 1665–1666, 1978.

434. Simenhoff ML, Guild WR, Dammin GJ. Acute diffuse interstitial nephritis. Am J Med 44: 618–625, 1968.

435. Jensen HA, Halveg AB, Saunamaki KI. Permanent impairment of renal function after methicillin nephropathy. Brit Med J 4: 406, 1971.

436. Aerenlund-Jensen H, Halveg AB, Saunamaki KI. Permanent impairment of renal function after methicillin nephropathy. Brit Med J 4: 406, 1971.

437. Woodroffe AJ, Thomson NM, Meadows R, Lawrence JR. Nephropathy associated with methicillin administration. Aust N Z J Med 256–261, 1974.

438. Pasternack A, Tallquist G, Kuhlback B. Occurrence of interstitial nephritis in acute renal failure. Acta Med Scand 187: 27–31, 1970.

439. Chazan JA, Garella S, Esparza A. Acute interstitial

nephritis. A distinct clinico-pathological entity? Nephron 9: 10–26, 1972.

440. Brass H, Lapp H, Heinz R. Akute interstitielle Nephritis-mögliche Ursache eines akuten Nierenversagens. Deutsch Med Wschr 99: 2335–2340, 1974.

441. Frommer P, Uldall R, Fay WP, Deveber GA. A case of acute interstitial nephritis successfully treated after delayed diagnosis. Can Med Ass J 121: 585–591, 1979.

442. Prescott LF, Wright N. The effects of hepatic and renal damage on paracetamol metabolism and excretion following overdosage. A pharmacokinetic study. Brit J Pharmacol 49: 602–613, 1973.

443. McJunkin B, Barwick KW, Little WC, Winfield JB. Fatal massive hepatic necrosis following acetaminophen overdose. JAMA 236: 1874–1875, 1976.

444. Wilkinson SP, Moodie H, Arroyo VA, Williams R. Frequency of renal impairment in paracetamol overdose compared with other causes of acute liver damage. J Clin Path 30: 141–143, 1977.

445. Mitchell JR, McMurtry RJ, Statham CN, Nelson SD. Molecular basis for several drug-induced nephropathies. Am J Med 62: 518–526, 1977.

446. Kleinman JG, Breitenfield RV, Roth DA. Acute renal failure associated with acetaminophen ingestion: Report of a case and review of the literature. Clin Nephrol 14: 201–205, 1980.

447. Cobden I, Record CO, Ward MK, Kerr DNS. Paracetamol-induced acute renal failure in the absence of fulminant liver damage. Brit Med J 284: 21–22, 1982.

448. Curry RW Jr, Robinson JD, Sughrue MJ. Acute renal failure after acetaminophen ingestion. JAMA 247: 1012–1013, 1982.

449. Prescott LF, Illingworth RN, Critchley JAJII, Stewart MJ, Adam RD, Proudfoot AT. Intravenous N-acetylcysteine: The treatment of choice for paracetamol poisoning. Brit Med J 2: 1097–1100, 1979.

450. Ganeval D, Grunfeld JP, Eloy L, Lacour B, Russo-Marie F, Noel LH, Anagnostopoulos T. Glaphenine-induced acute renal failure in the rat: A new experimental model. Am J Physiol 243: F416–F423, 1982.

451. Mirouze J, Barjon P, Mion Ch, Fourcade J, Monnier L, Marty L. Insuffisance rénale aiguë consécutive à l'absorption de glafénine. Thérapie 29: 587–592, 1974.

452. Peterfalvi M, Deraedt R, Pottier J, Vannier B, Boissier JR. Mécanisme des effets rénaux de hautes doses de glafénine chez le rat. Therapie 34: 377–391, 1979.

453. Vanholder R, Colardyn F, De Reuck J, Praet M, Lameire N, Ringoir S: Diquat intoxication. Am J Med 70: 1267–1271, 1981.

454. Malone JDG, Carmody M, Keogh B, O'Dwyer WF. Paraquat poisoning—A review of nineteen cases. J Irish Med Ass 64: 59–68, 1971.

455. Fitzgerald GR, Barniville G, Black J, Silke B, Carmody M, O'Dwyer WF. Paraquat poisoning in agricultural workers. J Irish Med Ass 71: 336–342, 1978.

456. Oreopoulos DG, Soyannwo MAO, Sinniah R, Fenton SSA, Mcgeon MG, Bruce JH. Acute renal failure in case of paraquat poisoning. Brit Med J 1: 749–750, 1968.

457. Editorial. Paraquat poisoning. Lancet 1: 1057, 1976.

458. Beebeejaun AR, Beevers G, Rogers WN. Paraquat poisoning: Prolonged excretion. Clin Toxicol 4: 397–407, 1971.

459. Vaziri ND, Ness RL, Fairshter RD, Smith WR, Rosen SM: Nephrotoxicity of paraquat in man. Arch Intern Med 139: 172–174, 1979.

460. Fitzgerald GR, Barniville G, Dickstein K, Carmody M, O'Dwyer W. Experience with Fuller's earth in paraquat poisoning. J Irish Med Ass 72: 149–152, 1979.

461. McCurdy DK, Frederick M, Elkinton JR. Renal tubular acidosis due to amphotericin B. N Engl J Med 278: 124–131, 1968.

462. Cronin RE. Antimicrobial agent nephrotoxicity. In Clinical Use of Drugs in Patients with Kidney and Liver disease, Anderson RJ, Schrier RW (eds). Philadelphia: W B Saunders, 1981, pp. 54–65.

463. Costantino D, Falzi G, Langer M, Rivolta E. Amanita-phalloides-related nephropathy. Contr Nephrol 10: 84–97, 1978.

464. Vercellone A, Piccoli G, Ragni R, Cavalli PL, Varese D, Zuccari G. La nefropatia da funghi. Min Nefrol 15: 31–48, 1968.

465. Walker DH, Mattern WD. Acute renal failure in Rocky Mountain spotted fever. Arch Intern Med 139: 443, 1979.

466. Chugh KS, Aikat BK, Sharma BK, Dash SC, Mathew MT, Das KC. Acute renal failure following snakebite. Am J Trop Med Hyg 24: 692–697, 1975.

467. Seedat YK, Reddy J, Edington DA. Acute renal failure due to proliferative nephritis from snake bite poisoning. Nephron 13: 455–463, 1974.

468. Shastry JCM, Date A, Carman RH, Johny KV. Renal failure following snake bite. Am J Trop Med Hyg 26: 1032–1038, 1977.

469. Dasilva OA, Lopez M, Godoy P. Bilateral cortical necrosis and calcification of the kidneys following snakebite: A case report. Clin Nephrol 11: 136–139, 1979.

470. Gjessing J. Renal failure in acute pancreatitis. Brit Med J 4: 359–360, 1972.

471. Goldstein DA, Llach F, Massry SG. Acute renal failure in patients with acute pancreatitis. Arch Intern Med 136: 1363–1365, 1976.

472. Gordon D, Calne RY. Renal failure in acute pancreatitis. Brit Med J 3: 801–802, 1972.

473. Seedat YK, Hitchcock PJ. Acute renal failure from Callilepsis laureola. S Afr Med J 45: 832–833, 1971.

474. Jones RH, Shuhaiber H, Noble C, Keats J, Parsons V. Primary meningococcal pericarditis complicated by acute renal failure. Thorax 34: 688–689, 1979.

475. Batey R, Scott J, Jain S, Sherlock S. Acute renal insufficiency occurring during intravenous desferrioxamine therapy. Scand J Haematol 22: 277–279, 1979.

476. Rossen B, Steiness I. The pathophysiology of acute renal failure after chlorprothixene overdosage. Acta Med Scand 209: 525–527, 1981.

477. Klintmalm GBG, Iwatsuki S, Starzl TE. Nephrotoxicity of Cyclosporin A in liver and kidney transplant patients. Lancet 1: 470–471, 1981.

478. Sweny P, Hopper J, Gross M, Varghese Z, Whiting PH. Nephrotoxicity of Cyclosporin A. Lancet 1: 663–664, 1981.

479. Calne RY, Rolles K, White DJG, Thiru S, Evans DE, McMaster P, Dunn DC, Craddock GN, Henderson RG, Aziz S, Lewis P. Cyclosporin A initially as the only immunosuppressant in 34 recipients of cadaveric organs: 32 kidney, 2 pancreases and 2 livers. Lancet 2: 1033–1036, 1979.

480. Calne RY. Cyclosporin. Nephron 26: 57–63, 1980.

481. Hamilton DV, Evans DB, Henderson RG, Thiru S, Calne RY, White DJG, Carmichael DJS. Nephrotoxicity and metabolic acidosis in transplant patients on cyclosporin. A Proc EDTA 18: 400–409, 1981.

482. Vidt DG, Bravo EL, Fouad FM. Captopril. N Engl J Med 306: 214–219, 1982.

483. Blumberg AL, Denny SE, Marshall GR, Needleman P. Blood vessel-hormone interactions: Angiotensin, bradykinin, and prostaglandins. Am J Physiol 232: H305–H310, 1977.

484. Swartz SL, Williams GH, Hollenberg NK, Levine L, Dluhy RG, Moore TJ. Captopril-induced changes in prostaglandin production. J Clin Invest 65: 1257–1264, 1980.

485. Moore TJ, Crantz FR, Hollenberg NK, Koletsky RJ, Leboff MS, Swartz SL, Levine L, Podolsky S, Dluhy RG, Williams GH. Contribution of prostaglandins to the antihypertensive action of captopril in essential hypertension. Hypertension 3: 168–173, 1981.

486. Johnston CI, Millar JA, McGrath BP, Matthews PG. Long-term effects of captopril (SQ14255) on blood-pressure and hormone levels in essential hypertension. Lancet 2: 493–496, 1979.

487. Farrow PR, Wilkinson R. Reversible renal failure during treatment with captopril. Brit Med J 1: 1680, 1979.

488. Woodhouse K, Farrow PR, Wilkinson R. Reversible renal failure during treatment with captopril. Brit Med J 2: 1146–1147, 1979.

489. Collste P, Haglund K, Lundgren G, Magnusson G, Ostman J. Reversible renal failure during treatment with captopril. Brit Med J 2: 612–613, 1979.

490. Grossman A, Eckland D, Price P, Edwards CRW. Captopril, reversible renal failure with severe hyperkalemia. Lancet 1: 712, 1980.

491. Hricik DE, Browning PJ, Kopelman R, Goorno WE, Madias NE, Dzau VJ. Captopril-induced functional renal insufficiency in patients with bilateral renal-artery stenoses or renal-artery stenosis in a solitary kidney. N Engl J Med 308: 373–376, 1983.

492. Curtis JJ, Luke RG, Whelchel JD, Diethelm AG, Jones P, Dustan HP. Inhibition of angiotensin-converting enzyme in renal-transplant recipients with hypertension. N Engl J Med 308: 377–381, 1983.

493. Hall JE, Guyton AC, Jackson TE, Coleman TG, Lohmeier TE, Trippodo NC. Control of glomerular filtration rate by renin-angiotensin system. Am J Physiol 233: F366–F372, 1977.

494. Hall JE, Coleman TG, Guyton AC, Balfe JW, Salgado HC. Intrarenal role of angiotensin II and [des-Asp^1] angiotensin II. Am J Physiol 236: F252–F259, 1979.

495. Graham JE. Efferent arterioles of glomeruli in the juxtamedullary zone of the human kidney. Anat Rec 125: 521–529, 1956.

496. Barahas L, Satta H. A three-dimensional study of the juxtaglomerular apparatus in the rat. Lab Invest 12: 257–269, 1963.

497. Andreucci VE, Dal Canton A, Corradi A, Stanziale R, Migone L. Role of the efferent arteriole in glomerular hemodynamics of superficial nephrons. Kidney Int 9: 475–480, 1976.

498. Navar LG, Lagrange RA, Bell PD, Thomas CE, Ploth DW. Glomerular and renal hemodynamics during converting enzyme inhibition (SQ20,881) in the dog. Hypertension 1: 371–377, 1979.

499. Brenner BM, Troy JL, Daugharty TM, Deen WM, Robertson CR. Dynamics of glomerular ultrafiltration in the rat. II Plasma flow dependence of GFR. Am J Physiol 223: 1184–1190, 1972.

500. Brunner HR, Gavras H, Waeber B, Kershaw GR, Turini GA, Vukovich RA, McKinstry DN, Gavras I. Oral angiotensin-converting enzyme inhibitor in long-term treatment of hypertensive patients. Ann Intern Med 90: 19–23, 1979.

501. Goldfinger D. Acute hemolytic transfusion reactions: A fresh look at pathogenesis and considerations regarding therapy. Transfusion 17: 85–98, 1977.

502. Birndorf N, Lopas H. Effects of red cell stroma-free hemoglobin solution on renal function in monkeys. J Appl Physiol 29: 573, 1970.

503. Relihan M, Litwin MS. Clearance rate and renal effects of stroma-free hemoglobin on acidotic dogs. Surg Gynecol Obstet 137: 73, 1973.

504. Schmidt PJ, Holland PV. Pathogenesis of the acute renal failure associated with incompatible transfusion. Lancet 2: 1169–1170, 1967.

505. Rock RC, Bove JR, Nemerson Y. Heparin treatment of intravascular coagulation accompanying hemolytic transfusion reactions. Transfusion 9: 57, 1969.

3. PREVENTION OF ISCHEMIC/TOXIC ACUTE RENAL FAILURE IN HUMANS

Vittorio E. Andreucci

1. Introduction

ARF is a preventable disease. Statistical evaluation of the frequency of ARF appears to support this view. Thus, during World War II, one in every 20 casualties developed ARF; during the Korean War, the incidence fell to one in every 800; during the Vietnam War, it further fell to one in every 1,800 casualities. The incidence of ARF in patients who have undergone cardiovascular surgery has recently fallen from 30 to 2.7% [1].

Undoubtedly early replacement of blood, fluid, and electrolytes plays a primary role in the prevention of ARF secondary to hemorrhage or to renal or extrarenal losses of salt and water. But this measure alone is not sufficient to reduce the incidence of ARF, particularly in severely ill patients and also in patients with mild infections.

Further general precautions should always be taken into consideration [1]:

a. Reduction in dosage of aminoglycosides in elderly patients (in whom creatinine clearance is presumably lowered) and in patients with pre-existent renal insufficiency.

b. Prevention of volume depletion in patients treated with nephrotoxic antibiotics or receiving radiocontrast media or undergoing general anesthesia.

c. Non use of long-term treatment with aminoglycosides, or aminoglycoside with cephalosporin, aminoglycoside with furosemide, or aminoglycoside with nephrotoxins

(such as radiocontrast media or methoxyflurane).

d. Maintenance of cardiac output, particularly in surgical patients (very important in open-heart surgery), by dopamine hydrochloride or volume expansion [1, 2].

e. Maintenance of a high urine output with alkalinization of urine when hyperuricemia is expected (such as during treatment of malignancies with cytotoxic drugs).

f. Caution in the concurrent use of aminoglycoside antibiotics and intravenous infusion of amino acids (in a program of parenteral nutrition) in severely ill patients; it has been recently demonstrated, in fact, that daily i.v. infusion of commercially available mixtures of amino acids (Freamine, Nephramine) in rabbits and rats treated with gentamicin or tobramycin increases severity and rapidity of onset of aminoglycoside-induced ARF [3].

g. Non use of nonsteroidal anti-inflammatory drugs in those clinical conditions in which vasoconstrictor forces are operative [4]: volume depletion, nephrotic syndrome, cirrhosis with ascites and congestive heart failure. These represent, in fact, clinical conditions of reduced effective blood volume in which indomethacin and other nonsteroidal anti-inflammatory drugs may cause ARF (see chapter 2, section 6).

But this list of precautions represents a simplification of a very complex problem, since ARF has usually a multifactorial etiology.

In many reports, while listing the different forms of ARF, only the main cause is usually indicated. This information is not correct. It is actually misleading. It has been clearly demonstrated, in fact, that an additive interaction usually occurs among different acute insults [5]. In particular, when a careful analysis of causes and risk factors was performed in 143 patients with ATN, it was observed that most patients without pre-existing renal disease had more than one insult [5]. The typical example is given by sepsis, which has been usually indicated as an important cause of ARF in man, with an incidence as high as 58% [6]. Actually, in patients without pre-existing renal disease, no causal relationship has been found between sepsis and ARF, unless other factors, such as volume depletion and/or hypotension and/or aminoglycoside nephrotoxicity, were associated [5].

This observation is obviously of great importance for the purpose of prevention. Thus, in septic patients it becomes crucial to prevent volume depletion and hypotension, and particular attention has to be paid when using aminoglycoside antibiotics.

The frequency of a single isolated acute insult is, on the other hand, greater in patients with pre-existing renal disease; in these patients, for instance, dehydration was the sole acute insult in 27% of the cases of ARF and hypotension in 23% [5]. These latter data stress the importance of preventing dehydration and hypotension in chronic uremic patients. Such prevention becomes crucial in the elderly, probably in relation to a greater incidence of hypertension in older patients; and chronic hypertension has been demonstrated to be a great risk factor when hypotension is one of the precipitating events [5].

Experimental studies in animals and/or clinical trials in humans have given some evidence in favor of a protective role of some drugs such as propranolol, clonidine, mannitol, and furosemide. In this chapter, we will first analyze these drugs and then suggest preventive measures against some forms of ARF. For prevention of other forms of ARF, the reader is referred to the specific chapters.

2. Propranolol

Many reports in recent years have given evidence of a partial protective effect of beta-adrenergic antagonists against post-ischemic ARF in experimental animals [7–14].

The mechanism of this protection, still a matter of debate, was initially attributed to the reduction in renin release that follows beta-adrenergic blockade [8]. But the degree of renal impairment could not be correlated with plasma renin activity, nor with renal renin content [9]. On the other hand, protection by beta blockers also occurs under angiotensin II receptor blockade by saralasin [8, 9].

Recent experimental studies in rats have clearly shown that the alleviation of ischemic ARF by propranolol and practolol is due to specific tubular beta-adrenergic blockade [15].

More recently, it has been demonstrated in rats with post-ischemic ARF that pretreatment with propranolol results in a minor increase in proximal intratubular pressure, a minor decrease in GFR, and no change in RBF; these data suggest a substantial relief of tubular obstruction by propranolol, which is presumably independent of its effect on renal hemodynamics [14]. The mechanism by which propranolol may reduce tubular obstruction following ischemia is not known; it has been attributed to metabolic effects within the cells, since the drug penetrates cells exerting an anesthetic effect; the latter may reduce the ischemic epithelial necrosis in proximal tubules [14].

There are no reports on beneficial effects of propranolol in ARF in humans.

3. Clonidine

The antihypertensive agent clonidine has been shown to partially protect experimental animals against post-ischemic ARF [16, 17]. The mechanism of this protection is not known. Clonidine has been shown to have many effects on the kidney undergoing ischemic insults: (a) it can reverse (rather than prevent) the podocyte changes (flattening of cell body and spreading of cytoplasm on glomerular capillaries with loss of foot processes) observed in post-ischemic ARF in transplanted human kidneys [18] and in rabbits following renal artery clamping [18, 19]; the reversion of these changes (which may represent the morphologic counterpart of a decrease in K_f) may imply an enhancing effect on K_f (see chapter 1); (b) it inhibits renin release [20]; (c) it decreases the renal responsiveness to vasopressin, thereby resulting in a diuretic effect [17]; and (d) it prevents the ischemic microvascular injury in the outer medulla [17]. It has been postulated that the latter effect is of primary importance in protection; better perfusion of the outer medulla in fact, would lessen desquamation of damaged tubular cells, thereby reducing tubular obstruction; decreased responsiveness of distal nephron to vasopressin induced by clonidine, by increasing tubular fluid flow rate, might further reduce tubular obstruction [17].

Unfortunately, there is no reported experience on possible protective effects of clonidine against ARF in humans.

4 Mannitol

4.1 OSMOTIC DIURESIS
The increase in urine output following the urinary excretion of nonreabsorbable (such as mannitol) or mildly reabsorbable (such as urea) solutes is called "osmotic diuresis." Osmotic diuretics are low-molecular-weight substances that are readily filtered by glomeruli and not reabsorbed (or only poorly reabsorbed) by renal tubules. Mannitol is the typical osmotic diuretic; it is a sugar (mol wt 182) that is distributed throughout the extracellular compartment once injected i.v. (usually for the therapeutic purposes); it is not metabolized, is freely filtered by glomeruli, and does not undergo tubular reabsorption (reabsorption is minimal). Similar behavior is exhibited by glucose when injected i.v. in large amounts; when the filtered load of this sugar exceeds, in fact, the reabsorptive capacity of proximal tubules, the nonreabsorbed amount will function as an osmotic diuretic. The same occurs in untreated diabetes mellitus with high blood levels of glucose. Even urea, which is only partially reabsorbed, may behave as an osmotic diuretic when injected i.v. in large amounts; the same occurs in patients with untreated chronic renal failure and high levels of plasma urea. In clinical practice, osmotic diuresis is also observed following the use of radiocontrast media, the unreabsorbable compounds employed for urographic and angiographic procedures.

4.2 MANNITOL INFUSION
A normal subject given 100 grams of mannitol i.v. will readily increase urine output up to 10 ml/min and sodium excretion up to 0.5 mmol/min; with larger amounts of mannitol, the fractional excretion of filtered water may reach 20 to 30%, and that of filtered sodium 10 to 15% [21]. This huge diuretic effect is due to a reduction in tubular reabsorption of water and salt, occurring both in proximal tubules and in loops of Henle (figure 3-1).

Three phenomena take place in proximal tubules following the i.v. injection of mannitol: First, a significant fall in water reabsorption: because of the intraluminal presence of osmotically active solute, in fact, water will not be reabsorbed in association with sodium, as usually occurs. Under such circumstances, since sodium continues to be removed from tubular fluid by active tubular transport, its concentration will fall as filtered fluid proceeds along the proximal tubule. But this phenomenon will lead to the second phenomenon, a decrease in net reabsorption of sodium: the active sodium transport is, in fact, progressively reduced since it has to occur against an increasing concentration gradient; the latter, on the other hand, will favor the passive backflux of sodium into the tubule. And third, the ECV expansion that follows the acute i.v. infusion of mannitol may further contribute to reducing proximal tubular reabsorption [21]. The combined result of these phenomena will be a distal delivery of a great amount of salt and especially of water.

A further reduction in tubular reabsorption occurs in the loop of Henle. Mannitol is known to increase renal medullary blood flow. The resulting wash-out effect on renal medulla will greatly reduce the medullary hypertonicity, thereby impairing the passive water reabsorption from the thin descending limb of the loop of Henle [21]. This factor, however, will also influence salt reabsorption. Evidence has been given, in fact, that sodium chloride reabsorption occurring in the thin ascending limb of Henle is a passive phenomenon: salt would move out of the tubular lumen down its concentration gradient [22]. The impaired water reabsorption in the thin descending limb will reduce or even abolish the favorable sodium concentration gradient in the thin ascending limb. The result will be a severe impairment in overall salt reabsorption in the loop of Henle, which is only blunted by a maintained or even increased active salt reabsorption in the thick ascending limb. [21].

In addition to the reduction in water and salt reabsorption in proximal tubules and loops of Henle, mannitol has been shown to increase the glomerular filtration rate [GFR] in experimental animals. The i.v. infusion of mannitol, in fact, by increasing the osmolality of extracellular fluid, causes an osmotic shift of water from cells (erythrocytes included) to the extracellular compartment with consequent ECV expansion, decline in blood viscosity, increase in cardiac output, decrease in renal renin release, lowering in renal vascular resistance, and increase in renal blood flow (RBF) (figure 3–1). The increase in GFR has been shown to result (a) from the increase in glomerular plasma flow and in glomerular capillary pressure (GCP) secondary to afferent arteriole dilation and (b) from the reduction in systemic oncotic pressure [23]. The increase in GFR will obviously contribute to the high water and salt excretion that follows mannitol infusion.

Because of the effects of mannitol on proximal tubular reabsorption and on medullary blood flow (with loss of medullary hypertonicity), after mannitol infusion urine osmolality tends to approach that of plasma (with a clear impairment of the renal capacity to concentrate and dilute urine) and urinary sodium concentration tends to be high (greater than 50 mmol/l). This should be taken into account when a patient with ARF is first observed by a nephrologist; the patient may have already been treated with mannitol or may have undergone radiographic procedures with radiocontrast compounds. Under such circumstances, urinary indexes for differentiating prerenal ARF from ATN become meaningless (see chapter 7).

4.3 HAZARDS OF MANNITOL INFUSION

As described above, the i.v. infusion of mannitol causes an osmotic shift of water from cells to extracellular compartment leading to ECV expansion, dilutional hyponatremia, hypochloremia, and expansion acidosis (due to bicarbon-

ate dilution). Thus, if the patient has oliguric ATN, the ECV expansion that may follow mannitol infusion (200 g mannitol may expand ECV by more than 2 liters) may cause pulmonary congestion or even pulmonary edema in the presence of heart disease [21]. But even when this complication does not occur, mannitol intoxication may be severe with a hyperosmolar state, severe dilutional hyponatremia, hypochloremia, and intracellular dehydration, which may cause the patient to be confused and disoriented with extremely dry tissues [24]. Under such circumstances, hyponatremia does not reflect hypoosmolality, but is instead associated with hyperosmolality, as may be calculated (see chapter 2/section 12.3) or directly measured.

Iatrogenic mannitol intoxication, which usually occurs in oliguric ATN, should be immediately treated by dialysis [24].

The effect of mannitol infusion on serum potassium is variable and seems to depend on the dose of mannitol, its infusion rate, and the insulin response. The abrupt rise in osmolality of extracellular fluid, in fact, causes not only water but also potassium flux out of the cells; should insulin response not occur (as it does not in diabetics, for instance), hyperkalemia results [23].

At the renal level the osmotic diuresis caused by mannitol (a) will reduce tubular reabsorption of filtered potassium and (b) will increase tubular secretion of potassium at its secretory sites in the distal nephron, as a result of increased distal delivery of sodium; the combined result will be a urinary loss of the cation.

Should the patient exhibit a clear increase in urine output and salt excretion after i.v. infusion of mannitol, adequate replacement of urinary loss of water and salt must be carefully performed in order to prevent volume depletion.

It should be stressed that the use of mannitol is hazardous in the condition of severe dehydration and/or acidosis.

4.4 PROPHYLAXIS OF ARF BY MANNITOL

A substantial body of evidence exists in experimental animals that mannitol prevents anuria and improves renal function when given prophylactically in many experimental models of ARF. This beneficial effect has been attributed (a) to increase in RBF and GCP and (b) to an increase in osmolar clearance [25, 26].

4.4.1 Increase in RBF and GRF After Mannitol Infusion

As mentioned, mannitol infusion has been shown to increase GFR by increasing RBF and GCP and by decreasing systemic oncotic pressure. This occurs even at normal renal perfusion pressure and has been attributed to ECV expansion.

Recent experimental studies in rats have demonstrated that the increase in RBF induced by mannitol is even greater in conditions of renal hypoperfusion [27] and that under such circumstances the improvement in RBF is due to a primary reduction in afferent arteriole resistance [27] with maintenance of glomerular filtration [28]. The afferent arteriole dilation is mediated, in large part, by an increase in prostaglandin (PGI_2) activity [29]. Pretreatment with indomethacin or meclofenamate (which block PG synthesis) greatly reduced the rise in RBF after mannitol in rats with hypoperfused kidney, while the renal response to mannitol was blunted by previous renal vasodilation by PGI_2 infusion; in contrast, pretreatment with converting enzyme inhibitor teprotide (SQ 20,881) or kallikrein inhibitor aprotinin failed to influence the effect of mannitol on RBF of hypoperfused rat kidney [29]. Blockade of PG synthesis, however, did not reduce the renal response to mannitol in rats with normal renal perfusion, suggesting that the rise in RBF after mannitol infusion under normal circumstances is not PG mediated [29].

These observations suggest that in condition of renal hypoperfusion, the benefical effect of mannitol on renal hemodynamics is not limited to the renal consequences of ECV expansion but is also due to increase in PG synthesis (figure 3–1).

4.4.2 The Protective Effect of the Increase in Osmolar Clearance

The increase in osmolar clearance (solute diuresis) rather than in urine output "per se" (water diuresis occurs more distally) has a further protective effect on renal function [25, 30], presumably by preventing tubular obstruction by cell debris or proteinaceous material (figure 3–1). This effect has been demonstrated by a variety of studies. Thus, "in vivo" microperfusion of proximal tubules in dogs with unilateral NE-induced ARF was followed by an increase in intratubular pressure behind the microperfusion site, suggesting tubular obstruction; this increase in tubular pressure was not observed in dogs pretreated with mannitol [26]. "In vitro" microperfusion of isolated tubular segments dissected from kidneys of rabbits with post-ischemic ARF has shown the formation of cellular debris with the onset of the microperfusion and a severe impairment of transport capacity of proximal tubules [31]. Pretreatment of rabbits with 5 g/dl (275 mmol/l) mannitol (or furosemide) resulted in preservation of tubular integrity (with no formation of cellular debris) and maintenance of normal (near normal with furosemide) epithelial function of proximal tubules [31].

Recent studies have given evidence of an increase in calcium content of mitochondria from the renal cortex of dogs with NE-induced ARF; this may result from impaired mitochondrial respiratory activity (mitochondrial oxygen uptake has been found impaired after ischemia) and might contribute, in the ischemic kidney, to tubular epithelial cell necrosis and afferent arteriole vasoconstriction (because of an increase in cytosolic calcium in the smooth muscle cells of afferent arterioles) [32]. This hypothesis is supported by the observation that verapamil (a blocker of slow-channel calcium influx into cells) prevents the fall in renal function in the ischemic experimental model of ARF [2]. Pretreatment of experimental animals with isotonic mannitol prevented both impairment of mitochondrial respiratory activity (mitochondrial oxygen uptake was no longer impaired, and calcium content of mitochondria was normal) and fall in renal function (renal vasoconstriction would not have occurred) [2, 32].

4.4.3 The Prophylaxis with Mannitol in Clinical Practice

Prophylactic use of mannitol has been suggested for preventing AFR in those high-risk clinical conditions in which renal impairment is predictable: general surgery in

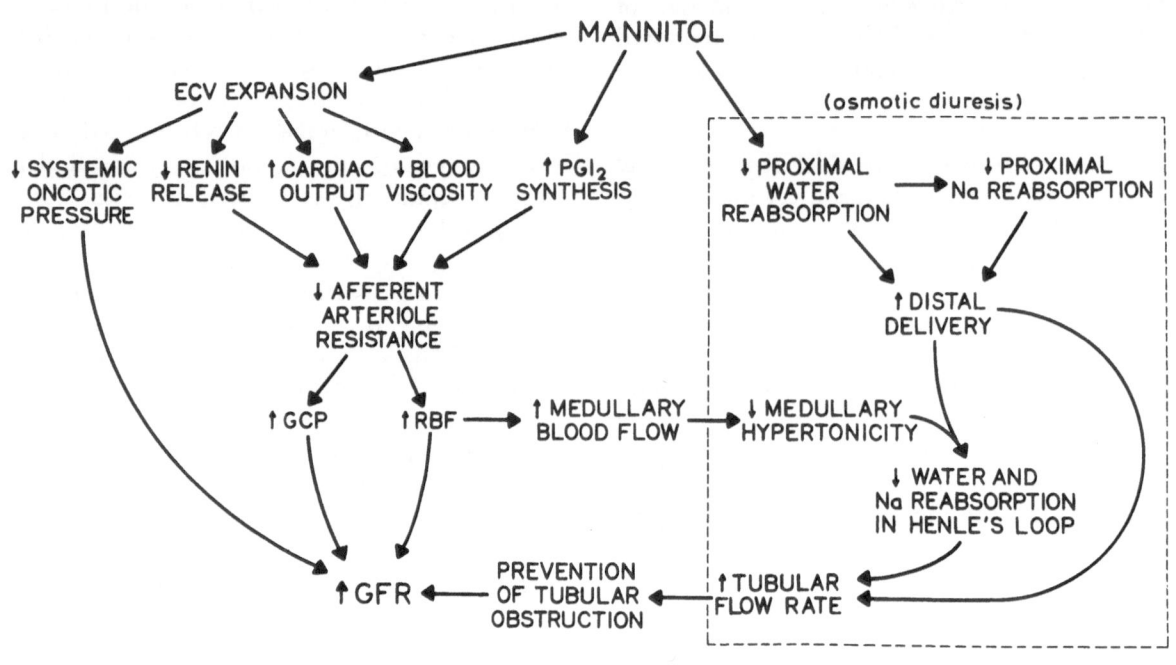

FIGURE 3–1. Effects of mannitol in preventing/treating acute renal failure.

high-risk patients and, in particular, cardiovascular surgery; shock; radiographic procedures with radiocontrast media; therapy with nephrotoxic drugs [33–41]. Thus, for instance, in a randomized study of 22 patients undergoing abdominal aorta resection, no oliguria occurred in mannitol-treated patients (25 grams of mannitol before and 40 grams during surgery); oliguria was observed in three untreated patients [35]. Similar beneficial effects have been obtained with mannitol in preventing radiocontrast-induced ARF and cisplatinum-induced ARF (see below).

Obviously, volume depletion should be corrected before mannitol infusion. Furthermore, urinary losses of salt and water during mannitol administration should be carefully replaced. It has been stated that negative salt balance during mannitol infusion is prevented by infusing 10 g/dl (550 mmol/l) mannitol in a half-normal saline solution (77 mmol/l NaCl) [42].

The following schedule has been suggested for prophylaxis: 250 ml of 20 g/dl (1,098 mmol/l) mannitol solution (i.e., 50 grams of mannitol) are infused i.v. over one hour; then a urine output of 50 ml/hour is maintained by

i.v. infusion of a solution with 275 mmol/l (5 g/dl) mannitol, 20 mmol/l of sodium chloride, and 2.33 mmol/l (1 g/l) of calcium gluconate [23].

For the use of mannitol in the prevention of ARF due to therapy with cisplatinum and diagnostic procedures with radiocontrast media, the reader is referred to the respective sections later in this chapter.

4.5 "REVASCULARIZATION" (REPERFUSION) SYNDROME: MANNITOL IN PREVENTION
There is some evidence that hypertonic mannitol is also effective in preventing the revascularization syndrome that follows vascular reconstruction (thromboembolectomy or arterial bypass) after acute ischemia of human limbs (usually the lower extremities) [43].

It is well known that reperfusion of acutely ischemic extremities is followed by a relatively high mortality. Actually, mortality seems to be greater after restoration of blood flow than before re-establishing circulation, suggesting that (a) reperfusion of ischemic muscles is associated with flushing out of metabolites (e.g., lactic acid) and substances (e.g., myoglobin), which may damage other organs such as kidney (ARF) and heart (myocardial depression), and lead to death [43–45]; and (b) metabolic activity of muscles does not return to normal immediately after muscle reperfusion [46] so that "toxins" may continue to be released into the general circulation.

Experimental data have demonstrated that, after reperfusion of ischemic limbs, blood flow is not restored to normal and that limb hypoperfusion is associated with increase in local vascular resistance, local edema, and high tissue pressures [43]. The latter phenomena may further reduce the local blood flow and favor thrombosis.

When hypertonic mannitol was injected intravenously prior to reestablishing blood flow (100 ml of 1,098 mmol/1, 20 g/dl mannitol as a bolus) and continued (i.v. infusion of 550 mmol/hour, 10 g/hour) for many hours (up to 24 hours), signs and symptoms of the reperfusion syndrome were not observed [43]. The important role of mannitol in preventing an increase of local vascular resistance, limb hypoperfusion, edema, and compartment syndrome was demonstrated by the rapid (within a few hours) swelling of the limb when mannitol was discontinued and a decrease in limb swelling when mannitol infusion was reinstituted [43].

5 Furosemide

Furosemide is the loop diuretic most often used, both in clinical practice [47–49] and in experimental models of ARF [50–52], to prevent or even reverse renal impairment. The results obtained by its use are controversial. Thus, while some authors have claimed shortening of ARF in humans by the use of this diuretic [47, 53], others have denied such beneficial results [48, 49, 54, 55]. Similarly, in experimental ARF, furosemide has been claimed to prevent ARF [51], to partially reverse renal impairment [50, 56], to increase urine output without affecting renal function [57, 58], to have no effect at all [56], or to be even harmful [51, 52, 59–62]. It appears

therefore worthwhile to review experimental and clinical studies reported in the literature on this contention.

5.1 FUROSEMIDE IN EXPERIMENTAL ARF

In unilateral norepinephrine (NE)-induced ARF in dogs, the administration of furosemide before or immediately after NE infusion, associated with complete replacement of urinary losses of water and salt, was followed by complete normalization of RBF (against a value 36% of control in untreated dogs) and clear improvement of renal function (inulin clearance 56% of control values against the 2% in dogs that did not receive furosemide) [63]. Under such circumstances, the protective effect of furosemide could not be attributed only to its vasodilatory properties, since in identical experimental conditions, intrarenal infusion of acetylcholine also normalized RBF but did not improve renal function. The dramatic increase in urine output and solute excretion observed under furosemide but not under acetylcholine appeared to support a primary protective role of high solute excretion; in other words, the inhibition of tubular reabsorption of salt and water induced by furosemide, by increasing the tubular flow rate, may have prevented or relieved the tubular obstruction (by cellular debris) that usually occurs after ischemic tubular necrosis (see chapter 1). The observation that chlorothiazide and benzolamide, which reduced RBF in the same experimental conditions, did not improve renal function despite the increase in solute excretion [30] would stress the need for both vasodilation and increase is osmolar clearance for obtaining protection, at least in this ischemic model of ARF.

A further demonstration of the beneficial effect of furosemide on ischemic ARF is given by microperfusion studies "in vitro": the microperfusion of isolated tubular segments dissected from kidneys of rabbits with post-ischemic ARF pretreated with furosemide (or 5 g/dl, 275 mmol/l, mannitol) did not exhibit cellular debris within the tubular lumen at the onset of the microperfusion nor the severe impairment in transport capacity of proximal tubules as observed instead in nonpretreated animals [31].

Other studies, however, have denied any protection by furosemide against ischemic ARF. Thus, in rats undergoing 45 minutes of bilateral warm ischemia, furosemide did not show any protective influence on GFR when given either before or after the ischemic insult, either in low or in high doses [56]. Similarly, in dogs with ischemic ARF due to renal artery clamping, the diuretic, given immediately after releasing the clamp, did not show beneficial effect on renal function, despite the increased urine output and sodium excretion [58].

Conflicting results have also been obtained in nephrotoxic models of ARF. Thus, furosemide given alone immediately after uranyl nitrate (UN) infusion in dogs did not protect the renal function of the animals despite reversal of renal vasoconstriction [64]. Under identical circumstances, while dopamine alone was also ineffective in protection, the combined administration of furosemide and dopamine induced (a) a marked renal vasodilation, (b) a greatly attenuated reduction in renal function, and (c) a brisk diuresis and natriuresis [64]. In other studies in rats, however, furosemide alone improved renal function when given either before or after UN administration, suggesting both a prophylactic and curative action of the diuretic in this model of ARF [56].

In the mercuric chloride model of ARF in rats the prophylactic use of furosemide was effective in protection only when very low doses (2 mg/Kg b.w.) of $HgCl_2$ were used [51]. No protection was observed when usual doses of $HgCl_2$ (4.7 mg/Kg b.w.) were employed. Under such circumstances, in fact, neither low doses nor high doses of furosemide given before [51] or early after [57] $HgCl_2$ injection in rats modified the decrement in GFR commonly observed in $HgCl_2$-induced ARF. In the same experimental model, when repeated doses of diuretic were given in order to evaluate the efficacy in shortening the duration of ARF, low repeated doses were ineffective while high repeated doses were even harmful. The worsening effect of these high doses, however, was due to volume depletion secondary to the saluretic effect of furosemide; it was, in fact, abolished by adequate replacement of urinary losses of sodium [57].

Bailey et al. [51] have demonstrated that prophylactic administration of furosemide conferred protection against the ARF induced in rats (a) by the combined administration of cephaloridine, furosemide, and 50 g/dl glycerol in subnephrotoxic doses and (b) by nephrotoxic doses of cephaloridine alone. When furosemide was administered together with cephaloridine, however, the severity of ARF was greatly potentiated [51]. This detrimental effect on renal function of furosemide when given at high doses in association with nephrotoxic antibiotics has been reported by others [59–62]. Since high doses of furosemide alone did not impair renal function of normal rats [57], any intrinsic toxicity of the diuretic was ruled out. Apparently, furosemide can potentiate, by a still undefined mechanism, the nephrotoxicity of some antibiotics and possibly of some other nephrotoxins. Thus, both prophylactic [51] and therapeutic [52] administration of furosemide has been shown to increase the severity of glycerol-induced ARF in rats. Surprisingly, in methemoglobin-induced ARF, the administration of diuretic after methemoglobin has been shown to improve GFR [50].

Taken together all these experimental studies suggest that furosemide may be effective in preventing and/or reversing some forms of ARF. They also provide some useful information with very important clinical implications:

a. Solute diuresis (such as that obtained by furosemide or mannitol) but not water diuresis (such as that obtained by i.v. infusion of glucose solutions) has a clear protective effect against ischemic ARF, provided that renal vasodilation is associated.

b. Protection by furosemide is exerted not only when given before but also immediately after the ischemic insult.

c. For this protection, it is essential that urinary losses of salt and water are replaced by i.v. infusion of isotonic saline.

d. Furosemide may potentiate the renal damage by nephrotoxic antibiotics when given concurrently.

5.2 THE MECHANISM OF PROTECTION

The protective effect exerted by furosemide on renal function as well as the therapeutic effect reported in some forms of ARF have been attributed to (a) renal vasodilation, (b) blockade of tubuloglomerular feedback, and (c) an increase in osmolar clearance.

5.2.1 Renal Vasodilation

Furosemide is known to cause renal vasodilation. This effect has been suggested as prostaglandin (PG) mediated [30], since it is completely blocked by indomethacin [65]. On the other hand, the administration of furosemide is followed by an increase in urinary excretion of PGs [66, 67], which is reversed by indomethacin [67]. However, experimental studies in animals failed to confirm an important role for the renal vasodilating effect of furosemide in preventing ARF [64]. Only with combined dopamine plus furosemide did a marked renal vasodilation and a clear improvement in GFR occur, which were significantly correlated to each other, suggesting some role of vasodilation in protection [64]. Renal vasodilation may increase not only RBF but also K_f through the increase in capillary surface area (see chapter 1).

It is interesting to note that in some cases of ATN in humans, combined dopamine and furosemide significantly increased urine output [68].

5.2.2 Blockade of Tubuloglomerular Feedback (TGF)

Microperfusion of the loop of Henle with furosemide has been shown to completely block TGF [69, 70]. This blockade is probably related to inhibition of active chloride transport at the macula densa level [70]. To the extent that TGF plays a major role in the pathogenesis of ARF (see chapter 1), blockade of TGF may represent the main protective mechanism of furosemide. Since renal vasoconstriction, which occurs in the early phase of ARF, may prevent adequate access of furosemide to the macula densa, the vasodilation induced by combined dopamine and furosemide may favor the delivery of the diuretic to the macula densa, thereby allowing its blocking effect on TGF [64].

5.2.3 Increase in Osmolar Clearance

As described above, an important role in protection is played by the increase in tubular flow rate that follows the inhibition of sodium chloride reabsorption in the loop of Henle. Since water diuresis resulting from inhibition of water reabsorption in the most distal part of the

nephron has no protective effect despite the increase in urine output, protection appears related to increase in osmolar clearance (solute diuresis) rather than in urine output [25, 30]. It has been suggested that the high tubular flow rate induced by furosemide will prevent (or reverse) tubular obstruction by flushing out cell debris and proteinaceous material and will maintain (or re-establish) the patency of renal tubules in a fashion similar to that obtained with mannitol [56, 64] (figure 1–2). It is therefore obvious that water diuresis is ineffective because it raises tubular flow rate too distally to adequately flush out all intratubular material. Consistent with this interpretation is the lack of protection of water diuresis (in water-drinking or diabetes insipidus rats) against glycerol-induced ARF [71, 72].

5.3 PROPHYLAXIS OF ARF IN HUMANS BY FUROSEMIDE

Mannitol has usually been preferred to furosemide as a prophylactic measure in high-risk patients. In a few reports on the use of furosemide in critically ill surgical patients, no clear benefit from diuretic prophylaxis has been demonstrated: furosemide did cause a marked increase in urine output and in salt excretion, but did not protect against ARF [73, 74].

As discussed in other sections of this chapter, furosemide has been suggested as an important measure for preventing ARF, which may follow severe hyperuricemia, therapy with cisplatinum, or diagnostic use of radiocontrast media.

The literature is more extensive on the therapeutic use of furosemide in oliguric ARF, for which the reader is referred to chapter 21.

6 Prevention of Radiocontrast-Induced ARF

The use of radiocontrast materials for diagnostic purposes is expected to increase in future years since contrast media are also required for modern radiographic techniques, such as computerized tomography and computerized intravenous arteriography.

In computerized tomography scanning, the contrast agent is used for image enhancement, which frequently allows the demonstration of lesions not visualized without contrast.

As far as computerized intravenous arteriography is concerned, the use of i.v. injection of contrast media rather than direct injection into extrarenal arteries is not expected to decrease their nephrotoxicity since these iodinate contrast media are not detoxicated by the liver or by the lung [75].

In outpatients with normal renal function, the slight subclinical impairment of renal function, which may occur (with a relatively low incidence) following the use of contrast media, will usually subside in 7 to 10 days without further problems. In these patients there is no need for routine evaluation of renal function after radiographic procedures [75].

However, special caution is mandatory in high-risk patients. As described in chapter 2, pre-existing impairment of renal function, diabetes mellitus, vascular diseases involving the kidneys, congestive heart failure, reduction in effective blood volume, dehydration, multiple myeloma, and advanced age represent predisposing factors in radiocontrast-induced ARF. They may be variously combined, thereby increasing the risk of renal function impairment. Grey-scale sonography and radionuclide scanning should be preferred whenever possible. Intravenous pyelography (IVP) will not usually provide useful information for management in diabetic patients unless they exhibit acute deterioration in renal function or recent symptoms suggesting reversible urologic problems. Sometimes tomography alone may be useful and sufficient for detecting the occurrence and even the cause of obstructive uropathy.

Should a radiocontrast procedure be unavoidable in high-risk patients, adequate hydration, saline infusion and/or alkalinization, and maintenance of solute diuresis by mannitol or furosemide have been suggested as preventive procedure.

6.1 HYDRATION

Even though there is no clear evidence that the incidence of contrast-induced ARF is reduced by hydration, free access to water should be permitted to all patients before radiocontrast procedures.

6.2 SALINE INFUSION

It has been claimed that adequate hydration with normal saline rather than water or dextrose solution prevents radiocontrast-induced ARF [76]. Thus, in a prospective study of 537 consecutive patients undergoing cerebral [295] and abdominal or peripheral [242] angiography followed by i.v. infusion of normal saline (250 ml/hr as flush solution during and 550 ml/hr after the procedure), no case of ARF (increase in BUN of 50% or 20 mg/dl and/or increase in serum creatinine by 88.4 μmol/1, 1 mg/dl) was observed within 24 hours of the angiographic procedure [76]. A very important drawback of this study, however, was the short duration of the postangiographic observation; it was limited to 24 hrs. It is, in fact, well known that serum creatinine reaches a peak most frequently on the third day (in some cases even on the seventh or eighth day) after the administration of the contrast medium (see chapter 2). Hence, this observation of a protective effect of saline infusion in patients undergoing angiography does not appear conclusive.

The results obtained by Shapiro's group in patients undergoing IVP who were similarly hydrated with i.v. saline solution are quite different [77]. In this study 40 patients with CRF were treated with i.v. infusion of 1,500 ml of 86 mmol/l (0.5 g/dl) NaCl solution in 278 mmol/l (5 g/dl) dextrose in the 12 to 16 hours preceding the IVP. The latter was performed by i.v. drip infusion of 300 ml of 30 g/dl sodium diatrizoate in 10 to 15 minutes. ARF (increase in serum creatinine of at least 25%) occurred within five days post-IVP in 28 patients with an overall incidence of 70%; as many as 11 out of the 12 diabetic patients developed ARF following the IVP; the incidence of ARF in nondiabetics was also very high (17 out of 28 cases) [77]. From this study, it appears that saline infusion by itself has no protective effect against radiocontrast nephrotoxicity.

6.3 MANNITOL AND FUROSEMIDE

The protective effects of mannitol (250 ml of 20 g/dl mannitol i.v. in 60 minutes) or furosemide (mg 4,000 divided by creatinine clearance at a rate of 100 mg/5 minutes) have been evaluated by Shapiro and his coworkers in two further groups of similarly hydrated patients (37 treated with mannitol and 17 with furosemide) [40, 41]. These two groups were matched with the previously described control group for age, sex, percent diabetics, renal function, proteinuria, urine output, and sodium excretion. The infusion of mannitol or furosemide was performed 60 minutes after the start of diatrizoate infusion and was followed by i.v. infusion of 77 mmol/l (0.45 g/dl) NaCl solution in 278 mmol/l (5 g/dl) dextrose, at a rate equal to the hourly urine output, for the next 24 hours. The incidence of radiocontrast-induced ARF fell from 70% of the control group (hydrated with i.v. saline) to 22% (8 out of 37 patients) in the mannitol group and to 18% (3 out of 17 patients) in the furosemide group [40, 41]. None of the patients had oliguria at any time; only three out of nine diabetics in the mannitol group and only one out of four diabetics in the furosemide group exhibited a significant nephrotoxic response to the contrast agents. No correlation was observed between the occurrence of ARF and baseline FE_{Na}; furthermore, the weight of the patients remained unchanged prior to and following IVP in all groups, thereby ruling out any ECV expansion in mannitol or furosemide treated patients (who underwent i.v. fluid infusion post-IVP to replace urinary losses) [40, 41].

The results of Shapiro's group on the protective effect of mannitol are consistent with a retrospective study by other authors [78]. When six patients wth CRF were infused intravenously with 5 g/dl mannitol solution over several hours within an hour of the radiocontrast procedure, no changes in serum creatinine were observed; but five control patients not given mannitol developed a significant increase in serum creatinine [78].

Taken together these interesting studies demonstrate that both mannitol and furosemide, given i.v. 60 minutes after the administration of radiocontrast agents, significantly protect patients with CRF against radiocontrast nephropathy. This protection may occur through a reversal of renal vasoconstriction and/or prevention of tubular obstruction [41] (see chapter 2).

6.4 RECOMMENDED PROTOCOL FOR PREVENTION OF ARF DUE TO UROGRAPHIC AND ANGIOGRAPHIC CONTRAST AGENTS IN HIGH-RISK PATIENTS

a. Even though the use of laxatives during routine preparation for IVP has not been shown to increase contrast-induced ARF, the association of laxatives and enemas in high-risk patients should be avoided in the 12 to 24 hours preceding radiocontrast procedures [79]. This precaution is important in patients with CRF, particularly in those who are already on a salt-restricted diet. Volume depletion should, in fact, be avoided before the study.

b. Minimal doses of contrast agent compatible with a satisfactory radiographic study should be used, allowing sufficient interval between doses to permit complete renal clearance. A contrast dose containing 0.75-1g iodine/kg b.w. has been suggested for IVP in CRF patients.

c. It is advisable to avoid, if possible, a second radiographic study in patients who have previously developed contrast nephropathy since these patients are particularly susceptible to a further episode on re-exposure to the same contrast agent. In patients who have, in their history, systemic reactions to contrast media, a steroid pretreatment has been suggested before contrast rechallenge; this may protect against anaphylactic reaction, but it has not been proven that this pretreatment will prevent ARF.

d. Mannitol should be infused intravenously according to one of the following protocols: First, the i.v. infusion, at a rate of 150 ml/hour, of a solution of mannitol (137 mmol, 25g) and sodium bicarbonate (100 mmol) in one liter of 278 mmol (5g/dl) dextrose; this infusion should start one-half to one hour prior to the contrast procedure [80]. Or second, the i.v. infusion of hypertonic mannitol (1,098 mmol/1, 20g/dl, 250 ml i.v. in 60 minutes), delaying its administration to one hour after the infusion of the contrast medium (30 g/dl sodium diatrizoate) in order to avoid the cumulative hyperosmotic effect of 30 g/dl sodium diatrizoate (943 mOsm/kg H_2O)

and 20 g/dl mannitol (1,098 mOsm/kg H_2O) [40].

Whatever the protocol, mannitol administration should be followed for the next 24 hours by infusion of half-normal saline (77 mmol/l, 0.45 g/dl NaCl) in 5 g/dl (278 mmol/l) dextrose, at a rate equal to the hourly urine output, in order to replace urinary losses of water and electrolytes.

e. Furosemide may replace mannitol, particularly in patients with heart failure. The dose of furosemide may be calculated by dividing mg 4,000 by the creatinine clearance in ml/min (e.g., 200 mg in a patient with creatinine clearance of 20 ml/min); the infusion should begin 60 minutes after the start of contrast infusion, with an infusion rate of 100 mg of furosemide/5 minutes [41]. Furosemide administration should be followed by continuous replacement of urinary losses of fluid and electrolytes for the next 24 hours (e.g., 77 mmol/l, 0.45 g/dl NaCl, in 278 mmol/l, 5 g/dl dextrose intravenously at a rate equal to the hourly urine output).

f. Any cause of volume depletion should be removed. Alternatively, any (renal or extrarenal) loss of fluid and electrolytes should be quantitatively replaced.

g. Serum creatinine should be measured every day at least for the following three days. This is particularly important when the patient has to face a further radiocontrast procedure, a surgical operation, or the use of nephrotoxic drugs.

6.5 RECOMMENDED PROTOCOL FOR PREVENTION OF ARF DUE TO ORAL CHOLECYSTOGRAPHIC AGENTS

a. Since there is no evidence that fluid restriction improves gallbladder visualization by oral cholecystography agents, fluid intake should be encouraged during the 12 to 24 hours preceding the radiographic procedure [79].

b. It is better to avoid the use of laxatives and enemas in the 36 hours preceding the cholecystographic procedure in order to avoid salt depletion [79].

c. Since ARF following oral cholecystographic

agents usually occurs after a second double-dose of the dye, it is suggested that this double-dose should be avoided. Should a satisfactory visualization not occur following a single dose, another single dose of the agent may be given 24 hours later [79].

d. Tomography of the gallbladder and common bile duct may sometimes obviate the use of additional doses of contrast agents [79].

e. Ultrasonic cholecystography may also prevent a further dose of oral cholecystographic agents following nonvisualization after the first dose [81].

7 Prevention of Cisplatinum-Induced ARF.

The widespread use of cisplatinum for treating solid tumors, such as testicular or bladder cancer, ovarian carcinoma, and tumors of neck and head (see chapter 1 and 2), and the high incidence of iatrogenic renal damage in treated patients requires well-defined precautions for reducing risk factors that may be involved in causing or increasing toxicity.

7.1 DRUG DOSAGE

It is well demonstrated that the nephrotoxic effects of cisplatinum are cumulative and that the severity of renal damage is directly proportional to the total dosage [82]. A single course with an overall dosage of 2 mg/kg b.w. (or 50–75 mg/m^2 body surface area) has been suggested as safe and adequate therapy; alternatively, 15 to 20 mg/m^2 body surface area/day repeated for 5 days may be used [83]. Higher doses will increase the frequency and severity of renal impairment. The rapidity of cisplatinum infusion seems to be an important factor; it has been stated that impairment of renal function is less frequent when the infusion rate of cisplatinum does not exceed 1 mg/kg b.w./hour [84, 85]. Fractionation of the total dose over five days does not seem to reduce the incidence of renal injury although it may delay it [86].

7.2 HYDRATION OF THE PATIENT

Adequate hydration of the patient (urine output should possibly exceed three liters daily) has been suggested for diluting urinary cisplatinum and consequently decreasing its nephrotoxicity [85] (see chapter 2). The intensive i.v. hydration may be carried out with 278 mmol/l (5 g/dl) dextrose solution, 150 to 200 ml/hour throughout the treatment and continued up to six hours after cisplatinum administration [85].

7.3 INFUSION OF SALINE SOLUTION

The i.v. infusion of isotonic saline solution is another very important precaution. It is based on the following reasons: (a) cisplatinum almost constantly causes vomiting, which may lead to salt depletion that potentiates cisplatinum nephrotoxicity, and platinum compounds should never be administered to patients with volume depletion; (b) ECV expansion will decrease proximal tubular reabsorption, thereby diluting cisplatinum already in the proximal tubular fluid (this will result in a minor toxicity on proximal and distal tubular cells); (c) saline infusion has been shown to decrease the renal tissue content of platinum and increase its urinary excretion; and (d) when saline solution is used as vehicle for cisplatinum administration, the nephrotoxicity of the drug is greatly reduced, presumably by preventing the aquation reaction in extracellular fluid (see chapter 2).

It has been suggested that the i.v. infusion of isotonic saline should be started 12 hours prior to cisplatinum administration, at an infusion rate of 100 ml/hour [86, 87]; cisplatinum may then be added to the infusion solution. Saline infusion should be continued for two to three days after cisplatinum therapy in order to maintain a urine volume of three to four liters/24 hours [83].

7.4 MANNITOL

Intravenous infusion of mannitol (5g/hour) during and up to six hours after cisplatinum administration has been suggested in order to reduce nephrotoxicity of the drug [39]. Mannitol has not been proven to give more protection than hydration and saline infusion; but since it will increase both the percentage of serum-free cisplatinum (i.e., unbound to a serum proteins) [88] and the urinary excretion of the drug [89], it is worthwhile adding this precaution, which does not impair the antineoplastic activity of the drug. Furthermore, its use may allow the administration of greater amounts of fluid, thereby offering better protection [85]. Thus mannitol administration should be followed by fluid replacement with one-half normal saline.

7.5 FUROSEMIDE

There is still controversy as to whether furosemide or other loop diuretics may have any role in reducing incidence and severity of cisplatinum nephrotoxicity. Promising results have been obtained in rats when furosemide was given prior to cisplatinum [90]. Only a few reports claim to have demonstrated some protective effect of furosemide in humans [91, 92]. When using diuretic therapy, however, it is important to provide adequate replacement of urinary losses of salt and water.

7.6 THE POSSIBLE PROTECTIVE ROLE OF GLUCOSE LOADING

It has been demonstrated that rats made diabetic by streptozotocin injection are completely protected against cisplatinum nephrotoxicity [93]. It is possible that this protection is related to the enhanced glucose reabsorption in proximal tubules. If this is the case, glucose load prior to and during cisplatinum treatment may protect patients against cisplatinum nephrotoxicity.

7.7 ASSOCIATION WITH OTHER NEPHROTOXIC DRUGS

Association with other nephrotoxic drugs must be avoided. This is particularly important for aminoglycosides; when associated with cisplatinum, these antibiotics caused a greater decrement in renal function [94].

7.8 RECOMMENDATION IN PATIENTS WITH PRE-EXISTENT RENAL INSUFFICIENCY

Although there is no experience concerning treatment of patients with pre-existent renal insufficiency, lower doses of cisplatinum should be used in these patients since the drug is excreted by the kidney. Only in the case of postrenal ARF due to urinary tract obstruction by platinum-sensitive tumor should a full-dose treatment be used. This treatment may lead to regression of the tumor, release of the obstruction, and improvement of renal function [85].

7.9 CAREFUL EVALUATION OF RENAL FUNCTION

Renal function should be carefully evaluated in all patients before, during, and after treatment. Serum creatinine by itself may be misleading in these patients with continuous loss of body muscle mass because of their malignant disease; the creatinine clearance will undoubtedly be a more accurate measure of renal function [85].

7.10 MAGNESIUM WASTING

It is not known how to prevent renal magnesium wasting during cisplatinum therapy. Serum magnesium concentration should be measured frequently during treatment and hypomagnesemia (and hypocalcemia) corrected by parenteral administration of magnesium (and calcium) salts (oral magnesium salts may cause diarrhea). Prophylactic magnesium salt administration should be avoided in view of the possibility of renal impairment by cisplatinum and the consequent danger of hypermagnesemia [85]. Hypokalemia is also corrected by potassium replacement.

8 Prevention of ARF Due to Fluorinated Inhalational Anesthetic Agents

General anesthesia may itself cause ARF (see chapter 2, section 11) or may contribute to the occurrence of postsurgical ARF (see chapter 2, section 2.5). Thus, it is important, first of all, to choose the least toxic anesthetic. Obviously, such anesthetic agents as enflurane, halothane, and isoflurane are preferable to methoxyflurane. The following guidelines may help in preventing renal toxicity.

a. Since the total dose of the anesthetic is an important factor for its nephrotoxicity, it is very important to limit the concentration of the anesthetic and the duration of the anesthesia as much as possible [95]. A light methoxyflurane anesthesia (exposure limited to 2 MAC-h) [96] for short periods has been shown to be nonnephrotoxic [97, 98].

b. Whenever possible other nephrotoxic agents, particularly aminoglycosides but also tetracyclines and penicillins, should be avoided preoperatively and in the immediate postoperative period [95].

c. Dehydration should be avoided by adequate fluid replacement during and after surgery or corrected immediately if occurring. Adequate water excretion during anesthesia would increase inorganic fluoride excretion and therefore protect against the nephrotoxicity of the anesthetic agent [99]. It should be borne in mind, however, that patients under intermittent positive pressure ventilation tend to retain sodium and water.

d. Careful attention should be paid to patients with hyperoxaluria or who have been treated for a long time with barbiturate or tolbutamide [95].

e. Methoxyflurane should be avoided in patients with renal disease [96, 100] and, possibly, in obese patients. The latter, in fact, absorb more drug and develop nephrotoxicity after a short exposure [101]. Previous recent exposure to fluorinated anesthetic agents should also represent a contraindication to methoxiflurane anesthesia.

f. Renal function and possibly serum fluoride levels should be regularly monitored in the postoperative period. The development of renal impairment may easily be missed in the early phase because ARF may be nonoliguric [95].

g. Should ARF occur following methoxyflurane anesthesia, hemodialysis should be performed as early as possible to prevent permanent damage [95] since both oxalic acid and fluoride are readily dialyzed [102].

h. Particular care should be given to the ventilation of the patient. It is well demonstrated, in fact, that mechanical ventilation and alteration in pulmonary gas exchange may impair renal function [100]. This is even more important in patients with chronic uremia.

It should be borne in mind that the oxygen carrying capacity of the blood of patients with renal failure is greatly reduced (usually half normal); thus, hypoxia should be avoided during and following anesthesia [103].

In renal failure patients, Mazze et al. [104] suggest the following protocol for general anesthesia: (a) induction by thiopentone, (b) succinylcholine for endotracheal intubation, (c) maintenance by halothane in a mixture of nitrous oxide and oxygen, and (d) intraoperative muscular relaxation by D-tubocurarine. In the same patients, Lawson [105] suggests (a) premedication with atropine and morphine in normal dosage; (b) induction by sodium thiopentone or nitrous oxide and oxygen; (c) maintenance by halothane or nitrous oxide and oxygen; and (d) muscular relaxation by tubocurare. According to Lawson [105], succinylcholine may cause a dangerous release of potassium from muscles. Muscle relaxants are potentiated by hypokalemia, by polymixin, and by aminoglycosides [105].

9   Prevention of Hyperuricemic ARF in Patients With Malignancies

Because of the rapid and massive production of uric acid in patients with malignancies (leukemias, lymphomas, multiple myeloma, large solid tumors), particularly during aggressive treatment (see chapter 2, section 13), adequate pretreatment of these patients should start two to three days before chemotherapy or radiation therapy in order to prevent acute uric acid nephropathy.

The following protocol is suggested:

a. *Allopurinol*. Starting two days before antitumor therapy, allopurinol (a xanthineoxidase inhibitor) should be given in a dosage of at least 300 mg daily in order to minimize uric acid production. There is apparently no risk of xanthine nephropathy secondary to the increase in xanthine following allopurinol administration.

b. *Hydration*. A high urine output (greater than three liters daily) should be obtained before and maintained throughout the period of antineoplastic therapy. This is achieved by i.v. infusion of saline (154 mmol/1, 0.9 g/dl NaCl solution) and/or 5

g/dl (278 mmol/l) glucose solution. Loop diuretics may also be used, provided that the amounts of water and salt excreted with urine are adequately replaced by i.v. infusions.

c. *Alkalinization*. The alkalinization of urine may be obtained, throughout the period of therapy, by i.v. infusion of isotonic (1/6 M, 167 mmol/1, 1.4 g/dl) sodium bicarbonate solution (e.g., 500 ml daily).

d. *Aluminum hydroxide*. Starting two days before antitumor therapy, aluminum hydroxide should be given orally (doses ranging from 1.5 to 5 grams daily) in order to prevent hyperphosphatemia (resulting from massive cell necrosis) and to minimize the risk of metastatic calcification and acute nephrocalcinosis (see chapter 2, section 15). The dosage of aluminum hydroxide should be adjusted according to the serum level of phosphate.

Adequate hydration, alkalinization, and administration of allopurinol and aluminum hydroxide should be pursued throughout antineoplastic therapy. Meanwhile, renal function and serum concentration of uric acid, calcium, and phosphate should be monitored carefully.

10   Precautions When Using Nephrotoxic Antibiotics

Any time physicians are forced to use antibiotics to treat infections, their choice should be based on benefit-toxicity ratio, especially in severely ill patients with uncertain or reduced renal function and potentially lethal infections. It should be borne in mind that many antibiotics are nephrotoxic and any further fall in renal function will increase their blood levels and consequently the exposure to their toxic effects.

The toxic effects of the antimicrobial drugs are also related to the conditions in which the drugs are administered, such as type of the underlying infection for which the antibiotic is required, possible alteration in renal blood flow occurred during the disease, pre-existent renal insufficiency, condition of dehydration and salt

134

depletion due to fluid loss (because of diarrhea, vomiting, sweating resulting from fever), or concomitant use of other nephrotoxic drugs [106].

As a general rule, nephrotoxic drugs (including antibiotics) should never be given to dehydrated and/or salt-depleted patients. Thus, at the first observation of an infected patient, severe fluid and electrolyte abnormalities should first be corrected; then antibiotics may be given; a few hours of delay in antimicrobial therapy will do no harm.

In patients with pre-existent renal insufficiency, the dosage of antibiotics should be adjusted to renal function. The latter is usually mirrored by the serum creatinine (S_{Cr}) level. The use of S_{Cr} for evaluating renal function, however, may lead to several types of errors [107]. First, slight rises (e.g., from 1 to 1.5 mg/dl, 88 to 133 µmol/l) in S_{Cr} are frequently and mistakenly ignored; they may represent a signficant fall in clearance (from 95 to 65 ml/min in the example above, if the patient is a 40-year-old male, 70 kg b.w.).

Second, the same S_{Cr} (e.g., 1 mg/dl, 88 µmol/l) may represent normal renal function (95 ml/min) in a 40-year-old man, 70 kg b.w. (normal muscle mass), but renal insufficiency (clearance 40 ml/min) in a 70-year-old woman, 50 kg b.w. (reduced muscle mass). It is therefore preferable to base the dosage schedule on creatinine clearance (rather than on S_{Cr}), which may be calculated as follows [108]:

$$\text{Creatinine clearance (ml/min)} = \frac{(140 - \text{age in years}) \times \text{kg b.w.}}{72 \times S_{Cr} \text{ (in mg/dl)}}$$

(The result should be multiplied by O.85 for female patients). Unfortunately for some drugs (e.g., netilmicin), no data are available on dosage based on creatinine clearance; even more precautions are necessary when using them.

And finally, S_{Cr} reflects renal function in steady-state conditions but not when rising each day as in ARF (see chapter 7, section 4); under such circumstances, the dosage of the antibiotic based on S_{Cr} (or on the relative calculated clearance) will be excessive [107].

11 Prevention of Aminoglycoside-Induced ARF

Undoubtedly, aminoglycosides are the typical nephrotoxic antibiotics. As a matter of fact, an experimental model of ARF has been created with one of them: gentamicin (see chapter 1, section 3).

ARF secondary to the use of aminoglycosides is seen very frequently in clinical practice (see chapter 2, section 7).

The severe toxicity of aminoglycosides has prompted research, in recent years, toward the discovery of new and less toxic cephalosporins and penicillin analogs for treating gram-negative bacterial infections [109]. The new synthetic penicillin piperacillin represents a successful example in this respect.

But the forecast for antibacterial drugs indicates that aminoglycosides will continue to play an important role in antibiotic therapy throughout the 1980s [109].

Recent experience with commercially available aminoglycosides and the expected appearance of newer aminoglycosides because of the predictable occurrence of resistant gram-negative bacteria have suggested some guidelines for the use of any antibiotic of this group, especially in severely ill patients in whom the underlying disease may enhance drug nephrotoxicity. These guidelines may refer to the modality of treatment and to patient's conditions.

11.1 MODALITY OF TREATMENT

When choosing treatment with aminoglycosides, we must be sure, first of all, that the risk of renal injury is adequately balanced by the benefits expected from therapy. We have, then, to bear in mind the following points.

11.1.1 Choice of the Aminoglycoside. The choice of the aminoglycoside should be based, for any one bacterial sensitivity, on the lower toxicity. Thus, since gentamicin and tobramycin have a similar spectrum of antibacterial activity, but the former has a greater cortical accumulation, prolonged excretion, and, apparently, greater ototoxicity and nephrotoxicity, it is advisable, whenever possible, to select tobramycin for sensitive bacterial infections [110]. The U.S. Federal Food and Drug Administration has warned about the toxicity of gentamicin by officially stating that nephrotoxicity is less frequent with tobramycin than with gentamicin [109]. Apparently, the nephrotoxicity of amikacin is similar to that of gentamicin [111–114]. Netilmicin, the new semisynthetic derivative of sisomicin, seems to be the least nephrotoxic aminoglycoside [115].

11.1.2 Daily Dosage of Aminoglycoside The daily dose of aminoglycoside must be adjusted (i.e., reduced) to the renal function. This is particularly important in elderly patients [116]. The dosage schedules shown in table 3–1 are suggested on the basis of data from recent literature [117–122] (see table 3–1: Gentamicin, Tobramycin, Sisomicin, Amikacin, Kanamicin, and Streptomycin).

Recent studies have demonstrated that minimum inhibitory serum concentrations of netilmicin for most negative bacilli are obtained, in subjects with normal renal function (creatinine clearance equal to or greater than 80 ml/min) with 2 mg/kg b.w. of the antibiotic every 8 to 12 hours i.m. or i.v. (i.v. infusion over 30 to 60 minutes); usually for urinary tract infections, a dose of 2 mg/kg b.w. every 12 hours i.m. is sufficient [123]. In patients with CRF, in order to achieve the minimum inhibitory serum concentrations of the drug, the interval between doses should be extended to three times the half-time ($T_{1/2}$) in hours. The following formula may be used for calculating $T_{1/2}$ in these patients [123]:

$$T_{1/2} \text{ (hours)} = 2.275$$
$$\times \text{ serum creatinine (mg/dl)} + 2.865.$$

For practical purpose, similar values of intervals in hours may be obtained by multiplying the serum creatinine (S_{Cr}, mg/dl) by 8. For high values of S_{Cr}, however, peak serum levels with a normal dose (2 mg/kg b.w.) are too high [123]. When S_{Cr} is greater than 6 mg/dl (530 μmol/l), therefore, it is suggested that half-dose (1 mg/kg b.w.) should be used at shorter intervals, calculated by multiplying S_{Cr} (mg/dl) $\times$ 4 (= intervals in hours). Since

these calculations are based on serum creatinine concentration (S_{Cr}) rather than on creatinine clearance (see section 10 in this chapter), they are valid only for adult patients with relatively normal muscle mass and with stable values of S_{Cr} (see chapter 7, section 4). Netilmicin is effectively removed by hemodialysis [124] and should be given after each dialysis session [123]. Table 3–1 gives the suggested dosages for netilmicin.

When deciding the doses of aminoglycoside antibiotics, we should bear in mind that they do not penetrate adipose tissue [125]. Thus, dosage should be related to the ideal rather than to the total body weight [121, 126]. Blouin et al. [127] have suggested, for instance, that tobramycin dosage in the obese patient should be based on 58% of the adipose weight of the patient.

Despite these dose adjustments to renal function, however, aminoglycoside nephrotoxicity remains high.

11.1.3 Frequency of Administration of the Aminoglycoside It has been demonstrated that the same daily dosage is less toxic in a single dose than in divided doses [128]. Thus, not only a greater efficacy of treatment but also a reduced toxicity of the drug are obtained with single doses at greater intervals rather than with divided doses at short intervals [116]. The suggested dosage schedules (table 3–1) take into consideration this important point.

11.1.4 Duration of Treatment The longer the duration of treatment, the greater the incidence of nephrotoxicity, presumably in relation to the increased renal cortical accumulation of the drug [129, 130]. Under normal circumstances, it takes 9 to 10 days of therapy for a clinical nephrotoxicity to develop [109]. The risk is increased and the time shortened by the coexistence of other predisposing factors.

In order to reduce the incidence and severity of nephrotoxicity, the course of therapy with aminoglycosides should be shortened as far as possible. For this reason, in cases of infection due to gram-negative bacilli, it has been suggested that an aminoglycoside should be given at first and then changed to a less toxic antibiotic (e.g., ampicillin) to which the microor-

TABLE 3–1. Recommended dosages of nephrotoxic antibiotics*

Gentamicin, Tobramycin, Sisomicin

GFR	DOSE (PARENTERAL USE)
>70 ml/min	1 mg/kg b.w. every 8–12 hours
50–70 ml/min	1 mg/kg b.w. every 12–16 hours
30–50 ml/min	1 mg/kg b.w. every 24 hours
10–30 ml/min	0.5 mg/kg b.w. every 24 hours
5–10 ml/min	0.5 mg/kg b.w. every 48 hours
Hemodialysis	1 mg/kg b.w. after each dialysis session

Amikacin, Kanamicin

GFR	DOSE (PARENTERAL USE)
>70 ml/min	7 mg/kg b.w. every 10–12 hours
50–70 ml/min	7 mg/kg b.w. every 12–14 hours
30–50 ml/min	7 mg/kg b.w. every 14–18 hours
10–30 ml/min	3.5 mg/kg b.w. every 9–20 hours
5–10 ml/min	3.5 mg/kg b.w. every 20–36 hours
Hemodialysis	3.5 mg/kg b.w. after each dialysis session

Streptomycin

GFR	DOSE (PARENTERAL USE)
>70 ml/min	1 g/day
30–70 ml/min	0,5 g/day
10–30 ml/min	0.25 g/day
<10 ml/min	0.25 g twice a week
Hemodialysis	0.25 g after each dialysis session

Netilmicin

GFR	DOSE (PARENTERAL USE)
≥80 ml/min	2 mg/kg b.w. every 8–12 hours

<80 ml/min	
up to S_{Cr} = 6 mg/dl	2 mg/kg b.w. at intervals in hours = S_{Cr} (mg/dl) × 8
for S_{Cr} > 6 mg/dl	1 mg/kg b.w. at intervals in hours = S_{Cr} (mg/dl) × 4
Hemodialysis	2 mg/kg b.w. after each dialysis session

Cefazolin

GFR	DOSE (PARENTERAL USE)
>50 ml/min	500 mg every 6 hours
30–50 ml/min	500 mg as loading dose; then 250 mg every 6 hours
5–30 ml/min	500 mg as loading dose; then 250 mg every 12 hours
Hemodialysis	500 mg as loading dose; then 250 mg after each dialysis session

Cephalothin

GFR	DOSE (PARENTERAL USE)
>30 ml/min	15–35 mg/kg b.w. every 4–6 hours
5–30 ml/min	20 mg/kg b.w. every 6–12 hours
Hemodialysis	2–4 g as loading dose; then 1 g after each dialysis session

Cephalexin

GFR	DOSE (ORAL USE)
>75 ml/min	500 mg every 6 hours
50–75 ml/min	500 mg every 8 hours
20–50 ml/min	500 mg every 12 hours
5–20 ml/min	500 mg every 24 hours
Hemodialysis	500 mg every 24 hours (after dialysis in the day of dialysis)

*Creatinine clearance (ml/min) $= \dfrac{(140 - \text{age in years}) \times \text{kg b.w.}}{72 \times S_{Cr} \text{ (in mg/dl)}}$ (the result should be multiplied by 0.85 for female patients)

ganism has been proven to be susceptible, even when initial aminoglycoside therapy appears satisfactory [131].

11.2 PATIENT'S CONDITION

11.2.1 Age of the Patient Undoubtedly the advanced age of the patient is an important predisposing factor to aminoglycoside nephro-

toxicity [130, 132, 133]. Thus, amikacin-induced ARF occurred in 7% of patients aged 16 to 30, but in 15% of those aged 46 to 60 and in 20% of those over the age of 75 [132]. Hence, even more care should be taken when treating old patients.

11.2.2 Renal Function One should never start a therapy with aminoglycosides without

TABLE 3–1. (Continued).

Cefamandole

GFR	DOSE (PARENTERAL USE)
>50 ml/min	0.5–1 g every 4–8 hours (maximum 2 g every 4 hours)
10–50 ml/min	125–500 mg every 4–8 hours
<10 ml/min	50–250 mg every 4–8 hours

Cephapirin

GFR	DOSE (PARENTERAL USE)
>10 ml/min	0.5–1 g every 6 hours or 30–80 mg/kg b.w./24 hours (in 4 divided doses)
<10 ml/min	0.5–1 g every 12 hours or 30–80 mg/kg b.w./24 hours

Cephradine

GFR	DOSE (ORAL OR PARENTERAL USE)
>50 ml/min	2–4 g/24 h or 50–100 mg/kg b.w./24 hours (in 2–4 divided doses)
10–50 ml/min	1–2 g/24 hours or 25–50 mg/kg b.w./24 hours
<10 ml/min	0.5–1 g/24 hours or 12.5–25 mg/kg b.w./24 hours

Cefadroxil

GFR	DOSE (ORAL USE)
>50 ml/min	500 mg every 6 hours
25–50 ml/min	500 mg every 8 hours
10–25 ml/min	500 mg every 24 hours
<10 ml/min	500 mg every 48 hours

Cefotaxime

GFR	DOSE (PARENTERAL USE)
>50 ml/min	15 mg/kg b.w. every 6 hours
30–50 ml/min	15 mg/kg b.w. every 6–8 hours
10–30 ml/min	15 mg/kg b.w. every 8–12 hours
<10 ml/min	15 mg/kg b.w. every 18–24 hours
Hemodialysis	15 mg/kg b.w. every 24 hours (after dialysis in the day of dialysis)

Cefoxitin

GFR	DOSE (PARENTERAL USE)
>50 ml/min	15 mg/kg b.w. every 3–6 hours
30–50 ml/min	15 mg/kg b.w. every 8–12 hours
10–30 ml/min	15 mg/kg b.w. every 12–24 hours
<10 ml/min	15 mg/kg b.w. every 24–36 hours
Hemodialysis	15 mg/kg b.w. or 1–2 g after each dialysis session

Colistin (Colomycin)

GFR	DOSE (PARENTERAL USE)
>80 ml/min	2.5 mg/kg b.w. every 12 hours
40–80 ml/min	1.5 mg/kg b.w. every 12 hours
5–40 ml/min	1.5 mg/kg b.w. every 18–36 hours
Hemodialysis	2 mg/kg b.w. every 12 hours

Vancomycin

GFR	DOSE (PARENTERAL USE)
>85 ml/min	30 mg/kg b.w./24 h (in divided doses)
60–85 ml/min	15–25 mg/kg b.w./24 hours
35–60 ml/min	10–15 mg/kg b.w./24 hours
20–35 ml/min	10–20 mg/kg b.w./48 hours
10–20 ml/min	6–10 mg/kg b.w./48 hours
<10 ml/min	4.5 mg/kg b.w./72 hours
Hemodialysis	1 g every 7–10 days

knowing the renal function of the patient. Serum creatinine should be measured immediately in order to decide the right dosage in relation to renal function according to the suggested dosage schedules. Renal function should then be monitored throughout the treatment (e.g., serum creatinine measured every other day) and even later (for at least one more week), since toxicity may occur more than four days after discontinuation of therapy [134].

A computer model has been proposed for prospective identification of the prenephrotoxic state during gentamicin therapy by monitoring the serum concentration of the drug throughout the treatment period [135]. Whether or not this approach is successful has not been established as yet [136]. However, since it is well established that renal damage may occur despite maintaining serum drug concentration within the accepted therapeutic range [111, 116, 137–140], in my opinion determination of serum drug concentration is unpractical and not necessary.

Pre-existing renal dysfunction is an important predisposing factor to aminoglycoside nephrotoxicity [55, 116, 132]. Thus, in a review by Lane et al. [132], the incidence of amikacin nephrotoxicity (i.e., deterioration in renal function) appeared proportional to the pretreatment level of serum creatinine, being 8.6% when pretreatment serum creatinine was less than 1.3 mg/dl, 15.9% when it was between 1.3 and 2.0 mg/dl, and 20.8% when it was greater than 2 mg/dl.

11.2.3 State of Hydration of the Patient
Dehydration and salt depletion represent predisposing factors to aminoglycoside nephrotoxicity [55, 109, 141–143]. In particular, salt depletion should be avoided prior to and during treatment or immediately and adequately corrected (with infusion of saline solutions rather than glucose solutions) if it occurs. Actually, ECV should be expanded whenever possible. There is, in fact, experimental evidence in rats that ECV expansion with isotonic sodium chloride or sodium bicarbonate will increase urinary excretion of gentamicin [144] and protect against its nephrotoxicity.

11.2.4 Metabolic Acidosis
There is evidence that metabolic acidosis is another predisposing factor to aminoglycoside nephrotoxicity [145]. Patients with chronic renal failure are usually in mild metabolic acidosis [122]; this will increase the risk of renal damage by aminoglycosides in these patients. But in all patients who experience a decrease of renal function due to the drug toxicity, the consequent occurrence of metabolic acidosis will create a vicious circle with progressively increasing impairment of renal function.

11.2.5 Potassium Depletion
Potassium depletion, experimentally induced in dogs by a low-potassium diet associated with the administration of DOCA, has been shown to increase gentamicin nephrotoxicity [146]. On the other hand, gentamicin may, by itself, cause potassium wasting [146], creating a vicious circle. Since potassium depletion may occur in severely ill patients through vomiting or diarrhea or in surgical patients through drainage from the gastrointestinal tract, any potassium loss in these patients should be monitored and adequately replaced.

11.2.6 Previous Exposure to Aminoglycosides
In contrast with the acquired insensitivity observed in experimental animals, as mentioned in chapter 2, the recent previous exposure of the patients to the same or different aminoglycosides represents a potentiating factor for aminoglycoside nephrotoxicity [132]. Thus, repetitive courses of these drugs should be avoided [131].

11.2.7 Concurrent Administration of Furosemide
Whenever aminoglycoside nephrotoxicity is suspected, neither furosemide nor other diuretics should be used. It has been, in fact, demonstrated that diuretics (furosemide in particular) potentiate aminoglycoside nephrotoxicity [109, 142, 147].

11.2.8 Concurrent Exposure to Other Nephrotoxic Agents
Recent or simultaneous exposure to other nephrotoxins—such as X-ray contrast media [116, 148], anesthetic agents [116, 149], cis-platinum [94], or other toxic antibiotics, cephalosporins in particular [55, 132]—should be avoided because of their demonstrated additive toxic effects.

11.2.9 Intravenous Infusion of Aminoacids
Even the i.v. infusion of amino acids in patients under treatment with aminoglycosides may represent a hazard [109].

It should be stressed that despite attention to these guidelines, aminoglycoside nephrotoxicity may occur during or even after completion of treatment [116, 137, 150]. Whether a mild, subclinical renal dysfunction or a nonoliguric ARF or a severe oliguric ARF occurs, it may depend on the coexistence of other undefined factors related to the clinical condition of the patients.

11.3 PREDICTABILITY OF AMINOGLYCOSIDE NEPHROTOXICITY

A low-molecular weight (11,800 daltons) protein, beta$_2$-microglobulin, is freely filtered by the glomerulus and then reabsorbed and catabolized by the epithelial cells of the proximal tubule; its enhanced urinary excretion has therefore been suggested as an index of proximal tubular damage [151, 152]. Several reports in the recent literature have suggested the usefulness of detecting an increased urinary excretion of beta$_2$-microglobulin for predicting a fall in renal function during aminoglycoside treatment [134, 153, 154]. The increased excretion of beta$_2$-microglobulin corresponds, in fact, to the described ultrastructural lesions occurring in the proximal tubular cells as early manifestations of aminoglycoside nephrotoxicity (see chapter 2). On the same basis, an enhanced urinary excretion of proximal tubular enzymes, such as N-acetyl-β-D-glucosaminidase (N.A.G.), alanine aminopeptidase (A.A.P.), and β-glucuronidase, has also been suggested as a useful although nonspecific predicting test [134, 155–158].

Sethi and Diamond [134] have described three different patterns of beta$_2$-microglobulin excretion in patients developing aminoglycoside nephrotoxicity: (a) a linear increase, (b) a single late peak, and (c) a double peak (while a single early peak was observed in five patients who did not develop any fall in renal function); this increase in beta$_2$-microglobulin preceded any rise in serum creatinine by four to five days. The authors therefore suggest that beta$_2$-microglobulin excretion should be monitored throughout aminoglycoside treatment in high-risk patients (beta$_2$-microglobulin can be easily measured by radio-immunoassay in any hospital laboratory with results available on the same day) [134].

12 Prevention of Renal Damage by Cephalosporins and Other Nephrotoxic Antibiotics

As widely discussed in chapter 2 (section 8), cephalosporins may cause severe renal damage. Nephrotoxicity is increased in humans by the combination of aminoglycosides with furose-

mide. Therefore, these combinations should be avoided. Nephrotoxicity caused by the various cephalosporins listed hereafter differ from that due to other antibiotics.

12.1 CEPHALORIDINE
The nephrotoxicity of cephaloridine has greatly limited its clinical use in humans [106, 159, 160]. In my opinion, cephaloridine should probably be avoided, particularly in patients with CRF [122].

12.2 CEFAZOLIN
Although cefazolin has not shown significant nephrotoxicity in humans [161, 162], it should be used with caution, especially in large doses, or in combination with aminoglycosides, or in patients with creatinine clearance less than 50 ml/min; in the latter condition, dosage should be reduced as shown in table 3–1 [122].

12.3 CEPHALOTHIN
Cephalothin is one of the least nephrotoxic cephalosporins (see chapter 2, section 8). On the basis of reported toxicity, cephalothin should be used at reduced dosage in patients with severely impaired renal function (GFR less than 30 ml/min) especially when associated with other nephrotoxic drugs [106]. Table 3–1 lists the doses that have been suggested [120, 122, 163, 164].

12.4 CEPHALEXIN
Reduced doses of this oral cephalosporin should be used when renal function is less than 75 ml/min. The recommended schedule is shown in table 3–1 [118, 120, 122].

12.5 CEFAMANDOLE
As mentioned in chapter 2 (section 8) cefamandole may cause ARF only at very high dosage. Thus, a considerable margin exists between therapeutic and nephrotoxic doses of this antibiotic. Table 3–1 gives the suggested schedule [165].

12.6 CEPHAPIRIN
For this antibiotic, no nephrotoxicity has been reported in humans. Dosage should be reduced

only in advanced renal failure. [165, 166]. Table 3-1 gives the recommended dosages.

12.7 CEPHRADINE

This antibiotic, available for oral or parenteral use, requires reduced doses when GFR is less than 50 ml/min [165]. See table 3-1 for recommended doses.

12.8 CEFADROXIL

Doses of cefadroxil should be reduced when GFR is less than 50 ml/min (see table 3-1), which allows adequate plasma and urinary concentration of the antibiotic [167].

12.9 CEFOTAXIME

Since nonrenal mechanisms of elimination of cefotaxime become important when renal function is reduced, only moderate reduction in dosage is necessary [168]. The dosage schedule shown in table 3-1 may be used [168, 169].

12.10 CEFOXITIN

For cefoxitin, the recommended dosage schedule is shown in table 3-1 [170].

12.11 COLISTIMETHATE OR COLISTIN (COLOMYCIN)

Cephalosporins seem to enhance the nephrotoxicity of colistin [131]. Their association, therefore, should be avoided. Table 3-1 gives the recommended dosage schedule for colistin patients with reduced renal function [118, 119, 122].

12.12 VANCOMYCIN

This antibiotic, which is very efficient for treating staphylococcal infections, is potentially nephrotoxic and ototoxic. Hearing loss has been observed only in patients with renal failure treated with high doses [131].

In order to reduce the risk of nephrotoxicity and ototoxicity, Moellering et al. [171] have recently constructed a nomogram for vancomycin dosage adjustment in patients with various degrees of renal failure. From that nomogram, the recommended dosage schedule shown in table 3-1 has been derived. Patients on RDT have been successfully treated with 1 gram intravenously every 7 to 10 days [131].

13 Prevention of Drug-Induced Acute Interstitial Nephritis (AIN)

Our experience in drug-induced AIN (see chapter 2, section 16) should warn all doctors about the use of drugs. We must remember that practically any drug can cause AIN. Thus, the occurrence of unexplained fever, skin rash, and/or hematuria during the administration of any drug must suggest its withdrawal since its continued use may lead to irreversible ARF.

13.1 PREVENTION OF RENAL DAMAGE BY HYPERSENSITIVITY REACTION TO RIFAMPICIN

As widely discussed in chapter 2 (section 16), discontinuation of treatment with rifampicin followed by resumption days to months later, or change of continuous daily medication into an intermittent regimen are the conditions that usually elicit the reaction to rifampicin. For this reason, when using rifampicin we prefer continuous daily therapy; the patient should be warned about the hazards of restarting therapy once it has been discontinued [172, 173]. Should we be forced, for any reason, to restart therapy after a preceding course, careful attention must be given to the first signs of intolerance; in this case rifampicin must be immediately withdrawn. Testing for circulating antirifampicin antibodies is not a useful screening since reaction may occur even in the absence of serum antibodies [174].

14 Prevention of Postsurgical ARF

Because of the high incidence of postsurgical ARF, particular attention should be addressed to all patients undergoing surgical operations. Problems concerning renal function may arise from anesthesia, fluid and electrolyte abnormalities, and prophylactic use of antibiotics.

14.1 ANESTHESIA

As widely discussed in chapter 2 (section 11), anesthesia may by itself cause ARF. In section 8 of this chapter, a detailed guidline for preventing renal damage by anesthetic agents was given.

14.2 HYDRATION BEFORE SURGERY

Adequate hydration with salt-containing solutions should precede surgical operation in order to prevent dehydration and salt depletion during and after operation. This precaution is important in patients with CRF who are particularly sensitive to dehydration because of their impaired ability to conserve sodium and water [175].

14.3 BLOOD, FLUID, AND ELECTROLYTE REPLACEMENT DURING AND AFTER SURGERY

During surgical intervention, blood loss should be adequately replaced. Adequate hydration, with salt-containing solutions, should be performed during operation to replace fluid losses that occur in all surgical operations. Furthermore, all salt and water losses through nasogastric and/or enteric drainage should be carefully monitored and precisely replaced.

14.4 ANTIMICROBIAL PROPHYLAXIS IN SURGERY

The use of prophylactic antibiotics in surgery has been a matter of debate for many years and is still controversial. Because of this division of opinion, it is the view of many physicians that antibiotic toxicity is an acceptable risk when infection is established but unacceptable when there is only the possibility of an infection [176].

14.4.1 Rationale for Antimicrobial Prophylaxis in Surgery Soon after the arrival of bacteria in host tissue, host defenses would immediately act against bacterial invasion to prevent the lesion; apparently, it takes 24 hours for the complete development of the classic inflammatory lesion, but only four hours for its establishment [176, 177]. Therefore, antimicrobial prophylaxis, in order to supplement host defenses, should cover the four hours after bacterial contamination [177]. On this basis, antimicrobial prophylaxis in surgery should be performed before rather than after the surgical operation. Clinical studies have, in fact, confirmed that only patients who received antibacterial prophylaxis were usually protected against postoperative infection of the wound; this did not occur when antibiotics were given after completion of the surgical operation [178, 179].

14.4.2 Hazards of Antimicrobial Prophylaxis The most common errors in antimicrobial prophylaxis include (a) its routine use in all surgical patients; (b) excessive dosage of antibiotics—it has been recently demonstrated that one dose of cephalothin, for instance, is as effective as 20 grams given prophylacticly for four days [180]; and (c) prolonged administration of prophylactic antibiotics [181].

The hazards of this procedure include (a) allergic drug reaction; (b) selection of resistant microorganisms with bacterial superinfection; (c) fungal superinfection; and (d) antibiotic toxicity, nephrotoxicity in particular.

14.4.3 Limits and Modality of Antibiotic Prophylaxis According to Nichols [182], who has recently reviewed this topic, antibiotic prophylaxis may be accepted only under the following conditions:

a. It is limited to patients at high risk for postoperative infections; these may include patients undergoing operations for bleeding or obstructing duodenal or gastric ulcer or malignancy; biliary tract operations when bile cultures are positive; surgical interventions of colon resection; those clean surgical procedures in which a prosthetic foreign body (e.g., cardiac valve, vascular graft, or total hip replacement) is implanted (infection in these cases would be catastrophic) [182]. Routine prophylaxis must be avoided.

b. It starts within one hour prior to operation, when the antibiotic agent is given intravenously, or within 24 hours before the operation with oral antibiotics as in operations of colon resection. This will allow high levels of the antibiotic agent in the wound during the operation.

c. It continues for no longer than 72 hours (i.e., it should last 24 to 72 hours) in order to reduce the risks of drug toxicity, bacterial resistance, and bacterial or fungal superinfection; on the other hand, prolonged treatment will not reduce the incidence of further infection.

Antibiotic agents should be given by fast i.v. injection (rather than by continuous i.v.

infusion or intermittent i.m. injection) in order to obtain more rapidly a high concentration of the drug in wound fluid [183].

Obviously, even when using antimicrobial prophylaxis, strict asepsis is absolutely necessary during and after the surgical operation.

14.5 TREATMENT OF INFECTIONS IN SURGICAL PATIENTS

Should infection occur in surgical patients and nephrotoxic antibiotics be unavoidable, their use requires all precautions as listed in sections 10, 11, 12, and 13 of this chapter.

Obviously, in all surgical patients, renal function should be carefully monitored before and for many days after operation.

References

1. Bichet DG, Burke TJ, Schrier RW. Prevention and pathogenesis of acute renal failure. Clin Exper Dial Apheresis 5: 127–141, 1981.
2. Schrier RW. Acute renal failure. JAMA 247: 2518–2525, 1982.
3. Solez K, Stout R, Bendush B, Silvia CB, Whelton A. Adverse effect of amino acid solutions in aminoglycoside-induced acute renal failure in rabbits and rats. In Acute Renal Failure, Eliahou HE (ed). London: John Libbey, 1982, pp. 241–247.
4. Levenson DJ, Simmons CE, Brenner BM. Arachidonic acid metabolism prostaglandins and the kidney. Am J Med 72: 354–374, 1982.
5. Rasmussen HH, Ibels LS. Acute renal failure. Am J Med 73: 211–217, 1982.
6. Balslow JT, Jorgensen HE. A survey of 499 patients with acute anuric renal insufficiency. Am J Med 34: 753–764, 1963.
7. Hermreck AS, Abrams JH, Joner RG. Mannitol and propranolol in treatment of ischemic renal failure. Improved survival rate and renal function. Surg Forum 24: 25–27, 1973.
8. Iaina A, Solomon S, Eliahou HE. Reduction in severity of acute renal failure in rats by beta-adrenergic blockade. Lancet II: 157–159, 1975.
9. Eliahou HE, Iaina A, Solomon S, Gavendo S. Alleviation of anoxic experimental acute renal failure in rats by beta-adrenergic blockade. Nephron 19: 158–166, 1977.
10. Solez K, Freshwater MF, Su CT. The effect of propranolol of post-ischemic acute renal failure in the rat. Transplantation 24: 148–151, 1977.
11. Solez K, D'Agostini RJ, Stawowy L, Freedman MT, Scott JR, Siegelman SS, Heptinstall RH. Beneficial effect of propranolol in a histologically appropriate model of post-ischemic acute renal failure. Am J Path 88: 163–192, 1977.
12. Eliahou HE, Iaina A, Solomon S, Oshman R, Serban I. Alleviation of acute anoxic renal failure in rats by beta$_1$-adrenergic blockade with practolol. Isr J Med Sci 14: 274–278, 1978.
13. Klein LA. Propranolol protection in acute renal failure. Invest Urol 15: 401–403, 1978.
14. Chevalier RL, Finn WF. Effects of propranolol on post-ischemic acute renal failure. Nephron 25: 77–81, 1980.
15. Iaina I, Serban I, Gavendo S, Kapuler S, Eliahou HE. Alleviation of ischemic acute renal failure by beta blockers: Specific tubular receptor blockade or membrane stabilising effect? Proc EDTA 17: 686–689, 1980.
16. Ideura T, Solez K, Heptinstall RH. Effect of clonidine on tubular obstruction in post-ischemic acute renal failure in the rabbit demonstrated using microradiography and microdinection. Am J Path 98: 123–150, 1980.
17. Solez K, Ideura T, Silvia CB, Hamilton B, Saito H. Clonidine after renal ischemia to lessen acute renal failure and microvascular damage. Kidney Int 18: 309–322, 1980.
18. Solez K, Racusen LC, Whelton A. Glomerular epithelial cell changes in early post-ischemic acute renal failure in rabbits and man. Am J Path 103: 163, 1981.
19. Racusen LC, Solez K, Whelton A. Glomerular prodocyte changes and increased permeability to protein in early post-ischemic acute renal failure. In Acute Renal Failure, Eliahou HE (ed). London: John Libbey, 1982, pp. 215–218.
20. Onesti G, Paz-Martinez V, Kim KE, Swartz C. Effect of clonidine on renin release. In Hypertension: Mechanisms and Management, Onesti G, Kim KE, Moyer JH (eds). New York: Grune and Stratton, 1973, pp. 405–409.
21. Gennari FJ, Kassirer JP. Osmotic diuresis. N Engl J Med 80: 714–720, 1974.
22. Kikko JP, Rector FC Jr. Countercurrent multiplication system without active transport in inner medulla. Kidney Int 2: 214–223, 1972.
23. Warren SE, Blantz RC. Mannitol. Arch Intern Med 141: 493–497, 1981.
24. Tiller DJ, Field M, Horvath JS, England J. Use of mannitol in renal failure. Med J Australia 2: 151, 1981.
25. Cronin RE, de Torrente A, Miller PD, Bulger RE, Burke TJ, Schrier RW. Pathogenic mechanisms in early norepinephrine-induced acute renal failure: Functional and histological correlates of protection. Kidney Int 14: 115–125, 1978.
26. Burke TJ, Cronin RE, Duchin KL, Peterson LN, Schrier RW. Ischemia and tubule obstruction during acute renal failure in dogs. Am J Physiol 238: F305–F314, 1980.
27. Johnston PA, Bernard DB, Donohoe JF, Perrin NS, Levinsky NG. Effect of volume expansion on hemodynamics of the hypoperfused rat kidney. J Clin Invest 64: 550–558, 1979.

28. Morris CR, Alexander EA, Bruns FJ, Levinsky NG. Restoration and maintenance of glomerular filtration by mannitol during hypoperfusion of the kidney. J Clin Invest 51: 1555–1564, 1972.

29. Johnston PA, Bernard DB, Perrin NS, Levinsky NG. Prostaglandins mediate the vasodilatory effect of mannitol in the hypoperfused rat kidney. J Clin Invest 68: 127–133, 1981.

30. Patak RV, Fadem SZ, Lifschitz MD, Stein JH. Study of factors which modify the development of norepinephrine-induced acute renal failure in the dog. Kidney Int 15: 227–237, 1979.

31. Hanley MJ, Davidson K. Prior mannitol and furosemide infusion in a model of ischemic acute renal failure. Am J Physiol 10: F556–564, 1981.

32. Schrier RW, Arnold PE, Burke TJ. Alterations in mitochondrial respiration and calcium movements in norepinephrine-induced acute renal failure: Modification by mannitol. In Acute Renal Failure, Eliahou HE (ed). London: John Libbey, 1982, pp. 21–22.

33. Barry KG, Cohen A, Knochel JP, Whelan TJ Jr, Beisel WR, Vargas CA, Le Blanc PC. Mannitol infusion. N Engl J Med 264: 967–971, 1961.

34. Etheredge EE, Levitin H, Nakamura K, Glenn WWL. Effect of mannitol on renal function during open-heart surgery. Ann Surg 161: 53–64, 1965.

35. Luck RJ, Irvine WT. Mannitol in the surgery of aortic aneurysm. Lancet 2: 409–411, 1965.

36. Byrne JJ. Shock. N Engl J Med 275: 659–660, 1966.

37. Mazze RI, Barry KG. Prevention of functional renal failure during anesthesia and surgery by sustained hydration and mannitol infusion. Anesth Analg 46: 61–68, 1967.

38. Dawson JL. Acute post-operative renal failure in obstructive jaundice. Ann R Coll Surg Engl 42: 163–181, 1968.

39. Hayes DM, Cvitkovic E, Golbey RB, Scheiner E, Helson L, Krakoff IH. High-dose cis-platinum diammine dichloride. Cancer 39: 1372–1381, 1977.

40. Anto HR, Chou SY, Porush JG, Shapiro WB. Infusion intravenous pyelography and renal function. Effects of hypertonic mannitol in patients with chronic renal insufficiency. Arch Intern Med 141: 1652–1656, 1981.

41. Porush JG, Chou SY, Anto HR, Oguagha C, Shapiro WB, Faubert PF. Infusion intravenous pyelography and renal function: Effects of hypertonic mannitol and furosemide in patients with chronic renal insufficiency. In Acute Renal Failure, Eliahou HE (ed). London: John Libbey, 1982, pp. 161–167.

42. Gann DS, Wright HK, Newsome HH. Prevention of sodium depletion during osmotic diuresis. Surg Gynecol Obstet 119: 265–268, 1964.

43. Buchbinder D, Karmody AM, Leather RP, Shah DM. Hypertonic mannitol. Arch Surg 116: 414–421, 1981.

44. Haimovici H. Myopathic-nephrotic-metabolic syndrome associated with massive acute arterial occlusions. J Cardiovasc Surg 14: 589–593, 1973.

45. Blaisdell FW, Steele M, Allen RE. Management of acute lower extremity arterial ischemia due to embolism and thrombosis. Surgery 84: 822–834, 1978.

46. Anderson J, Eklof B, Hegler P. Metabolic changes in blood and skeletal muscle in reconstructive aortic surgery. Ann Surg 189: 283–289, 1979.

47. Cantarovich F, Galli C, Benedetti L, Chena C, Castro L, Correa C, Perez Loredo J, Fernandez JC, Locatelli A, Tizado J. High-dose furosemide in established acute renal failure. Brit Med J 4: 449–450, 1973.

48. Ganeval D, Kleinknecht D, Gonzales-Duque LA. High-dose furosemide in renal failure. Brit Med J 1: 244–245, 1974.

49. Epstein M, Schneider NS, Befeler B. Effect of intrarenal furosemide on renal function and intrarenal hemodynamics in acute renal failure. Am J Med 58: 510–516, 1975.

50. Montoreano R, Mouzet MT, Cunarro J, Ruiz-Guinazu A. Prevention of the initial oliguria of acute renal failure by the administration of furosemide. Postgrad Med J (Suppl) 47: 7–10, 1971.

51. Bailey RR, Natale R, Turnbull DI, Linton AL. Protective effect of furosemide in acute tubular necrosis and acute renal failure. Clin Sci Mol Med 45: 1–17, 1973.

52. Greven J, Klein H. Renal effects of furosemide in glycerol-induced acute renal failure of the rat. Pflügers Arch 365: 81–87, 1976.

53. Kjellstrand CM. Ethacrynic acid in acute tubular necrosis. Nephron 9: 337–348, 1972.

54. Kleinknecht D, Ganeval D, Gonzales-Duque LA, Fermanian J. Furosemide in acute oliguric renal failure. A controlled trial. Nephron 17: 51–58, 1976.

55. Andreucci VE, Dal Canton A. Can acute renal failure in humans be prevented? Proc EDTA 17: 123–132, 1980.

56. Mason J, Kain H, Welsch J, Schnermann J. The early phase of experimental acute renal failure. VI The influence of furosemide, Pflügers Arch 392: 125–133, 1981.

57. Ufferman RC, Jaenike JR, Freeman RB, Pabico RC. Effects of furosemide on low-dose mercuric chloride acute renal failure in the rat. Kidney Int 8: 362–367, 1975.

58. Papadimitriou M, Milionis A, Sakellariou G, Metakas P. Effect of furosemide on acute ischemic renal failure in the dog. Nephron 20: 157–162, 1978.

59. Dodds MG, Foord RD. Enhancement by potent diuretics of renal tubular necrosis induced by cephaloridine. Brit J Pharmacol 40: 227–236, 1970.

60. Lawson DH, Macadam RF, Singh H, Gavras H, Linton AL. The nephrotoxicity of cephaloridine. Post-grad Med J (Suppl) 46: 36–38, 1970.

144

61. Lawson DH, Macadam RF, Singh H, Gavras H, Hartz S, Turnbull D, Linton AL: Effect of furosemide on antibiotic-induced renal damage in rats. J Infect Dis 126: 593–600, 1972.

62. Linton AL, Bailey RR, Turnbull DI. Relative nephrotoxicity of cephalosporin antibiotics in an animal model. Can Med Ass J 107: 414–416, 1972.

63. de Torrente A, Miller PD, Cronin RE, Paulsen PE, Erickson AL, Schrier RW. Effects of furosemide and acetylcholine in norepinephrine-induced acute renal failure. Am J Physiol 235: F131–F136, 1978.

64. Lindner A, Cutler RE, Goodman WG. Synergism of dopamine plus furosemide in preventing acute renal failure in the dog. Kidney Int 16: 158–166, 1979.

65. Williamson HE, Bourland WA, Marchand GR, Farley DB, Van Orden DE. Furosemide-induced release of prostaglandin E to increase renal blood flow. Proc Soc Exp Biol Med 150: 104–106, 1975.

66. Ciabattoni G, Pugliese F, Cinotti GA, Stirati G, Ronci R, Castrucci G, Pierucci A, Patrono C. Characterization of furosemide activation of the renal prostaglandin system. Eur J Pharmacol 60: 181–187, 1979.

67. Dusing R, Nicholas V, Glanzer K, Kipnowski J, Kramer HJ. Prostaglandins participate in the regulation of NaCl absorption in the diluting segments of the nephron in vivo: Effects of furosemide. Renal Physiol 5: 115–123, 1982.

68. Graziani G, Cairo G, Tarantino F, Ponticelli C. Dopamine and furosemide in acute renal failure. Lancet II: 1301, 1980.

69. Wright FS, Schnermann J. Interference with feedback control of glomerular filtration rate by furosemide, triflocin, and cyanide. J Clin Invest 53: 1695–1708, 1974.

70. Schnermann J, Briggs J. Concentration-dependent sodium chloride transport as the signal in feedback control of glomerular filtration rate. Kidney Int 22 (Suppl 12): S82–S89, 1982.

71. Wilson DR, Thiel G, Arce ML, Oken DE. Glycerol-induced hemoglobinuric acute renal failure in the rat: III Micropuncture study of the effects of mannitol and isotonic saline on individual nephron function. Nephron 4: 337–355, 1967.

72. McDonald FD, Thiel G, Wilson DR, Dibona GF, Oken DE. The prevention of acute renal failure in the rat by long-term saline loading: A possible role of the renin-angiotensin axis. Proc Soc Exp Biol Med 131: 610–614, 1969.

73. Yeboah ED, Petrie A, Pead JL. Acute renal failure and open-heart surgery. Brit Med J 1: 415–418, 1972.

74. Lucas CE, Zito JG, Carter KM, Cortex A, Stebner FC. Questionable value of furosemide in preventing renal failure. Surgery 82: 314–320, 1977.

75. D'Elia JA, Gleason RE, Alday M, Malarick C, Godley K, Warram J, Kaldany A, Weinrauch LA. Nephrotoxicity from angiographic contrast material. A prospective study. Am J Med 72: 719–725, 1982.

76. Eisenberg RL, Bank WO, Hedgock MW. Renal failure after major angiography can be avoided with hydration. Am J Roentgenol 136: 859–861, 1981.

77. Shafi T, Chou SY, Porush JG, Shapiro WB. Infusion intravenous pyelography and renal function: Effects in patients with chronic renal insufficiency. Arch Intern Med 138: 1218–1221, 1978.

78. Old CW, Lehrner LM. Prevention of radiocontrast-induced acute renal failure with mannitol. Lancet 1: 885, 1980.

79. Krumlovsky FA, Simon N, Santhanam S, Del Greco F, Roxe D, Pomaranc MM. Acute renal failure. Association with administration of radiographic contrast material. JAMA 239: 125–127, 1978.

80. Ng RCK, Suki WN. Treatment of acute renal failure. In Acute Renal Failure, Brenner BM, Stein JH (eds). New York: Churchill Livingstone, 1980, pp. 229–273.

81. Bartrum RJ Jr, Crow HC, Foote SR. Ultrasonic and radiographic cholecystography. N Engl J Med 296: 538–541, 1977.

82. Rossof AH, Slayton RE, Perlia CP. Preliminary clinical experience with cis-diamminedichloroplatinum (II) (NSC 119875, CACP). Cancer 30: 1451–1456, 1972.

83. Madias NE, Harrington JT. Platinum nephrotoxicity. Am J Med 65: 307–314, 1978.

84. Hill JM, Loeb E, Maclellan A. Clinical studies of platinum coordination compounds in the treatment of various malignant diseases. Cancer Chemother Rep 59: 647–651, 1975.

85. Blackley JD, Hill JB. Renal and electrolyte disturbances associated with cisplatinum. Ann Intern Med 95: 628–632, 1981.

86. Einhord LH, Donohue J. Cis-diamminedichloroplatinum, vinblastine, and bleomycin combination chemotherapy in disseminated testicular cancer. Ann Intern Med 87: 293–298, 1977.

87. Einhorn LH, Williams SD. The role of cis-platinum in solid-tumor therapy. N Engl J Med 300: 289–291, 1979.

88. Belt RJ, Himmelstein KJ, Patton TF, Bannister SJ, Sternson LA, Repta AJ. Pharmacokinetics of non-protein bound platinum species following administration of cis-dichlorodiammine platinum (II). Cancer Treat Rep 63: 1515–1521, 1979.

89. Cvitkovic E, Spaulding J, Bethune V, Martin J, Whitmore WF. Improvement of cis-dichlorodiammineplatinum (NSC 119875): Therapeutic index in an animal model. Cancer 39: 1357–1361, 1977.

90. Ward JM, Grabin ME, Berlin E, Young DM. Prevention of renal failure in rats receiving cis-diamminedichloroplatinum (II) by administration of furosemide. Cancer Res 37: 1238–1240, 1977.

91. Chary KK, Higby DJ, Henderson ES. A phase I study of high-dose cis-diamminedichloroplatinum II (NSC 119875) with forced diuresis. J Clin Hematol Oncol 7: 633–641, 1977.

92. Gonzales-Vitale JC, Hayes DM, Cvitkovic E, Sternberg SS. The renal pathology in clinical trials of cis-platinum (11) diammine-dichloride. Cancer 39: 1362–1371, 1977.

93. Vaamonde LA, Teixeira RB, Morales J, Roth D, Kelley J, Alpert H, Pardo V. A new model for studying drug-induced acute renal failure: The rat with untreated diabetes mellitus. In Acute Renal Failure, Eliahou HE (ed). London: John Libbey, 1982, pp. 96–101.

94. Dentino ME, Luft RC, Yum MN, Einhorn LH. Long-term effect of cis-diamminedichloride platinum on renal function and structure in man. Cancer 41: 1274–1281, 1978.

95. Churchill D, Knaack J, Chirito E, Barre P, Cole C, Muehrcke R, Gault MH. Persisting renal insufficiency after methoxyflurane anesthesia. Am J Med 56: 575–582, 1974.

96. Cousins MJ, Mazze RI. Methoxyflurane nephrotoxicity. A study of dose response in man. JAMA 225: 1611–1616, 1973.

97. Hetrick WD, Wolfson B, Garcia DA, Siker ES. Renal response to "light" methoxyflurane anesthesia. Anesthesiology 38: 30–32, 1973.

98. Tobey RE, Clubb RJ. Renal function after methoxyflurane and halothane anesthesia. JAMA 223: 649–652, 1973.

99. Schiffl H, Binswanger U. Renal handling of fluoride in healthy man. Renal Physiol 5: 192–196, 1982.

100. Bevan DR. Renal Function in Anesthesia and Surgery. London: Academic Press, 1979.

101. Young SR, Stoelting RK, Peterson C, Madura JA. Anesthetic biotransformation and renal function in obese patients during and after methoxyflurane. Anesthesiology 42: 451–457, 1975.

102. Taves DR, Gillies AJ, Freeman RB, Fry BW. Toxicity following methoxyflurane anesthesia. JAMA 214: 91–97, 1970.

103. Briggs JD. Renal transplantation. In Acute Renal Failure, Chapman A, (ed). Edinburgh: Churchill Livingstone, 1980, pp. 149–171.

104. Mazze RI. Critical care of the patient with acute renal failure. Anesthesiology 47: 138–148, 1977.

105. Lawson DH. Drug therapy in acute renal failure. In Acute Renal Failure, Chapman A (ed). Edinburgh: Churchill Livingstone, 1980, pp. 125–148.

106. Appel GB, Nev HC. The nephrotoxicity of antimicrobial agents. N Engl J Med 296: 663–670, 722–728, and 784–787, 1977.

107. Rose BD. Acute renal failure. In Pathophysiology of Renal Disease, Rose BD (ed). New York: McGraw-Hill, 1981, pp. 55–95.

108. Cockcroft DW, Gault MH. Prediction of creatinine clearance from serum creatinine. Nephron 16: 31–41, 1976.

109. Whelton A, Solez K. Aminoglycoside nephrotoxicity. A tale of two transports. J Lab Clin Med 99: 148–155, 1982.

110. Kumin GD. Clinical nephrotoxicity of tobramycin and gentamicin JAMA 244: 1808–1810, 1980.

111. Smith CR, Baughman KL, Edwards CQ, Rogers JF, Leitman PS. Controlled comparison of amikacin and gentamicin. N Engl J Med 296: 349–353, 1977.

112. Lau WK, Young LS, Black RE, Winston DJ, Linne SR, Weinstein RJ, Hewitt WL. Comparative efficacy and toxicity of amikacin/carbenicillin versus gentamicin/carbenicillin in leukopenic patients: A randomized prospective trial. Am J Med 62: 959, 1977.

113. Keating MJ, Bodey GP, Valdivieso M, Rodriguez V. A randomized comparative trial of three aminoglycosides: Comparison of continuous infusion of gentamicin, amikacin and sisomycin combined with carbenicillin in the treatment of infections in neutropenic patients with malignancies. Medicine 58: 159, 1979.

114. French MA, Cerra FB, Plaut ME, Schentag JJ. Amikacin and gentamicin accumulation pharmacokinetics and nephrotoxicity in critically ill patients. Antimicrob Agents Chemother 19: 147, 1981.

115. Herting RL, Lane AZ, Lorber RR, Wright JJ. Netilmicin: Chemical development and overview of clinical research. Scand J Infect Dis 23 (Suppl): 20–29, 1980.

116. Cronin RE. Aminoglycoside nephrotoxicity: Pathogenesis and prevention. Clin Nephrol 11: 251–256, 1979.

117. Reidenberg MM: Renal Function and Drug Action. Philadelphia: WB Saunders, 1971.

118. Curtis JR, Williams GB. Clinical Management of Chronic Renal Failure. Oxford: Blackwell Scientific Publications, 1975.

119. Cutler RE, Christopher TG. Drug therapy during renal insufficiency and dialytic treatment. In Clinical Aspects of Uremia and Dialysis, Massry SG, Sellers AL (eds). Springfield: CC Thomas, 1976, pp. 427–452.

120. Anderson RJ, Gambertoglio JG, Schrier RW. Clinical Use of Drugs in Renal Failure. Springfield: CC Thomas, 1976.

121. Sarubbi FA, Hull JH. Amikacin serum concentrations: Prediction of levels and dosage guidelines. Ann Intern Med 89: 612–618, 1978.

122. Andreucci VE. Chronic renal failure. In The Treatment of Renal Failure, Castro JE (ed). Lancaster: MTP Press Limited, 1982, pp. 33–167.

123. Humbert G, Leroy A, Fillastre JP, Oksenhendler G. Pharmacokinetics of netilmicin in the presence of normal or impaired renal function. Antimicrob Agents Chemother 14: 40–44, 1978.

124. Kahlmeter G. Netilmicin: Clinical pharmacokinetics and aspects on dosage schedules. An overview. Scand J Infect Dis 23 (Suppl): 74–81, 1980.

125. Bennett WM. Drugs and the kidney. In Contemporary Nephrology, Klahr S, Massry SG (eds). New York: Plenum Medical Book Company, 1981, Volume 1, pp. 657–694.

126. Hull JH, Sarubbi FA. Gentamicin serum concentration: Pharmacokinetic predictions. Ann Intern Med 85: 183–189, 1976.

127. Blouin RA, Mann HJ, Griffen WO, Bauer LA, Record KE. Tobramycin pharmacokinetics in morbidly obese patients. Clin Pharmacol Ther 26: 5, 1979.

128. Plamp C, Bennett W, Gilbert D, Porter G. The effect of dosage regimen on experimental gentamicin nephrotoxicity: Dissociation of peak serum levels from renal failure. Clin Res 26: 125A, 1978.

129. Schentag JJ, Jusko WJ. Renal clearances and tissue accumulation of gentamicin. Clin Pharmacol Ther 22: 364–370, 1977.

130. Appel GB, Neu HC. Gentamicin in 1978. Ann Intern Med 89: 528–538, 1978.

131. Cronin RE. Antimicrobial agent nephrotoxicity. In Clinical Use of Drugs in Patients with Kidney and Liver Disease, Anderson RJ, Schrier RW (eds). Philadelphia: WB Saunders, 1981, pp. 54–65.

132. Lane AZ, Wright GE, Blair DC. Ototoxicity and nephrotoxicity of amikacin. Am J Med 62: 911–918, 1977.

133. Kaloyanides GJ, Pastoriza-Munoz E. Aminoglycoside nephrotoxicity. Kidney Int 18: 571–582, 1980.

134. Sethi K and Diamond LH. Aminoglycoside nephrotoxicity and its predictability. Nephron 27: 265–270, 1981.

135. Colburn WA, Schentag JJ, Jusko WJ, Gibaldi M. A model for the prospective identification of the pre-nephrotoxic state during gentamicin therapy. J Pharmacokinet Biopharm 6: 179–186, 1978.

136. Bennett WM, Luft F, Porter GA. Pathogenesis of renal failure due to aminoglycosides and contrast media used in roentgenography. Am J Med 69: 767–774, 1980.

137. Wade JC, Smith CR, Petty BG, Lipsky JJ, Conrad G, Ellner J, Lietmann PS. Cephalothin plus an aminoglycoside is more nephrotoxic than methicillin plus an aminoglycoside. Lancet II: 604–606, 1978.

138. Smith CR, Lipsky JJ, Laskin OL, Hellman DB, Mellits ED, Longstreth J, Lietman PS. Double-blind comparison of the nephrotoxicity and auditory toxicity of gentamicin and tobramycin. N Engl J Med 302: 1106–1109, 1980.

139. Trollfors B, Alestig K, Krantz I, Norrby R. Quantitative nephrotoxicity of gentamicin in nontoxic doses. J Infect Dis 141: 306–309, 1980.

140. Fong IW, Fenton RS, Bird R. Comparative toxicity of gentamicin versus tobramycin: A randomized prospective study. J Antimicrob Chemother 7: 81–88, 1981.

141. Bennett WM, Hartnett MN, Gilbert D, Houghton D, Porter GA. Effect of sodium intake on gentamicin nephrotoxicity in the rat. Proc Soc Exp Biol Med 151: 736–738, 1976.

142. Adelman RD, Spangler WL, Beasom F, Ishizaki G, Conzelman GM. Furosemide enhancement of experimental gentamicin nephrotoxicity. Comparison of functional and morphological changes with activities of urinary enzymes. J Infect Dis 140: 342–352, 1979.

143. Bennett WM. Aminoglycoside nephrotoxicity. Experimental and clinical considerations. Mineral Electrolyte Metab 6: 277–286, 1981.

144. Senekjian HO, Knight TF, Weinman EJ. Micropuncture study of the handling of gentamicin by the rat kidney. Kidney Int 19: 416–423, 1981.

145. Hsu CH, Kurtz TW, Easterling RE, Weller JM. Potentiation of gentamicin nephrotoxicity by metabolic acidosis. Proc Soc Exp Biol Med 146: 894–897, 1974.

146. Brinker K, Cronin R, Bulger R, Southern P, Henrich W. Potassium depletion risk factor for and consequence of gentamicin nephrotoxicity. Kidney Int 16: 849, 1979.

147. de Rougemont D, Oeschger A, Konrad L, Thiel G, Torhorst J, Wenk M, Wunderlich P, Brunner FP. Gentamicin-induced acute renal failure in the rat. Effect of dehydration, DOCA-saline and furosemide. Nephron 29: 176–184, 1981.

148. Barshay ME, Kaye JH, Goldman R, Coburn JW: Acute renal failure in diabetic patients after intravenous infusion pyelography. Clin Nephrol 1: 35–39, 1973.

149. Mazze RI, Cousins M. Combined nephrotoxicity of gentamicin and methoxyflurane anesthesia in man. Brit J Anaesth 45: 394–397, 1973.

150. Gary NE, Buzzco L, Salaki J. Gentamicin-associated acute renal failure. Arch Intern Med 136: 1101–1104, 1976.

151. Hall PW, Vasiljevic. Beta$_2$-microglobulin excretion as an index of renal tubular disorders with special reference to endemic Balkan nephropathy. J Lab Clin Med 81: 897–904, 1973.

152. Fredriksson A. Renal handling of beta$_2$-microglobulin in experimental renal disease. Scand J Clin Lab Invest 35: 591–600, 1975.

153. Schentag JJ, Sutfin TA, Plaut ME, Jusko WJ. Early detection of aminoglycoside nephrotoxicity with urinary beta$_2$-microglobulin. J Med 9: 201–210, 1978.

154. Schentag JJ, Plaut ME. Patterns of urinary beta-2-microglobulin excretion by patients treated with aminoglycosides. Kidney Int 17: 654–661, 1980.

155. Luft FC, Patel V, Yum MN, Patel B, Kleit SA. Experimental aminoglycoside nephrotoxicity. J Lab Clin Med 86: 213–220, 1975.

156. Patel V, Luft FC, Yum MN, Patel B, Zeman W, Kleit SA. Enzynuria in gentamicin-induced kidney damage. Antimicrob Agents Chemother 7: 364–369, 1975.

157. Wellwood JM, Lovell D, Thompson AE, Tighe JR. Renal damage caused by gentamicin. A study of the effects on renal morphology and urinary enzyme excretion. J Path 118: 171–182, 1976.

158. Ninane G. Cefotaxime and nephrotoxicity. Lancet 1: 332, 1979.

159. Foord RD. Cephaloridine, cephalothin and the kidney. J Antimicrob Chemother 1: 119–133, 1975.
160. Tune BM, Fravert D. Mechanisms of cephalosporin nephrotoxicity: A comparison of cephaloridine and cephaloglycin. Kidney Int 18: 591–600, 1980.
161. Turck M, Clark RA, Beaty HN. Cefazolin in the treatment of bacterial pneumonia. J Infect Dis 128:S382–S385, 1973.
162. Reinarz JA, Kier CM, Guckian JC. Evaluation of cefazolin in the treatment of bacterial endocarditis and bacteremias. J Infect Dis 128: S392–S395, 1973.
163. Seldin DW, Carter NW, Rector FC Jr. Consequences of renal failure and their management. In Disease of the Kidney, Strauss MB, Welt LG (eds). Boston: Little, Brown, 1971 (2nd ed), pp. 211–272.
164. Blythe WB. The management of intercurrent medical and surgical problems in the patient with chronic renal failure. In Strauss and Welt's Diseases of the Kidney, Earley LE, Gottschalk CW (eds). Boston: Little, Brown, 1979 (3rd ed), pp. 517–537.
165. Anderson RJ, Schrier RW. Clinical use of drugs in patients with kidney and liver disease. Philadelphia: WB Saunders, 1981.
166. Coggins CH, Bennett WM, Singer I. Drugs and the kidney. In Pathophysiology of Renal Disease, Rose BD (ed). New York: McGraw-Hill, 1981, pp. 711–732.
167. Cutler RE, Blair AD, Kelly MR. Cefadroxil kinetics in patients with renal insufficiency. Clin Pharmacol Ther 25: 514–521, 1979.
168. Bergan T, Wiik Larsen E, Brodwall EK. Pharmacokinetics of a new cephalosporin, cefotaxime (HR 756) in patients with different renal function. Chemotherapy 28: 85–104, 1982.
169. Fillastre JP, Leroy A, Humbert G, Godin M. Pharmacokinetics of cefotaxime in subjects with normal and impaired renal function. J Antimicrob Chemother 6 (Suppl): S103–S111, 1980.
170. Humbert G, Fillastre JP, Leroy A, Godin M, Van Winzum C. Pharmacokinetics of cefoxitin in normal subjects and in patients with renal insufficiency. Rev Infect Dis 1: 118–125, 1979.
171. Moellering RC, Krogstad DJ, Greenblatt DJ. Vancomycin therapy in patients with impaired renal function—A nomogram for dosage. Ann Intern Med 94: 343–346, 1981.
172. Flynn CT, Rainford DJ, Hope E. Acute renal failure and rifampicin danger of unsuspected intermittent dosage. Brit Med J 1: 482, 1974.
173. Rothwell DL, Richmond DE. Hepatorenal failure with self-initiated intermittent rifampicin therapy. Brit Med J 2: 481–482, 1974.
174. Girling DJ, Mitchison DA, Fox W. Sensitivity to rifampicin. Brit Med J 2: 114, 1974.
175. Tasker PRW, Mac Gregor GA, De Wardener HE. Prophylactic use of intravenous saline in patients with chronic renal failure undergoing major surgery. Lancet II: 911–912, 1974.
176. Ronald AR. Pros and Cons of antimicrobial prophylaxis in surgery. Can J Surg 24: 113–115, 1981.
177. Burke JF. The effective period of preventive antibiotic action in experimental incisions and dermal lesions. Surgery 50: 161–168, 1961.
178. Fullen WD, Hunt J, Altemeier WA. Prophylactic antibiotics in penetrating wounds of the abdomen. J Trauma 12: 282–289, 1972.
179. Stone HH, Hooper CA, Kolb LD, Geheber CE, Dawkins EJ. Antibiotic prophylaxis in gastric, biliary and colonic surgery. Ann Surg 184: 443–452, 1976.
180. Conte JE Jr, Cohen SN, Benson BR, Elashoff RM. Antibiotic prophylaxis and cardiac surgery. A prospective double-blind comparison of single-dose versus multiple-dose regimens. Ann Intern Med 76: 943–949, 1972.
181. Shapiro MB, Townsend TR, Rosner B, Kass EH. Use of antimicrobial drugs in general hospitals. Pattern of prophylaxis. N Engl J Med 301: 351–355, 1979.
182. Nichols RL. Use of prophylactic antibiotics in surgical practice. Am J Med 70: 686–692, 1981.
183. Alexander JW, Alexander NS. The influence of route of administration on wound fluid concentration of prophylactic antibiotics. J Trauma 16: 488–495, 1976.

4. PATHOLOGY OF ACUTE RENAL FAILURE

Steen Olsen

1 Introduction

As appears from the chapter headings of this book, acute renal failure (ARF) may be due to a multitude of causes. Not surprisingly, therefore, the histopathology of ARF reflects a corresponding heterogeneity. However, this is not to say that the histopathology of the various types always gives clues to the underlying pathogenetic mechanisms. On the contrary, the acute decrease in renal function often cannot be explained by the structural alterations. Exceptions to this are some types associated with anatomical changes that are obviously not compatible with normal glomerular perfusion such as bilateral occlusion of the main renal arteries, some glomerular diseases, and widespread vascular thrombotic occlusion.

While it is thus the opinion of this author that histopathology has not yet provided conclusive pathogenetic insight, as regards the most frequent types, the morphological picture characteristic for a type must of course be taken into consideration when pathophysiological hypotheses are discussed. Another reason why knowledge of the histopathology is important is that it may have diagnostic implications.

The following account is mainly based on the information provided by renal biopsy specimens. Without doubt the introduction of the percutaneous biopsy method [1] has presented a much more secure base for our knowledge of renal structure than autopsy specimens. On the other hand, it should be stressed that biopsy material is influenced by preparation artifacts.

V.E. Andreucci (ed.), ACUTE RENAL FAILURE.
All rights reserved. Copyright © 1984.
Martinus Nijhoff Publishing, Boston/The Hague/
Dordrecht/Lancaster.

This may be of less importance regarding lesions such as necrosis and inflammation, but may have profound implications for quantitative data obtained by morphometry. It is therefore necessary to be cautious in drawing conclusions from measurements such as the size of tubular cells and tubular luminal diameter [2].

ARF may be prerenal, renal, and postrenal. This review will deal mainly with the renal (or parenchymatous) forms, and the classification will be based on morphology (table 4–1) [2].

The literature on the pathology of ARF is very large, particularly on the subject of drug-induced lesions. Although the reference list does not claim to be exhaustive, it contains some recent review articles, which may be consulted for more detailed reference to the literature.

2 Prerenal ARF

Experience from autopsy specimens of patients dying with prerenal ARF have not indicated structural damage, which can be separated from known autolytic changes. Since there is no indication for renal biopsy in this situation, no structural lesions are known. If the glomerular hypoperfusion is due to bilateral occlusion of the main renal artery and if this occlusion is not surgically removed, total necrosis of the kidney will result.

3 Postrenal ARF

This type of renal failure is due to obstruction of the urinary tract. No discussion of the numerous causes of this shall be presented here. An acute obstruction may sometimes give rise

TABLE 4–1. Types of acute renal failure classified according to renal morphology

Morphologic class (the most important structural lesions)	Clinicopathological examples
ARF DUE TO GLOMERULAR AND/OR VASCULAR LESIONS	
1. Glomerulonephritis	Acute postinfectious glomerulonephritis (anuric type)
	Extracapillary glomerulonephritis (crescentic)
2. Arteriolar microangiopathy	Hemolytic uremic syndrome
	Thrombotic, thrombocytopenic purpura
	Scleroderma
	Malignant hypertension
	Postpartum renal failure
3. Arteriolar and glomerular capillary thrombosis	Disseminated intravascular coagulation
ARF WITHOUT PROMINENT GLOMERULAR OR VASCULAR LESIONS	
1. Extensive tubular necrosis	Toxic and drug-induced (dose-related) ARF (e.g., by $HgCl_2$ or aminoglycosides in high doses)
2. "Shock kidney," vasomotor nephropathy (mild structural lesions: tubular dilatation, casts, scattered tubular necroses)	ARF following shock, sepsis, hemolysis, myolysis, etc.
	Some drug-induced or toxic conditions associated with hypovolemia and hypersensitivity type (e.g., barbiturates, morphine derivatives, etc.)
3. Interstitial cellular ifiltration	Acute drug-induced interstitial nephritis (AIN) of hypersensitivity type (e.g., methicillin)
	Acute interstitial nephritis associated with sepsis
	Malignant lymphoma and leucemia
	Acute (bilateral) pyelonephritis
4. ARF with extensive tubular obstruction	Methoxyfluorane-induced ARF
	Uric acid deposition in malignant lymphoreticular diseases
	ARF in myeloma with protein casts
5. ARF with normal structure	ARF in nephrotic patients with minor glomerular abnormalities
	Some toxic or drug-induced conditions

to dilatation of tubular lumina and glomerular urinary space, but these changes are not always present. If the obstruction is of more than a few days duration, PAS-positive material (probably Tamm-Horsfall's protein) may accumulate in distended periarterial lymph vessels and in adjacent interstitial tissue.

4   Parenchymatous ARF

4.1   VASCULAR AND GLOMERULAR DISEASE

Several vascular diseases may be associated with extensive arteriolar and glomerular thrombosis. These are the visceral form of sclerodermia, thrombotic thrombocytopenic purpura, hemolytic uremic syndrome, malignant hypertension and the nonhypertension-associated diffuse arteriolar necrosis, and thrombosis seen postpartum and rarely in other situations. In these conditions, there is such widespread arteriolar and glomerular thrombotic occlusion that it is easy to understand an effective perfusion pressure cannot be maintained [3]. The same can be said of the disseminated intravascular coagulation occurring in sepsis or other situations. The end result of this (and sometimes of some of the conditions mentioned above) may be bilateral cortical necrosis.

Although ARF may occur in virtually all types of glomerulonephritis, it is most often seen in acute poststreptococcal glomerulonephritis and particularly in crescentic glomerulonephritis [4–6]. Ganeval et al. [7] studied 790 patients treated for ARF and found indication for renal biopsy in 93. Predominantly,

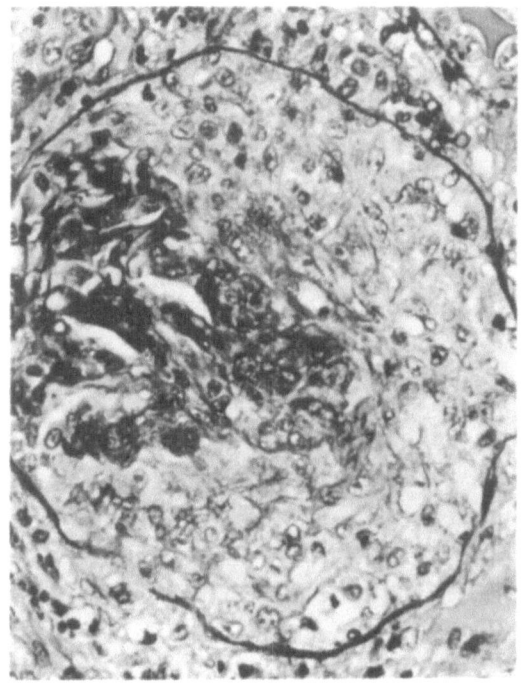

FIGURE 4–1. Crescentic glomerulonephritis. From a patient with rapidly progressive glomerulonephritis and anuria. The capillary tuft (on the left) is strongly compressed by the large cellular crescent, which obstructs the urinary space. If virtually 100% of glomeruli are affected as it occurred in this case, no glomerular filtration is possible (PAS-hematoxylin × 450).

glomerular lesions were seen in 32 of these. The diagnosis may be suggested by the clinical presentation, but in many patients the diagnosis depends on renal biopsy.

Histologically, the glomerular morphology belongs to one of the several types of glomerulonephritis [8], which shall not be discussed in detail here. The glomerular lesions often seem to explain the oliguria. The compression of the tuft by cellular proliferation and accumulation of fibrin in the urinary space in the crescentic types with 100% glomerular involvement can thus be so severe that any significant degree of glomerular filtration is precluded (figure 4–1). Glomerular thrombosis may also contribute to the glomerular hypoperfusion in these cases.

In acute complex nephritis of the endocapillary type—for example, that due to streptococcal infection—the glomerular lesions are less severe. Nevertheless, thin silver-stained sec-

tions may in such cases show that almost all glomerular capillary lumina are occluded by proliferating and swollen mesangial and endothelial cells (figures 4–2 and 4–3). It should, however, be noted that there are patients who have renal failure but no glomerular tuft compression or obstruction. The last mentioned cases must be explained by other pathogenetic mechanisms, possibly identical with those operative in ischemic ARF (see also chapters 13 and 14).

4.2 ARF WITH EXTENSIVE TUBULAR NECROSIS

This is the classical example of a toxic nephropathy, e.g., due to poisoning with mercuric chloride. Most descriptions of this morphological type of ARF have been based on autopsy tissue that introduces the risk of misinterpreting autolytic changes. The existence of the type is, however, well documented by the few reported biopsies as well as by some autopsy specimens taken out early after death. The interpretations are also reinforced by animal experiments with comparable doses. The functional effects and the severity of histological damage in this type of ARF are strongly dose-related, in contradistinction to other drug-induced types, e.g., hypersensitivity-mediated interstitial nephritis.

Mercuric chloride ($HgCl_2$, corrosive sublimate) in sufficient doses induces a severe proximal tubular necrosis [9] with acute anuric renal failure. The initial phase is characterized by tubular cell necrosis and desquamation from the basement membrane. The necrotic remnants of the tubular cells can be seen in the lumina of proximal as well as distal tubules and collecting ducts. Later on, if the patient survives, the tubular basement membranes are covered by regenerating, flat, or cubical epithelium with strongly basophilic cytoplasm. Gradually, this type of epithelium takes on a normal structure. Potassium bichromate and uranyl nitrate have also strong tubulotoxic effects.

Other agents, which may cause extensive tubular necrosis, are diethylene-glycol and ethylene glycol as well as carbon tetrachloride. The latter may, however, also give rise to the

152

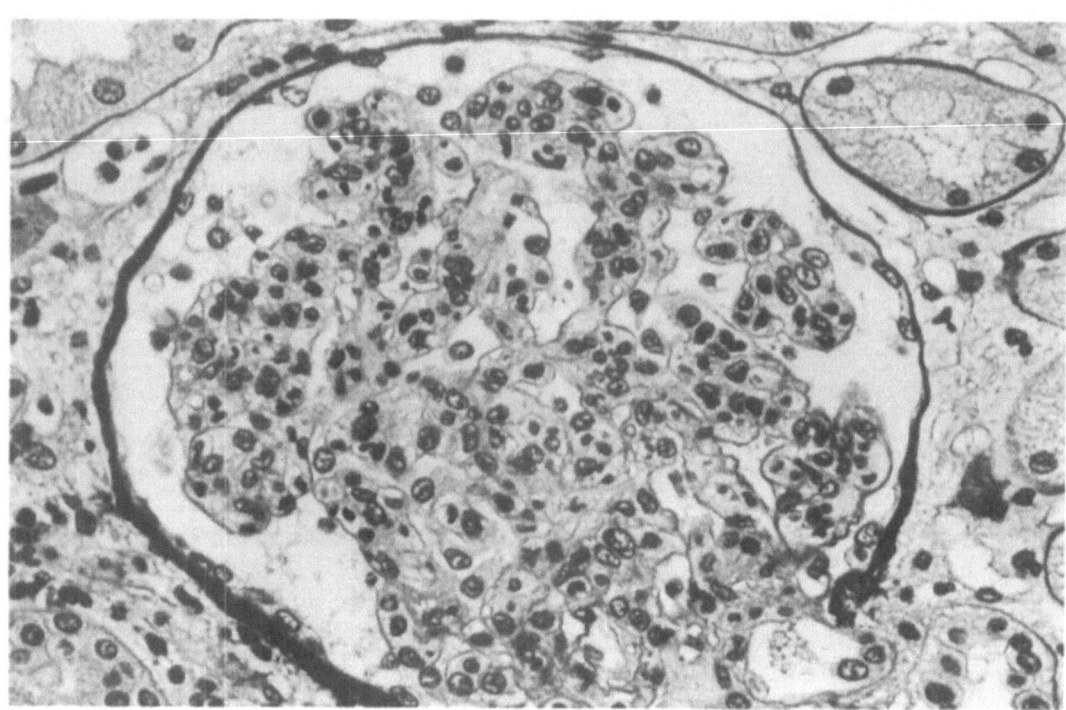

FIGURE 4–2. Acute anuric glomerulonephritis of the endocapillary type. There is global, mesangial, and endothelial proliferation with scattered polymorphonuclear leucocytes (silver methenamine-hematoxylin ×500).

"ischemia" type of ARF. Some antibiotics have also been reported to cause extensive tubular necrosis: cephaloridine in high doses [10], bacitracin [11]. While the aminoglycosides [12] may cause dose-related focal necrosis of the proximal tubules, it is rare that they produce confluent necrosis of lengthy segments like those seen in mercuric chloride poisoning (figures 4–4 and 4–5). A possible exception is neomycin, which proved to be so nephrotoxic that it was withdrawn from parenteral use soon after its introduction. Autopsy studies have given evidence of extensive tubular necrosis following this drug.

Based on autopsy studies and microdissection, it appears that nephrotoxins affect specific segments of the nephron [13]. While potassium bichromate affects the first segment of the proximal contorted tubule, uranyl nitrate, carbon tetrachloride, ethylene glycol, diethylene glycol, as well as kanamycin and gentamicin in high doses affect the whole proximal convoluted tubule. Mercury, some mushroomtoxins, and cephaloridine lead to necrosis of the third segment, that is, to the straight part of the proximal tubule.

Calcification of the necrotic tubular epithelium is a well-known sequela to mercuric chloride poisoning. It may also occur after some drugs (bacitracin, amphotericin) and following treatment with streptozotocin, a β-cell poison (figure 4–6) [14].

4.3 ISCHEMIC ARF (ACUTE TUBULAR NECROSIS, ATN)

This frequent type of ARF presents some problems of nomenclature [12]. The most frequently used term for many years has been, and is still, acute tubular necrosis (ATN). Our group [2, 14–17] has persistently objected to this since tubular cellular necroses are rare and probably without pathogenetic significance. One more reason why this nomenclature seems inappropriate is that another situation exists, a situation characterized by extensive tubular necroses as discussed above. The name we have used formerly, acute tubulo-interstitial nephropathy, can, on the other hand, scarcely be

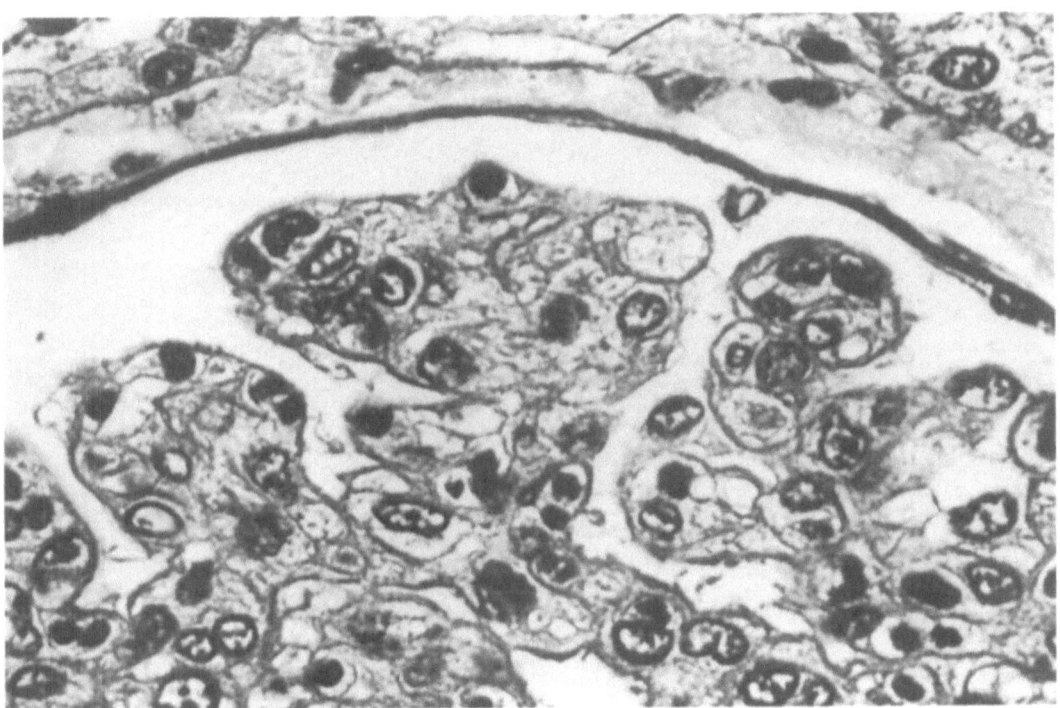

FIGURE 4–3. Acute anuric glomerulonephritis. Higher magnification from the same biopsy as figure 4–2. The swollen endothelial cells are totally obstructing the capillary lumina, and no glomerular filtration seems possible (PAS-hematoxylin × 1,100).

sustained since, logically, it also would cover the methicillin type of ARF. Since circulatory shock and hypovolemia have often been present, the term *ischemic ARF* is used in the present context. This type of ARF can also be due to septic abortion and follow large surgical interventions [18]. Recent experience points toward drugs as the most common eliciting factor (e.g., barbiturate poisoning, sulfonamides, antibiotics). In a comparatively large proportion of cases, no responsible factor can be found.

The histopathology of the ischemic type of ARF as it appears in the renal biopsy is dominated by tubular changes, but they are usually rather weak or moderate. In fact, one of the most impressive features of this type is the contrast between the complete breakdown of the renal function and the comparatively weak morphological lesions [15–17]. The most constant alteration (figures 4–7 to 4–11) is a dila-

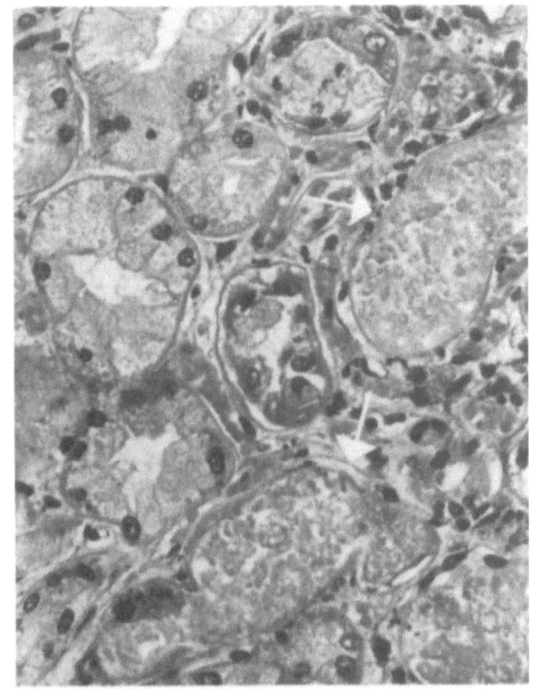

FIGURE 4–4. Extensive tubular necrosis. Kanamycin poisoning. Tubular segments show total cellular disintegration (arrows) (H & E. × 500).

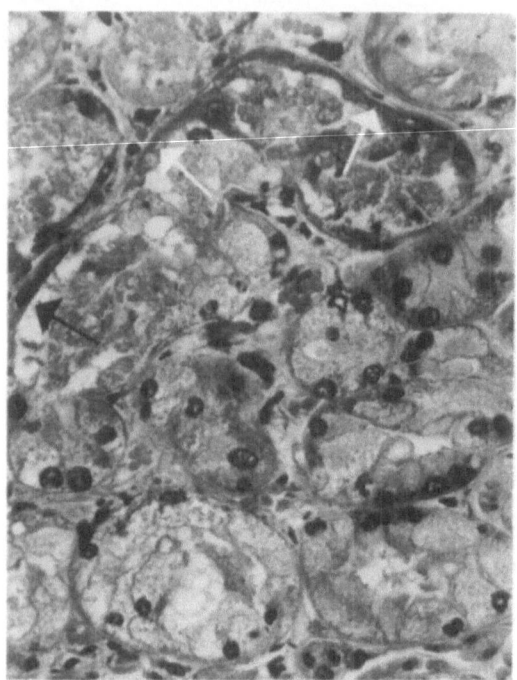

FIGURE 4–5. Extensive tubular necrosis. From the same biopsy as in figure 4–4. A field with large areas of regenerative epithelium (arrows) beneath the granular remnants of necrotic proximal epithelium (H & E × 500).

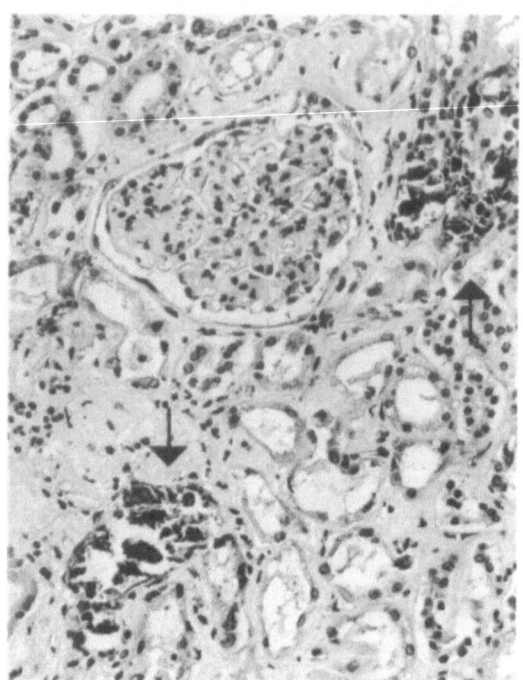

FIGURE 4–6. Calcification following tubular necrosis. Autopsy specimen from a patient who developed ARF following treatment with streptozotocin (a potent β-cell poison used in this patient with the aim of destroying tumor tissue from a metastasizing islet cell tumor in the pancreas). Two areas of calcified proximal tubules (arrows). Other tubules are covered by degenerative type of epithelium (H & E × 175).

tation of the distal convoluted tubules with flattening of the tubular epithelium. The lumina may be empty but often contain casts consisting of a granular brownish or reddish material (H&E staining). They are most prominent in ARF following hemo- and myolysis. The proximal tubules sometime show slight dilatation with a weak flattening of the cells. The proximal tubular cells may show severe hydropic change with swollen cytoplasma (figures 4–12 and 4–13). This lesion is, however, only present in patients who have been treated with i.v. dextran, sucrose, or other hyperosmotic fluids. Kaliopenic vacuolation (rather large vacuoles) may occur in patients with hypokalemia. Single cell necroses may be present, mostly in distal tubules, but this lesion will be discussed in more detail below. Solez and co-workers [19] have pointed out that there is a loss of PAS-positive tubular brush border. The interstitium may be moderately edematous, and a slight focal infiltration with mononuclear cells

(mostly lymphocytes) may be present. The glomeruli and vessels appear light-microscopically normal. The venae rectae in the outer zone of the medulla may be dilated and contain immature cells, mostly lymphocytes and plasma cells. Morphometric measurements [20] have shown swollen proximal tubular epithelium and widening of the interstitial space due to edema.

Light microscopy of autopsy specimens deviate from the picture described above. The proximal convoluted tubules are widely open [20], which is in contrast to biopsies from patients without ARF but also to the collapsed state of normal postmortem tubules. The occurrence of tubular epithelial necrosis in this type of ARF is a special problem. It has already been touched on in the remarks above about nomenclature. We have always stressed that

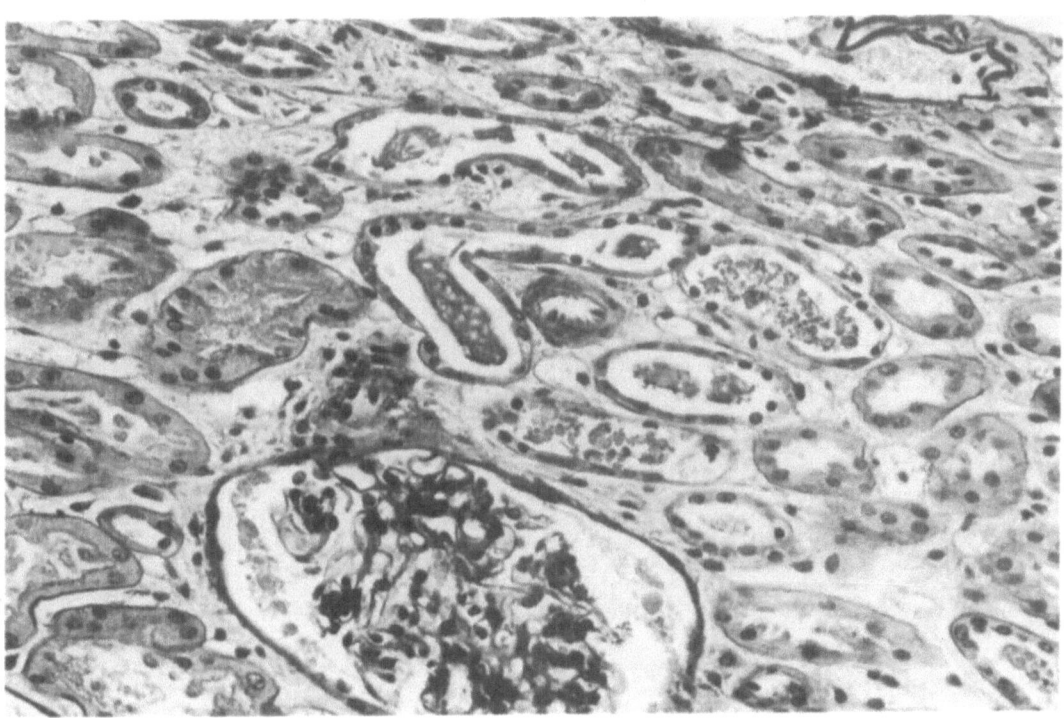

FIGURE 4–7. Ischemic ARF. This biopsy was taken in a polyuric phase. There is no cellular necrosis but severe distal tubular dilatation and finely granular casts (arrows) (PAS-hematoxylin × 200).

cellular necroses are few and focal (15–17, 21, 22). The widely held view that extensive necroses are present had its origin in a mixing together of this type with that of severe toxic renal damage (e.g., due to mercuric chloride) but also in an uncritical interpretation of autopsy specimens with autolysis.

On the other hand, that focal necroses are present is unquestionable (figure 4–9). As pointed out by Solez and co-workers [19], it is difficult to communicate an idea of the extent of tubular necrosis by using common words such as "gross," "extensive," "patchy," "focal," etc. Furthermore, pathologists who recognize only dead cells will note less necrosis than investigators who also noted focal absence of cells (denudation of the basement membrane). In the light of this discussion, this author has reinvestigated the problem in his earlier series as well as in recent biopsies. From this reinvestigation, it appears that small, focal tubular necroses evidently are present in

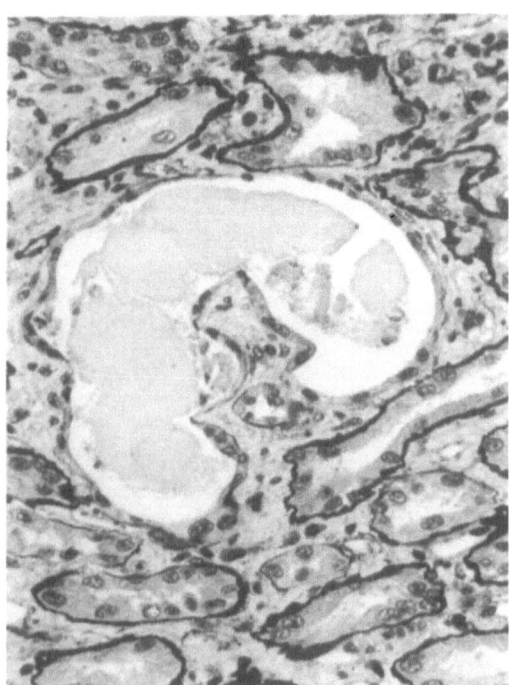

FIGURE 4–8. Ischemic ARF. Strongly dilated convoluted distal tubule forming a "pretzel"-like structure, which is very characteristic for this type of ARF. There is no necrosis, the tubular cells are very thin but cover the whole circumference without defects (silver methenamine-hematoxylin × 250).

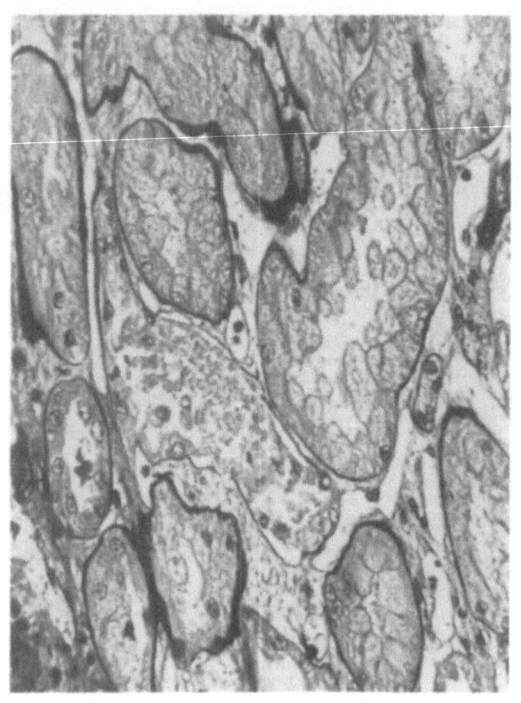

FIGURE 4–9. Ischemic ARF. In the center of the picture, a tubule (the type cannot be identified) with necrosis and cellular desquamation. This is a rare phenomenon in this type of ARF. Patchy necroses are nearly always unicellular. From a case of ARF following sepsis (silver methenamine-hematoxylin).

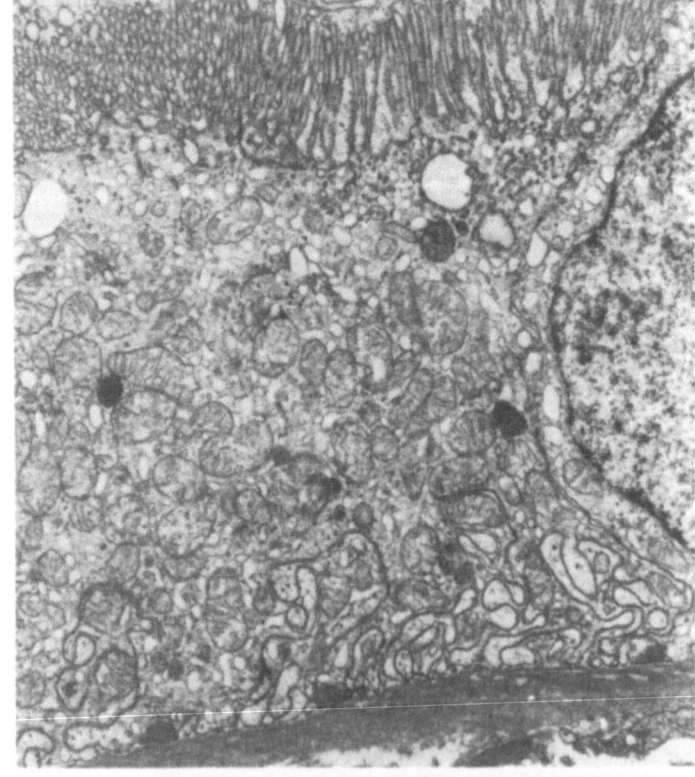

FIGURE 4–10. Ischemic ARF. Electron micrograph (×20,000) showing proximal tubular cell with well-preserved brush border.

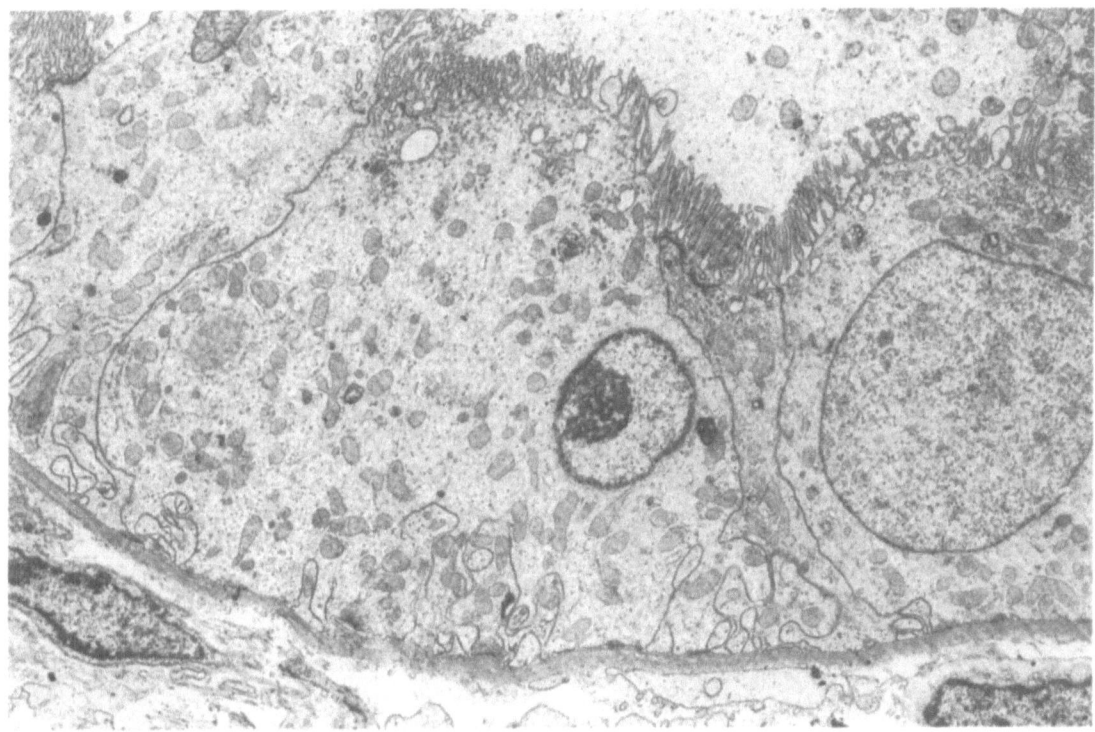

FIGURE 4–11. Ischemic ARF. Other proximal tubules show atrophic brush border. In some areas, there was no brush border present. The basal infoldings are scanty, but since it is impossible to identify the exact location of the segment, this may be without significance. No cellular necroses are present (× 20,000).

most biopsies from this type of ARF. They can appear in two forms. One of these is that pointed out by Solez and co-workers [19]: a short denuded part of the tubular basement membrane (tubular cell "nonreplacement"). The other type is even more characteristic. It appears as small foci of degenerated or necrotic tubular epithelial cells, usually associated with local disruption of the tubular basement membrane and surrounded by a small collection of mononuclear cells in the interstitium as well as in between the (often desquamated) epithelial cells. This lesion, which we have called "focal tubulo-interstitial lesion" is present in the ischemic type of ARF and even more in interstitial nephritis [23]. Focal tubulointerstitial lesion is, however, not specific for ARF; it can also be found in several types of acute and chronic renal disease (e.g., glomerulonephritis) without ARF.

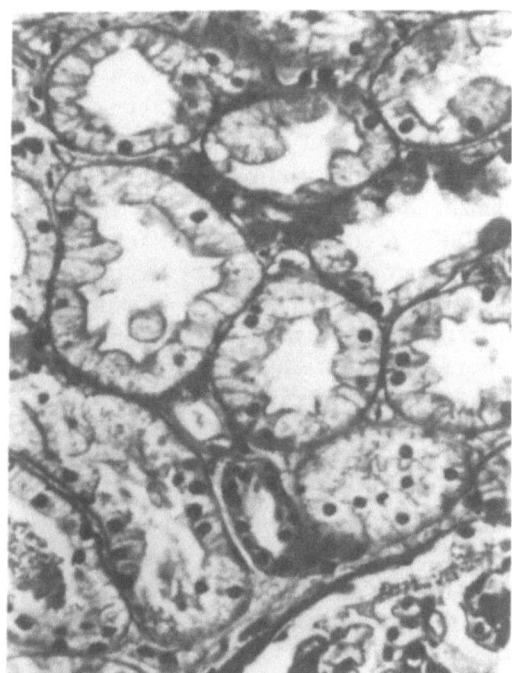

FIGURE 4–12. Ischemic ARF. Hydropic degeneration of proximal tubular epithelium. This phenomenon is not associated with ARF, but is caused by infusion of osmotic active solutions, in this case dextran (PAS-hematoxylin × 500).

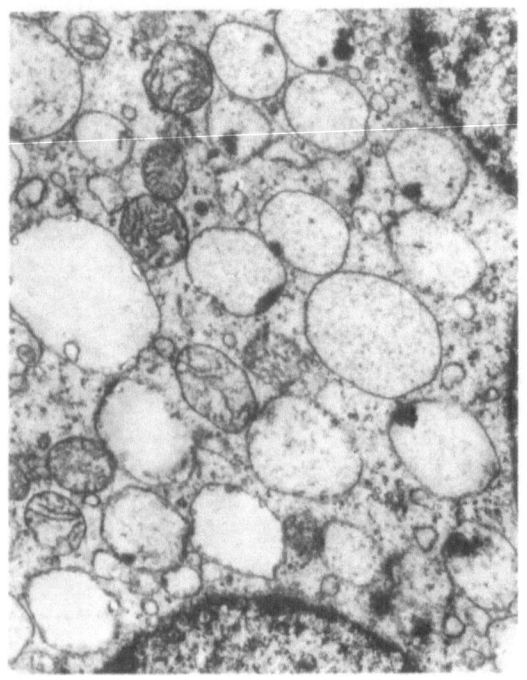

FIGURE 4–13. Ischemic ARF. This electron micrograph shows cytoplasm from hydropic changed proximal epithelium following dextran. There are a multitude of expanded lysosomes with electron lucent content as well as small accumulations of electron dense matter, probably dextran ($\times 35,000$).

Ultrastructural studies of tubular structure [21, 24, 25] have confirmed the relative rarity of tubular necroses (figures 4–10, 4–11, and 4–14). Early investigations by electron microscopy [21] showed preserved proximal brush border, but recent work [26] including blind, semiquantitative technique [24] has demonstrated that the brush border is in fact partially absent, thus confirming previous light microscopy observations [19, 25]. The decrease of proximal brush border is so marked that proximal tubules may easily be mistaken as distal [24]. The basal infoldings are decreased in number and height [21, 24]; this has also been confirmed by use of a systematic, semiquantitative technique [24].

Dilated, distal tubules have flat epithelial cells with increased number of lysosomes. Glomerular ultrastructure is normal [27] with the only exception being the large cytoplasmic extensions from the podocytes were present in

some patients. The significance of this phenomenon is not clear.

Immunofluorescent microscopy has not revealed immunoglobulins or complement in the glomeruli [19, 26].

The question of the significance for the renal failure and for the oliguria (if present) of the various histopathological lesions has recently been investigated. Solez et al. [19] studied a biopsy series semiquantitatively in order to see if one or more of the histopathological lesions were present in ARF but not in patients who had recently recovered from ARF. Most of the changes that were assessed (e.g., leucocyte aggregation in the vasa recta, tubular dilatation, casts, interstitial inflammation, and edema) were in fact more severe in ARF than in controls, but they persisted in the recovery group, for which reason it was considered unlikely that they play any role in causing renal failure. Only patchy tubular necrosis and loss of brush border were significantly more severe in ARF than in the recovery phase. It was therefore

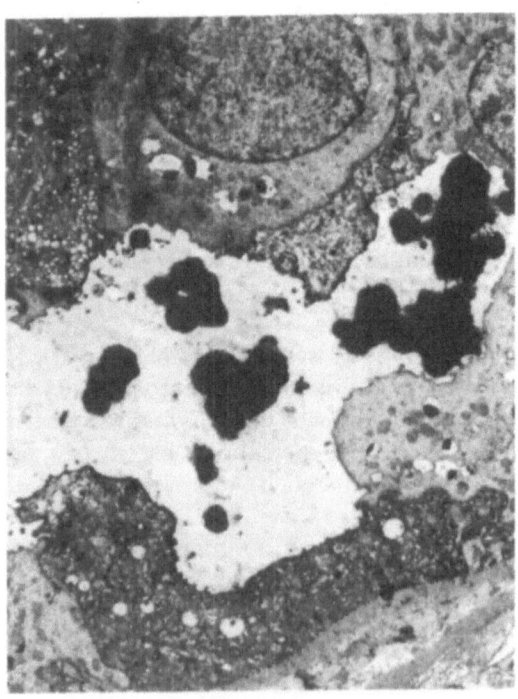

FIGURE 4–14. Ischemic ARF. Distal tubule with electron dense, granular cast. One epithelial cell is necrotic (bottom); another, partly represented in the upper left, is probably also ($\times 8,000$).

proposed that these lesions might be the cause of ARF [19].

The present author found by electron microscopy that the severe reduction of the basal infoldings in the anuric period is significantly less pronounced in recovery [24], and this is probably also valid for the brush border disappearance. These observations seem to point toward a primary lesion taking place in structures concerned with transcellular transport, although other interpretations are still possible.

4.4 INTERSTITIAL NEPHRITIS

The term interstitial nephritis is applied to renal diseases with no primary glomerular affection but with severe inflammatory changes in the interstitial tissue [28]. This rather ill-defined group of diseases is usually referred to as acute and chronic pyelonephritis, chronic analgesic nephropathy, and acute interstitial nephritis due to an allergic reaction against certain drugs. The last mentioned types (for which the term *acute interstitial nephritis*, AIN, will be used) is exemplified by the ARF due to methicillin [29–34] (see also chapter 2, section 16). The typical clinical picture is that of a patient who some days or a couple of weeks after treatment with the drug develops fever and a skin rash. Within a few days, the renal function decreases and oliguric or nonoliguric ARF develops. There may be eosinophilia. The patient may need dialysis but usually recovers, and only rarely a permanent impairment of the renal function follows. Histologically (figures 4–15, 4–16, and 4–17), the renal biopsy shows severe interstitial inflammatory infiltration, most typically with lymphocytes (the designation "acute" is appropriate for this condition despite the predominant mononuclear infiltration since the clinical course is acute). The infiltration is present in all parts of the cortex, it is somewhat patchy, and the medulla may also be involved, but not always and to a much lesser degree. Besides small and large lymphocytes, histiocytes are also present in a considerable number. Plasma cells and polymorphonuclear leucocytes are rare. Some cases have been described in which eosinophils were present in a large number, but this is a rare type. There is a severe interstitial edema. Focal tubulo-interstitial lesions [23] are very conspicuous. They appear as small foci of tubules with rupture of the basement membrane, degeneration or necrosis of the tubular epithelium, which is often desquamated, and infiltration of the tubular wall with mononuclear cells (figure 4–17). It is unclear exactly what part of the tubules are affected due to the severe degenerative alterations of the tubular cells. We have formerly considered this lesion to be exclusively distal, but have more recently gained the opinion that proximal tubules may also be affected. The tubules outside these foci are usually normal, and it is particularly important to note that they lack the tendency to distal dilatation as well as the haemcasts characteristic for the ischemic type of ARF. Morphometry has demonstrated a considerable expansion of the interstitial space (in fact this disease has the largest interstitium of all types of ARF) as well as a comparatively slight distension of the distal tubular lumen. The proximal tubular cell volume and the size of

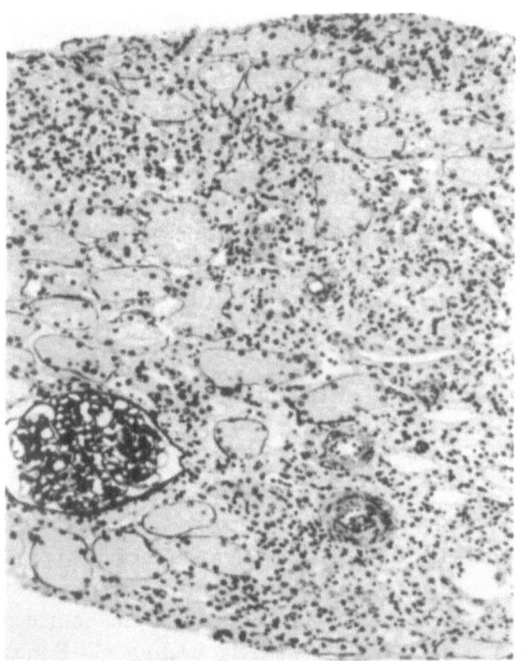

FIGURE 4–15. Acute interstitial nephritis following methicillin. Low-power micrograph showing interstitial infiltration with mononuclear cells (silver methenamine-hematoxylin ×175).

the proximal lumen are normal [2]. The remarkable distension of the interstitial space might give rise to the assumption that compression of the tubules was the direct cause of anuria or oliguria. We therefore measured the relative interstitial volume in a series of biopsies from patients with ARF, including many with acute interstitial nephritis [25]. Although the mean interstitial volume was greater in patients with oliguria (43.6%) than in those with nonoliguric ARF (35.0%) and patients in recovery (38.4%), the large dispersion of the values excluded this hypothesis since normal as well as strongly increased values occurred in all three groups. These data demonstrate that a functioning kidney with production of a normal amount of urine may be compatible with an expansion of the interstitial space to about 60% of the total kidney volume.

Glomerular structure is normal. Arteries and arterioles are normal or show slight thickening of their walls, which is probably unrelated to the acute disease. The intertubular capillaries are dilated, and some contain lymphocytes. Immunofluorescent microscopy has usually been negative [32], but some cases have been described in which antibodies and complement were present in tubular basement membranes [31, 33, 35]. Electron microscopical studies are scarce [26, 29] and have usually confirmed the lymphocytic composition of the inflammatory infiltrate. No deposits are present in the glomerulus or in or near the tubular basement membranes.

Although methicillin has been the most frequent responsible agent during later years, this drug is by no means the sole offender. The list of other drugs implicated is long. The most frequently cited in the literature are ampicillin, cephalosporins, rifampicin, sulfonamides, phenindione, and allopurinol [12, 30, 34]. Acute interstitial nephritis has been known long before the antibiotic era [36, 37]. It was then associated with diphtheria, scarlet fever, and sepsis.

The possibility that the disease may be brought about by sepsis or other infections makes it sometimes uncertain whether the infection for which the patients were treated or the drug was responsible. Our report on a series of cases occurring in patients without in-

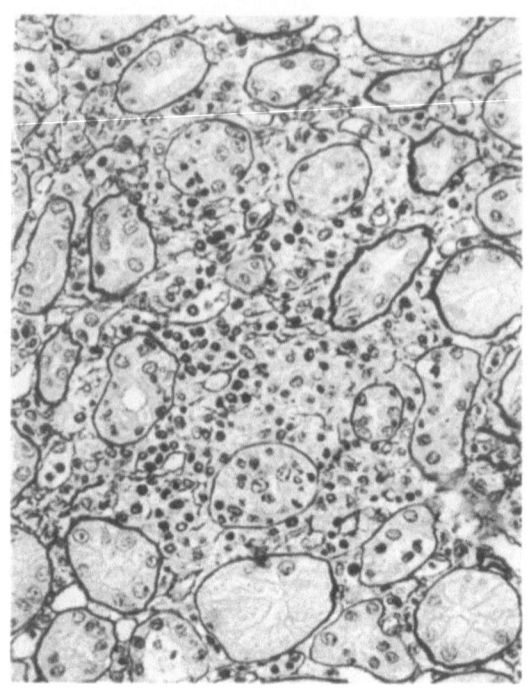

FIGURE 4–16. Acute interstitial nephritis following methicillin. Higher magnificaton from the same biopsy as in figure 4–15. There is strong expansion of the intertubular space due to the inflammatory infiltrate (silver methenamine-hematoxylin × 200).

fection but treated prophylactically demonstrates, however, unmistakably that drugs may be the responsible factor [32].

The pathogenesis is not known. Two reports [31, 32] showing the presence of penicilloyl hapten and IgG in the tubular basement membranes were interpreted as indicating an antitubular antibody reaction. Most cases are, however, negative (as indicated above), and other mechanisms must be sought.

Acute renal failure may occur in patients with bilateral acute or subacute pyelonephritis [18, 38]. The biopsy shows a diffuse infiltration with leucocytes, mainly polymorphonuclear neutrophils, as well as leucocyte casts. Microabscesses may be present. The prognosis depends on successful removal of the source of infection, which is usually urological. Repeat biopsies in cases with persisting renal failure have shown transition to the picture of chronic pyelonephritis with interstitial fibrosis, infiltration with mononuclear cells, and nephronic atrophy [38].

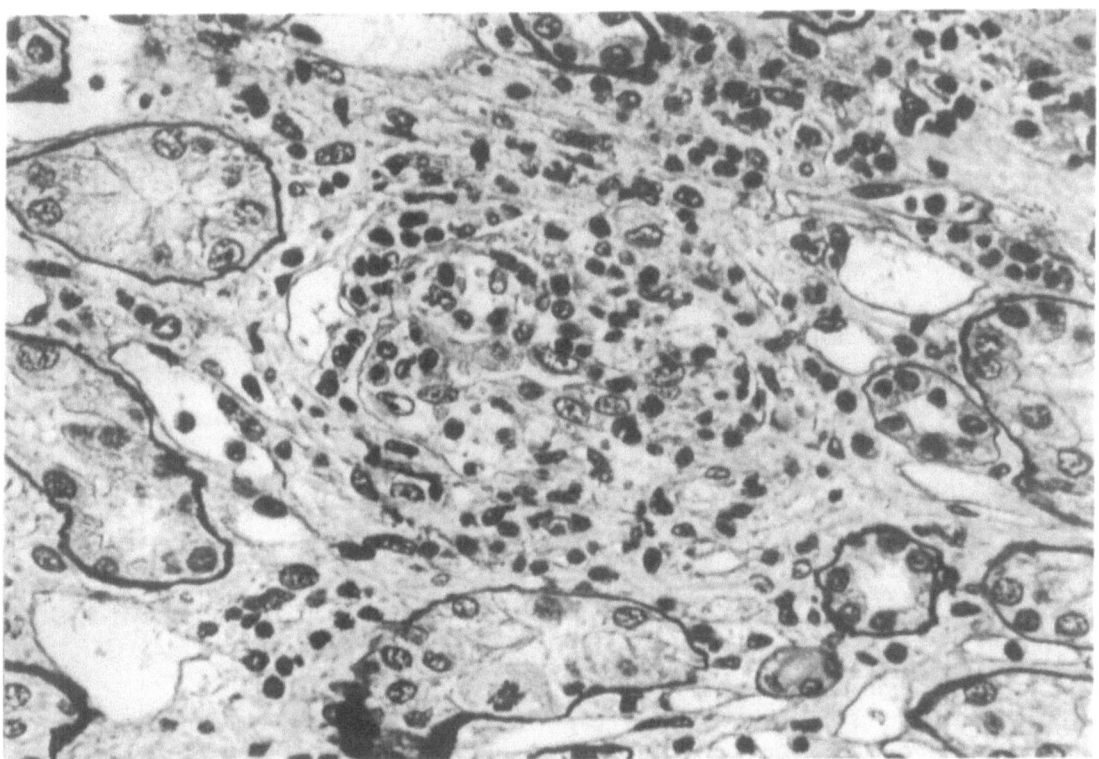

FIGURE 4-17. Acute interstitial nephritis following meth-icillin. Centrally, there are cellular remnants of a dis-rupted tubule with disappearance of the basement mem-brane and infiltration with lymphocytes around and between the epithelial cells (focal tubulo-interstitial le-sion) (silver methenamine-hematoxylin × 500).

4.5 ARF WITH EXTENSIVE TUBULAR OBSTRUCTION

It appears from the discussion above that casts in the renal tubules are frequent in ischemic ARF (ATN). Their presence in polyuric ARF and in the period of restitution following ARF, however, does make it improbable that they have causative importance for the decrease of renal function.

There are, however, some forms of ARF in which material in the tubules or collecting ducts is so abundant that the possibility of an obstruction becomes possible.

To this category belongs the acute methoxy-fluorane nephropathy [39] (see chapter 2, sec-tion 11). This drug which was formerly much used for anesthesia, could give rise to anuric or polyuric ARF. Extensive deposition of calcium oxalate crystals was present in the renal tu-bules. Obstruction could be of importance in the anuric cases, but scarcely in polyuria, and the ARF might also be due to the action of fluoride, which (together with oxalate) is a me-tabolite of methoxyfluorane. In ethylene glycol poisoning (see chapter 2, section 12), there is also heavy deposition of oxalate crystal in the tubules.

Tubular crystalline deposits may occur in pa-tients with leucemia or malignant lymphomas treated with cytotoxic drugs. Also in these cases, there can be other causes for the renal failure, e.g., an action of the elevated serum uric acid (see chapter 2, section 13).

Reactions to sulfonamides with ARF are usually associated with a morphologic picture of the ischemic type of ARF or AIN, and it is unlikely that the rather small number of crys-tals deposited in such cases are of causal impor-tance.

4.6 ARF WITH NORMAL KIDNEY STRUCTURE

It is of considerable theoretical interest that this severe functional disorder may exist without any light microscopical or electron microscopi-cal lesions (figure 4-18).

This situation is sometimes met with in patients with minimal change nephrotic syndrome [5, 40] (see chapter 13, section 2). In most of these patients, recovery of renal function occurred after diuretic therapy. It has been suggested that this complication may be due to a reversible alteration in glomerular hemodynamics related to fluid retention [40]. With the exception of the interstitial edema noted in many of the biopsies, there were no glomerular, tubular, or other lesions by light or electron microscopy. It should particularly be noted that no evidence of tubular necrosis was present. Normal renal structure in ARF has also been reported in some cases of acute poisoning with lithium [2] and diphenhydramine [14].

4.7 TRANSPLANT ARF

Acute decrease in graft function is a complication that may happen at any moment of the life of the graft although it occurs most frequently during the first weeks. The renal failure may be due to rejection or to other causes (see chapter 20).

The most frequent causes of early graft failure are acute rejection, primary graft anuria, and vascular occlusion. More rare causes are transmission of glomerulonephritis, hyperacute rejection, pyelonephritis, and ureteral obstruction.

In the present context, only hyperacute rejection, acute rejection, and primary graft anuria shall be discussed. For a more extensive presentation of the pathology of graft disease, the reader is referred to a recent review [41].

The term *primary graft anuria* refers to the situation wherein the function of the graft does not begin immediately following opening of the anastomoses but only after a period that may extend to several weeks. This phenomenon is practically only seen in cadaver kidneys. The cause of this lack of function is not entirely clear, but must be sought in conditions affecting the kidney during the disease of the donor, the period between cardiac arrest and nephrectomy, as well as during the warm and cold ischemia. The histopathology of this condition is only poorly known since biopsies are usually not performed until several days (or more) have

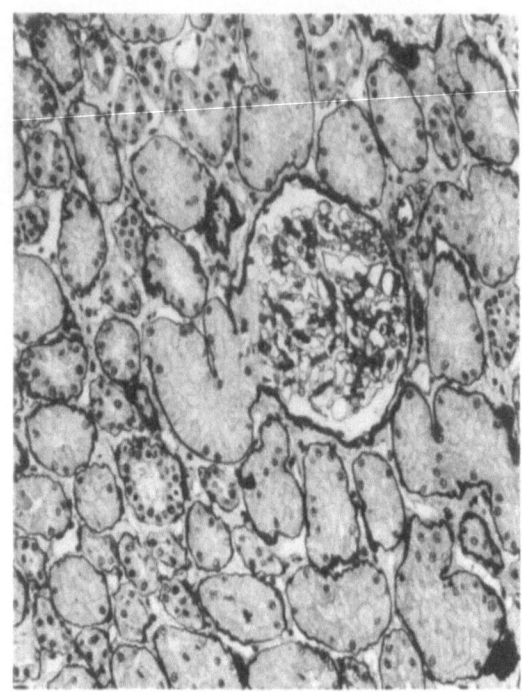

FIGURE 4–18. ARF with normal renal structure. The renal failure, which was reversible, followed intoxication with diphenhydramin. Light microscopically as well as electron microscopically, there was normal structure (silver methenamine-hematoxylin × 200).

elapsed. This means that the picture may be complicated to an unknown degree of alterations due to incompatibility or to actual rejection, which may be difficult to recognize when it occurs in a nonfunctioning graft.

Some cases present a histopathological picture resembling that of ischemic anuria (as described above). There is, however, usually more focal tubular necrosis and often a rather severe interstitial edema, and there may be a slight mononuclear cell infiltration. Late biopsies from patients with established function have shown patchy tubular epithelial calcification as a sequel to the necroses of the tubules.

Solez et al. [42] have recently described a peculiar change in one-hour biopsies from renal transplants in patients who later showed clinical signs of primary transplant anuria. They observed by scanning electron microscopy podocyte cell bodies and major processes that covered the foot processes. The physiological significance of the phenomenon is still unclear, but it may be related to a decrease in glomerular permeability. It is possible that the cytoplasmic expansion of podocytes seen in some patients with ischemic ARF (in native kidneys) described above [27] is related to this phenomenon. Hyperacute rejection is a graft failure occurring very early (i.e., often a few minutes) after opening of the anastomoses. It is elicited by pre-existing humoral antibodies against the graft, due to pregnancies or multiple transfusions [43]. Very early biopsies show leucocyte accumulation in the glomerular capillaries. Soon after an extensive glomerular capillary and arteriolar thrombosis occur (figures 4–19 and 4–20); if the graft is left in situ, it will develop total cortical necrosis with a gross pathology as well as histopathology identical with that known from disseminated intravascular coagulation. A similar picture may develop after machine perfusion.

The acute allograft rejection may occur as a graft failure as early as a week after transplantation, but it is not restricted to the early post-

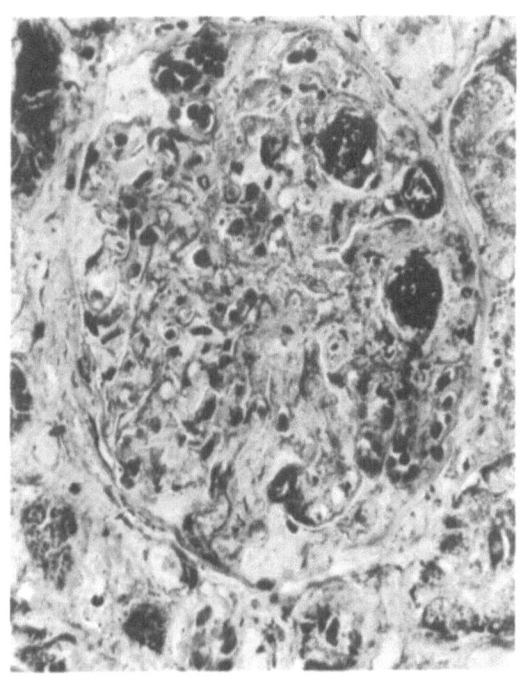

FIGURE 4–20. Hyperacute rejection. The same specimen as in figure 4–19 in larger magnificaton. Glomerular capillary thrombosis stained black with Weigert's stain for fibrin (× 500).

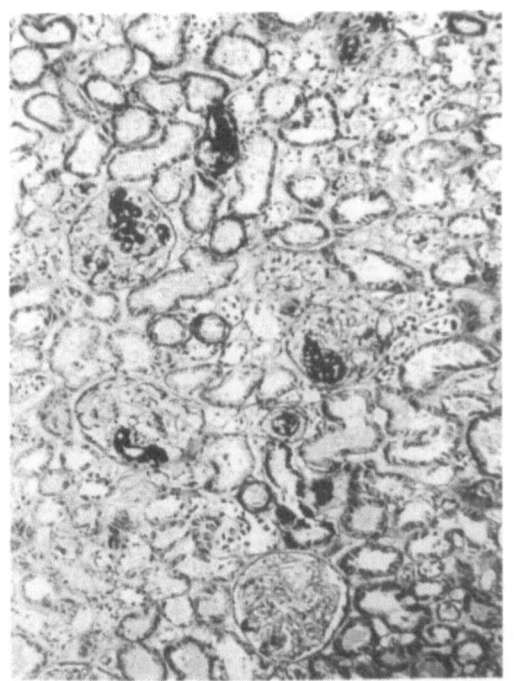

FIGURE 4–19. Hyperacute rejection. Virtually all glomeruli have capillary thrombosis (stained black). There is widespread cortical necrosis. Graftectomy specimen (Weigert's stain for fibrin × 175).

transplant period, and may set in after several years of function. The histopathology of acute rejection is dominated by interstitial and vascular phenomena [41, 44]. Interstitial edema and a patchy infiltration with mononuclear cells (lymphocytes, histiocytes, plasma cells) is most marked in the inner cortex, but can be seen in all parts of the parenchyma. The infiltrate is most marked around small veins. Many mononuclear cells are also present in the lumina of dilated intertubular capillaries, and they may be seen passing through the wall of the vessel.

Medium-sized and small arteries show edema and mononuclear cell infiltration of the intima, and the lumen of the vessels may be much narrowed or totally obstructed (figures 4–21 and 4–22). Fibrin may appear in the intima as well as the media. The glomeruli may show moderate mesangial hypercellularity and endothelial swelling. In more severe cases of acute rejection, vascular thrombosis affecting glomerular capillaries (figure 4–23) and small arteries and

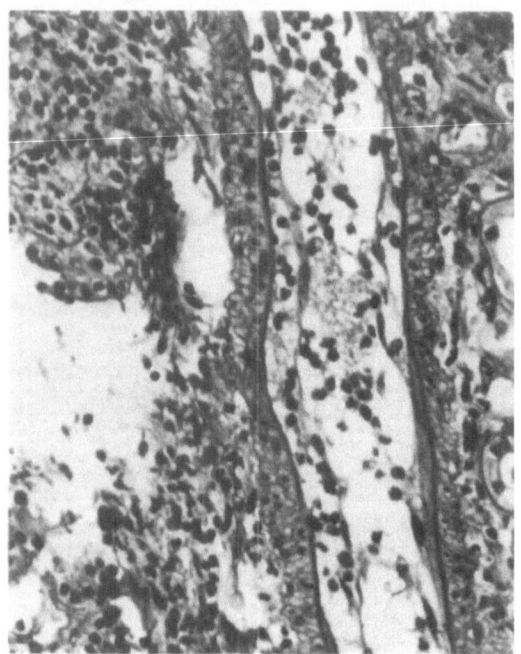

FIGURE 4–21. Acute rejection. Small artery with edema and lymphocyte infiltration in the swollen intima. There is severe interstitial lymphocyte infiltration to the left (PAS-hematoxylin × 800).

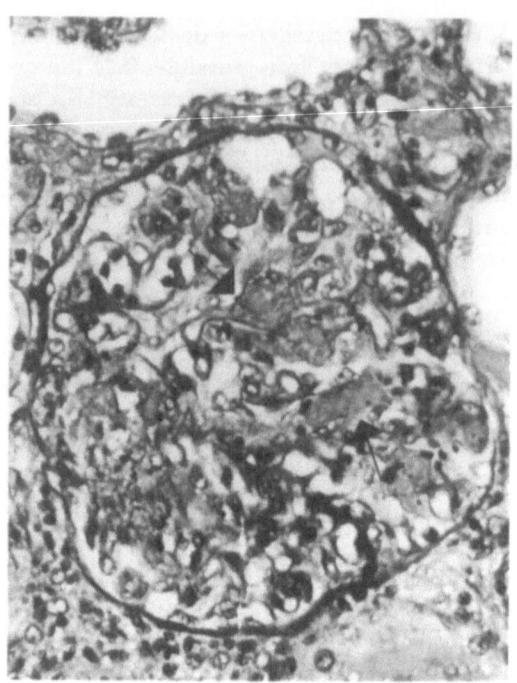

FIGURE 4–23. Acute rejection. Glomerulus with capillary thrombosis (arrows) and moderate cellular proliferation of the tuft (PAS-hematoxylin × 450).

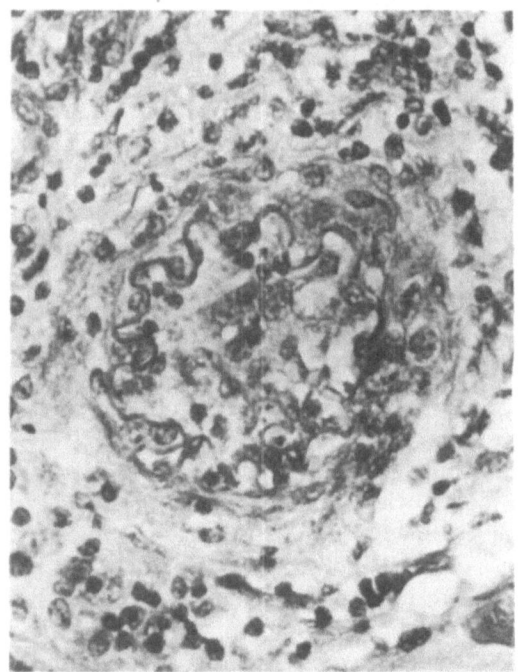

FIGURE 4–22. Acute rejection. Arteriole with total occlusion of the lumen due to endothelial proliferation. This may lead to multiple, small cortical infarctions (PAS-hematoxylin × 800).

veins may complicate the picture. In such cases, there are multiple small cortical infarcts with tubular wall necrosis and interstitial hemorrhage. The terminal stage of a severe acute rejection may be complicated with thrombotic occlusion of the main renal vessels, eventually leading to total graft necrosis.

Not all histopathological lesions have any impact on graft survival. Interstitial cellular infiltration may be severe, but its degree is not related to graft survival. Vascular thrombosis and focal tubular cell necrosis, on the other hand, indicate a poor prognosis for long-term graft function [45].

The renal failure in hyperacute as well as acute rejection can be related to the widespread vascular obstruction due to intimal swelling and/or thrombosis, but it is also possible that other mechanisms are responsible. Interstitial edema and the cellular infiltrate have probably no importance since renal function is maintained in other conditions with severe expansion of the interstitial volume (e.g., leucemic infiltration and methicillin nephropathy in the recovery phase).

References

1. Iversen P, Brun C. Aspiration biopsy of the kidney. Am J Med 11: 324–330, 1951.
2. Olsen S. Renal histopathology in various forms of acute anuria in man. Kidney Int. 10: S-2–S-8, 1976.
3. Mattern WD, Sommers SC, Kassirer JP. Oliguric renal failure in malignant hypertension. Am J Med 52: 187–197, 1972.
4. Leonard CD, Nagle RB, Striker GE, Cutter RE, Schribner BH. Acute glomerulonephritis with prolonged anuria. Ann Intern Med 73: 703–711, 1970.
5. Peters K, Boulton-Jones M, Sissons JGP, Brown C, Cameron JS, Ogg SC. Acute renal failure and glomerulonephritis. In Acute Renal Failure, Flynn CY (ed). Lancaster: Medical and Technical Publishing Co, 1974, pp. 69–82.
6. Beaufils M, Morel-Maroger L, Sraer J-D, Kanfer A, Kourilsky O, Richet G. Acute renal failure of glomerular origin during visceral abscesses. N Engl J Med 295: 185, 1976.
7. Ganeval D, Daniel F, Lhoste F, Boucard P. Problèmes diagnostiques et thérapeutiques au cours de l'insufficance rénale. In Actualité Néphrologiques de l'Hopital Necker. Paris: Flammation, 1976, pp. 305–327.
8. Churg J. Renal Disease. Classification and Atlas of Glomerular Diseases. Tokyo: Igaku-Shoin, 1982.
9. Heptinstall RH. Pathology of the Kidney (2nd ed). Boston: Little, Brown and Co. 1974, vol. II, pp. 802–807.
10. Rosenthal T, Boichis H. Nephrotoxicity of cephaloridine. Br Med J 4: 115, 1971.
11. Genkins G, Uhr JW, Bryer MS. Bacitracin nephropathy. Report of a case of acute renal failure and death. JAMA 155: 894–897, 1954.
12. Olsen S, Solez K. The pathology of drug nephrotoxicity in humans. In The Aminonucleosides, Neu HC, Whelton A (eds). New York: Marcel Decker, 1982, chapter 15.
13. Darmady EM, McIlver AG. Renal Pathology. Butterwords: London, 1980, pp. 209–218.
14. Brun C, Olsen S. Atlas of renal biopsy. Munksgaard: København, 1981.
15. Brun C. Acute Anuria. Copenhagen: Munksgaard, 1954.
16. Brun C. The renal lesion in acute tubulo-interstitial nephropathy. In Acute Renal Failure, Flynn CT (ed). Lancaster: Medical and Technical Publishing Co, 1974, pp. 46–53.
17. Brun C, Munck O. Lesions of the kidney in acute renal failure following shock. Lancet I: 603–607, 1957.
18. Balsløv JT, Jørgensen HE. A survey of 499 patients with acute anuric renal insufficiency. Am J Med 34: 753–764, 1963.
19. Solez K, Morel-Maroger L, Sraer J-D. The morphology of "Acute tubular necrosis" in man: Analysis of 57 renal biopsies and a comparison with the glycerol model. Medicine 58: 362–376, 1979.
20. Bohle A, Jahnecke J, Meyer D, Schubert GE. Mor-
phology of acute renal failure: Comparative data from biopsy and autopsy. Kidney Int 10: S-9–S-16, 1976.
21. Olsen S. Ultrastructure of the renal tubules in acute renal insufficiency. Acta pathol microbiol scand sect A 71: 203–218, 1967.
22. Olsen S. Some observations on the structure and ultrastructure in the acute anuria kidney. In Pathogenesis and Clinical Findings with Renal Failure, Gessler U, Schröder K, Weidiger H (eds). Stuttgart: Georg Thieme Verlag, pp. 63–72.
23. Olsen S, Hansen ES, Jepsen FL. The prevalence of focal tubulo-interstitial lesions in various renal diseases. Acta pathol microbiol scand sect A 89: 137–145, 1981.
24. Olsen S, Olsen H. A second look on the ultrastructure in acute renal failure. In Solez K and Whelton A, Acute Renal Failure. New York: Marcel Dekker, 1983 (in press).
25. Olsen S. Renal histopathology in drug-induced and toxic acute renal failure. Acute Renal Failure, pp. 189–199, Karger, Basel, 1982.
26. Jones D. Ultrastructure of human acute renal failure. Lab Invest 46: 254–264, 1982.
27. Olsen S, Skjoldborg H. The fine structure of the renal glomerulus in acute anuria. Acta pathol microbiol scand sect A 70: 205–214, 1967.
28. Heptinstall RH. Interstitial nephritis. A brief review. Amer J Pathol 83: 214–236, 1976.
29. Galpin JE, Shinaburger JH, Stanley TM, Blumenkrantz MJ, Bayer AS, Friedman GS, Montgomery JZ, Genze LB, Coburn JW, Glassock RJ. Acute interstitial nephritis due to methicillin. Am J Med 65: 756–765, 1978.
30. Linton AN, Clark WF, Dredger AA, Turnbull DI, Lindsay RM. Acute interstitial nerphritis due to drugs. Ann Int Med 93: 735–741, 1980.
31. Baldwin DS, Levine BL, McCluskey RT, Galto GR. Renal failure and interstitial nephritis due to penicillin and methicillin. N Engl J Med 279: 1245–1252.
32. Olsen S, Asklund M. Interstitial nephritis with acute renal failure following cardiac surgery. Acta Med Scand 199: 305–310, 1976.
33. Border WA, Lehman DH, Egon SD, Sass HJ, Glode JE, Wilson CB. Antitubular basement-membrane antibodies in methicillin-associated interstitial nephritis. N Engl J Med 291: 381–384, 1974.
34. Laberke HG. Acute interstitial nephritis, nephrotoxic lesions, analgetic nephropathy. In Current Topics in Pathology, vol. 69, p. 185–215, 1980, Drug-Induced Pathology, Grundmann, E (ed). Berlin, Heidelberg, New York: Springer-Verlag.
35. Hansen ES, Tauris P. Methicillin-induced nephropathy. Acta Pathol Microbiol Scand Sect A 84: 440–442, 1976.
36. Councilman WT. Acute interstitial nephritis. J Exp Med 3: 393–427, 1898,
37. Zollinger MU. Interstitial nephritis. In The Kidney, Mostofi FK, Smith DE (eds). Baltimore: Williams & Wilkins, 1966, pp. 269–281.
38. Richet G, Mayaud C. The course of acute renal fail-

ure in pyelonephritis and other types of interstitial nephritis. Nephron 22: 124–127, 1978.

39. Aufderheide AC. Renal tubular calcium oxalate crystal deposition. Arch Pathol 92: 162–166, 1971.

40. Lowenstein J, Schacht RG, Baldwin DS. Renal failure in minimal change nephrotic syndrome. Am J Med 70: 227–233, 1981.

41. Olsen S. Pathology of renal allograft rejection. In Churg G, Spargo B, Mostofi FK, Abell MR, Kidney Disease: Present Status. Baltimore: Williams & Wilkins, 1979, pp. 327–355.

42. Solez K, Racusen LC, Whelton A. Glomerular epithelial cell changes in early post-ischemic acute renal failure in rabbits and man. Am J Pathol 103: 163–173, 1981.

43. Kissmeyer-Nielsen F, Olsen S, Posborg Petersen V, Fjeldborg O. Hyperacute rejection of kidney allografts, associated with pre-existing humoral antibodies against donor-cells. Lancet II: 662–665, 1966.

44. Busch GJ, Reynolds ES, Galvanek EG, Braun WE, Dammin GJ. Human renal allografts. The role of vascular injury in early graft failure. Medicine 50: 29–83, 1971.

45. Kiaer H, Hansen HE, Olsen S. The predictive value of percutaneous biopsies from human renal allografts with early impaired function. Clin Nephrol 13: 58–63, 1980.

5. ENDOCRINE SYSTEM IN ACUTE RENAL FAILURE

Franciszek Kokot

1 Introduction

Occurrence of endocrine abnormalities in acute renal failure (ARF) may be expected for the following reasons: (a) The kidney is an important endocrine organ, in which erythropoietin angiotensin I and II, active vitamin D metabolites, kinins, and prostaglandins are synthesized. (b) The kidney is an important excretory and biodegrading organ for hormones. (c) The kidney is the target organ of several hormones involved in the regulation of its excretory and endocrine functions. (d) ARF is caused by different etiological factors or is accompanied by deep alterations of the internal environment, which per se may influence secretion control of hormones, their transport, transformation, degradation, and binding to target cells.

There exist several differences between ARF and chronic renal failure (CRF), which may influence the function of endocrine organs in different ways. Among them the following are to be mentioned: (a) In contrast to CRF, in ARF the amount of active renal parenchyma is relatively well preserved [1–4]. (b) Etiological and pathogenetic factors involved in ARF are different from those of CRF [5–7]. (c) ARF is characterized by oliguric and polyuric phases that may influence endocrine organs in different ways. (d) In ARF severity of reduction of renal blood supply and glomerular filtration rate and the degree of tubular obstruction and/or back-leakage across the damaged tubule vary from one case to another; these may influence the endocrine and biodegrading function of the

V.E. Andreucci (ed.), ACUTE RENAL FAILURE.
All rights reserved. Copyright © 1984.
Martinus Nijhoff Publishing, Boston/The Hague/
Dordrecht/Lancaster.

kidneys to differing degrees. In contrast to ARF, in end-stage renal failure, the severity of reduced renal function is much more homogeneous. (e) Finally, the nutritional and therapeutic management of ARF differs from that of CRF.

2 Endocrine Abnormalities in ARF

2.1 ADENOHYPOPHYSIS

2.1.1 Growth hormone (HGH, Somatotrophin)
In patients with ARF during the oliguric phase, significantly elevated basal as well as insulin-induced HGH levels are found [8]. Postdialysis HGH secretion nearly normalizes despite maintaining resistance to the hypoglycemic effect of insulin [8]. Fasting, environmental and physical stress, protein and calorie undernutrition, and disturbances of the water-electrolyte and acid-base metabolism could be excluded as potential factors involved in the pathogenesis of abnormal HGH secretion in ARF [8]. Since the half-life of HGH estimated in CRF after somatostatin secretion is normal [9], it seems barely true that impaired renal clearance of this hormone is responsible for its elevated plasma level in ARF. Thus, it follows that increased plasma levels of HGH in ARF are rather due to enhanced secretion of this hormone. In turn, increased secretion of HGH could be caused by an enhanced cellular influx of calcium ions stimulated by the existing secondary hyperparathyroidism [10, 11] or by other factors.

The pathophysiological role of elevated plasma HGH levels in ARF is still a subject for speculation. That this hormone is involved in the pathogenesis of carbohydrate intolerance [12, 13] and increased lipolysis, which are commonly observed in ARF, cannot be excluded [8]. As HGH exerts a stimulatory effect on intestinal calcium absorption [14] and 1,25-dihydroxycholecalciferol $(1,25\text{-}(OH)_2D_3)$ biosynthesis [15, 16], increased HGH secretion could be regarded as a purposeful mechanism counteracting hypocalcemia usually present in ARF.

2.1.2 Prolactin (LtH)

Basal plasma prolactin (LtH) levels are significantly increased in patients with ARF both in the oliguric and polyuric phases [17, 18]. After chlorpromazine administration, an exaggerated increase of plasma prolactin can be observed, while ingestion of α-bromocriptine is followed by a moderately delayed decline of plasma levels of this hormone [17]. In patients with ARF, in the oliguric phase, administration of luliberin (LH-RH) is followed by an unexpected significant increase of plasma prolactin concentration [18]. Abnormal responsiveness of serum LtH to thyroliberin (TRH) has also been reported [10]. Plasma prolactin levels found in the oliguric phase are positively correlated to plasma estradiol but negatively to plasma testosterone levels [18]. In contrast to other authors [10, 11, 19], we could not find a significant correlation between plasma LtH and PTH levels [18]. From the results obtained in our laboratory [17], it seems that hyperprolactinemia in ARF is due to increased secretion rather than to decreased renal biodegradation of this hormone. Estrogens [20] and PTH [21] are undoubtedly among the potential factors stimulating prolactin secretion; as blood levels of these hormones are elevated in ARF [18], their role in the pathogenesis of hyperprolactinemia is very suggestive. This does not exclude participation of other factors (e.g., LH-RH, TRH, etc.) in the pathogenesis of increased prolactin secretion. As reduced binding of LtH to renal receptors has been reported in experimentally induced ARF [22], it seems that hyperprolactinemia in ARF may be due to renal hyporesponsiveness to this hormone.

The pathophysiologic importance of hyperprolactinemia in ARF is not clear. The existence of a negative correlation between plasma prolactin and testosterone levels [18] suggests that hypersecretion of LtH may be involved in the pathogenesis of depressed function of the Leydig cells. As prolactin exerts a stimulatory effect on $1,25\text{-}(OH)_2 D_3$ biosynthesis [23], involvement of prolactin in the re-establishment of normocalcemia in patients with ARF is probable.

2.2 NEUROHYPOPHYSIS: VASOPRESSIN (ADH)

In oliguric patients with ARF, basal ADH levels are sevenfold as high as in normals [24]. After morphine administration, an absolute increase of plasma ADH levels was observed with a peak value appearing at 30 minutes (in normals it occurs at 60 to 90 minutes after morphine administration) [24]. In the polyuric phase, the morphine-induced ADH curve approaches normal [24]. In patients with ARF, ADH plasma levels are not related to plasma osmolality.

As plasma ADH levels in CRF are only twice as high as in normals [25], it seems unlikely that elevated ADH levels in ARF are due to impaired renal ADH biodegradation. Participation of enhanced angiotension II levels (which are very often present in patients with ARF) [26–29], in the pathogenesis of elevated ADH levels is very suggestive but not yet proved.

From results obtained in experimental ARF [30, 31], it seems that elevated ADH plasma levels may be contributory to the development and maintenance of ARF in man.

2.3 HORMONES OF THE PITUITARY/ THYROID AXIS

In oliguric patients with ARF, the following abnormalities in the function of the pituitary-thyroid axis were found: elevated [32] or normal thyrotropin (TSH) levels, decreased thyroxine (T_4) and triiodothyronine (T_3) levels [32], but elevated [32] or normal reverse T_3 (rT_3) levels [33]. During the polyuric phase, TSH plasma levels are elevated [32] or normal [33], while T_4, T_3, and rT_3 are usually normal [32]. Moreover, a blunted response to thyroliberin (TRH) was reported in oliguric patients with ARF [33]. In these patients, plasma thyroxine binding globulin (TBG) levels are normal [33], while the T_3-binding index (T_3I) and the index of free thyroxine (FT_4I) are significantly elevated [32].

Most of the above described abnormalities in thyroid function in ARF are very similar to those found in CRF [34–38] or in systemic nonthyroid diseases [39], suggesting that they are not related to the acute uremic state. As rT_3 is biologically inactive but capable of blocking the T_3 effect at the subcellular level, it seems that depressed T_4 and T_3 and elevated rT_3 levels [32] are purposeful adaptive mechanisms counteracting the catabolic constellation existing in patients with ARF.

2.4 HORMONES INVOLVED IN THE CALCIUM-PHOSPHATE METABOLISM

2.4.1 Parathyroid Hormone (PTH) Secondary hyperparathyroidism is one of the main endocrine abnormalities encountered in ARF [40–48] and is inversely related to the degree of hypocalcemia [43, 44, 46] and responsive to the suppressive action of calcium ions [43]. Elevated PTH plasma levels persist into the early polyuric phase [46, 47]. Peak levels of PTH coincide usually with the nadir of 25-hydroxy-cholecalciferol (25-(OH) D_3) concentrations [47, 48]. In hypercalcemic patients with ARF, normal [49], elevated [40, 41, 50–52], as well as undetectable [53] PTH plasma levels have been reported. Plasma PTH levels are not related to plasma calcitonin levels [54]. In contrast to other authors [10, 11, 19], we could not find any significant relationship between either plasma PTH and testosterone levels or plasma PTH and prolactin levels [18]. Restoration of normal renal function is regularly followed by the return to normal of PTH levels [46–48].

Secondary hyperparathyroidism in ARF seems to be due predominantly to hypocalcemia [43, 44, 46]. Retention of phosphates by failing kidneys [55], resistance to the skeletal action of PTH [46], deficiency of active vitamin D metabolites [45, 47, 48, 56, 57], and hypercalcitoninemia [54] are probably contributing to the stimulation of the parathyroid

glands. As skeletal extraction of PTH and cAMP release by the bone cells are not impaired [58], it seems that skeletal resistance to PTH is probably due to a defect located beyond the generation of cAMP. As no correlation exists between PTH and plasma creatinine levels [47], it seems unlikely that impaired renal PTH degradation is contributing to the elevated plasma levels of this hormone.

Increased PTH secretion seems to be a purposeful mechanism counteracting the existing hypocalcemia. It may be that hypersecretion of PTH, by promoting the cellular Ca influx, may also contribute to elevated HGH and prolactin secretion [59].

2.4.2 Calcitonin (CT) In oliguric ARF, plasma CT levels are moderately or extremely elevated [60]. Following intravenous calcium administration, there is a similar absolute increase in serum concentrations of CT as in normals [54]. No correlation was found between plasma PTH and CT levels [54]. In contrast, a significant positive correlation between plasma CT and calcium and a negative one between plasma CT and creatinine have been reported [60]. In contrast to healthy subjects and polyuric patients with ARF, no correlation was found between plasma CT and gastrin levels in patients with oliguric ARF [61].

Elevated CT plasma levels seem to be due not only to reduced degradation of this hormone by the failing kidneys [54] but also to its increased secretion triggered by phosphates [62] and enterohormones [63, 64]. These substances are known stimulants of CT secretion.

The pathophysiological importance of hypercalcitoninemia in ARF is not clear. CT could antagonize the osteolytic effect of PTH and contribute to the skeletal resistance to the calcemic action of PTH [46] and to hypocalcemia existing in patients with ARF.

2.4.3 Active Metabolites of Vitamin D: 25-(OH) D_3 and 1,25-(OH)$_2$ D_3 Significantly reduced plasma levels of 25-(OH) D_3 [45, 47, 48] and 1,25-(OH)$_2$ D_3 [45] have been reported in ARF. The nadir of plasma 25-(OH) D_3 level coincides with the peak of plasma PTH concentration [47, 48]. In oliguric patients, the apparent half-life of 25-(OH) D_3 is three to five times shorter than in healthy subjects [47, 48]. In polyuric patients, normal 25-(OH) D_3 [45, 47, 48] but elevated 1,25-(OH)$_2$ D_3 levels [45] have been reported.

According to the results of our own investigations, the significant decline of plasma 25-(OH) D_3 levels in oliguric patients seems to be caused neither by an insufficient dietary supply of vitamin D nor by an altered 25-(OH) D_3 binding capacity of serum proteins [47, 48]. Rather an increased turnover rate seems to be the predominant factor responsible for depressed plasma 25-(OH) D_3 levels. Whether the same mechanism is also responsible for depressed 1,25-(OH)$_2$ D_3 levels remains to be elucidated.

2.5 ADRENAL CORTEX: CORTISOL

Basal plasma cortisol levels are usually normal during both the oliguric and polyuric phases [64, 65]. After ACTH administration, a normal or exaggerated response of cortisol secretion is observed [65]. These findings suggest the presence of a normal pituitary-adrenal feedback in patients with ARF.

2.6. RENIN-ANGIOTENSIN SYSTEM

In oliguric patients with noninflammatory ARF, plasma renin activity (PRA) [28, 29, 66–73] and plasma angiotensin II levels [26–29] are abnormally high, while plasma aldosterone levels are normal or moderately increased [28, 65, 69]. Moreover, in these patients plasma renin concentrations and angiotensin II levels are significantly correlated [28]. Plasma renin substrate is usually elevated [28]. In contrast to normals, no significant correlation is found between plasma aldosterone and PRA, plasma renin concentration [28, 69], angiotensin II [28], and potassium levels [28, 69]. In inflammatory ARF, PRA is usually normal [67]. In most patients with ARF, a "physiological" reaction of PRA to weight loss [68] and a normal response of aldosterone secretion to ACTH administration [65] can be found. The cause of the dissociation of the physiological relationship between PRA and plasma aldosterone in ARF is not clear. Presence of significantly raised plasma levels of angiotensin II

but normal or only moderately elevated plasma aldosterone suggests impaired adrenocortical responsiveness to angiotensin II.

The importance of enhanced activity of the renin-angiotensin system in the development and maintenance of ARF is a subject of still unsolved controversy [5–7, 74–78]. As no correlation was found between plasma prolactin and PRA or plasma aldosterone levels (personal unpublished data), prolactin as a potential modulator of aldosterone biosynthesis [79] seems unlikely.

2.7 PITUITARY-GONADAL AXIS IN MAN

In oliguric patients with ARF, basal plasma lutropin (LH) levels are significantly elevated, displaying a normal or even exaggerated response to luliberin (LH-RH) administration [18]. In contrast to LH, basal plasma FSH levels are unexpectedly significantly elevated only during the polyuric phase [19]. After LH-RH administration, an exaggerated and prolonged response of plasma FSH is found [18]. Contrary to our results, depressed basal plasma FSH levels were reported by other investigators in oliguric ARF [19].

Oliguric ARF is characterized by significantly depressed plasma testosterone levels [18, 19], which are neither responsive to LH-RH [18] nor to human chorionic gonadotropin (HCG) [24] administration. These results suggest the presence of hyporesponsive Leydig cells. During the polyuric phase, plasma testosterone levels are normal or only moderately depressed [18].

In oliguric male patients, basal plasma estradiol levels are moderately though significantly higher than in normals [18], but not in the polyuric phase.

In contrast to healthy subjects, both in oliguric and polyuric patients, no correlation was found between plasma LH and testosterone levels [18]. As already mentioned, in oliguric patients, plasma testosterone levels are negatively related to plasma prolactin levels [18]. In contrast to other authors [11], we did not find a significant correlation between plasma PTH and testosterone levels [18].

From the results obtained in our laboratory, it seems that elevated basal plasma gonadotropin levels in patients with ARF are caused by increased secretion rather than by impaired renal biodegradation of these hormones [18]. Presence of significantly elevated plasma LH and depressed testosterone levels suggests the intactness of the physiological feedback between plasma testosterone and hypothalamic LH-RH secretion and hyporesponsiveness of Leydig cells to LH. As a significant inverse correlation was found between plasma prolactin and testosterone [18], it seems very likely that increased prolactin secretion is involved in the pathogenesis of depressed Leydig cell function. Increased estradiol levels [18] could also contribute to the hyporesponsiveness of Leydig cells to LH in male patients. As a positive correlation was found between plasma prolactin and estradiol levels [18], it seems that increased estrogen secretion may depress testicular function indirectly by stimulating prolactin secretion.

Function of the pituitary-gonadal axis in women with ARF remains to be investigated.

2.8 PANCREATIC HORMONES

2.8.1 Insulin
In oliguric and polyuric patients with ARF, basal plasma levels of immunoreactive insulin (IRI) are normal or only moderately elevated [12]. After i.v. administration of glucose, an excessive response of plasma IRI levels has been reported [12]. Hemodialysis does not affect the glucose induced plasma IRI curve despite significant improvement of glucose tolerance [12]. Stress, starving, potassium depletion, and acidosis could be excluded as potential diabetogenic factors [12]. It seems very likely that increased levels of HGH [8] and free fatty acids [8] may be involved in the pathogenesis of glucose intolerance and ineffective hyperinsulinism in patients with ARF. As basal IRI levels are usually normal or only moderately elevated in oliguric ARF, it seems unlikely that impaired renal clearance of insulin is the predominant factor responsible for elevated glucose-induced levels of this hormone. It follows that ineffective hyperinsulinism in ARF is probably due to insulin receptor or postreceptor defects caused by uremia.

2.8.2 Glucagon
In contrast to CRF in oliguric and polyuric patients with ARF, basal plasma glucagon levels are usually normal or only moderately elevated [24]. After administration of a test meal, a normal or sometimes blunted response of plasma glucagon is found [24]. In contrast to these findings, a sharp rise of plasma glucagon was reported in experimental ARF caused by bilateral ureteral ligation [80].

From data obtained in man, it seems that glucagon is not an important factor in glucose intolerance of patients with ARF.

2.8.3 Pancreatic Polypeptide (PP)
Both in oliguric and polyuric patients with ARF, basal plasma PP levels are significantly elevated. After administration of a test meal, a "normal" absolute increase of plasma PP is found [24]. As basal plasma PP levels in the polyuric phase are equal to or even higher than those in the oliguric phase [24], it seems barely probable that they are due to impaired renal clearance of this hormone. The pathophysiological importance of abnormal plasma PP levels remains to be elucidated.

2.8.4 Gastrin
In oliguric ARF, basal plasma gastrin levels are significantly increased [81-84] and decline during the polyuric phase [82-84]. In some patients, normal plasma gastrin levels have been reported while in others extremely elevated values were found [82]. Administration of a test meal [83] or of calcium [84] is followed by a normal absolute increase of gastrinemia although the gastrin curves are located significantly above the normal range. In contrast to normal and polyuric patients, oliguric patients show no significant correlation between plasma gastrin and calcitonin levels [61].

As both normal and highly elevated levels of plasma gastrin were reported in ARF [82], it seems that hypergastrinemia, if present, is not due to impaired renal degradation of this hormone; it could be related to the increased leakage in the gastric mucosa of H^+ ions (unpublished personal data), which, by increasing the pH of the gastric juice [82], is triggering gastrin secretion. As experimental ARF induced by ligation of the ureters is not accompanied by hypergastrinemia [85], it seems that presence of elevated plasma gastrin levels in man are not directly related to the uremic state.

The pathophysiological importance of elevated plasma gastrin levels as well as of the dissociation of the physiological calcitonin-gastrin relationship remain to be elucidated.

2.9 RENAL HORMONES

In addition to the renin-angiotensin system and the active metabolite of vitamin D, prostaglandins and erythropoietin represent the other known renal hormones.

2.9.1 Prostaglandins Investigations on prostaglandins in patients with ARF are scarce, although there exists a vast literature on renal vasodilating and natriuretic prostaglandins and on the existence of a positive feedback interplay between renin and prostaglandin secretion. The role of prostaglandins in the pathogenesis of ARF has been advocated by some authors [86, 87] but denied by others [78, 88, 89]. Inhibition of prostaglandin synthesis promotes the development of ARF in patients with increased PGE secretion, in patients who are dependent on prostaglandins for maintenance of renal function, and in patients with pre-existant renal diseases, particularly lupus [90]. Moreover, increased renal venous levels of the potent vasoconstrictor product of cyclooxygenase activity, tromboxane, have been reported in experimental ARF and in vitro perfused hydronephrotic kidneys [91]. Unexpectedly, reduction of renal vascular resistance and restoration of normal renal blood flow by prostaglandin administration did not alter the glomerular filtration rate in ARF [88, 89]. Moreover, infusion of prostaglandin E_1 into the renal artery of an anuric patient was not followed by an increase of urine output despite a twofold increase in renal blood flow [4]. From the above facts, it follows that the role of prostaglandins in the development and maintenance of ARF is far from being elucidated.

2.9.2 Erythropoietin In most patients with ARF, plasma erythropoietin is absent or markedly depressed and not related to the degree of anemia and severity of uremia [92]. These data call in question the importance of this hormone in the pathogenesis of anemia in patients with ARF.

2.10 BRADYKININ

In healthy subjects, activation of the renin-angiotensin system evoked by sodium depletion or upright posture is accompanied by a parallel rise in plasma bradykinin [93].

Significantly depressed bradykinin levels have been reported in patients who develop functional renal failure in the course of hepatic cirrhosis, despite normally raised PRA and angiotensin II concentrations [29]. As bradykinin is a potent stimulant of prostaglandin synthesis [94], deficiency of this diuretic and natriuretic nonapeptide may contribute to the development and/or maintenance of some forms of ARF.

3 Conclusion

Endocrine abnormalities in ARF are the result of interaction of two factors influencing the endocrine organs: first, the cause of ARF, which per se may change the control of secretion, transport, peripheral transformation, or binding to target cells of hormones; and second, the impaired function of the kidney as an endocrine, target, excretory, and degradating organ of hormones. In ARF, the following endocrine abnormalities may be found: increased growth hormone secretion, enhanced but not autonomous secretion of prolactin, elevated plasma vasopressin levels, depressed plasma T_3 and T_4 concentrations but raised rT_3 and TSH levels, hypercalcitoninemia, secondary hyperparathyroidism, reduced plasma levels of active vitamin D metabolites [25-(OH) D_2, 1,25-(OH)$_2$ D_3], elevated plasma LH, FSH and estradiol concentrations, but reduced levels of testosterone, hyporesponsiveness of Leydig cells to human chorionic gonadothropin, increased activity of the renin-angiotensin system, but dissociation of the physiological relationship between the renin-angiotensin axis and aldosterone secretion, hypergastrinemia, dissociation of the gastrin-calcitonin relationship, and hyperinsulinism. Glucocorticoid and glucagon secretion are not altered markedly in ARF. Secretion of erythropoietin, kallikrein, and vasodilatory prostaglandins seems to be reduced, while that of vasoconstrictive tromboxanes elevated.

It remains to be elucidated to what extent endocrine abnormalities in ARF are life-saving adaptations or coincidental side effects of acute uremia.

References

1. Hollenberg NK, Adams DF, Oken DE, Abrams HL, Merrill JPT. Acute renal failure due to nephrotoxins. Renal hemodynamic and angiographic studies in man. N Engl J Med 282: 1329–1334, 1970.
2. Hollenberg NK, Epstein M, Rosen SM, Basch RI, Oken DE, Merrill JP. Acute renal failure in men. Evidence for preferential renal cortisol ischemia. Medicine 47: 455–474, 1968.
3. Hollenberg NK, Sandor T, Controy M, Adams DS, Solomon HS, Abrams HL, Merrill JP. The transit of radioxenon through the oliguric human kidney: Analysis by the method of maximum likelihood. Kidney Int 3: 177–185, 1973.
4. Reubi FC, Vorburger C. Renal hemodynamics in acute renal failure after shock in man. Kidney Int 10: S137–S143, 1976.
5. Börner H, Klinkmann H. Pathogenesis of acute noninflammatory renal failure. Nephron 25: 261–266, 1980.
6. Kokot F. Die Pathophysiologie des akuten, nichtentzündlichen Nierenversagens. Z Ges Inn Med 33:329–335, 1978.
7. Levinsky NG. Pathophysiology of acute renal failure. N Engl J Med 296: 1453–1458, 1977.
8. Kokot F, Kuska J. Influence of extracorporeal dialysis on insulin-induced human growth hormone secretion in patients with acute renal failure. Nephron 12: 241–248, 1974.
9. Pimstone BL, Le Roith D, Epstein S, Kronheim S. Disappearance rates of plasma growth hormone after intravenous somatostatin in renal and liver diseases. J Clin Endocrinol Metab 41: 392–395, 1975.
10. Levitan D. Human and animal studies of the function of hypothalamic-pituitary-gonadal (H-P-G) axis during acute renal failure. In Acute Renal Failure, Eliahou HE (ed). London: John Libbey, 1982, p. 301.
11. Massry SG, Goldstein DA, Procci WR, Kletzky OA. On the pathogenesis of sexual dysfunction of the uremic male. Proc EDTA 17: 139–145, 1980.
12. Kokot F, Kuska J. Influence of hemodialysis in glucose utilization and insulin secretion in patients with acute renal failure. Eur J Clin Invest 3: 105–111, 1973.
13. Sagild U. Glucose tolerance in acute renal failure. Acta Med Scand 172: 405–411, 1962.
14. Henneman PH, Forbes AP, Moldawer M, Dempsey EF, Caroll EL. Effects of human growth hormone in man. J Clin Invest 39: 1223–1238, 1960.
15. Eskildsen PC, Sørenson OH, Bishop JE, Norman AW. Acromegaly and vitamin D metabolism: Effect of bromocriptine treatment. J Clin Endocrinol Metab 49: 484–486, 1979.
16. Spanos E, Barett D, MacIntyre I, Pike JW, Safilian EF, Haussler MR. Effect of growth hormone on vitamin D metabolism. Nature 273: 246–247, 1978.
17. Grzeszczak W, Kokot F, Dulawa J. Prolactin secretion in patients with acute chronic renal failure. Arch Immunol Ther Exp (in press).
18. Kokot F, Mleczko A, Pazera A. Parathyroid hormone and prolactin and function of the pituitary gonadal axis in male patients with acute renal failure. Kidney Int (in press).
19. Levitan D, Moser S, Goldstein DA, Kletzky O, Massry SG. Disturbances in the function of the hypothalamic-pituitary gonadal (H-P-G) axis during acute renal failure in the male. Kidney Int 19: 131, 1981.
20. Ferland L, Kabris F, Kelly PA, Raymond V. Interactions between hypothalamic and peripheral hormones in the control of prolactin secretion. Fed Proc 39: 2917–2920, 1980.
21. Isaac R, Merceron RE, Caillens G, Raymond JP, Ardaillou R. Effect of parathyroid hormone on plasma prolactin in man. J Clin Endocrinol Metab 47: 18–23, 1978.
22. Dobbie JW, Mountjoy D, Cowden EA, Allison MEM, Ratcliffe JG. Prolactin status in experimentally induced acute renal failure in the rat. Nephron 27: 316–319, 1981.
23. Spanos E, Colston KW, Evans IMS, Galante LS, McAuley SJ, McIntyre I. Effect of prolactin on vitamin D metabolism. Mol Cell Endocrinol 5: 163–167, 1967.
24. Kokot F. The endocrine system in patients with acute renal failure. Proc EDTA 18: 617–629, 1981.
25. Horky K, Sramkova J, Lachmanova, Tomasek R, Dvorakowa J. Plasma concentrations of antidiuretic hormone in patients with chronic renal insufficiency on maintenance dialysis. Horm Metab Res 11: 241–246, 1979.
26. Massani ZM, Finkielman S, Worcel M, Agrest A, Paladini AC. Angiotensin blood levels in hypertensive and nonhypertensive diseases. Clin Sci 30: 473–483, 1966.
27. Ochoa E, Finkielman S, Agrest A. Angiotensin blood levels during the evolution of acute renal failure. Clin Sci 38: 225–231, 1970.
28. Paton AM, Lever AF, Cliver NWJ, Medina A, Briggs JD, Morton JJ, Brown JJ, Robertson JIS, Fraser R, Tree M, Gavras H. Plasma angiotensin II, renin substrate and aldosterone concentrations in acute renal failure in man. Clin Nephrol 3: 18–23, 1975.

29. Wong PY, Talamo RC, Wiliams GH. Kallikrein-kinin and renin-angiotensin systems in functional renal failure of cirrhosis of the liver. Gastroenterology 73: 1114–1118, 1977.

30. Hofbauer KG, Konrads A, Bauereiss K, Möhring J, Gross F. Vasopressin and renin in glycerol-induced acute renal failure in the rat. Circ Res 41: 424–428, 1977.

31. Iaina A, Omdorff M, Gaveno S, Solomon S. ADH effect in development of ischemic acute renal failure. Proc Soc Exp Biol Med 163: 206–211, 1980.

32. Bodziony D, Kokot F, Czekalski S. Thyroid function in patients with acute renal failure. Intern Urol Nephrol 13: 81–88, 1981.

33. Kapstein EM, Levitan D, Feinstein EI, Nicoloff JT, Massry SG. Thyroid hormone indices in acute renal failure. Kidney Int 19: 129, 1981.

34. Czekalski S, Burton ST, Malczewska E, Kosowicz J, Baczyk K. Comparison of serum levels of thyroid hormones T_4, T_3, rT_3 in dialyzed and nondialyzed uremics. Proceeding of the Second Int Congress for Artificial Organs, New York City, 1981, pp. 98–100.

35. Gomez-Pan A, Alvarez-Ude F, Yeo PPB, Hall R, Evered DC, Kerr DNS. Function of the hypothalamo-hypophysial-thyroid axis in chronic renal failure. Clin Endocrinol 11: 567–574, 1979.

36. Lim VS, Tang VS, Katz A, Refetoff S. Thyroid dysfunction in chronic renal failure. J Clin Invest 60: 522–534, 1977.

37. Spector DA, Davis PJ, Helderman JH, Bell B, Utiger RD. Thyroid function and metabolic state in chronic renal failure. Ann Intern Med 85: 724–730, 1976.

38. Weissel M, Stummvoll MK, Wolf A, Fritzsche H. Thyroid hormone in chronic renal failure. Ann Intern Med 86: 664–665, 1977.

39. Bravermann LE, Vagenakis AG. The thyroid. Clin Endocrinol Metab 8: 621–639, 1979.

40. Black AMS. Calcium, phosphate and parathyroid disturbances in acute renal failure. Anaesth Intensive Care 6: 342–349, 1978.

41. Fuss M, Bagon J, Dupont E, Manderlier T, Brauman H, Corvilain J. Parathyroid hormone and calcium blood levels in acute renal failure. With special reference to one patients developing transient hypercalcemia. Nephron 20: 196–202, 1978.

42. Fuss M, Bergans A, Geurts J, Brauman H, Corvilain J. Effect of rapid variation of renal function on plasma calcitonin and parathyroid hormone in man. Acta Endocrinol 92: 130–137, 1979.

43. Kokot F, Kuska J. Influence of extracorporeal dialysis on parathyroid hormone secretion in patients with acute renal failure. Nephron 16: 302–309, 1976.

44. Kovithavongs T, Becker FO, Ing TS. Parathyroid hyperfunction in acute renal failure. Serial studies in man. Nephron 9: 349–255, 1972.

45. Llach F, Felsenfeld AJ, Haussler MR. The pathophysiology of altered calcium metabolism in rhabdomyolysis-induced acute renal failure. Interactions of parathyroid hormone 25-hydroxycholecalciferol and 1,25-dihydroxycholecalciferol. N Engl J Med 305: 117–123, 1981.

46. Massry SG, Arieff AI, Coburn JW, Palmieri G, Kleeman CR. Divalent ion metabolism in patients with acute renal failure: Studies on the mechanism of hypocalcemia. Kidney Int 5: 437–445, 1974.

47. Pietrek J, Kokot F, Kuska J. Kinetics of serum 25-hydroxyvitamin D in patients with acute renal failure. Am J Nutr 31: 1919–1926, 1978.

48. Pietrek J, Kokot F, Kuska J. Serum 25-hydroxyvitamin D and parathyroid hormone in patients with acute renal failure. Kidney Int 13: 178–185, 1978.

49. Turbkington RW, Delcher HK, Neelon PA. Hypercalcemia following acute renal failure. J Clin Endocrinol 28: 1224–1226, 1964.

50. Leonard CD, Eichner ER. Acute renal failure and transient hypercalcemia in idiopathic rhabdomyolysis. J Am Med Assoc 211: 1539–1540, 1970.

51. Weinstein RS, Rudson JB. Parathyroid hormone and 25-hydroxycholecalciferol levels in hypercalcemia of acute renal failure. Arch Intern Med 140: 410–411, 1980.

52. Wu BC, Pillary VKG, Hawker CD, Armbruster KFW, Shapiro MS, Ing TS. Hypercalcemia in acute renal failure of acute alcoholic rhabdomyolysis. South Afr J 46: 1631–1633, 1972.

53. De Torrente A, Berl T, Cohn PD, Kawamoto E, Hertz P, Schrier RW. Hypercalcemia of acute renal failure. Clinical significance and pathogenesis. Am J Med 61: 119–123, 1976.

54. Kokot F, Kuska J, Sledziński Z, Pietrek J, Baczyński R. Serum calcitonin levels in patients with acute renal failure. Water Mineral Metab 4: 43–48, 1980.

55. Sommerville PJ, Kaye M. Evidence that resistance to the calcemic action of parathyroid hormone in rats with acute uremia is caused by phosphate retention. Kidney Int 16: 552–560, 1979.

56. Sommerville PJ, Kaye M. Resistance to parathyroid hormone in renal failure: Role of vitamin D metabolites. Kidney Int 14: 245–254, 1978.

57. Massry SG, Stein R, Garty J, Arieff AI, Coburn JW, Normann AW, Friedler RM. Skeletal resistance to the calcemic action of parathyroid hormone in uremia: Role of $1,25(OH)_2D_2$. Kidney Int 9: 467–474, 1976.

58. Ølgaard K, Schwartz J, Finco D, Martin K, Korkor A, Font EB, Arbelaez M, Klahr S, Slatopolsky E. The extraction of PTH (1–34) and the generation of cAMP by isolated perfused bones from acutely uremic dogs. Kidney Int 19: 210, 1981.

59. Gautvik KM, Tashjian AH Jr. Effects of cations and colchicine on the release of prolactin and growth hormone by functional pituitary tumor cells in culture. Endocrinology 93: 793–799, 1979.

60. Ardaillou R, Beaufils M, Nivez M-P, Isaac R, Mayard C, Sraer J-D. Increased plasma calcitonin in early acute renal failure. Clin Sci Mol Med 49: 301–304, 1975.

61. Kokot F, Kuska J, Mleczko Z, Szczechowska E, Pazera A. Uber die Beziehung zwischen Gastrin- und Kalzitonin-Sekretion bei Kranken mit akuter und chronischer Niereninsuffizienz. Dtsch Gesundh-Wesen 36: 429–432, 1981.
62. Heynen G, Franchimont P. Human calcitonin and serum phosphate. Lancet I: 267, 1974.
63. Hennesy JF, Gray TK, Cooper CW, Ontjes DA. Stimulation of thyrocalcitonin by pentagastrin and calcium in two patients with medullary carcinoma of the thyroid. J Clin Endocrinol Metab 36: 200–203, 1973.
64. Melvin KEW, Voelkel EF, Tashjian AH Jr: Medullary carcinoma of the thyroid: Stimulation by calcium and glucagon of calcitonin secretion. In Taylor and Foster, Calcitonin 1969, Proc 2nd Int Symp, London, Heineman Medical, 1969, pp. 487–496.
65. Dulawa J, Kokot F, Grzeszczak W. Function of the adrenal cortex in acute renal failure (in press).
66. Brown JJ, Gleadle RI, Lawson DH, Lever AF, Linton AL, Mac Adam RF, Prentice E, Robertson JIS, Tree M. Renin and acute renal failure: Studies in man. Br Med J 1: 253–258, 1970.
67. Kokot F, Kuska J. Plasma renin activity in acute renal insufficiency. Nephron 6: 115–127, 1969.
68. Kokot F, Kuska J. Plasma renin activity in patients with acute and chronic renal insufficiency treated by hemodialysis. Proc. EDTA 8: 542–545, 1971.
69. Kokot F, Kuska J. Die Aldosteronämie bei Kranken mit akuter Niereninsuffizienz. Z Ges Inn Med 31: 144–148, 1976.
70. Mydlik M, Langos, Novotny J, Blazicek P, Derzsiova K, Takac M. Plasmaticka reninova aktivita pri akutnej oblickovej nedostatocnosti. Vnitr Lek 24: 1–10, 1978.
71. Schröder E, Herms W, Wetzels E, Dume T, Grabensee B. Plasma-Renin bei akuter und chronischer Niereninsuffizienz und Hämodialyse. Dtsch Med Wochenschr 94: 2262–2267, 1967.
72. Stone RA, Tisher CC, Hawkins HK, Robinson RR. Juxtaglomerular hyperplasia and hyperreninemia in progressive systemic sclerosis complicated by acute renal failure. Am J Med 56: 119–123, 1974.
73. Tu WH. Plasma renin activity in acute tubular necrosis and other renal disease with hypertension. Circulation 31: 686–695, 1965.
74. Blachley JD, Henrich WL. The diagnosis and management of acute renal failure. Semin Nephrol 1: 11–19, 1981.
75. Kleinknecht D. Donnes recentes sur la physipathologie des nephrites tubulares aique. Pathol Biol (Paris) 29: 197–205, 1980.
76. Schrier RW, Burke TJ, Conger JD, Arnold PE. Newer aspect of acute renal failure. Proc 8th Int Congr Nephrol Athens, 1981 pp 63–69.
77. Stein JH, Patak RV, Lifschitz MD. Acute renal failure: Clinical aspects and pathophysiology. Contrib Nephrol 14: 118–141, 1978.
78. Thurau K, Boylan JW, Mason J. Pathophysiology of acute renal failure. In Renal Disease, Black D, Jones NF (eds). Oxford; Blackwell Scientific Publication, 1979, pp. 64–92a.
79. Birkhäuser M, Riondel A, Valloton MB. Bromocriptine-induced modulation of plasma aldosterone response to acute stimulation. Acta Endocrinol 91: 294–302, 1979.
80. Bilbrey GL, Faloona GR, White MG, Knochel JP, Borroto J. Hyperglucagonemia in renal failure. J Clin Invest 53: 841–847, 1974.
81. Dent RI, Hirsch, James JH, Fischer JE. Hypergastrinemia in patients with acute renal failure. Surg Forum 23: 312–313, 1972.
82. Falcao NA, Wesdorf RIC, Fischer JE. Gastrin levels and gastric acid secretion in anephric patients and in patients with chronic and acute renal failure. J Surg Research 18: 107–111, 1975.
83. Kokot F, Król Z, Makowski C, Bodziony D. Serumgastrin bei Patienten mit akuten Nierenversagen. Z Ges Inn Med 34: 753–755, 1979.
84. Kuska J, Kokot F, Gerlach J. Zachowanie się gastrynemii po stymulacji jonami wapnia u chorych z ostrą i przewlekłą niewydolnością nerek. Pol Arch Med Wewn 63: 149–155, 1980.
85. Davidson WO, Moore TC, Shipey W, Convaloff AJ. Effect of bilateral nephrectomy and bilateral ureteral ligation on serum gastrin levels in the rat. Gastroenterology 66: 522–525, 1974.
86. Oken DE. Role of prostaglandins in the pathogenesis of acute renal failure. Lancet 1: 1319–1322, 1975.
87. Vincenti F, Goldberg LI. Combined use of dopamine and prostaglandin A_1 in patients with acute renal failure and hepatorenal syndrome. Prostaglandins 15: 463–472, 1978.
88. Mauk RH, Patak RV, Fadem SZ, Lifschitz MF, Stein JH. Effect of prostaglandin E administration in a nephrotoxic and a vasoconstrictor model of acute renal failure. Kidney Int 12: 122–130, 1977.
89. Robinson PJA, Gaunt A, Leung WK, Ima G, McLachlan MSF. Failure of prostaglandin A_1 to modify renal diatrizoate uptake in experimental acute renal failure. Invest Radiol 13: 150–154, 1978.
90. Henrick WL, Blachley JD. Acute renal failure with prostaglandin inhibitors. Semin Nephrol 1: 57–60, 1981.
91. Morrison AR, Thornton F. Thromboxane A_2-major prostaglandin of human hydro-nephrotic kidney. Kidney Int 19: 224, 1981.
92. Agranenko VA, Komarov LS, Chizhova AI. Erythropoietin and ceruloplasmin in acute renal insufficiency (in Russian). Ter Arkh 40: 77–81, 1968.
93. Wong PY, Talamo RC, Wiliams GH, Colman RW. Response of kallikrein-kinin and renin-angiotensin systems to saline infusion and upright posture. J Clin Invest 55: 691–698, 1975.
94. Nasjletti A, Malik KU. Renal kinin-prostaglandin relationship implications for renal function. Kidney Int 19: 860–868, 1981.

6. COAGULATION SYSTEM IN ACUTE RENAL FAILURE

Alain Kanfer

Intravascular coagulation (IC) undoubtedly takes place in many forms of acute renal failure (ARF), although its pathogenetic role and importance are still a matter of debate. Conversely, acute uremia per se provokes disturbances of the hemostatic system, with concomitant bleeding and a hypercoagulable tendency. In this chapter, we will deal successively with these two aspects.

1. Intravascular Coagulation and ARF

The precise significance of IC in ARF is not clearly established, and a reappraisal seems timely. Indeed, in the sixties and the early seventies, IC was generally held to be an intermediary mechanism pathophysiologically important in most types of ARF [1, 2]. In subsequent years, IC tended to become neglected and in several recent reviews on the pathogenesis of ARF, it is not even mentioned [3–6]. Historically, generalized Shwartzman phenomenon was the first condition that led to consideration of a causal relationship between IC and ARF. Postpartum bilateral cortical necrosis, hyperacute allograft rejection, and the hemolytic uremic syndrome were then admittedly thought to be human counterparts of experimental Shwartzman reaction. In these relatively uncommon diseases, it seems reassuring and

probably correct to ascribe renal insufficiency to the gross and conspicuous thrombosis of renal microvasculature. However in the much more frequent cases of ARF due to acute tubular necrosis, microthrombi are seldom seen, and a role for IC in this situation relies only on indirect arguments.

1.1 INTRAVASCULAR COAGULATION: DEFINITION, DIAGNOSIS

IC is defined as the formation and presence of thrombin in circulating blood. Nonroutinely, thrombin may be found directly by radioimmunologic or chromogenic assay [7, 8]. Usually, diagnosis of IC relies on the demonstrable effects produced by active circulating thrombin, i.e. (a) activation and consumption of platelets, factor V, and factor VIII; (b) transformation of fibrinogen to fibrin monomers and fibrin, with hypofibrinogenemia; (c) presence of fibrinous and platelet thrombi; (d) release into the circulating blood of fibrin degradation products (FDP) resulting from secondary, purely local, fibrinolysis (euglobulin lysis time being normal) [9–11]. Clinical and experimental conditions associated with IC are multiple and often complicated; unfortunately, there is not a unique diagnostic criterion. A diagnosis of IC is made or presumed in either of the two following circumstances: (a) evidence of overt consumption coagulopathy, indicating acute disseminated intravascular coagulation (DIC), although massive local IC may lead to similar systemic hemostatic disturbances; (b) presence of high levels of blood FDP and/or fibrin monomers (assessed by ethanol-gelation test or protamine test), associated with histological demonstration of fibrin thrombi, indicating

The author is indebted to Professor G. Richet for helpful criticism.
The author wishes to dedicate this work to the memory of Professor Francois Josso.

progressive (subacute) IC, which may be disseminated or localized.

1.2 INTRAVASCULAR COAGULATION AND EXPERIMENTAL ARF

Various methods can induce IC and ARF in experimental animals [12]: (a) infusion of thrombin [12–14); (b) infusion of thromboplastin, thus activating the extrinsic coagulation pathway; (c) repeated or protracted injection of endotoxin (generalized Shwartzman reaction) [15, 16] and injection of immune complexes [17], these two methods triggering intrinsic coagulation pathway through Hageman factor and platelet activation [18–21]; (d) injection of glycerol, with release of a procoagulant intraerythrocytic phospholipid component due to hemolysis [22, 23].

Each of these protocols for experimental ARF leads to (a) intrarenal (glomerular and arteriolar) deposition of fibrin or fibrin derivatives, (b) renal lesions with tubular necrosis or bilateral cortical necrosis, and (c) acute renal insufficiency. Renal damage is correlated, on the one hand, with the degree of fibrin deposition and, on the other hand, with the severity of renal failure [13, 16]. The pathogenetic role of IC is further emphasized by the efficacy of heparin in preventing renal cortical necrosis of the Shwartzman phenomenon [24].

However, for fibrin deposition to persist and renal damage and failure to occur, activation of the coagulation system must be associated with other factors; in their absence thrombin-induced fibrin deposition is only transient [25]. Thus, a synergistic interaction of fibrinolysis inhibition and vasoactive phenomena with intravascular coagulation "per se" is of prime importance.

Inhibition of fibrinolysis, as induced by epsilon-aminocaproic acid or spontaneously occurring in pregnant animals, is necessary to obtain renal damage after infusion of thrombin [13]; it allows the Shwartzman phenomenon to occur after one single endotoxin injection [12], and it aggravates renal damage of glycerol hemoglobinuric ARF [22].

Renal cortical fibrinolytic activity is probably important in the genesis of the Shwartzman phenomenon since it decreases after the first injection of endotoxin, the lowest activity being correlated with the most severe renal damage [16, 26]. The basic pathophysiological importance of vascular factors in IC-induced renal lesions is demonstrated by the following facts; (a) the concomitant injection of angiotensin or norepinephrine is essential to produce intrarenal fibrin deposits and renal failure following thrombin infusion [12]; (b) the Shwartzman phenomenon is prevented by alpha-blocking agents [27, 28]; (c) suppression of renin-angiotensin system by salt loading or saralasin injection prevents the onset of ARF after the injection of thrombin or glycerol [14, 29]. Finally, depending on the experimental protocols, IC is apt to induce various renal injuries, with slight as well as massive thrombosis leading to acute tubular necrosis (ATN) or acute cortical necrosis (ACN), suggesting the absence of a clear-cut limit between these two lesions.

1.3 INTRAVASCULAR COAGULATION AND HUMAN ARF DUE TO ACUTE TUBULAR NECROSIS (ATN) OR ACUTE (BILATERAL) CORTICAL NECROSIS (ACN)

1.3.1 Clinical Presentation Acute DIC with overt consumption coagulopathy is present in 5 to 30% of patients affected with ARF, the prevalence of DIC being especially high in obstetric ARF [30–35]. The main conditions leading to this clinical association are shown in table 6–1. The well-known severity of such situations is due to both the hemorrhagic and

TABLE 6–1. Main causes of association of disseminated intravascular coagulation and acute renal failure

Obstetric conditions
Preeclamptic toxemia, eclampsia
Abruptio placenta
Amniotic embolism
Intrauterine fetal death
Septic abortion
Puerperal sepsis
Septicemias
Intravascular hemolytic anemias
Acute leukemias
Disseminated cancers
Acute pancreatitis

thrombotic consequences of IC. Thus, in patients having ARF with DIC, severe protracted circulatory shock, mucocutaneous hemorrhages and necrosis, and arterial occlusions are strikingly frequent features [30, 32, 34]; moreover, pulmonary edema or acute cor pulmonale during the so-called "obstetric shock" is probably due to (or at least favored by) the pulmonary vasoconstriction triggered by circulating fibrinopeptides, fibrin-monomers, and FDP [36–38]. Finally, DIC aggravates the outcome of patients with ARF by increasing the frequency of lasting renal sequelae (chronic post-ARF) [31] and mortality (at least in obstetric conditions) [32]. Persisting renal insufficiency might be due to partial bilateral cortical necrosis, at times demonstrated by arteriography or renal biopsy [31, 39].

1.3.2 Pathophysiologic Role of Intravascular Coagulation in Human ARF
Presumption of a pathogenetic role of IC in ATN or ACN depends on the answers to the following questions: (a) May (disseminated) IC appear as the single (or main) cause preceding the onset of ARF? (b) Do serum and urinary FDP indicate intrarenal IC? (c) Is there compelling histological evidence of IC in such cases? (d) Is it possible to correlate IC phenomena with acute renal dysfunction?

1.3.2.1 DIC PRECEDING ARF. DIC precedes the onset of ARF in the absence of any other known cause of renal insufficiency (such as shock or nephrotoxins) in some instances: severe infections [10], neoplastic diseases [11, 40], acute pancreatitis [41], preeclamptic toxemia and abruptio placentae [39, 42–44]. Table 6–2 summarizes the clinical features of four

obstetric patients in whom DIC appeared as the main factor of ARF; microangiopathic hemolytic anemia was probably a direct consequence of DIC [11].

1.3.2.2 SIGNIFICANCE OF FIBRIN/FIBRINOGEN DEGRADATION PRODUCTS (FDP) IN ARF. More than half of the patients with ARF have high serum and urinary FDP levels [45–48] even in the absence of consumption coagulopathy; the meaning of this anomaly is still subject to controversy [48, 49].

Systemic fibrino (geno) lysis being excluded in ARF-euglobulin lysis time is normal [32, 34]—serum FDP arise from local lysis of fibrin deposits; a renal origin is demonstrated is some patients by an FDP level higher in renal vein than in renal artery [34]. Urinary FDP might theoretically reflect (a) lysis of intrarenal fibrin deposits, or (b) filtration of serum FDP through glomeruli, or (c) filtration of fibrinogen then destroyed by urokinase. The latter hypothesis is unlikely since urine urokinase activity is low or abolished during ARF [50]. Moreover, DIC per se is accompanied by urinary excretion of low molecular weight FDP (E product), while in ARF (with or without DIC) urine contains mainly high molecular weight FDP, probably indicating intrarenal lysis and "active" renal disease [47].

1.3.2.3 HISTOLOGICAL EVIDENCE OF INTRAVASCULAR COAGULATION IN ARF. In ATN intra-arteriolar and intraglomerular fibrin deposits are occasionnaly found [2, 45, 51, 52]. There is no agreement concerning actual frequency of this finding: the high incidence (about 40% of the patients have renal biopsy) observed by Clarkson et al. [45] and Conte et al. [34] has not been confirmed in a recent study of Solez et al.

TABLE 6–2. Acute renal failure related to disseminated intravascular coagulation in four pregnant patients

Patient no.	Age (years)	Onset of ARF (weeks of pregnancy)	Toxemia	Hemolytic anemia	Platelets (× 1,000/mm^3)	Factor V plasma level (%)	Fibrinogen plasma level (g/liter)	Renal pathology	Outcome
1	24	32	+	+ schistocytes	60	28	2,40	Acute tubular necrosis	Recovery
2	27	29	+	+	54	41	4,10	–	Recovery
3	21	32	+	+ schistocytes	60	42	1,50	Acute tubular necrosis	Recovery
4	25	35	–	+	65	35	0,90	–	Recovery

[53], showing renal fibrin in only 7% of the patients.

In ACN, on the contrary, massive fibrinous thrombosis of microvasculature and glomeruli is present in the vast majority of patients [39, 54].

1.3.2.4 CORRELATIONS BETWEEN INTRAVASCULAR COAGULATION, RENAL LESIONS, AND ARF   In ACN, parenchymal destruction is best explained by massive reduction or abolition of cortical blood flow [39].

The pathogenicity of microvascular thrombosis in this condition is strongly suggested by the parallelism in the severity of renal thrombi, glomerular destruction, and renal functional impairment [39]. In ATN, the pathophysiologic role of IC is not well defined.

According to Vassalli and Richet [55], the same etiologic circumstances may lead either to ATN or to ACN.

Probably in both conditions, cortical ischemia (due to vasoconstriction) is the initial event. In patients having ATN, serum and urinary FDP and occasional renal fibrin deposits or platelet aggregates indicate minor intravascular coagulation, which may add some degree of mechanical obstruction to the reversible functional vasomotor disturbance characteristic of this situation; in patients with ACN, massive intravascular thrombosis occurs and leads to irreversible parenchymal destruction and cortical necrosis.

Several causal factors might account for the extensive character of IC in cortical necrosis: inhibition of fibrinolysis induced by pregnancy or antifibrinolytic drugs; DIC of abrupt onset; protracted shock with stasis favoring local thrombosis; hypercoagulability of pregnancy or post-operative period; severe metabolic acidosis with decrease of glomerular fibrinolytic activity [56].

1.3.3 Therapy of ARF Associated With DIC

So far there is no definite proof that heparin therapy is beneficial in ARF associated with DIC [57]; thus, treatment of the underlying disorder is apt to reverse "per se" hemostatic disturbances [32]; nevertheless, heparin therapy has been said to reduce the incidence of ultimate renal sequels following an episode of

DIC [31, 34]. Finally, management of ARF with DIC might rely on the following somewhat subjective principles:

a. heparin is not indicated when the underlying disease or condition (e.g., shock, sepsis, pre-eclamptic toxemia) is curable by etiologic treatment; moreover, anticoagulant therapy is obviously dangerous when a local cause of bleeding is present (e.g., peptic ulcer, recent operation).

b. heparin must be given when a therapeutic maneuver may trigger or aggravate intravascular coagulation: uterine curettage, chemotherapy of acute promyelocytic leukemia (platelet transfusion must also be given in this case).

c. a trial of heparin therapy may also be undertaken when underlying disease is not rapidly accessible to efficient treatment as during certain neoplastic diseases and hemolytic anemias.

1.4 INTRAVASCULAR COAGULATION AND THE HEMOLYTIC UREMIC SYNDROME (HUS)

HUS is defined as the association of acute uremia and microangiopathic hemolytic anemia; arteriolo-glomerular thrombi are a constant finding on renal examination [58–61]. In infancy and childhood, the syndrome appears quite often to be idiopathic, although in some cases a viral etiology is likely [60]. In adults, HUS is not infrequently associated with or preceded by widely different conditions, such as pregnancy, oral contraceptive treatment, malignant hypertension, or scleroderma [62, 63]. All etiologic forms of HUS share the same hematologic and pathologic features indicating intravascular coagulation, while pathogenesis probably varies with the underlying disorder.

1.4.1 Pathologic Features of Intravascular Coagulation in HUS

Subendothelial fibrin deposits or thrombi are constant findings in HUS [61, 64, 65]. Immunofluorescent studies reveal that fibrin or fibrin derivatives are associated with the presence of factor VIII-antigen [66]; intravascular platelet aggregates may be shown by electron microscopy [67]. Lesions may predominate either in glomeruli or in arterioles, the latter localization pointing to a poorer prognosis [64]. Admittedly, glomerular ischemia, arteriolar occlusive endothelial proliferation, and cortical necrosis are direct consequences of intravascular coagulation.

1.4.2 Hematologic Signs of Intravascular Coagulation in HUS

Thrombocytopenia affects more than two-thirds of patients [58–60, 63]. Platelet life span is shortened [68]. Platelet aggregability is diminished, probably because of previous exhaustion in renal microvasculature [69]. FDP are almost always found in serum and urine of patients with HUS [48, 58, 60, 63]. Concentrations of coagulation factors, especially fibrinogen, are generally normal in HUS [64], and the half-life of labeled fibrinogen is also normal or minimally shortened [68, 70]. Interestingly, however, at the very initial phase of the disease or later accompanying deterioration of renal function, hypofibrinogenemia, decrease of factor V and VIII [60, 71, 72], and decrease of circulating antithrombin III [73] may be observed. Finally, a complete picture of DIC is present in some cases.

Circulatory fibrinolytic activity is normal in HUS [58]; on the contrary, local parietal fibrinolytic activity of thrombosed microvessels is diminished or even absent [74].

1.4.3 Pathophysiology of Intravascular Coagulation in HUS

The mechanism(s) triggering intravascular coagulation in the HUS is not known. Most probably, the etiologic diversity of the disease is associated with various pathogenetic pathways. For instance, "primum movens" of intravascular coagulation might be the vascular lesions in malignant hypertension or a preexistent blood hypercoagulability in pregnancy or during oral contraception. In any case, acute hemolytic anemia contributes to thrombin formation by releasing intraerythrocytic procoagulant phospholipid [75].

Cure or improvement of cases of HUS by exchange transfusion, plasmapheresis, or plasma infusion led to the hypothesis that deficiency of some plasma component(s) was implicated in the pathogenesis of the disease [76, 77]. Recently, in a few patients with HUS, Remuzzi et al. [77, 78] reported preliminary results

showing absence of a plasma factor stimulating endothelial synthesis of prostacyclin, a factor present in normal controls; moreover patients' vascular specimens lacked prostacyclin (antiaggregant) activity, this anomaly being reversed after plasma infusion; finally catabolism of circulating prostacyclin was found increased [79]. Similar results were obtained in some patients by other authors [80, 81]. Thus, HUS might be characterized by prostacyclin-thromboxane imbalance in favor of the latter, with subsequent enhancement of in vivo platelet aggregation. This attractive theory has to be confirmed in additional cases, more especially as the abnormalities cited above and plasma infusion efficiency are inconstant and still a matter of controversy [82].

1.5 INTRAVASCULAR COAGULATION AND ARF OF TRANSPLANT REJECTION

1.5.1 Hyperacute rejection

1.5.1.1 HUMAN DATA. In hyperacute rejection, arising a few hours or even a few minutes after transplantation in patients presensitized against donors' antigen, the pathogenetic role of intravascular coagulation is indisputable. Indeed, the hallmark of this situation is massive thrombosis of graft arteries, arterioles, and peritubular and glomerular capillaries, eventually leading to cortical necrosis of the transplanted kidney. Thrombi are made of fibrin and platelet aggregates [83–86]. In this situation, platelets and factors II, V, VIII, and fibrinogen are sequestered in the allograft to such an extent that systemic depletion of clotting factors may occur, thus mimicking DIC [84].

1.5.1.2 EXPERIMENTAL DATA Xenografts (pig to dog), and allografts implanted in animals presensitized against donors' lymphocytes or skin, are hyperacutely rejected. As in humans, massive thrombosis and cortical necrosis of the transplant occurs, with local consumption of platelets and coagulation factors [87–89]. Moreover, in the rabbit, reduction of graft cortical fibrinolytic activity is correlated with the onset of cortical necrosis [90], suggesting a pathogenetic role for impaired local fibrinolysis in perpetuation of thrombosis.

1.5.1.3 MECHANISMS OF VASCULAR THROMBOSIS IN HYPERACUTE REJECTION. Graft vascular endothelium is the target of complement dependant cytotoxic antibodies in hyperacute rejection. The endothelial lesion is apt to trigger several reactions leading to intravascular coagulation: release of factor VIII/von Willebrand factor provoking platelet adhesion [91]; release of thromboplastin; activation of Hageman factor and aggregation of platelets, owing to their contact with subendothelial structures (collagen, basement membrane).

1.5.2 Human Acute Allograft Rejection By comparison with hyperacute rejection, the role of intravascular coagulation in acute rejection of renal transplant is much less clear-cut; notably, overt consumption coagulopathy is not a feature of this condition [92].

1.5.2.1 HISTOLOGICAL FINDINGS. Glomerular capillary lumens are often filled with platelet clumps and fibrin deposits; in some cases, such abnormalities are mild and are found only by electron microscopy [85, 93]. Immunopathologic studies disclose deposition of fibrin and factor VIII-Ag in glomeruli and renal arterial vessel walls [66]. Interestingly, the platelets are intact during a reversible rejection crisis, while membrane disruption and platelet degranulation are present in the case of an irreversible rejection. Renal cortical fibrinolytic activity, measured by a fibrin-slide method, is diminished or even abolished, the lowest activity being associated with the most severe (irreversible) renal lesion [94, 95].

1.5.2.2 LABORATORY DATA. FDP are almost always found in the urine of patients acutely rejecting renal transplant [47, 48, 96–98]. FDP concentration may reach 50 to 100 mg/liter; concomitantly, urine may contain factor VIII antigen. Urinary FDP may be simply markers of ATN during the first two weeks following transplantation; then their predictive value for diagnosis of rejection during this period is questionable [48, 97, 98]; afterward, there is a close correlation between appearance of urinary FDP and the onset of acute rejection; urinary FDP may even announce the rejection episode since they are sometimes found several days before clinical signs. Therefore, it has been recommended to search systematically and regularly for their presence in transplanted patients [98].

An increase of serum FDP levels is less consistently found during acute allograft rejections [46, 47, 97, 99]; again, the diagnostic value of this abnormality appears greater when found more than two weeks after transplantation [99]. Numerous laboratory data militate for the participation of platelets in the pathogenesis of acute rejection, in keeping with the histological findings cited above: (a) radio-labeled platelets accumulate in the rejected kidney [100–102]; (b) platelet survival is shortened [70] (c) activation of circulating platelets occurs, as indicated by release of platelet-factor 4 and enhanced bioavailability of platelet factor 3 [103, 104] (table 6–3); (d) urinary immunoreactive thromboxane B2 is increased [105]. Each of these abnormalities disappears when the rejection episode is reversed by successful steroid treatment.

1.5.2.3 PATHOPHYSIOLOGY. Most probably, intrarenal immunological injury triggers activa-

TABLE 6–3. Platelet factor 3 (PF 3) activities (thrombin generation test)*, expressed in NIH thrombin units during 4 renal allograft rejection crises in three patients

| Incubation time (min) | Patients with rejection crisis | | Statistical analysis | | | |
	AT THE ONSET (1)	AFTER SUCCESSFUL TREATMENT (2)	Control (c)	1 VS 2	1 VS C	2 VS C
10	17.25 ± 0.8	10 ± 0.9	8.9 ± 0.5	$p < 0.005$	$p < 0.01$	ns
12	18.4 ± 1.7	11.2 ± 1.1	9.4 ± 0.5	$p < 0.01$	$p < 0.01$	ns

*Thrombin generation test: Platelets (120,000/µl) were added to a plasma substrate deprived of PF 3 activity; after recalcification thrombin generated, at any given incubation time depends on PF 3 activity from platelets; using fibrinogen clotting time, thrombin generated was measured at intervals of 2 min. (2 to 14 min.) (see text).

Source: Reprinted with permission of *Transplantation* [ref. 104].

tion of the coagulation system and platelets. Thus, immune complexes may activate Hageman factor [21]; also, they induce profound complement-dependant platelet changes: availability of procoagulant factor 3 [19], platelet aggregation with subsequent release of histamine and serotonin [20, 106], and release of platelet factor 4. Renal cortical ischemia is a major finding of renal failure in acute allograft rejection [107]; conceivably, the coagulation system may participate in this abnormality via serotonin-induced vasoconstriction and mechanical obstruction by fibrin and platelet thrombi.

1.5.3 Anticoagulant Therapy in Renal Transplant Rejection Heparin therapy prevents the onset of hyperacute rejection in presensitized dogs [88]. So far, however, there is no proof of such a favorable effect in man [83, 84]. The same holds for anticoagulant or antiplatelet therapy given for acute rejections; indeed, in such cases increasing dosage of corticosteroid drugs alone is sufficient to reverse the rejection episode. In a controlled study, the course of renal transplants and notably the incidence of rejection episodes were similar in the group of patients receiving dipyridamole and prednisone by comparison to patients receiving only prednisone [103]. This fact (and also the steroid-induced recovery of platelet abnormalities) brings evidence that activation of platelets is a secondary event, depending on the immunological injury, and is reversible along with it.

2 Hemostasis and Fibrinolysis Disturbances in ARF

2.1 THE BLEEDING TENDENCY
In 20 to 60% of all cases, acute uremia whatever its cause—consumption coagulopathy being excluded—is accompanied by hemorrhagic symptoms such as ecchymotic purpura and mucocutaneous and gastrointestinal bleeding; hemorrhages contribute to or directly cause death in a variable proportion of patients (probably close to 10%) [108–111]. The basic defect underlying the hemorrhages of acute uremia is thrombocytopathy, bleeding time

being prolonged while the platelet number is normal in a vast majority of patients. Bleeding time is especially prolonged in patients who bled; relevantly, it is negatively correlated with hemoglobin concentration [108]. Analysis of platelet dysfunction in ARF indicates decrease of platelet adhesivity [108, 109], aggregability [112], and factor 3 availability [113]; recently, an imbalance has been reported between diminished platelet thromboxane synthesis and increased vascular production of prostacyclin, which might play a role in genesis of thrombocytopathy [114]. Indeed, pathophysiology of bleeding tendency of ARF, though not completely elucidated, is at least in part caused by elevated plasma levels of "uremic toxins." There is a negative correlation between blood urea and creatinine concentration and platelet adhesivity [108]. Infusion of urea prolongs bleeding time and diminishes platelet adhesivity in normal volunteers [108]. Moreover, phenols, phenolic acids, and guanidinosuccinic acid, whose plasma levels are greatly elevated in acute uremia, inhibit platelet aggregability in vitro" [115, 116]. Finally, according to the toxin hypothesis, it is not surprising that dialysis treatment reduces or even reverses uremic platelet abnormalities [113] and bleeding tendency; likewise, prophylactic hemodialysis decreases the incidence and severity of hemorrhages (notably gastrointestinal) during ARF [110].

2.2 DISORDERS OF COAGULATION FACTORS AND FIBRINOLYSIS SYSTEM: THE HYPERCOAGULABILITY OF ACUTE UREMIA
Factor VIII coagulant activity is enhanced, up to two- to threefold above the normal level [109]; likewise, hyperfibrinogenemia is noted in most patients with ARF [109]. Fibrinolytic activity is diminished, as shown by decreased lysis of fibrin slides by plasma of acutely uremic patients [109]; also, levels of circulating inhibitors of fibrinolysis are increased: urokinase inhibitors, on the one hand [109], and "slow" plasma antiplasmin on the other hand [117]. We have demonstrated the latter abnormality in most of 20 patients affected with ARF independently of the cause of ARF and of the presence or absence of DIC (figure 6–1).

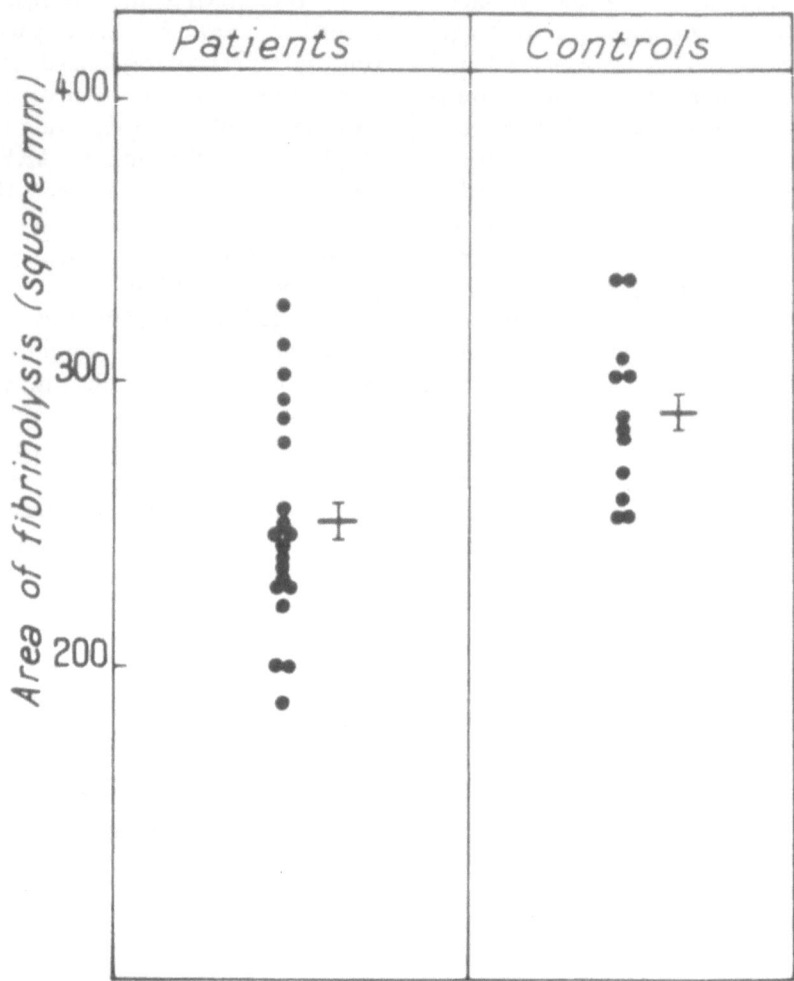

FIGURE 6–1. Plasma antiplasmin activity in 20 patients with acute renal failure. Lysis of fibrin plates by human plasmin was measured in the presence of patients' and controls' plasma. The area of lysis is negatively correlated with antiplasmin activity. Mean value of the lysed area of patients was significantly ($p < 0.001$) less than that of controls (250.5 ± 5 vs 289 ± 6 mm^2). (Reprinted with permission of *British Medical Journal* [ref. 117].)

The significance of coagulation-fibrinolysis system anomalies in ARF is uncertain. They are probably related to the conditions associated with or preceding ARF as much as to acute uremia "per se"; thus, postoperative or posttraumatic period, protracted infections, or inflammatory diseases increase the levels of coagulation factors and fibrinolysis inhibitors. In any case, such potential hypercoagulability could favor the occurrence of extrarenal thrombotic episodes that complicate the course of some 10% of patients having ARF [110, 118] and also act as a nonspecific phenomenon facilitating onset or perpetuation of renal intravascular coagulation.

References

1. Kincaid-Smith P. Coagulation and renal disease. Kidney Int 2: 183–190, 1972.
2. Wardle EN. Fibrin in renal disease: Functional considerations. Clin Nephrol 2: 85–92, 1974.
3. Levinsky NG. Pathophysiology of acute renal failure. N Engl J Med 196: 1453–1458, and 1977.
4. Hostetter TH, Wilkes BM, Brenner BM. Mecha-

nisms of impaired glomerular filtration in acute renal failure. In Acute Renal Failure, Brenner BM, Stein JH. (eds). New York; Churchill Livingstone, 1980, pp. 52–78.

5. Schrier RW, Gardenswartz MH, Burke TJ. Insuffisance rénale aiguë: Pathogénie, diagnostic et traitement. In Actualités Néphrologiques de l'hopital Necker. Paris; Flammarion, 1980, pp. 205–230.

6. Levinsky NG, Alexander EA, Venkatachalam MA. Acute renal failure. In The Kidney, Brenner BM, Rector FC Jr (eds). Philadelphia: WB Saunders, 1981, pp. 1181–1236.

7. Shuman MA, Majerus PW. The measurement of thrombin in clotting blood by radioimmunoassay. J Clin Invest 58: 1249–1258, 1976.

8. Herrmann RP, Bailey PE. Plasma thrombin assay using a chromogenic substrate in disseminated intravascular coagulation due to snake bite envenomation. Thrombos Haemostas 41: 544–552, 1979.

9. Colman RW, Robboy SJ, Minna JD. Disseminated intravascular coagulation: An approach. Amer J Med 52: 679–689, 1972.

10. Siegal T, Seligsohn U, Aghai E, Modan M. Clinical and laboratory aspects of disseminated intravascular coagulation: A study of 118 cases. Thrombos Haemostas 39: 122–134, 1978.

11. Spero JA, Lewis JH, Hasiba U. Disseminated intravascular coagulation findings in 346 patients. Thrombos Haemostas 43: 28–33, 1980.

12. Whitaker AN. Acute renal failure in disseminated intravascular coagulation. Progr Biochem Pharmacol 9: 45–64, 1975.

13. Whitaker AN, Bunce I, Nicoll P, Dowling SV. Interaction of angiotensin with disseminated intravascular coagulation. A possible mechanism in the genesis of acute renal failure. Amer J Path 72: 1–12, 1973.

14. Rammer L, Gerdin B. Protection against the impairment of renal function after intravascular coagulation by increased ingestion of sodium chloride. Nephron 14: 433–441, 1975.

15. Beller K. The role of endotoxin in disseminated intravascular coagulation. In Disseminated Intravascular Coagulation, Mammen EF, Anderson GF, Barhartt MI (eds). Stuttgart: FK Schattauer, 1969, pp. 124–149.

16. Graeff H, Mitchell PS, Beller FK. Fibrinolytic enzyme system of the kidney related to renal function after infusion of endotoxin in rabbits. Lab Invest 19: 169–173, 1968.

17. Lee L. Antigen-antibody reaction in the pathogenesis of bilateral renal cortical necrosis. J Exp Med 117: 365–376, 1963.

18. Semeraro N. Interactions of platelets, leucocytes and endothelium with bacterial endotoxins: Possible relevance to kidney disorders. In Hemostasis, Prostaglandins and Renal Disease, Remuzzi G, Mecca G, de Gaetano G (eds). New York: Raven Press, 1980, pp. 99–116.

19. Robbins J, Stetson CA. An effect of antigen-antibody interaction on blood coagulation. J Exp Med 109: 1–8, 1959.

20. Mueller-Eckhardt C, Luscher EF. Immune reactions of human blood platelets. Thrombos Diathes Haemorrh 20: 155–167, 1968.

21. Kaplan AP, Gigli I, Austen KF. Immunologic activation of Hageman factor and its relationship to fibrinolysis, bradykinin generation and complement. J Clin Invest 50: 51, 1971.

22. Wardle N, Wright NA. Intravascular coagulation and glycerin hemoglobinuric acute renal failure. Arch Pathol 95: 271–275, 1973.

23. Carvalho JS, Carvalho ACA, Vaillancourt RA, Page LB, Colman RW, Landewehr DM, Oken DE. The pathogenetic significance of intravascular coagulation in experimental acute renal failure. Nephron 22: 484–491, 1978.

24. Corrigan JJ. Effects of anticoagulating and non-anticoagulating concentration of heparin on the generalized Shwartzman reaction. Thrombos Diathes Haemorrh 24: 136–145, 1970.

25. Margaretten W, Csavossy I, McKay DG. An electron microscopic study of thrombin-induced disseminated intravascular coagulation. Blood 29: 169–181, 1967.

26. Bergstein JM, Michael AF. Renal cortical fibrinolytic activity in the rabbit following one or two doses of endotoxin. Thrombos Diathes Haemorrh 29: 27–32, 1973.

27. Muller-Berghaus G, McKay DG. Prevention of the generalized Shwartzman reaction in pregnant rats by adrenergic blocking agents. Lab Invest 17: 276–280, 1967.

28. Bolton WK, Atuk NO. Study of chemical sympathectomy in endotoxin-induced lethality and fibrin deposition. Kidney Int 13: 263–270, 1978.

29. Stahl E, Gerdin B, Rammer L. Protective effect of angiotensin II inhibition on acute renal failure after intravascular coagulation in the rat. Nephron 29: 250–257, 1981.

30. Haanen C, Holdrinet A, Wijdeweld P. Intravascular clotting and acute renal failure. In Pathogenesis and clinical findings with renal failure, Gessler U, Schroeder K, Weindinger H (eds). Stuttgart: Georg Thieme, 1971, pp. 132–139.

31. Zech P, Beruard M, Ducluzeau R, Moskovtchenko JF, Berthet P, Traeger J. Evolution des insuffisances renales aigues avec coagulation intravasculaire. J Urol Nephrol (Paris), 78: 337–341, 1972.

32. Kleinknecht D, Kanfer A, Josso F. Intravascular coagulation and heparin therapy in acute renal failure: A reappraisal. Europ J Clin Biol Res 17: 695–700, 1972.

33. Josso F, Cosson A, Girot R, Gazengel C. Coagulation intravasculaire et nephropathies. In Actualités Néphrologiques de l'Hopital Hecker. Paris: Flammarion, 1973, pp. 181–200.

34. Conte J, Delsol J, Mignon-Conte M, Ton-That H, Suc JM. Insuffisance rénale aigue et coagulation in-

travasculaire. In Actualités Néphrologiques de l'Hopital Necker. Paris: Flammarion, 1973, pp. 202–206.

35. Larcan A, Lambert H, Laprevote-Heully MC, Alexandre P, Gerbaux A. Insuffisances rénales aigues et coagulopathies de consommation au cours de l'état gravido-puerpéral. Sem Hop, Paris, 54: 595–601, 1978.

36. Schneider CL, Engstrom RM. Experimental pulmonary arterial occlusions: Acute cor pulmonale simulating "obstetrical shock" of late pregnancy. Amer J Obstet Gynec 68: 691–705, 1954.

37. Bayley T, Clements JA, Osbahr AJ. Pulmonary and circulatory effects of fibrinopeptides. Circ Res 21: 469–485, 1967.

38. Manwaring BA, Thorning D, Curreri PW. Mechanism of acute pulmonary dysfunction induced by fibrinogen degradation product D. Surgery 84: 45–54, 1978.

39. Kleinknecht D, Grunfeld JP, Cia-Gomez P, Moreau JF, Garcia-Torres R. Diagnostic procedures and long-term prognosis in bilateral renal cortical necrosis. Kidney Int 4: 390–400, 1973.

40. Gralnick HR, Marchesis, Givelber H. Intravascular coagulation in acute leukemia: Clinical and subclinical abnormalities. Blood 40: 709–707, 1972.

41. Kleinknecht D, Verger D, Mignon F, Richet G. Insuffisance rénale et pancréatite aigue. Signification des dépôts fibrinoïdes intraglomérulaires. Ann Med Int 121: 17–28, 1970.

42. Pritchard JA, Weisman R, Ratnoff OD, Vosburgh GJ. Intravascular hemolysis, thrombocytopenia and other hematologic abnormalities associated with severe toxemia of pregnancy. N Engl J Med 250: 89–98, 1954.

43. Vardi J, Fields GA. Microangiopathic hemolytic anemia in severe pre-eclampsia. Amer J Obstet Gynec 119: 617–622, 1974.

44. Grunfeld JP, Ganeval D, Bournerias E. Acute renal failure in pregnancy. Kidney Int 18: 179–191, 1980.

45. Clarkson AR, McDonald MK, Fuster V, Cash JD, Robson JS. Glomerular coagulation in acute ischemic renal failure. Quart J Med 39: 585–599, 1970.

46. Haanen C, Novakova I, Wijdeveld P, Van Lieberger F. Significance of fibrin split products in patients with renal failure. Scand J Haemat Suppl 13: 345–350, 1971.

47. Hedner U, Nilsson IM. Clinical experience with determination of fibrinogen degradation products. Acta Med Scand 189: 471–477, 1971.

48. Hedner U, Nilsson IM. Maladies du rein et produits de dégradation de la fibrine. In Actualités Néphrologiques de l'Hopital Necker, Paris: Flammarion, 1973, pp. 257–285.

49. Donati MB, Molla A, Michiesen P, Vermylen J. Measurement of urinary fibrinogen related material: Methodological aspects. J Lab Clin Med 83: 921–936, 1974.

50. Vreeken J, Boom-Gaard J, Deggeler K. Urokinase excretion in patients with renal disease. Acta Med Scand 180: 15–157, 1966.

51. Koffler D, Paronetto F. Fibrinogen deposition in acute renal failure. Amer J Path 49: 383–395, 1966.

52. Benshay Z. Contributions to renal pathology through the use of electron microscope. Israel J Med Sci 3: 191–198, 1967.

53. Solez K, Morel-Maroger L, Sraer JD. The morphology of "acute tubular necrosis" in man: Analysis of 57 renal biopsies and a comparison with the glycerol model. Medicine 58: 362–376, 1979.

54. Antonovych T. Bilateral cortical necrosis. In Controversies in Nephrology, Schreiner GE (eds). Washington DC: Georgetown University, 1979, pp. 513–519.

55. Vassalli P, Richet G. Nécrose corticale et Insuffisance rénale aigue des états de choc. In Comptesrendus du 1er Congrès International de Néphrologie, Richet G (ed). Basel: Karger, 1961, pp. 236–302.

56. Sraer JD, Blanc E, Delarue F, Kanfer A, Ardaillou R, Richet G. Effect of calcium and hydrogen ion on the fibrinolytic activity of isolated renal glomeruli from rat. Kidney Int 15: 238–245, 1979.

57. Corrigan JJ, Jordan CM. Heparin therapy in septicemia with disseminated intravascular coagulation. N Engl J Med 283: 778–782, 1970.

58. Clarkson AR, Lawrence JR, Meadows R, Seymour AE. The hemolytic uremic syndrome in adults. Quart J Med 39: 227–244, 1970.

59. Sraer JD, Morel-Maroger L, Beaufils P, Ardaillou N, Helenon C, Richet G. Les insuffisances renales aigues d'origine vasculaire. J Uron Néphrol (Paris) 78: 317–329, 1972.

60. Gianantonio CA, Vitacco M, Mendilaharzu F, Gallo GE, Sojo ET. The hemolytic-uremic syndrome. Nephron 11: 174–192, 1973.

61. Goldstein MH, Churg J, Strauss L, Gribetz D. Hemolytic-uremic syndrome. Nephron 23: 263–272, 1979.

62. Editorial. Hemolytic uremic syndrome of young women. Lancet 1: 943–944, 1976.

63. Kanfer A, Morel-Maroger L, Solez K, Sraer JD, Richet G. The value of renal biopsy in hemolyticuremic syndrome in adults. In Hemostasis, Prostaglandins and Renal Disease, Remuzzi G, Mecca G, de Gaetano G (eds). New York: Raven Press, 1980, pp. 399–406.

64. Morel-Maroger L, Kanfer A, Solez K, Sraer JD, Richet G. Prognostic importance of vascular lesions in acute renal failure with miroangiopathic hemolytic anemia (hemolytic-uremic syndrome): Clinicopathologic study in 20 adults. Kidney Int 15: 548–558, 1979.

65. Levy M, Gagnadoux MF, Habib R. Pathology of hemolytic uremic syndrome in children. In Hemostasis, Prostaglandins and Renal Disease, Remuzzi

G, Mecca G, de Gaetano G (eds). New York Raven Press, 1980, pp. 383–397.

66. Hoyer JR, Michael AF, Hoyer LW. Immunofluorescent localization of antihemophilic factor antigen and fibrinogen in human renal diseases. J Clin Invest 53: 1375–1384, 1974.

67. Ford PM, Levison DA, Down PF, Mc Connel JB. Clinicopathological spectrum of late post-partum renal failure: Two contrasting cases. J Clin Path 29: 101–110, 1976.

68. Metz J. Observations on the mechanism of the hematological changes in the hemolytic uremic syndrome of infancy. Brit J Haemat 23 (suppl): 53–59, 1972.

69. Kaplan BS, Fong JSC. Platelet aggregation in hemolytic uremic syndrome. Lancet 1: 46, 1980.

70. George CRP, Slichter SJ, Quadracci LJ, Striker GE, Harker LA. A kinetic evaluation of hemostasis in renal disease. N Engl J Med 291: 1111–1115, 1974.

71. Avalos JS, Vitacco M, Molinas F, Penalver J, Gianantonio CA. Coagulation studies in the hemolytic-uremic syndrome. J Pediat 76: 538–548, 1970.

72. Willoughby MLN, Murphay AV, Mc Morris S, Jewell FG. Coagulation studies in the hemolytic uremic syndrome. Arch Dis Child 47: 766–771, 1972.

73. Brandt P, Jesperson J, Gregersen G. Post-partum hemolytic-uremic syndrome treated with antithrombin-III. Nephron 27: 15–18, 1981.

74. Kwan HC. Role of fibrinolysis in thrombotic thrombocytopenic purpura. Semin Thrombos Hemostas 6: 395–400, 1980.

75. Josso F, Dosne AM. Les syndromes de défibrination experimentaux. Nouv Rev Fr Hemat 8: 35–44, 1968.

76. Remuzzi G, Misiani R, Marchesi D, Livio M, Mecca G, de Gaetano G, Donati MB. Hemolytic-uremic syndrome: Deficiency of plasma factor(s) regulating prostacyclin activity. Lancet 2: 871–872, 1978.

77. Remuzzi G, Misiani R, Marchesi D, Livio M, Mecca G, de Gaetano G, Donati MB. Treatment of the hemolytic uremic syndrome with plasma. Clin Nephrol 12: 279–284, 1979.

78. Donati MB, Misiani R, Marchesi D, Livio M, Mecca G, Remuzzi G, de Gaetano G. Hemolytic uremic syndrome, Prostaglandins and plasma factors. In Hemostasis, Prostaglandins and Renal Disease, Remuzzi G, Mecca G, de Gaetano G (eds). New York: Raven Press, 1980, pp. 283–290.

79. Remuzzi G, Imberti L, de Gaetano G. Prostacyclin deficiency in thrombotic microangiopathy. Lancet 2: 1422–1423, 1981.

80. Machin SJ, Defreyn G, Chamone DAF, Vermylen J. Plasma 6-Keto-PGF-1-alpha levels after plasma exchange in thrombotic thrombocytopenic purpura. Lancet 1: 661, 1980.

81. Chen YC, McLeod B, Hall ER, Wu KN. Accelerated prostacyclin degradation in thrombotic thrombocytopenic purpura. Lancet 2: 267–269, 1981.

82. Lee SH, Wainscoat JS, Zeitlin H, Bolton FG, Leaver HA, Seawright A, Preece JM. Prostacyclin and thromboxane A2 in thrombotic thrombocytopenic purpura. Brit Med J 283: 1351–1352, 1981.

83. Myburgh JA, Cohen I, Gecelter I, Myers AM, Abrahams C, Furman KI, Goldberg B, van Blerk PJP. Hyperacute rejection in human-kidney allografts-Shwartzman or Arthus reaction? N Engl J Med 281: 131–135, 1969.

84. Starzl TE, Boehmig HJ, Amemiya H, Wilson CB, Dixon FJ, Giles GR, Simpson KM, Halfrimson CG. Clotting changes, including disseminated intravascular coagulation, during rapid renal-homograft rejection. N Engl J Med 283: 384–390, 1970.

85. Kincaid-Smith P. The pathogenesis of the vascular and glomerular lesions of rejection in renal allografts and their modification by antithrombic and anticoagulant drugs. Austral Ann Med 19: 1–14, 1970.

86. Callard P, Bedrossian J, Idatte JM, Belair MF, Grossetete J, Mandet Ch, Bariety J. Les lésions artérielles au cours des phénomènes de rejets des allogreffes rénales. In Actualités Néphrologiques de l'Hopital Necker. Paris: Flammarion, pp. 165–185.

87. Rosenberg JC, Hawkins E, Mammen E, Palutke M, Riddle J, Rosenberg B. Hyperacute rejection of heterografts: Studies of pig to dog renal transplants. In Coagulation Problems in Transplanted Organs, von Kaulla KN (ed). Springfield: Charles C Thomas, 1972, pp. 107–155.

88. Beleil OM, Lecky JW, Stanley TM, Mittal KK, Olmsted WW, Kaufman JJ. Protective value of heparin in hyperacute rejection of renal allografts in presensitized dogs. Invest Urol 10: 318–326, 1973.

89. Shons AR, Najarian JS. Modification of xenograft rejection by aspirin, dextran, and crinanserin: The importance of platelets in hyperacute rejection. Transplant Proc 6: 435–440, 1974.

90. Myhre-Jensen O, Lund B. Fibrinolytic activity of renal transplants in rabbits; relation to graft thrombosis and necrosis. Acta Path Microbiol Scand Section A 80: 651–658, 1972.

91. Ruggeri ZM. Endothelium, Factor VIII, von Willebrand Factor and renal diseases. In Hemostasis Prostaglandins and Renal Disease, Remuzzi G, Mecca G, de Gaetano G. New York: Raven Press, 1980, pp. 11–20.

92. Colman RW, Braun WE, Busch GJ, Dammin GJ, Merrill JP. Coagulation studies in the hyperacute and other forms of renal allograft rejection. N Engl J Med 281: 685–691, 1969.

93. Porter KA, Dossetor JB, Marchioro TL, Peart WS, Rendall JM, Starzl TE, Terasaki PI. Human renal transplants. Lab Invest 16: 153–181, 1967.

94. Bergstein JM, Michael AF. Cortical fibrinolytic activity in normal and diseased human kidneys. J Lab Clin Med 70: 701–709, 1972.

95. Morozumi K, Yoshida A, Fujinami T, Watanabe Y. Studies on local fibrinolytic activity of the kidney in rejection of human renal allograft. Abstract of 8th International Congress of Nephrology, Athens, 1981, p. 470.

96. Antoine B, Neveu T, Ward PD. La fibrinurie au cours de la transplantation rénale chez l'homme. Rev Fr Et Clin Biol 14: 744–754, 1969.

97. Shah BC, Ambrus JL, Mink IB, Albert DJ, Sampson D, Murphy GP. Fibrin degradation products in renal parenchymal disease states and renal transplant patients. Transplantation 14: 705–710, 1972.

98. Hulme B, Pitcher PM. Rapid latex-screening text for detection of fibrin/fibrinogen degradation products in urine after renal transplantation. Lancet 1: 6–10, 1973.

99. Bennett NM, Bennett D, Holland NH, Luke RG. Serum fibrin degradation products in the diagnosis of transplantation rejection. Transplantation 14: 311–316, 1972.

100. Hardman MR, Eitjes-van Overbeek, van Velzen AJM. Early detection of kidney transplant rejections with autologous radiolabeled blood cells: Preliminary results. In Hemostasis, Prostaglandins, and Renal Disease, Remuzzi G, Mecca G, de Gaetano G. New York: Raven Press, 1980, pp. 363–367.

101. Nicolls FA, Mac Leod A, Smith F. Indium-labeled platelet scanning after renal transplanation. Kidney Int 19: 619, 1981.

102. Leithner C, Sinzinger H, Schwaez M. Prostacyclin reduces platelet deposition and prolongs platelet life span in transplant rejection. Abstracts of the 8th International Congress of Nephrology, Athens, 1981, p 453.

103. Anderson M, Dewar P, Fleming LB, Hacking PM, Morley AR, Murray S, Swinney J, Taylor RMR, Uldall PR, Wardle EN. A controlled trial of dipyridamole in human renal transplantation and an assessment of platelet function studies in rejection. Clin Nephrol 2: 93–99, 1974.

104. Kanfer A, Delarue F, Languille T. Transient platelet factor 3 activation during human renal allograft rejection. Transplantation 18: 78–81, 1974.

105. Foegh ML, Zmudka M, Cooley C, Winchester JF, Hekfrich GB, Ramwell PW, Schreiner GE. Urine i-TXB$_2$ in renal allograft rejection. Lancet 2: 431–434, 1981.

106. Humphrey JH, Jaques R. The release of histamine and 5-hydroxy-tryptamine (serotonin) from platelets by antigen-antibody reactions (in vitro). J Physiol 128: 9–27, 1955.

107. Hollenberg NK, Retik AB, Rosen SM, Murray JE, Merrill JP. The role of vasoconstriction in the ischemia of renal allograft rejection. Transplantation 6: 59–69, 1968.

108. Eknoyan G, Wacksman SJ, Glueck HI, Will JJ. Platelet function in renal failure. N Engl J Med 280: 677–681, 1969.

109. Larsson SO, Hedner U, Nilsson IM. On coagulation and fibrinolysis in acute renal insufficiency. Acta Med Scand 189: 443–451, 1971.

110. Kleinknecht D, Jungers P, Chanard J, Barbanel C, Ganeval D. Uremic and non uremic complications in acute renal failure: Evaluation of early and frequent dialysis on prognosis. Kidney Int 1: 190–196, 1972.

111. Conger JD. A controlled evaluation of prophylactic dialysis in post-traumatic acute renal failure. J Trauma 15: 1056–1063, 1975.

112. Castaldi PA, Rozenberg MC, Stewart JH. The bleeding disorder of uremia. Lancet 2: 66–69, 1966.

113. Rabiner SF, Hrodek O: Platelet factor 3 in normal subjects and patients with renal failure. J Clin Invest 47: 901–902, 1968.

114. Remuzzi G, Marchesi D, Cavenaghi AE, Livio M, Donati MB, de Gaetano G, Mecca G. Bleeding in renal failure: A possible role of vascular prostacyclin (PGI$_2$). Clin Nephrol 12: 127–131, 1979.

115. Rabiner SF, Molinas F. The role of phenol and phenolic acids on the thrombocytopathy and defective platelet aggregation in patients with renal failure. Amer J Med 49: 346–351, 1970.

116. Horowitz HI, Stein IM, Cohen BD, White JG. Further studies on the platelet-inhibiting effect of guanidinosuccinic acid and its role in uremic bleeding. Amer J Med 49: 336–345, 1970.

117. Kanfer A, Vandewalle A, Beaufils M, Delarue F, Sraer JD. Enhanced antiplasmin activity in acute renal failure. Brit Med J 4: 195–197, 1975.

118. Mc Murray SD, Luft FC, Maxwell DR, Hamburger RJ, Futty D, Swed JJ, Lavelle KJ, Kleit SA. Prevailing patterns and predictor variables in patients with acute tubular necrosis. Arch Intern Med 138: 950–955, 1978.

7. CLINICAL DIAGNOSIS OF ACUTE RENAL FAILURE

Vittorio E. Andreucci,

Stefano Federico,

Bruno Memoli,

Mario Usberti

1 Introduction

For practical purposes, we may define acute renal failure (ARF) as any abrupt elevation of serum creatinine (S_{Cr}) above 177 µmol/l (2 mg/dl) or, in patients with stabilized chronic renal failure (CRF) a sudden increase in S_{Cr} by 50% of the baseline value. This renal shutdown may occur with complete anuria or oliguria or with preserved urine output (nonoliguric ARF).

Since ARF is a syndrome of multiple etiologies, a careful history, an accurate physical examination, and a critical evaluation of laboratory biochemical data may greatly help in suggesting the correct diagnosis.

Undoubtedly, the main difficulty when dealing with a patient with acute impairment of renal function is the differentiation of prerenal (functional) ARF from acute tubular necrosis (ATN) or any other acute nephropathy once postrenal ARF has been ruled out.

The patient with ARF should be classified as early as possible in one of the following categories: acute obstructive uropathy (postrenal ARF) (chapter 19); functional ARF (prerenal ARF) (chapter 2); the so-called acute tubular necrosis (ATN) in both varieties of oliguric (chapter 2) and nonoliguric ATN (chapter 10); acute interstitial nephritis (AIN) (chapter 2); acute glomerulopathy (chapter 13); acute vascular nephropathy (chapter 14); myoglobinuric ARF (chapter 12); hepatorenal syndrome (chapter 11); leptospirosis (chapter 15); hemolytic uremic syndrome (chapter 16). For specific forms of ARF, the reader is referred to the respective chapter.

In this chapter only the general diagnostic criteria will be reviewed.

2 History and Physical Examination

The history uncovers factors that may help in classifying the cause of renal shutdown. Thus, for instance, a recent history of hemorrhage, burns, fluid loss (vomiting, diarrhea, gastric and/or enteric drainage, profuse sweating, diuretic therapy), especially if the patient is thirsty, insufficient or absent salt ingestion, myocardial infarction, low-output heart failure, hypotension, and sepsis, may each draw our attention to possible prerenal ARF; all the above conditions are, in fact, potentially responsible for a reduction in effective arterial blood volume. The use of nephrotoxic drugs, recent blood transfusions, muscular trauma, or exposure to radiocontrast media or to anesthetics may instead suggest ATN. Historical evidence of urinary tract obstruction (see chapter 19) points toward postrenal failure.

Physical examination may uncover signs of dehydration (ECV depletion): shriveled and dry tongue, poor skin turgor, dry axillas, soft eyeballs, hypotension with resting tachycardia or normal blood pressure in a previously hypertensive patient, postural accentuation of supine tachycardia and hypotension (suggesting a fall in blood volume by approximately 10%) [1].

As mentioned in chapter 2, symptoms of fever, skin rash, and/or arthralgia associated with ARF in patients under treatment with any drug should suggest drug-induced acute interstitial nephritis (AIN).

3 Urine Volume

Complete anuria (usually a few milliliters of urine) occurs rarely and is characteristic of bilateral complete ureteral obstruction (see chapter 19), renal cortical necrosis, bilateral renal artery occlusion, or acute glomerulonephritis.

We usually call anuria a urine volume of less than 50 ml daily and oliguria a volume of less than 500 ml daily, that is, less than 20 ml/hour if we record hourly urine output as is advisable in severely ill patients. In prerenal ARF, oliguria is the combined result of reduced glomerular filtration and increased tubular reabsorption, which represents the physiologic response of intact renal parenchyma to hypoperfusion secondary to a decrease in effective blood volume. Oliguria in ATN is the expression of reduction in glomerular filtration.

In nonoliguric ARF, urine output is greater than 500 ml/24 hours (see chapter 10).

3.1 URINE OSMOLALITY (U_{Osm}) AND URINE SPECIFIC GRAVITY

In prerenal ARF, the increased release of ADH leads to a urine osmolality (U_{Osm}) which is usually at least 50 mOsm/kg water greater than that of plasma, with a urine to plasma osmolality ratio (U/P_{Osm}) [2] greater than 1.15; in ATN, urine approximately isosmolar with plasma (U/P_{Osm} equal to or less than 1.1) is produced even if the patient is dehydrated [3]. There are, however, exceptions to this general rule. Thus, it has been demonstrated that only when U_{Osm} is greater than 500 mOsm/kg H_2O is there a strong possibility of a potentially reversible prerenal ARF, whereas a U_{Osm} less

than 350 mOsm/kg H_2O strongly suggests ATN [4].

Urine specific gravity is of limited usefulness since it is influenced by several factors. Thus, each g/dl of urinary protein will increase the urine density by 3 units, and each g/dl of glucose by 4 units (without affecting appreciably urinary osmolality) [1]. Nevertheless, in prerenal ARF urine specific gravity is greater than 1,013, whereas in ATN it is usually 1,008–1,012.

The isosthenuria of ATN has been attributed to a decreased sensitivity of collecting tubules to ADH. Microperfusion of isolated tubular segments dissected from kidneys of rabbits with post-ischemic ARF, in fact, has demonstrated a reduced ability of cortical collecting tubules to respond to ADH-mediated osmotic water flow [5].

3.2 URINARY SEDIMENT

Urinary sediment may be of great importance in the diagnosis of ARF. Dirty brown, coarsely granular casts, free tubular epithelial cells, and epithelial cellular casts have been defined as characteristic elements of urinary sediment both in oliguric and nonoliguric forms of ATN. Modest leucocyturia and microhematuria are also observed, but RBC casts and hem-pigmented casts are unusual in ATN unless hemoglobinuria or myoglobinuria is present.

Free erythrocytes and in casts are common in acute glomerulonephritis and in vasculitis, particularly when associated with heavy proteinuria (greater than 2 to 3 g/24 hours) and hypertension. Isolated hematuria may occur in vasculitis or in urinary tract obstruction.

The occurrence of mild proteinuria, microscopic hematuria, and leucocyturia with many eosinophils in the urinary sediment may suggest AIN (see chapter 2).

When numerous leucocytes, both free and in casts, are observed in urinary sediment, they are suggestive of pyelonephritis (bacteria are also present) or acute papillary necrosis.

The presence of an indwelling bladder catheter, however, may itself cause hematuria and leucocyturia, making these findings meaningless for diagnostic purposes.

3.3 URINARY SODIUM CONCENTRATION (U_{Na}), FRACTIONAL EXCRETION OF SODIUM (FE_{Na}), AND RENAL FAILURE INDEX (RFI)

In prerenal ARF, kidneys retain sodium avidly because of tubular overreabsorption. Thus, a urinary sodium concentration (U_{Na}) less than 20 mmol/liter strongly suggests prerenal ARF; a U_{Na} greater than 40 mmol/liter is typical of ATN [4, 6]; values of U_{Na} between 20 and 40 may occur in all types of ARF [4]. Fractional excretion of filtered sodium (FE_{Na}) has been found to be less than 1% in 94% of patients with prerenal ARF [4, 7, 8] while it is greater than 1% in ATN [4]. It has been stated that most patients with ATN have a FE_{Na} equal to or greater than 6%, many have values between 3 and 6%, and only a minority have values 2 to 3% [9].

The tendency to lose sodium despite salt depletion in ATN has been attributed to an impaired transport capacity particularly of proximal tubules, but also of the thick ascending limb of the loops of Henle; this has been demonstrated by microperfusion of isolated tubular segments dissected from kidneys of rabbits with post-ischemic ARF [5].

FE_{Na} may be easily calculated from urine and plasma concentrations of sodium (U_{Na} and P_{Na}) and creatinine (U_{Cr} and P_{Cr}) determined in simultaneously collected "spot" samples of blood and urine:

$$FE_{Na} (\%) = \frac{U_{Na} \times P_{Cr}}{P_{Na} \times U_{Cr}} \times 100,$$

since

$$FE_{Na} = \frac{Na \text{ excreted}}{Na \text{ filtered}} \times 100 = \frac{U_{Na} \times V}{P_{Na} \times GFR} \times 100$$

$$= \frac{U_{Na} \times V}{P_{Na} \times (U_{Cr} \times V/P_{Cr})} \times 100 = \frac{U_{Na} \times P_{Cr}}{P_{Na} \times U_{Cr}} \times 100.$$

(Concentrations of creatinine and sodium in serum and plasma are assumed to be equal).

If we consider that P_{Na} varies within fairly narrow limits, P_{Na} may be disregarded. The resulting formula has been called "renal failure ratio" or "renal failure index" (RFI) and is actually dependent on FE_{Na} [6]:

$$RFI = \frac{U_{Na}}{U_{Cr}/P_{Cr}}.$$

The RFI, like FE_{Na}, is of important diagnostic value in differentiating prerenal ARF from ATN. It has been found to be less than 1.0 in 85% of patients with prerenal ARF, while no patients with ATN had an RFI of less than 1.98 [4, 6].

Both FE_{Na} and RFI (since plasma sodium concentration is usually available, it is not necessary to calculate RFI once FE_{Na} is known) are easily calculated without the need to measure urine volume, a very difficult procedure in oliguric patients. Two conditions that are characterized by a reduced tubular reabsorption of sodium may make these urinary tests meaningless for diagnosing prerenal ARF: chronic uremia (in which homeostasis is maintained by an increased FE_{Na}) and the use of powerful/loop or osmotic diuretics.

Salt-losing nephritis may itself cause prerenal ARF, in which, obviously, FE_{Na} is greatly increased (figure 2–1).

4 Creatinine Concentration in Serum and in Urine

Usually renal function is evaluated as creatinine clearance. But it is more practical to measure serum creatinine (S_{Cr}) alone, which is much better than BUN as an index of renal function since it is not significantly influenced by protein intake or by the catabolic state of the patient.

Creatinine clearance may be calculated from the value of S_{Cr} according to the following formula [10]:

$$\text{Creatinine clearance (ml/min)} = \frac{(140 - \text{age in years}) \times \text{kg body weight}}{72 \times S_{Cr} \text{ (in mg/dl)}}.$$

For female patients the obtained value should be multiplied by 0.85.

It should be pointed out that in some conditions, S_{Cr} becomes a poor index of renal function, unless adequate precautions are taken:

a. After a meal with cooked meat or its broth, normal subjects may exhibit an increase in S_{Cr} that is not an expression of reduced renal function. Cooked meat and its broth, in fact, contain enough creatinine to raise S_{Cr} 70.7 to 88.4 μmol/l (0.8 to 1.0 mg/dl) [11]. This will double the S_{Cr} of a normal man. Thus, S_{Cr} should be measured in blood samples obtained in a fasting condition.

b. Both cimetidine and trimethoprim may cause a slight increase in S_{Cr} without changing the GFR [12, 13]. Apparently, this is due to competitive inhibition of creatinine secretion by the proximal tubules.

c. S_{Cr} may be falsely elevated with most assay systems when determined in blood samples taken soon after cefoxitin administration [14]. It has therefore been suggested that S_{Cr} should be determined at least two hours after the infusion of cefoxitin in normal subjects and at least six hours after cefoxitin in moderate renal failure; in severe renal failure, S_{Cr} determination is inaccurate during therapy with cefoxitin because of the very long half-life of the drug [14].

It should be borne in mind that S_{Cr} depends on muscle mass and exhibits diurnal variations even in normal subjects [15]. If glomerular filtration suddenly stops, the rise in S_{Cr} does not continue to reflect changing GFR but the rate of release of creatinine from muscles; in this state the increment will be 88-177 μmol/l/day (1–2 mg/dl/day); an increment of less than 88 μmol/l/day (1 mg/dl/day) suggests a less severe impairment of renal function; increments greater than 265 μmol/l/day (3 mg/dl/day) suggest rhabdomyolysis [1].

As mentioned above, in prerenal ARF an increased tubular reabsorption of ultrafiltrate occurs. Since creatinine is not reabsorbed by renal tubules, its urine concentration will be increased. Because of this, it has been suggested that the urine-to-plasma-creatinine ratio (U/P_{Cr}) should be used to differentiate prerenal ARF from ATN [16]. A ratio greater than 40 is usually observed in prerenal ARF [4, 6] and also in acute glomerulonephritis [4], indicat-

ing, in both conditions, the preservation of tubular function; a ratio less than 20 is suggestive of ATN [4, 6, 16].

5 Beta$_2$-Microglobulin Concentration in Plasma and Urine

Beta$_2$-microglobulin is a low-molecular weight (11,800 daltons) protein, which is freely filtered by the glomeruli and then almost completely (99.9%) reabsorbed and catabolized by the epithelial cells of proximal tubules. Its enhanced urinary excretion has therefore been suggested as an index of proximal tubular damage [17, 18] while its plasma concentration has been used as a highly suitable index of renal function [19–21]. Actually, plasma concentrations of beta$_2$-microglobulin have been found to correlate more closely with GFR than do plasma creatinine concentrations; in particular the former were found increased because of reduction of GFR below 80 ml/min/1.73m^2 even when the latter were still within normal ranges [20, 21].

Plasma beta$_2$-microglobulin concentration is stable throughout the day [21, 22] (whereas plasma creatinine concentration exhibits diurnal variations even in normal subjects) [15]; it may be measured by radioimmunoassay in very small blood samples (only 10 to 20 μl of plasma are required), which may be obtained by finger prick; it increases, even without renal function impairment, in patients with liver, malignant, or immune disease [21]. On the basis of these properties, beta$_2$-microglobulinemia may be used for the early detection of renal impairment during treatment with nephrotoxic drugs and for monitoring renal function when GFR is already reduced.

On the other hand, as mentioned in chapter 2, the increase in urinary excretion of beta$_2$-microglobulin has been suggested as a useful text for predicting a fall in renal function during aminoglycoside treatment.

6 Blood Urea Nitrogen (BUN)

Urea is the main end product of nitrogen metabolism. It is a diamide of carbonic acid

$(CO(NH_2))$ and is derived from protein catabolism. Urea concentration in blood is frequently determined by measuring the amount of blood urea nitrogen (BUN) (concentration of urea nitrogen in blood, plasma, and serum are assumed to be equal) [23]. Since the urea molecule (mol wt 60) contains two nitrogen atoms (atomic weight of $N = 14$; for two atoms the weight is 28), blood urea may be calculated by multiplying BUN by two (since 28 is approximately half of 60) [23].

When renal perfusion is reduced (as occurs in prerenal ARF), the consequent decrease in GFR leads to a reduction in tubular fluid flow rate; in this condition, tubular reabsorption of urea increases, leading to a disproportionate rise in BUN as compared to S_{Cr}. Thus, the ratio BUN/S_{Cr}, which is usually 10:1 to 15:1, will exceed 20:1, unless urea production is reduced by a low protein intake or concomitant severe hepatic disease [24].

However, BUN is elevated in all other types of ARF; this rise is proportional to the fall in GFR so that the BUN/S_{Cr} ratio is maintained around 10:1 to 15:1. The usual rise of BUN in ATN is of the order of 7 mmol/l/day (20 mg/dl/day). Increase in protein intake or in catabolic rate may induce a greater increase in BUN, which may lead to a BUN/S_{Cr} ratio greater than 20:1. Particularly in nonoliguric ARF, the rate in BUN increase is related more to the catabolic rate than to the degree of renal impairment [3]. In hypercatabolic conditions (burns, traumatic injuries, heat stroke, and complications of ARF, such as fever, sepsis, gastrointestinal bleeding, blood sequestration, extensive tissue necrosis), the rise in BUN may reach 18–21 mmol/l/day (50–60 mg/dl/day) [3].

Since a BUN/S_{Cr} ratio greater than 20:1 may be observed even in postrenal ARF because of increased urea reabsorption both from tubules (due to a reduced tubular fluid flow rate) and from pelves, ureters, and bladder (because of prolonged contact time), this ratio is suggestive but not diagnostic of prerenal ARF. [24]. In normal subjects, the urine-to-plasma-urea-nitrogen ratio (U/P_{UN}) is greater than 14 [1]. It has been demonstrated that in ATN, since

urinary excretion of urea is decreased and BUN is increased, the U/P_{UN} ratio is reduced [25], usually to less than 8 or even less than 3. In prerenal ARF, since the percentage of glomerular ultrafiltrate that is reabsorbed by tubules (because of their preserved functional integrity) exceeds the percentage of the reabsorbed urea, the U/P_{UN} is usually greater than 8 [4]. It should be noted that values of this ratio greater than 8 are also observed in acute glomerulonephritis [4].

An isolated increase in BUN may be observed in some normal subjects without renal disease and with normal renal function. Preliminary clearance studies performed in a number of these subjects in our unit appear to support the hypothesis that this phenomenon is due to urea overreabsorption in the distal nephron (presumably in the collecting duct); the urea nitrogen appearance (UNA, net urea nitrogen production) in these subjects is, in fact, perfectly normal [26].

Finally, it is interesting to note that in patients with CRF loop diuretics cause an isolated increase in BUN without affecting GFR. We have recently demonstrated that this phenomenon is accounted for by an increase in urea reabsorption in the distal nephron (presumably in the inner medullary collecting duct), secondary to diuretic-induced ECV depletion [27].

7   Serum Uric Acid

With the exception of acute uric acid nephropathy (UAN) in which hyperuricemia may be strikingly severe (see chapter 2), serum uric acid in ARF is mildly elevated, usually not exceeding 0.71 mmol/l (12 mg/dl) [28]. Urinary excretion of uric acid in ARF is reduced because of the fall in GFR, but less than would be predicted from impairment of renal function, thereby reflecting the relative preservation of uric acid tubular secretion; thus, the uric-acid-clearance-to-creatinine-clearance ratio may rise as GFR falls [29], but not as much as in UAN (see chapter 2). Thus, it has been demonstrated that urinary uric acid/creatinine concentration is greater than 1 only in UAN, being less than 1 (as in normal subjects) in ARF due to other causes [30].

8 Serum Sodium Concentration and ECV

8.1 HYPOVOLEMIC HYPONATREMIA

The normal osmolality (number of solute particles per unit of solvent) in ECV (in which sodium accounts for virtually all osmotically active solutes) is maintained by the combined actions of thirst, ADH secretion, and renal concentrating-diluting mechanism, which modify the volume of water in which solutes (mainly sodium) are dissolved [31]. Mild primary deficit of sodium, by causing hypotonicity in ECV, inhibits thirst and ADH secretion, leading to an immediate equivalent renal loss of water; thus, isotonicity is promptly re-established at the cost of a mild ECV contraction. Therefore, mild salt depletion is not reflected by changes in serum sodium concentration. If hyponatremia is observed in these circumstances, it indicates changes in hydration (i.e., water in excess of sodium) secondary either to increase in water intake or to i.v. infusion of salt-free solutions. This is usually an iatrogenic hyponatremia that requires water restriction rather than salt administration for correction (see chapter 21).

When salt depletion is particularly severe and ECV contraction assumes more significant proportions, the initial priority of maintaining a normal osmolality in ECV is sacrificed in order to minimize ECV contraction. In these circumstances, the three water-retaining forces are stimulated (rather than inhibited, as usually expected) and hyponatremia occurs, reflecting severe hypovolemia [31, 32]. It is therefore not surprising that in prerenal ARF, secondary to ECV depletion, hyponatremia is observed. The loss of sodium-containing fluid through the gastrointestinal tract (vomiting, diarrhea, gastrointestinal drainage), the skin (severe sweating) or the kidneys (e.g., in salt-losing nephritis) stimulates the hypothalamic-renal factors leading to renal retention of ingested water. If salt-free solutions are given by mouth and/or by i.v. infusion, this replacement of sodium-

rich fluid by water will worsen hypotonicity and hyponatremia [31].

8.2 HYPERVOLEMIC HYPONATREMIA

Increased tubular reabsorption of salt and water also occurs in those edematous states, which are characterized by a decrease in effective arterial blood volume. The effective arterial blood volume may be defined as the relative fullness of the arterial tree as determined by cardiac output, peripheral vascular resistance, and total blood volume. The effective arterial blood volume is usually diminished in congestive heart failure (because of a reduced cardiac output), in cirrhosis with ascites (because of a reduction in total peripheral resistance), and in nephrotic syndrome or severe burns (because of reduced total blood volume secondary to protein losses). In these circumstances in which ECV is expanded (with edema and/or ascites) but effective arterial blood volume is reduced, the disproportionate retention of ingested water leads to hypervolemic hyponatremia [31]. Renal hypoperfusion causes prerenal ARF (see chapters 1 and 2), with oliguria, high urine osmolality, and low FE_{Na} (see below), which are reversed by hemodynamic improvement and re-expansion of effective arterial blood volume (see chapter 21).

8.3 HYPOVOLEMIC HYPERNATREMIA

Frequently, ECV depletion, which may cause prerenal ARF, results from losses of hypotonic body fluids with sodium concentration below that of plasma [31]. This is the case with fluid loss by vomiting or nasogastric suction (normal gastric juice contains an average of 60 mmol/l of Na with a range of 30 to 90 mmol/l), diarrhea, or intestinal drainage (normal small bowel juice: mean Na = 105 mmol/l with range 72–158; normal ileal fluid: mean Na = 129 mmol/l range 90–140; normal cecal fluid: mean Na = 80 mmol/l with range 50–116), excessive sweating (sweat: mean Na = 45 mmol/l with range 18–97) [33]. Should these losses remain either unreplaced or partially replaced by relatively hypertonic solutions (e.g., normal saline: Na = 154 mmol/l), hypernatremia will occur [31], which may be worsened by associated conditions of water loss such as increase in insensible water loss (for example, for hyperpnea caused by metabolic acidosis) or diabetes insipidus.

This hypovolemic hypernatremia can be corrected by hypotonic saline solutions (e.g., half-normal saline or even more diluted solutions).

8.4 HYPERVOLEMIC HYPERNATREMIA

Hypervolemic hypernatremia is usually iatrogenic. Thus, it may occur in patients with metabolic acidosis treated with i.v. infusion of hypertonic solutions of sodium bicarbonate [31]. Obviously, it is a condition that should be prevented by correcting metabolic acidosis with isotonic or hypotonic solutions of sodium bicarbonate.

9. Serum Potassium Concentration

Serum potassium concentration in ARF may vary with external and internal potassium balance.

9.1 HYPERKALEMIA

Undoubtedly, in ARF the danger of death derives mainly from hyperkalemia. Thus, a blood sample must be immediately taken to measure serum potassium concentration when a patient first presents with suspected ARF.

Particularly in oliguric ARF, hyperkalemia occurs because of potassium retention. This may be even more severe when impaired potassium excretion is associated with excessive potassium administration as potassium intake, stored blood transfusion, i.v. infusion of potassium-rich solutions, or K-penicillin administration (K-penicillin contains 1.7 mmol of K^+/ 10^6 units of the antibiotic).

Redistribution of potassium from the intracellular space to the extracellular fluid may further increase serum potassium concentration. This occurs in metabolic acidosis, which is commonly observed in ARF, and in hypercatabolic states, such as in postsurgical or posttraumatic ARF.

In diabetic patients, sudden hyperglycemia (as occurs following i.v. infusion of glucose solutions without insulin) may cause fatal hyperkalemia due to cellular water (containing potassium) movement to the extracellular fluid in response to the osmotic effect of hyperglycemia; this life-threatening hyperkalemia is not observed in nondiabetic subjects because secretion of aldosterone and insulin is stimulated by hyperglycemia and hyperkalemia and this leads to cellular re-entry of potassium [31, 34]. Hyperkalemia due to cellular leak of potassium may follow excessive administration of digitalis, which inhibits Na-K-ATPase [31].

Serum potassium may be spuriously elevated because of test-tube phenomena; this pseudo-hyperkalemia, however, is not harmful to the patient and may be due to (a) test-tube hemolysis, (b) strangulation of the patient's arm during blood sampling, and (c) release of potassium from white blood cells and platelets during coagulation in the test tube (this factor is important when white blood cells exceed 5×10^5/ mm^3 or platelets exceed $7.5 \times 10^5/mm^3$) [31]. Even when a pseudohyperkalemia is suspected, it is mandatory to institute immediately emergency therapy (e.g., i.v. bicarbonate infusion) and possibly to evaluate an ECG for signs of hyperkalemia while awaiting a further laboratory measurement of potassium (possibly plasma potassium) in a fresh blood sample; the danger of sudden death is too high to take the chance and wait without therapeutic measures.

9.2 HYPOKALEMIA

Hypokalemia may be observed even in oliguric ARF. It is usually due to potassium losses through vomiting or nasogastric suction (normal gastric juice contains an average of 9 mmol/l of K with a range of 5-15 mmol/l) [31, 33], intestinal drainage (normal small bowel juice: mean K = 5 mmol/l with range 3.5-7; normal ileal fluid: mean K = 11 mmol/l with range 6-30; normal cecal fluid: mean K = 21 mmol/l with range 11-28) [33], diarrhea (in diarrheal states, stool may contain 10 to 100 mmol/l of K; gastrointestinal potassium wasting is enhanced by secondary hyperaldosteronism) [31], severe sweating (sweat: mean K = 4.5 mmol/l with range 1-15 being increased by hyperaldosteronism) [33]. It should be stressed that in normal subjects the potassium depletion that follows gastric losses is mainly due to renal potassium wasting stimulated by the secondary metabolic alkalosis and volume depletion. Volume depletion, in fact, will cause renal retention of sodium and chloride while alkalosis will favor tubular secretion of potassium; the result will be hyperkaliuria with hypochloriduria [31, 35].

The above conditions causing potassium losses may, on occasion, exhibit normokalemia or even slight hyperkalemia because of simultaneous severe metabolic acidosis with a consequent redistribution of potassium from the intracellular space to the extracellular fluid. In these circumstances, potassium depletion should be identified because the correction of metabolic acidosis without potassium supplements may lead to fatal hypokalemia.

10 Acid-Base Balance

The evaluation of acid-base status may help in determining the etiology of prerenal ARF. Thus, metabolic alkalosis may indicate vomiting, nasogastric suction, diuretic treatment; metabolic acidosis may indicate CRF, diarrhea, intestinal fistulas, adrenal insufficiency and (in diabetic ketoacidosis) glucose-induced osmotic diuresis [24]. It should be stressed, however, that once renal shutdown has occurred (as in ATN), acid retention will invariably lead to metabolic acidosis, which may be blunted by persisting vomiting or nasogastric suction. In these circumstances, the anion gap (i.e., the amount of the undefined anions that in addition to bicarbonate and chloride counterbalances sodium's positive charge; calculated as $[Na^+] - ([HCO_3^-] + [Cl^-])$) is clearly increased (normal value = 12 ± 2 mmol/l). In prerenal ARF secondary to diarrhea or intestinal fistulas, the anion gap may be normal, the lost bicarbonate being replaced by chloride overreabsorbed by proximal tubules of the hypoperfused kidneys (hyperchlemic acidosis).

Any cause of overproduction of organic or inorganic acids in ATN will worsen the metabolic acidosis; this occurs, for instance, in hypercatabolic states, in lactic acidosis, and in diabetic ketoacidosis. Severe metabolic acidosis with serum bicarbonate levels as low as 2 mmol/l has been reported in rhabdomyolysis-induced ARF and attributed to a large loading of hydrogen ions and their associated anions released from tissue destruction [36].

11 Serum Calcium Concentration

11.1 HYPOCALCEMIA

Hypocalcemia is a frequent biochemical feature of the oliguric phase of ARF and is responsible for the secondary hyperparathyroidism commonly observed in this condition (see chapter 5). The fall in serum calcium concentration appears secondary to phosphate retention due to the severe impairment of renal function [37] as occurs in CRF [23], low blood levels of 25OHD [38] and 1,25(OH)$_2$D [39], and a skeletal resistance to the calcemic actions of PTH [39].

Undoubtedly, marked hypocalcemia is a typical feature of the oliguric phase of ARF associated with rhabdomyolysis (see chapter 12); in this condition, in fact, the severe hyperphosphatemia is the combined result of both phosphate retention (due to the renal shutdown) and phosphate release (due to excessive breakdown of skeletal muscles); calcium salt deposition occurs in traumatized muscles, leading to a severe fall in serum calcium concentration [40, 41].

Finally, hypocalcemia with hyperphosphatemia may be observed in patients with acute lymphoblastic leukemia and ARF (secondary to acute nephrocalcinosis), which follows cytolytic therapy [42, 43] (see chapter 2).

It should be stressed that a reduction in total serum calcium may occur as result of hypoalbuminemia. Since 1 g/dl of serum albumin binds 0.8 mg/dl (0.2 mmol/l) of calcium, the component of hypocalcemia due to protein depletion may be easily calculated (as grams of serum albumin decrement times 0.8) [31].

Hypocalcemia may also result from binding of calcium by citrate (derived, for instance, from blood transfusion) or by oxalate (following ethylene glycol intoxication) [31].

11.2 HYPERCALCEMIA

Hypercalcemia is a typical biochemical feature of the diuretic phase of rhabdomyolysis-induced ARF (see chapter 12). Resolution of soft-tissue calcification, which occurred during the oliguric phase, increased calcium resorption from bone, and increase in gut calcium absorption have all been implicated as contributing factors to this hypercalcemia. In such patients, PTH plasma levels have been found normal, elevated, or undetectable (see chapter 5); the blood levels of 25OHD elevated or normal; those of $1,25(OH)_2D$ elevated (see chapter 12)

It has to be stressed that hypercalcemia may occur as late as 55 days after the onset of the diuresis; thus, determination of serum calcium should be included in the follow-up after rhabdomyolysis-induced ARF.

The occurrence of hypercalcemia in the oliguric phase of rhabdomyolysis-induced ARF is a very rare but extremely severe observation since the simultaneous occurrence of hyperphosphatemia may cause acute calcium deposition in vital organs. This hypercalcemia does not seem to depend on increase in PTH secretion but has been associated with increased blood levels of $25OHD_3$ [44].

It has been recently proposed that hypercalcemia in ARF may not be dissimilar from immobilization hypercalcemia, and its occurrence in the diuretic phase of ARF may be related to the immobilization time rather than to diuresis [45] (see chapter 12).

12 Anemia and Granulocytosis

A moderate to severe normocytic, normochromic anemia is regularly seen in all types of ARF. Hemoglobin values as low as 3.7–4.3 mmol/l (6–7 g/dl) and an hematocrit of 0.20–0.25 are frequently observed. Mild but continuous hemorrhage (for instance, in the gastrointestinal tract), increased hemolysis, and decreased erythropoiesis have been suggested as causative factors. As mentioned in chapter 6, a bleeding tendency is undoubtedly frequent. A relative proerythroblastosis with a decrease in RBC precursors (and increase in granulocytopoiesis) in the bone marrow has been reported with a rise in the myeloid/erythroid ratio [46]. This finding is suggestive of a suppressed maturation of erythrocytes probably due to uremic "toxins." Plasma erythropoietin has been re-

ported as either absent or markedly depressed (see chapter 5). Bone marrow regains a normal erythropoietic activity in the diuretic phase of ARF when a reticulocyte response is observed.

Granulocytosis is another frequent finding in ARF, even when no infection is present, particularly in rhabdomyolysis-induced ARF (see chapter 12). The occurrence of an increase in blood eosinophil count (greater than $0.7 \times 10^9/1$) suggests AIN (see chapter 2).

13 Differential Diagnosis Between Prerenal ARF and ATN

The differential diagnosis between prerenal ARF and ATN is frequently difficult. In the former condition, the preserved capacity to retain sodium and concentrate urine indicates a complete integrity of tubular function; in the latter, sodium is usually lost and the urine is not concentrated, suggesting a severe impairment of tubular function.

Several factors, however, may interfere with this general rule. Thus, when prerenal ARF occurs in elderly patients [9] and in patients with pre-existent CRF and/or a chronic nephropathy with urinary salt leaks (the so-called "salt-losing nephritis" usually secondary to chronic urinary obstruction, polycystic kidney disease, phenacetin nephropathy, or chronic pyelonephritis with urinary infection) [23], sodium may be lost despite salt depletion. Similarly, the administration of loop diuretics or the induction of osmotic diuresis by mannitol or by radiocontrast media may significantly increase sodium excretion interfering with the renal capacity to retain sodium in a state of severe dehydration or renal hypoperfusion. On the other hand, it should be borne in mind that high urinary sodium concentration and isosthenuria may occur in other forms of ARF, such as postrenal ARF, renal cortical necrosis, acute interstitial nephritis, and glomerular diseases.

With the aim of helping in differentiating prerenal ARF from ATN, several diagnostic indexes (see above) have been proposed. But the limits of these indexes, as listed in table 7–1, should not be regarded as inviolative; the farther a value of each index strays from the stated limits, the less likely is the corresponding di-

TABLE 7-1. Diagnostic indexes for differentiating prerenal ARF and ATN

	Prerenal ARF	ATN
Urine-specific gravity	>1013	<1013
U_{Osm} (mOsm/kg water)	>500	<350
U/P_{Osm}	>1.15	≤1.1
U/P_{Cr}	>40	<20
U/P_{UN}	>8	<3
BUN/S_{Cr}	≥20:1	<20:1
U_{Na} (mmol/l)	<20	>40
FE_{Na} (%)	<1	>3
RFI	<1	>4

U = urine; P = plasma; B = blood; Osm = osmolality; Cr = creatinine; UN = urea nitrogen; FE_{Na} = Fractional excretion of sodium; RFI = renal failure index.

agnosis to be correct [9]. It has been stated that FE_{Na} and RFI are the best urinary tests for this purpose [4].

A more recent study on nonoliguric ARF, however, has demonstrated that in sodium-avid states, such as severe hepatic dysfunction (cirrhosis with ascites), low values of urinary sodium concentration (less than 20 mmol/1), FE_{Na} (less than 1%), and RFI (less than 1) may coexist with a diagnosis of nonoliguric ATN, based on typical urinary sediment, isosthenuria, and U/P creatinine ratio less than 20 [47]. Similar findings have been reported in patients with nonoliguric ATN secondary to extensive burns [48, 49], nephrotic syndrome [50], and low-output cardiac failure following heart surgery [51]. The common denominator of these sodium-avid states is a decrease in effective arterial blood volume, which can fully account for tubular sodium overreabsorption, probably in the distal tubule [47, 48], in residual nephrons the tubular function of which is still preserved [49, 52]. These observations appear to support the assumption that sodium retention may clearly differentiate functional (prerenal) ARF from ATN only when oliguria is present [48].

Thus, for the diagnosis of prerenal ARF, all the tests listed in table 7−1 should be performed and evaluated in association with the following criteria: (a) the daily urine volume should be less than 500 ml; (b) the impairment of renal function should have occurred in association with volume depletion, transient hy-

potension, or congestive heart failure, that is, with a condition that may cause renal hypoperfusion; (c) no cellular casts should be observed on urinalysis; and (d) renal function should be normalized within 24 to 72 hours after correction of volume depletion, hypotension, or congestive heart failure. It should be mentioned that elderly patients with prolonged salt depletion may not respond promptly to fluid administration and may remain oliguric for up to 24 hours, even when a prerenal ARF is undoubtedly present [9]; after volume replacement, however, they frequently exhibit a prompt diuretic response to loop diuretics or mannitol [9].

The early renal functional changes of hepatorenal syndrome (HRS) are indistinguishable from prerenal ARF; but in HRS, the expansion of ECV is not successful in reversing the renal impairment (see chapter 11).

13.1 NONOLIGURIC PRERENAL ARF
Things become more difficult when prerenal ARF occurs in a nonoliguric form. Thus, patients with volume-compromised hemodynamic state have been reported in the recent literature with nonoliguric ARF with a low RFI (less than 1.0), a normal urinary sediment, and other signs compatible with the diagnosis of prerenal ARF, including the prompt recovery of renal function after correction of impaired hemodynamics [53]; the nonoliguric state in these patients, in the absence of diabetes melitus or solute diuresis, has been attributed to a concentrating defect [47].

On the other hand, in elderly subjects, as well as in hypertensives and in patients with CRF, the ability to concentrate urine is frequently reduced; should prerenal ARF occur in these subjects, U/P_{Osm} and U/P_{Cr} would be lower than expected [9].

13.2 ACUTE REJECTION AFTER RENAL TRANSPLANTATION
After renal transplantation, early postoperative graft failure creates the practical problem of differentiating between prerenal ARF, acute rejection, and ATN. While referring the reader to chapter 20, it is worthwhile to mention that since acute rejection starts with a re-

duction in renal perfusion while tubular function integrity is preserved, the clinical pattern of the early phase of acute rejection is quite similar to that of prerenal ARF: oliguria, high U_{Osm}, low U_{Na}, and, in particular, low values of FE_{Na}. This may help to rule out ATN and diagnose acute rejection once systemic factors such as volume depletion and/or hypotension are excluded [54].

13.3 ACUTE GLOMERULONEPHRITIS

Urinary diagnostic indexes (U_{Osm}, U_{Na}, U/P_{UN}, U/P_{Cr}, RFI, and FE_{Na}) in patients with acute glomerulonephritis have been demonstrated to be similar to the values observed in prerenal ARF [4]. This observation suggests that tubular function integrity is preserved in acute glomerulonephritis.

Thus, the above diagnostic indexes appear quite useful for differentiating this disease from oliguric ATN (see chapter 13).

References

1. Bastl CP, Rudnick MR, Narins RG. Diagnostic approaches to acute renal failure. In Acute Renal Failure, Brenner BM, Stein JH (eds). New York; Churchill Livingstone, 1980, pp. 17–51.
2. Eliahou HE, Bata A. The diagnosis of acute renal failure. Nephron 2: 287–295, 1965.
3. Oken DE. Clinical aspects of acute renal failure (vasomotor nephropathy). In Pediatric Kidney Disease, Edelman CM (ed). Boston: Little, Brown and Company, 1978, pp. 1108–1119.
4. Miller TR, Anderson RJ, Linas SL, Henrich WL, Berns AS, Gabow PA, Schrier RW. Urinary diagnostic indices in acute renal failure. A prospective study. Ann Intern Med 89: 47–50, 1978.
5. Hanley MJ, Davidson K. Prior mannitol and furosemide infusion in a model of ischemic acute renal failure. Am J Physiol 10: F-556–564, 1981.
6. Handa SP, Marrin PAF. Diagnostic indices in acute renal failure. Can Med Ass J 96: 78–82, 1967.
7. Espinel CH. The FE_{Na} test. JAMA 236: 579–581, 1976.
8. Espinel CH, Gregory AW. Differential diagnosis of acute renal failure. Clin Nephrol 13: 73–77, 1980.
9. Oken DE. On the differential diagnosis of acute renal failure. Am J Med 71: 916–920, 1981.
10. Cockcroft DW, Gault MH. Prediction of creatinine clearance from serum creatinine. Nephron 16:31–41, 1976.
11. Jacobsen FK, Christensen CK, Mogensen CE, Andreasen F, Heilskov NSC. Pronounced increase in serum creatinine concentration after eating cooked meat. Brit Med J 1: 1049–1050, 1979.
12. Berglund F, Killander J, Pompeius R. Effect of trimethoprim-sulfamethoxazole on the renal excretion of creatinine in man. J Urol 114: 802, 1975.
13. Dubb JW, Stote RM, Familiar RG, Lee K. Alexander F. Effect of cimetidine on renal function in normal man. Clin Pharmacol Ther 24: 76, 1978.
14. Saah AJ, Hoch TR, Drusano GL. Cefoxitin falsely elevates creatinine levels. JAMA 247: 205–206, 1982.
15. Pasternak A, Kuhlback B. Diurnal variation of serum and urine creatine and creatinine. Scand J Clin Lab Invest 27: 1–7, 1971.
16. Bull GM, Joekes AM, Lowe KG. Renal function studies in acute tubular necrosis. Clin Sci 9: 379–404, 1950.
17. Hall PW, Vasiljevic. Beta$_2$-microglobulin excretion as an index of renal tubular disorders with special reference to endemic Balkan nephropathy. J Lab Clin Med 81: 897–904, 1973.
18. Fredriksson A. Renal handling of beta$_2$-microglobulin in experimental renal disease. Scand J Clin Lab Invest 35: 591–600, 1975.
19. Wibell L, Evrin PE, Berggard I. Serum B$_2$-microglobulin in renal disease. Nephron 10: 320–331, 1973.
20. Kult J, Lammilein Ch, Rocken A, Heidland A. Beta-2-Mikroglobulin im Serum-ein Parameter des Glomerulofiltrates. Dtsch Med Wochenschr 99: 1686–1688, 1974.
21. Viberti GC, Keen H, Mackintosh D. Beta$_2$-microglobulinemia: A sensitive index of diminishing renal function in diabetics. Brit Med J 282: 95–98, 1981.
22. Kawai T, Kin K. Diurnal variation of serum B$_2$-microglobulin in normal subjects. N Engl J Med 293: 879–880, 1975.
23. Andreucci VE. Chronic renal failure. In The Treatment of Renal Failure, Castro JE (ed). Lancaster: MTP Press Limited, 1982, pp. 33–167.
24. Rose BD. Acute renal failure. In Pathophysiology of Renal Disease, Rose BD (ed). New York: McGraw-Hill, 1981, pp. 55–95.
25. Perlmutter M, Grossman SL, Rothenberg S. Urine-serum urea nitrogen ratio. JAMA 170: 1533–1537, 1959.
26. Conte G, Dal Canton A, Terribile M, Capuano A, Cianciaruso B, Genualdo R, Russo D, Andreucci VE. Iperazotemia persistente in soggetti con normofunzione renale, Nefrologia, Dialisi, Trapianto (Wichtig Editor Milan, Italy) 1983, pp. 367–368.
27. Dal Canton A, Fuiano G, Conte G, Terribile M, Sabbatini M, Cianciaruso B, Andreucci VE. Why diuretic treatment increases azoteuria. Proc EDTA 19: 744–748, 1982.
28. Rose BD. Tubulointerstitial diseases. In Pathophysiology of Renal Disease, Rose BD (ed). New York: McGraw-Hill, 1981, pp. 295–345.
29. Yu TF, Berger L. The Kidney in Gout and Hyper-

uricemia. Mount Kisco, NY: Futura Publishing, 1982.

30. Kelton J, Kelley WN, Holmes EW. A rapid method for the diagnosis of acute uric acid nephropathy. Arch Intern Med 138: 612–615, 1978.

31. Narins RG, Jones ER, Stom MC, Rudnick MR, Bastl CP: Diagnostic strategies in disorders of fluid electrolyte and acid-base homeostasis. Am J Med 72: 496–520, 1982.

32. Morgan DB, Thomas TH. Water balance and hyponatremia. Clin Sci 56: 517–522, 1979.

33. Arieff AI. Principles of parenteral therapy. In Clinical Disorders of Fluid and Electrolyte Metabolism, Maxwell MH, Kleeman CR (eds). New York: McGraw-Hill, 1972, pp. 567–589.

34. Goldfarb S, Cox M, Singer I, Goldberg M. Acute hyperkalemia induced by hyperglicemia: Hormonal mechanisms. Ann Intern Med 84: 426–432, 1976.

35. Seldin DW, Rector FC Jr. The generation and maintenance of metabolic alkalosis. Kidney Int 1: 305–321, 1972.

36. McCarron DA, Elliott WC, Rose JS, Bennett WM. Severe mixed metabolic acidosis secondary to rhabdomyolysis. Am J Med 67: 905–908, 1979.

37. Meroney WH, Herndon RF. The management of acute renal insufficiency. JAMA 155: 877–883, 1954.

38. Pietrek J, Kokot F, Kuska J. Serum 25-hydroxyvitamin D and parathyroid hormone, in patients with acute renal failure. Kidney Int 13: 178–185, 1978.

39. Massry SG, Arieff AI, Coburn JW, Palmieri G, Kleeman CR. Divalent ion metabolism in patients with acute renal failure: Studies on the mechanism of hypocalcemia. Kidney Int 5: 437–445, 1974.

40. Meroney WH, Arney GK, Segar WE, Balch HH. The acute calcification of traumatized muscle, with particular reference to acute posttraumatic renal insufficiency. J Clin Invest 36: 825–832, 1956.

41. Akmal M, Goldstein DA, Telfer N, Wilkinson E, Massry SG. Resolution of muscle calcification in rhabdomyolysis and acute renal failure. Ann Intern Med 89: 928–930, 1978.

42. Vanhille P, Raviart B, Tacquet A, Jovet JP, Huart JJ, Bauters F, Goudemand M. Insuffisance rénale aiguë par hyperphosphatémie majeure an cours de leucémies aiguës lymphoblastiques. Nouv Presse Med 8: 3977–3979, 1979.

43. Kaplan BS, Hebert D, Morrell RE. Acute renal failure induced by hyperphosphatemia in acute lymphoblastic leukemia. Can Med Ass J 124: 429–431, 1981.

44. Feinstein EI, Akmal M, Goldstein DA, Telfer N, Massry SG. Hypercalcemia and acute widespread calcification during the oliguric phase of acute renal failure due to rhabdomyolysis. Mineral Electrolyte Metab 2: 193–200, 1979.

45. Zabetakis PM, Singh R, Michelis MF, Murdaugh HV. Acute renal failure. Bone immobilization as cause of hypercalcemia. NY State J Med 79: 1887–1891, 1979.

46. Pasternack A, Wahlberg P. Bone marrow in acute renal failure. Acta Med Scand 181: 505–511, 1967.

47. Diamond JR, Yoburn DC. Nonoliguric acute renal failure. Arch Intern Med 142: 1882–1898, 1982.

48. Vertel RM, Knochel JP. Nonoliguric acute renal failure. JAMA 200: 598–602, 1967.

49. Danovitch G, Carvounis C, Wlinstein E, Levenson S. Nonoliguric acute renal failure. Isr J Med Sci 15: 5–8, 1979.

50. Counahan R, Cameron JS, Ogg CS, Spurgeon P, Williams DG, Winder E, Chantler C. Presentation, management, complications, and outcome of acute renal failure in childhood: Five years' experience. Brit Med J 1: 599–602, 1977.

51. Hilberman M, Myers BD, Carrie BJ, Derby G, Jamison RL, Stinson EB. Acute renal failure following cardiac surgery. J Thorac Cardiovasc Surg 77: 880–888, 1979.

52. Schrier RW, Gardenswartz MH, Burke TJ. Acute renal failure: Pathogenesis, diagnosis and treatment. Adv Nephrol 10: 213–240, 1981.

53. Miller PD, Krebs RA, Neal BJ, McIntyre DO. Polyuric prerenal failure. Arch Intern Med 140: 907–909, 1980.

54. Hong CD, Kapoor BS, First MR, Pollak VE, Alexander JW. Fractional excretion of sodium after renal transplantation. Kidney Int 16: 167–178, 1979.

8. RENAL BIOPSY IN ACUTE RENAL FAILURE: ITS INDICATIONS AND USEFULNESS

Olivier Kourilsky,

Liliane Morel-Maroger,

Gabriel Richet

Acute tubular necrosis (ATN) is the most common form of ARF. Less often, ARF results from arterial, glomerular, or interstitial lesions. These forms of ARF may regress, but may also lead to chronic renal failure (CRF). Progression to CRF may sometimes be prevented by appropriate therapeutic measures, especially if they are undertaken early, for often the lesions only become irreversible later in the course of the illness. These treatments are potentially expensive and hazardous. Thus, they must rely on precise and early identification of the anatomical lesions, their mechanism, and their cause. The situation may be highly complex since the same etiology can produce different forms of ARF, each of which requires its own treatment. In order to guide the therapy and in the absence of the usual contraindications (which are often temporary), early renal biopsy should be considered in ARF whenever the diagnosis of ATN appears doubtful and/or the etiology equivocal.

1 Distribution of the Lesions Displayed by Renal Biopsy in ARF

It is difficult to state precisely the respective frequencies of the renal lesions responsible for ARF because of differences in patient popula-tions and sometimes in the diagnostic attitude in the numerous intensive care units and nephrological centers. Approximately, ATN accounts for 80% of ARFs, acute glomerulonephritis for 5 to 10%, acute vascular nephritis for 5 to 10%, acute interstitial nephritis for 3 to 5%, with wide variations from one center to another. Renal biopsy is therefore performed in a limited number of cases. Even in Hôpital Tenon, where the diagnostic attitude may be considered as active, only 178 (20%) of the 889 patients treated by dialysis for ARF between 1966 and 1980 underwent a renal biopsy [1]. The distribution of lesions is shown in Table 8–1. The distribution observed by Bonomini et al. [2] was different, but they performed renal biopsy in 65% of 317 patients with ARF; in particular, the incidence of ATN was 61.5%.

2 Contribution of Renal Biopsy to the Etiological Diagnosis of ARF

2.1 ATN

The contribution of renal biopsy is obvious in this group since it represents nearly one-third of the biopsied patients in our series. In 25 cases, biopsy was performed either because of lack of precise etiology or protracted renal failure. In 29 other cases, the clinical diagnosis had been toxic or immunotoxic interstitial nephritis (10 cases), vascular nephritis (1 case),

V.E. Andreucci (ed.), ACUTE RENAL FAILURE.

All rights reserved. Copyright © 1984.

Martinus Nijhoff Publishing. Boston/The Hague/

Dordrecht/Lancaster.

TABLE 8-1. Distribution of renal lesions in 178 patients with ARF biopsied at Hôpital Tenon between 1966 and 1980

Condition	No./% patients
Acute tubular necrosis (ATN) (54; 30%)	
Pure	29 (16%)
With interstitial reaction	25 (14%)
Acute vascular nephritis (45; 25%)	
Thrombotic microangiopathy (TMA)	25 (14%)
Malignant nephroangiosclerosis (NAS)	17 (9%)
TMA or NAS	3 (9%)
Acute glomerulonephritis (46; 26%)	
Extracapillary glomerulonephritis[b]	26 (24%)
Membranoproliferative glomerulonephritis	3
Endocapillary glomerulonephritis[c]	9
Focal and segmental glomerulonephritis[d]	5
Others[e]	3
Acute interstitial nephritis (16; 9%)	
With polymorphs	8
With round cells	7
Necrotic tuberculosis	1
Cortical necrosis (5; 3%)	
Myeloma kidney (8; 4)	
Miscellaneous[f] (4)	

[a]Three had previously unknown glomerulonephritis.
[b]Ten with linear IgG deposition in glomerular basement membranes, 7 with polyarteritis nodosa, 1 with Wegener granulomatosis, 2 with polymorphs in the interstitium.
[c]Three with cryoglobulinemia.
[d]Four with polymorphs in the interstitium.
[e]Two unclassified glomerulonephritis (one with mesangial IgA deposition), and one amyloidosis associated with acute tubule-interstitial lesions.
[f]Including two with massive neoplastic cell infiltration.

or glomerulonephritis (18 cases). In the latter group, atypical renal signs (proteinuria >2 g/day, macroscopic or microscopic hematuria, hypertension), and, in certain cases, extrarenal symptoms suggestive of systemic disease had been noted. Besides their practical importance (see section 3), these findings demonstrate the (rare) possibility of atypical forms of ATN that can be recognized only by renal biopsy.

2.2 ACUTE VASCULAR NEPHRITIS
Acute vascular nephritis is nearly always diagnosed clinically. In our experience, serious complications of renal biopsy occurred only in this group, despite previous arteriography when necrotizing angiitis was suspected: extensive perirenal hematoma in four patients, lead-

ing to partial or total nephrectomy in three. This should weigh heavily against biopsy in such patients.

2.3 ACUTE GLOMERULONEPHRITIS
Acute glomerulonephritis is most often recognized clinically. On the other hand, in our series, renal biopsy confirmed the diagnosis in only 43 of the 75 patients considered as having glomerulonephritis on clinical grounds. Furthermore, the precise histological pattern, which affects both prognosis and therapy, cannot be anticipated. Renal biopsy is therefore highly justified in patients with ARF and with symptoms suggestive of glomerular disease.

2.4 ACUTE INTERSTITIAL NEPHRITIS (AIN)
The clinical diagnosis is very difficult (see chapter 2, section 16). Only 9 of our 16 patients with AIN were recognized clinically. Only 7 of our 18 patients clinically diagnosed as AIN had interstitial lesions on the renal biopsy. Moreover, the biopsy allows the identification of the cellular infiltrate: polymorphonuclear leucocytes with microabscesses suggesting infectious interstitial nephritis, or mononuclear cells (lymphocytes, plasma cells, eosinophils) suggesting immunotoxic interstitial nephritis. Therapeutic implications are opposite (see section 3).

2.5 OTHER LESIONS
Cortical necrosis is rare. The diagnosis was confirmed by renal biopsy in only 2 of 18 patients in our series. ARF may be the presenting feature in some patients with multiple myeloma [3]; histological evaluation in patients with multiple myeloma and ARF is useful for prognosis and therapy since lesions different from myeloma kidney, such as ATN, may be encountered. Massive infiltration of the kidney by neoplastic cells can be recognized in certain patients with lymphomas [4].

3 Contribution of Renal Biopsy to Prognosis and Treatment of ARF
In our series, the results of renal biopsy influenced our therapeutic attitude in the great majority of cases [1]. In some cases, an appropri-

ate therapy was started or continued; in others, useless and potentially harmful therapy was withdrawn or discarded. Furthermore, renal biopsy was helpful to establish a prognosis.

The histological recognition of ATN leads to the immediate exclusion of any treatment other than symptomatic.

Despite the high incidence (9%) of severe complications of renal biopsy in patients with acute vascular nephritis [1], this investigation may be considered when the patient is seen early, in order to appreciate the extent of proliferative endarteritic lesions [5].

In acute glomerulonephritis, appropriate treatment can be given according to the histological pattern displayed by renal biopsy. Drugs are withheld in the presence of pure endocapillary or advanced extracapillary glomerulonephritis with sclerosis. Extracapillary glomerulonephritis with fresh cellular crescents is not a homogenous group. It may be associated with either arterial lesions, such as those found in polyarteritis nodosa and Wegener's granulomatosis, or with deposits in the mesangium and polymorphonuclear cells in the interstitium suggesting an infectious cause, or not associated with any particular histological or clinical pattern. Each of these cases requires different and sometimes opposite therapeutic measures. Membranoproliferative and focal and segmental glomerulonephritis are frequently associated with mesangial C3 deposits and related to infection [6].

In AIN, the identification of the cellular infiltrate may lead to many decisions, that are frequently opposite: administration of antibiotics and elimination of the source of infection in acute pyelonephritis (either hematogenic or resulting from urinary tract obstruction); withdrawal of the responsible drug in immunotoxic interstitial nephritis (see chapter 2, section 16).

Thus, renal biopsy may be considered as a guide in the treatment of certain cases of "medical" acute renal failure. This is particularly illustrated by ARF associated with acute infection. Septicemia, for example, may lead to ATN from shock, to glomerular ischemia or necrosis from angiitis, to glomerulonephritis with complement and sometimes immunoglob-

TABLE 8–2. Results of renal biopsy in 56 patients with acute infection and ARF seen in Hôpital Tenon between 1966 and 1980

Condition	No. of patients
Acute tubular necrosis (septicemia, 18; pulmonary infection, 5)	23
Acute vascular nephropathy (septicemia)	2
Acute glomerulonephritis Extracapillary, 5 Membranoproliferative, 3 Endocapillary, 3 Focal and segmental, 3 Miscellaneous, 3 (Septicemia, 9; pulmonary infection, 5; nasopharyngeal infection, 3)	17
Acute interstitial nephritis With polymorphonuclear cells, 7 With round cells, 3 With ruberculous granulomata, 1 (Septicemia 8: with urinary infection, 5; pulmonary infection, 2; tuberculosis, 1)	11
Cortical necrosis (Septicemia, 1; pulmonary infection, 1)	2
Myeloma kidney (Pulmonary infection)	1

ulin deposits, or even to pyelonephritis. Acute immunotoxic interstitial nephritis may be induced in such circumstances by antibiotics. The diversity of lesions clearly appears in our series of 56 patients with an acute infection and ARF (table 8–2). Each form requires its own treatment.

4 Conclusion

The mortality rate of ARF is still high, more than 50% in a recent study [7]. "Medical" ARFs are at least as frequent as "surgical" ARFs, and their mortality rate is hardly lower. Furthermore, 9.9% of the survivors have chronic renal failure, which requires dialysis in nearly half of them. That is, 30 to 40 new patients require a maintenance hemodialysis in France every year after a ARF.

According to these considerations, effective medical management should take into account the following points: (a) when there is doubt over the diagnosis of ATN, patients with ARF should immediately be transferred to a specialized renal unit; (b) this unit should be located in a hospital having the necessary facilities for dealing with extrarenal complications, which may dominate the immediate and short-term prognosis; (c) the unit should have an easy access to all immunological, toxicological, and histopathological examinations and to any other necessary complementary procedures. These facilities are indispensable in identifying the exact type of ARF. The most rewarding investigation in "parenchymatous" ARF is early renal biopsy. This should not be done routinely because it carries a risk; on the other hand, any delay in taking the biopsy diminishes the therapeutic potential. Biopsy should be considered every time the diagnosis of ATN is doubtful for one or more of the following reasons: progressive ARF; equivocal case history (absence of cause or multiple possible etiology); atypical renal signs (hematuria, abundant proteinuria, hypertension, edema); extrarenal manifestations suggestive of systemic disease (prolonged fever; arthralgia; inflammatory edema; lesions of the skin, lung, and endocardium; etc.); prolonged renal failure. The contraindications (hemorrhagic syndrome, hypertension) can be controlled and hence are most often temporary. The decision to biopsy permits the possibility of early pathogenetic treatment, which is alone capable of reducing mortality and the incidence of subsequent chronic renal failure.

References

1. Duhoux P, Kourilsky O, Kanfer A, Sraer JD, Morel-Maroger L, Richet G. Les insuffisances rénales aiguës nécessitant un traitement étiopathogénique. Utilité de la biopsie rénale précoce. In Séminaires d'Uro-Néphrologie, la Pitié-Salpêtriére: 7e série, Küss R, Legrain M (eds). Paris: Masson, 1981, pp. 226–240.
2. Bonomini V, Baldrati L, Scolari MP, Stefoni S, Vangelista A. Acute renal failure: 10 years experience. In Acute Renal Failure, Eliahou HE (ed). London: John Libbey, 1982, pp. 149–151.
3. Border WA, Cohen AH. Renal biopsy diagnosis of clinically silent multiple myeloma. Ann Intern Med 93: 43–46, 1980.
4. Kanfer A, Vandewalle A, Morel-Maroger L, Feintuch MJ, Sraer JD, Roland J. Acute renal insufficiency due to lymphomatous infiltration of the kidney. Cancer 38: 2588–2592, 1976.
5. Morel-Maroger L, Kanfer A, Solez K, Sraer JD, Richet G. Prognostic importance of vascular lesions in acute renal failure with microangiopathic hemolytic anemia (hemolytic-uremic syndrome). Clinicopathologic study in 20 adults. Kidney Int 15: 548–558, 1079.
6. Beaufils M, Morel-Maroger L, Sraer JD, Kanfer A, Kourilsky O, Richet G. Acute renal failure of glomerular origin during visceral abscesses. N Engl J Med 295: 185–189, 1976.
7. Chapman A. Etiologie et pronostic actuel de l'insuffisance rénal aliguë en France. Résultats d'une çanquête. In L'insuffisance Rénal Aiguë Monographie de la Société de Réanimation de Langue Française. Paris, L'Expansion, 1978, pp. 37–54.

9. RENAL RADIOLOGY AND ACUTE RENAL FAILURE

Vittorio E. Andreucci,

Antonio Dal Canton,

Alfredo Capuano,

Vittorio Iaccarino,

Luigi Cirillo

1 Excretion Urography or Intravenous Pyelography (IVP)

Patients with ARF require early diagnosis of the type of ARF and of the exclusion of surgically correctable causes such as renal artery occlusion or urinary tract obstruction.

For a long time, radiocontrast urographic agents have been used only to opacify the hollow structures of the urinary tract—i.e., calyces, pelves, and ureters—and the terms *urography* and *intravenous pyelography* (IVP) testify to the initial aim of this radiographic procedure [1]. It is today commonly accepted that high-dose IVP and renal arteriography provide very useful information on gross structural or functional alterations of the kidneys through the different patterns of the "nephrogram."

1.1 NORMAL UROGRAPHIC NEPHROGRAM
The nephrogram represents the radiographic shadow of the renal parenchyma opacified by radiocontrast media. Fast i.v. injection of a contrast agent is followed, within a minute or so, by visualization of the peripheral renal cortex, which is more densely opacified than the medulla. Despite the considerable blood vol-

ume of the kidney, it is the concentrated contrast material within the tubules that is mostly responsible for the radiographic density of the nephrogram. A volume of glomerular ultrafiltrate (containing the contrast) equal to the plasma volume of the kidney is, in fact, formed in less than half a minute after the i.v. injection of the contrast [1]; then, as the filtrate enters the proximal convoluted tubules, the unreabsorbable contrast is greatly concentrated by the isosmotic tubular reabsorption, making the very dense radiographic image of the renal cortex. As the filtrate then enters the loop of Henle and collecting tubules, the corticomedullary distinction is obliterated. The normal nephrogram begins to fade 30 minutes after contrast injection; sometimes a faint nephrogram may be seen at six hours or even later [2]. The pyelogram reaches its maximal density usually 10 minutes after contrast injection.

Thus, during IVP there is no "vascular phase"; the time in which the amount of contrast material in the vascular bed is greater than in the tubules is so short that a "vascular phase" cannot be detected.

Other factors in addition to the tubular concentration of the contrast material may influence the density of the nephrogram: the shape of the kidney (density varies with the thickness of the renal parenchyma), the amount of overlying tissue (a large amount will decrease density), and the kV and the mA of the x-ray beam (which are inversely related with the density of the nephrogram) [1]. All these factors should be taken into consideration in evaluating the nephrogram.

Acute hypotension may occur after the injection of contrast media with a fall in GFR and severe oliguria: lower tubular flow rate causes an early dense nephrogram [3]. This will readily disappear with the correction of hypotension and re-establishment of urine output.

1.2 UROGRAPHIC NEPHROGRAM IN ARF
By studying the density/time pattern of the urographic nephrogram in ARF, we may differentiate the different forms of ARF [4], as shown in table 9–1.

1.2.1 Urographic Nephrogram in ATN An immediate, persistent nephrogram, the density of which is high and does not change during the whole radiographic study (i.e., up to 24 hours) has been reported as typical of ATN, occurring with an incidence of 86% [2] or 61% [5] according to different groups. This nephrographic pattern is observed both in the oliguric phase (figure 9–1) and in the early diuretic (recovery) phase of ATN [2] (figure 9–2). A pyelogram is usually observed in those patients with urine output greater than one liter daily

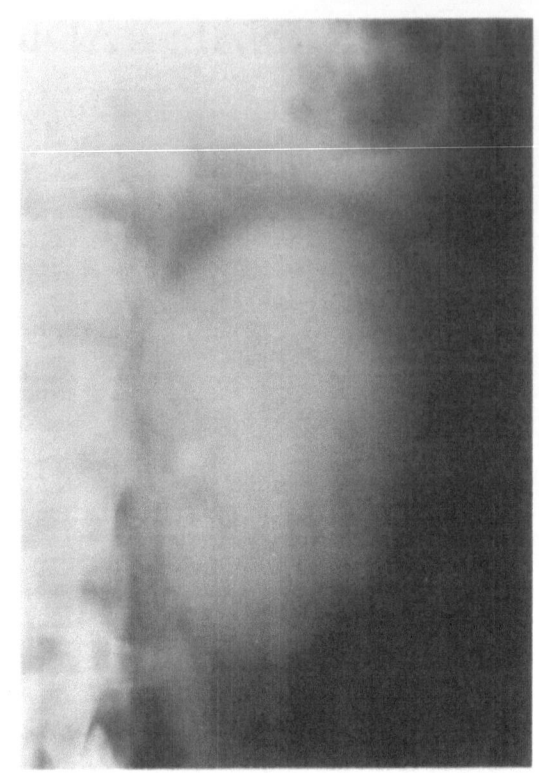

FIGURE 9–1. Nephrotomogram in the oliguric phase of a patient with ATN. A faint pyelogram is observed.

TABLE 9–1. Patterns of urographic nephrogram in ARF

DENSE PERSISTENT NEPHROGRAM
    Rapid onset
        ATN (uncomplicated)
        Acute oliguric pyelonephritis
    Slow onset
        Postrenal ARF
        ATN in pre-existing renal disease
        Systemic hypotension
        Partial acute occlusion of the renal artery
        Renal vein thrombosis
        Acute glomerulonephritis

ABSENT NEPHROGRAM
    Complete acute occlusion of renal artery
    Complete acute obstruction of the urinary tract (some time after the occlusion)
    ATN (rarely)

FAINT NONHOMOGENOUS NEPHROGRAM
    Acute (bilateral) cortical necrosis (ACN)

(figure 9–2); in oliguric patients, no pyelogram or only a very faint pyelogram is more frequent [2] (figure 9–1).

This radiographic pattern suggests that glomerular filtration is preserved so that the radiocontrast medium is filtered by glomeruli and enters the proximal convoluted tubules. The excessive density of the nephrogram has been attributed to an increase in "permeability" of the damaged tubular wall to radiocontrast medium so that the volume of distribution of the contrast agent is increased [3].

Another less frequent nephrographic pattern, the incidence of which may vary from 14% [2] to 27% [5], is that of a nephrogram of low density at onset that becomes increasingly dense over the next 24 hours. This pattern seems to occur in ATN patients with severe pre-existing renal disease [2]. It suggests a reduced renal cortical perfusion leading to severely reduced (but not abolished) glomerular

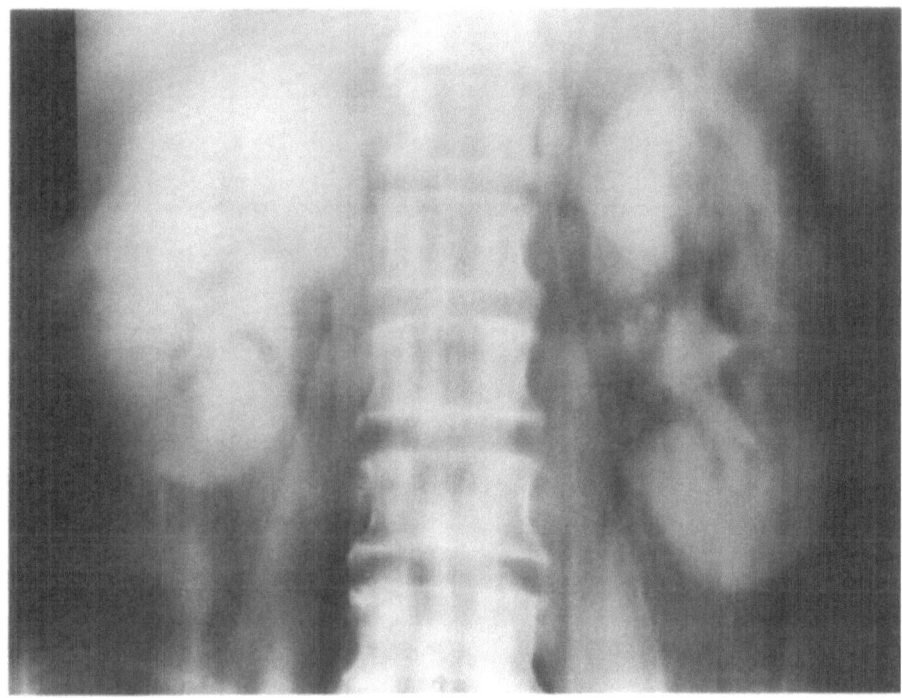

FIGURE 9–2. Intravenous pyelography with nephrotomography in the early diuretic (recovery) phase of ATN.

filtration, similar to the findings of systemic hypotension or intratubular obstruction [1]. Because of the reduced GFR, the contrast medium enters the tubules more slowly; this accounts for the early low density of the nephrogram. Since the flow rate of tubular fluid along the nephron is reduced, however, proximal tubular reabsorption is increased, leading to an increasing density of the nephrogram with time. The persistence of the renal shadow is due to the markedly reduced urine output; the filtration rate of the contrast agent, in fact, exceeds the rate at which the agent is excreted with urine [3].

Only a few patients with ATN (12% incidence in the quoted series) [5] exhibit a very poor or no appreciable nephrogram [5]. In these patients there is no glomerular filtration.

The occurrence of a dense nephrogram on IVP in patients with oliguric ARF following abdominal aortic surgery (e.g., for repair of an aortic aneurysm) permits the differentiation of ATN from renal artery occlusion [5].

1.2.2 Urographic Nephrogram in Acute Oliguric Pyelonephritis An immediate, persistent (up to 24 hours) nephrogram with unchanged density with time (similar to the typical nephrogram of ATN) is observed in severe oliguric pyelonephritis [2].

1.2.3 Urographic Nephrogram in Acute Glomerulonephritis In ARF due to acute glomerulonephritis, a faint nephrogram at onset that gradually became more dense over the next 24 hours with no pyelogram has been reported [2].

1.2.4 Urographic Nephrogram in Acute (Bilateral) Cortical Necrosis (ACN) It has long been believed that the IVP was of no value in patients with ACN. In recent years, however, the use of high-dose IVP with tomography has been shown to be of value for an early diagnosis of ACN [6–8]. The resulting nephrogram has been reported as similar in appearance, even though diminished in extent, to the angiographic pattern (see below): faint opacification of the central portion as well as the margin of each kidney, with a nonopacified zone of the cortex in between [8]. A similar nephrogram

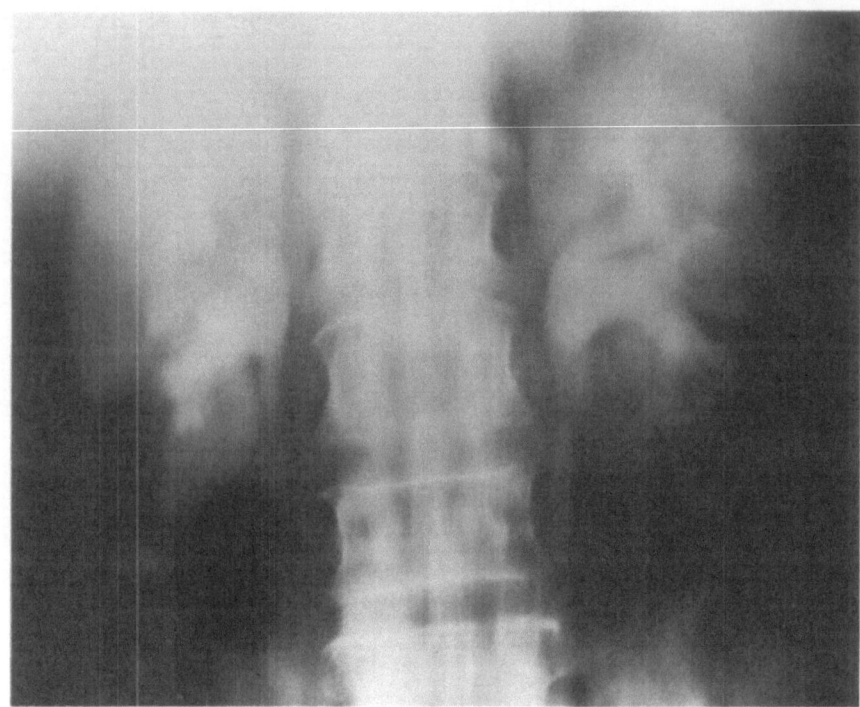

FIGURE 9–3. Intravenous pyelography with nephrotomography in a patient with postrenal ARF. Twenty-four hours after radiocontrast injection, the nephrograms have become very dense. Pyelograms outline dilated calyces and pelves.

may be seen only after an incomplete embolic obstruction of the renal artery; in this case, however, the lesion is usually unilateral while ACN affects both kidneys, albeit not to the same extent [8].

The opacification of the viable renal parenchyma in ACN may be due partly to filtered contrast in the tubular lumen of the remnant nephrons that are still functioning, in cases in which the disease is patchy; but it may be also due to the whole body opacification effect, particularly in those cases with more extensive necrosis [8].

Undoubtedly, the demonstration of bilateral renal cortical "tramline" calcification of abdominal film tomograms will clearly confirm a provisional diagnosis of ACN that is suspected on the basis of the clinical picture. But this radiographic appearance is limited to a minority of patients [9, 10] and occurs quite late, i.e., not earlier than four weeks after the onset of ARF [8].

1.2.5 Urographic Nephrogram in Postrenal ARF
An abnormally long-lasting urographic nephrogram is typically observed in postrenal ARF:

the nephrogram is slow to develop but becomes increasingly dense, even more dense than normal, over a period of time (up to 24 hours) [1, 4] (Figure 9–3). In this condition of obstruction of the urinary tract, glomerular filtration is maintained while tubular flow is greatly reduced or even stopped; the tubular reabsorption of filtrate greatly concentrates nonreabsorbable solutes, including contrast agents, so that a dense, late (24 hours) nephrogram will be observed, which might be associated in nonanuric patients with a normal early pyelogram [3]. The striations sometimes observed radiating from the medulla toward the renal margin represent the collecting tubules (the so-called medullary rays) filled with concentrated radiopaque material [1].

The obstructive situation will be confirmed by the pyelogram (figure 9–3) outlining the dilated calyces, pelves, and ureters; if the early pyelogram is of feeble density, late 24-hour

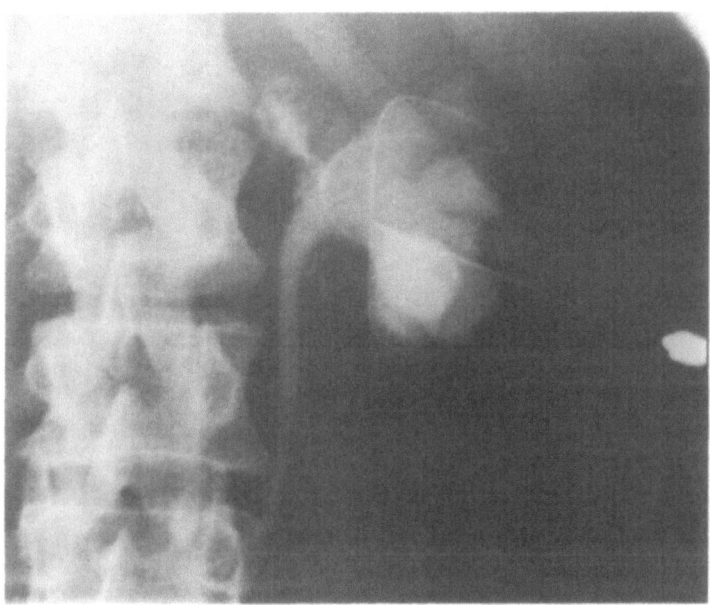

FIGURE 9–4. Antegrade percutaneous pyelography in a patient with postrenal ARF. The dilated pelvis of the left kidney was punctured with a fine-gauge Chiba needle and radiocontrast injected through the needle. (A percutaneous pyelostomy tube was then inserted.)

tomograms may emphasize the radiographic density [5]. In the presence of a dense nephrogram, the pelvicalyceal system should be outlined at some stage, at least partially; otherwise, obstruction can be ruled out [11] (See also chapter 19.)

1.3 SUGGESTIONS FOR IVP IN ARF

a. Prerenal ARF should be excluded before deciding to carry out an IVP. In patients with severe salt and water retention (usually oliguric overhydrated patients), dialysis should be performed prior to IVP. In nonoliguric patients with severe uremia for whom dialysis is indicated, IVP is better deferred until uremia has been controlled [12], not only to improve the general condition of the patients but also to obtain better results from the IVP. The osmotic diuresis associated with uremia (which is reduced by dialysis), in fact, greatly contributes to impairing urine concentration and, consequently, radiographic density, as demonstrated in patients with CRF [13].

b. Fluid restriction should be avoided prior to IVP. Since it is a routine procedure to keep patients with normal renal function deprived of fluids, specific instructions should be given to the nursing staff to avoid fluid restriction.

c. Control plain radiograph of the abdomen and plain film tomography may be helpful prior to IVP for defining site, size, and shape of the kidneys; for detecting nephrocalcinosis or small renal stones; and for comparing later nephrograms.

d. Rapid (over a period of a few minutes) i.v. injection of the contrast medium is preferred to continuous i.v. infusion for optimal nephrographic appearances.

e. The dosage of the contrast agent suggested in ARF is 2.2 ml/Kg b.w. of 45 to 50% diatrizoate. This corresponds to about 1g iodine/Kg b.w.

f. Radiographs should be taken immediately after the radiocontrast injection, and then at 5, 10, 30, and 60 minutes. Late radiographs should be taken at 6 and 24 hours.

g. Early tomograms should be obtained soon after the injection. Tomography is an essential part of the whole radiographic procedure in ARF patients.

h. Films should be exposed at low kilovoltage

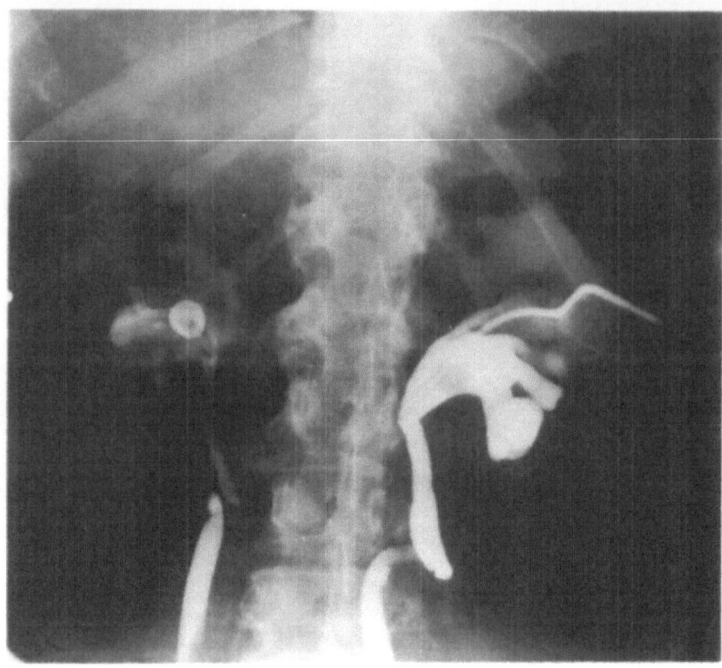

(60 to 70 kV usually in adults) [4] to maximize the minimal differences in nephrogram density.

FIGURE 9–5. Antegrade percutaneous pyelography in a
patient with postrenal ARF due to carcinoma of the bladder. Film was made after bilateral percutaneous pyelosto-
mies.

1.4 ANTEGRADE PERCUTANEOUS PYELOGRAPHY

Antegrade percutaneous pyelography may be
preferred to retrograde pyelography (see chapter
19) in unilateral nonvisualization of the ureter
on IVP and in oliguric ARF, when ultrasonography or computerized tomography has revealed dilated ureter(s) [14]. It is a safe procedure performed by percutaneous puncture of
the renal pelvis with a fine-gauge (22-gauge)
Chiba needle under ultrasound control (figure
9–4).

After puncturing, the pressure in the renal
pelvis may be measured first; the mean normal
value of this pressure is 0.98 kPa (10 cm H_2O)
and becomes elevated usually in the early stage
of complete obstruction and for much longer in
incomplete obstruction. Then, radiocontrast is
injected through the needle; the pelvis and the
ureter will be outlined down to the level of the
obstruction. In order to evaluate the degree of
obstruction, fluid may be injected into the pelvis, at different flow rates, measuring the intra-

pelvic pressure and evaluating radiologically
the degree of pelvic distension (normal unob-
structed ureters tolerate a flow of at least 10
ml/min without change in pressure and volume) [14].

In a case of complete obstruction, X-ray performed hours later will show persisting dense
pyelogram with distended pelvis [14]. A percutaneous pyelostomy tube may be inserted
(figure 9–5).

2 Renal Arteriography

Aortography or selective renal arteriography is
less frequently indicated in ARF. The main indication for renal arteriography is the suspicion
of complete or partial occlusion of the renal artery by embolization (in patients with a past
history of myocardial infarction, valvular disease, or atrial fibrillation) or thrombosis (in patients with vascular disease, which may affect
aorta and/or renal arteries). In these cases, the

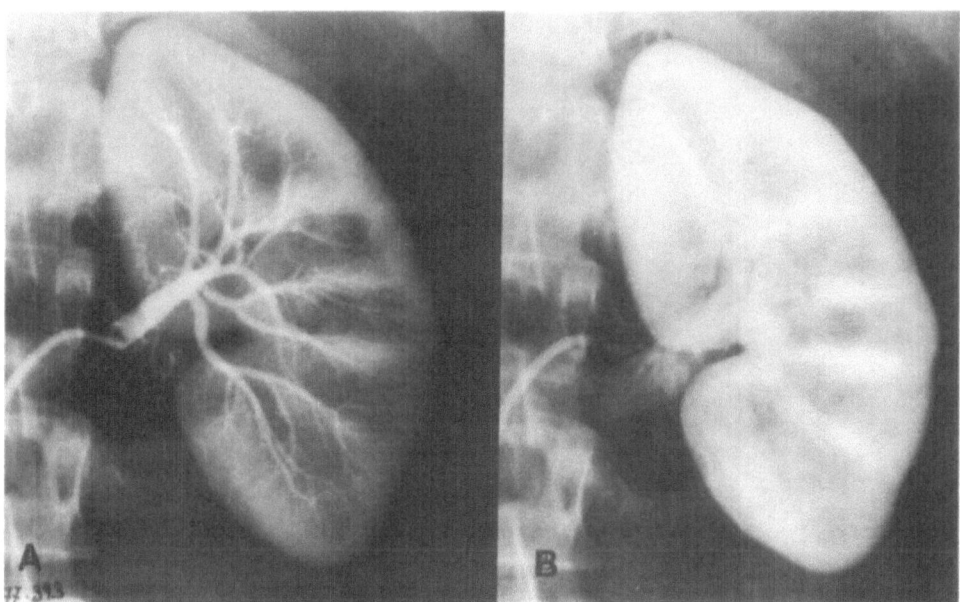

FIGURE 9–6. Selective renal arteriogram in a normal subject. A. Vascular phase: the whole tree of the kidney (including fifth-order vessels) is clearly visualized. B. Nephrogram: dense opacification of the renal cortex with a clear corticomedullary demarcation. Faint opacification of the renal vein is seen.

arterial occlusion is bilateral, unless the patient has only one functioning kidney.

Renal arteriography may also be useful in identifying small vascular aneurysms in patients with suspected polyarteritis nodosa and in making an early diagnosis of ACN (see below).

2.1 THE "VASCULAR PHASE" AND THE ARTERIOGRAPHIC NEPHROGRAM IN NORMAL SUBJECTS

After renal artery catheterization, a bolus injection of 6 to 8 ml of radiocontrast (e.g., Renografin 60%) is immediately followed by the "vascular phase" of the selective renal arteriography (figure 9–6A). In normal subjects, the whole arterial tree of the kidneys, including the vasculature distal to the arcuate and subarcuate arteries in the renal cortex ("fifth-order vessels") is clearly visualized [15].

The "capillary phase" is the moment when the contrast bolus reaches the glomeruli; part (20%) of the contrast material enters the tu-

bular lumen where it is concentrated by tubular reabsorption (generating the arteriographic nephrogram) (figure 9–6 B) and then excreted; the remnant moves in the postglomerular peritubular capillaries, enters the cortical and medullary interstitium, and then diffuses back into the capillary blood, finally leaving the kidney through the renal vein. Thus, the rapid decrease in density of the arteriographic nephrogram is accounted for by the removal of radiocontrast material both by urinary excretion and by blood flow [1].

Actually, the nephrographic phase of renal or aortic arteriography (but not of IVP) has a biphasic behavior, which has been attributed to biphasic changes in RBF: an early renal shadow appears in a few seconds following radiocontrast injection (in association with the acute peak blood concentration of the contrast agent) and then rapidly subsides; within a few minutes a dense renal shadow is formed, which represents the normal nephrogram [3].

2.2 THE "VASCULAR PHASE" AND THE ARTERIOGRAPHIC NEPHROGRAM IN ARF

2.2.1 ATN In oliguric patients with post-ischemic or nephrotoxic ARF, the "fifth-order vessels" cannot be visualized on selective renal

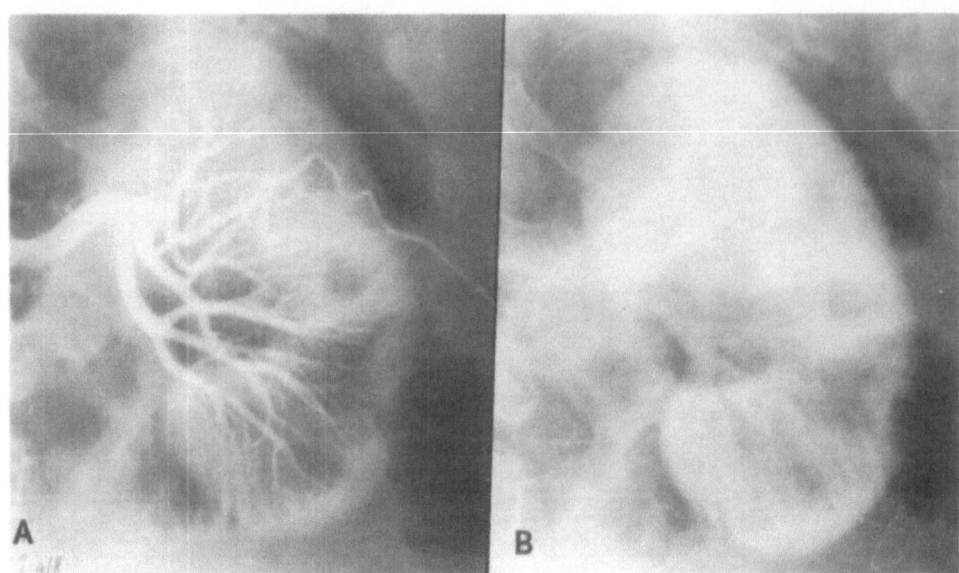

arteriography [15, 16] (figure 9–7A). Furthermore, arcuate vessels ("fourth-order vessels") constantly, and interlobar vessels very frequently (in 80% of the cases), exhibit a distinct reduction in caliber and a rapid, regular tapering attenuation [15, 16] (figure 9–8A). Sometimes, stretching and straightening of renal vessels is observed and is attributed to edema of the kidney [15].

A reduced density of the arteriographic nephrogram is quite typical, particularly in the cortical portion of the kidney (figure 9–8B) with the consequent obliteration of corticomedullary demarcation [15, 16] (figures 9–7B and 9–8B). Transit time of contrast medium through the kidney is greatly prolonged [15].

The whole arteriographic pattern has been attributed to a homogeneous reduction in renal cortical blood flow. When, in fact, epinephrine was injected intra-arterially in man in doses adequate to cause diffuse renal vasoconstriction, a homogenous reduction in renal cortical perfusion was observed on renal arteriography, which appeared to mimic the arteriographic pattern of ARF [15]. The reduced cortical perfusion reduces the glomerular filtration of contrast material, accounting for the faint arteriographic nephrogram.

During recovery of renal function, ARF patients exhibit a patchy and then diffuse reappearance of vessels beyond the arcuate and subarcuate arteries in the renal cortex while the arteriographic nephrogram gradually recovers the increased density of the cortical zone.

2.2.2   Acute (Bilateral) Cortical Necrosis (ACN)
At an early stage of ACN, a typical radiographic pattern is obtained during renal arteriography [9, 10, 17]: delayed and incomplete filling of interlobular arteries with poor arborization; complete filling of capsular arteries; early venous filling; poor (patchy or even absent) opacification of renal cortex during the nephrographic phase (the extent of opacification being inversely proportional to the severity of the cortical necrosis) in contrast to the clear opacification of the renal margin (since subcapsular cortex is supplied by capsular arteries) and medulla (since the blood supplied by renal arteries is shunted to the medulla in the juxtaglomerular region) [8–10, 17] (figure 17–1).

3.   Digital Subtraction Angiography (DSA)

In recent years much attention has been given to the improvement of angiographic procedures.

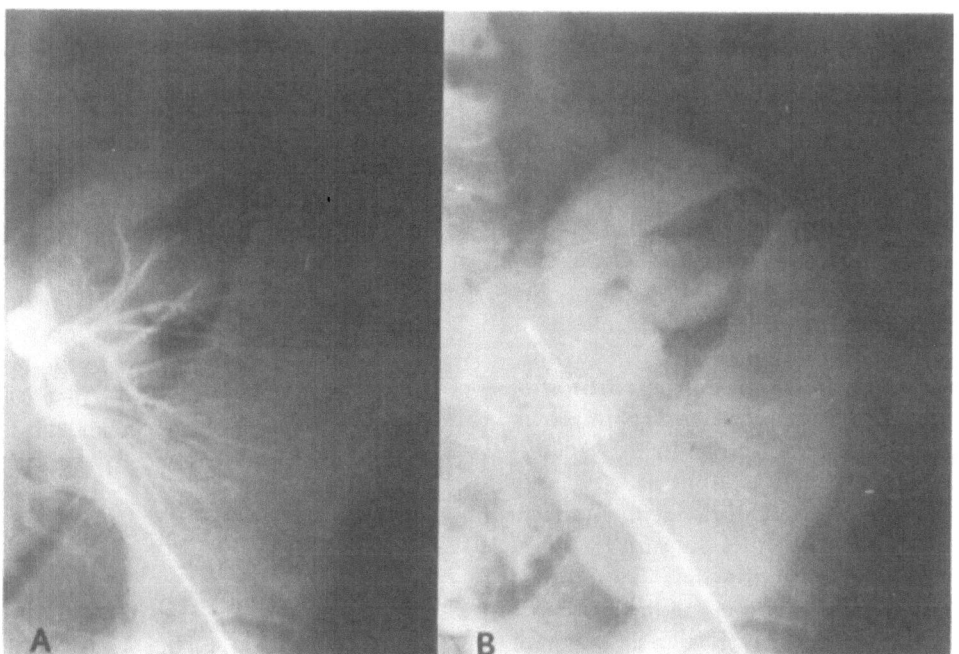

FIGURE 9–8. Selective renal arteriogram in oliguric transplanted kidney with ATN. A. Vascular phase: reduction in caliber and rapid, regular tapering attenuation of interlobar vessels; fourth- and fifth-order vessels cannot be visualized. B. Nephrogram: reduced density of the nephrogram with obliteration of corticomedullary demarcation.

Digital subtraction angiography (DSA) is a new computer-assisted technique that integrates digital data collection and computer processing in order to produce a medical image [18]. The basic principles of this technique may be summarized as follows. The televised fluoroscopic images are converted into digital data. The baseline image, obtained before arrival of contrast material, is digitally subtracted from the succeeding contrast image; hence, the contrast-filled structures are made free of the background and therefore visible, particularly after the enhancement of the final image. Subtraction and enhancement are performed in real time, i.e., rapidly enough for clinical examination [18].

DSA permits direct visualization of heart and blood vessels following i.v. injection of a small quantity of contrast. Thus, as little as 40 ml of meglumine ioxithalamate (Telebrix 38) injected i.v. (into the basilic vein of the arm) at a rate of 12 ml/sec has been shown to clearly

visualize a subtotal occlusion with a poststenotic dilatation of the renal artery; good correlation was then observed between DSA and the conventional angiography, which was performed just before the transluminal angioplasty [19]. Similarly, excellent diagnostic information may be obtained by this technique in other arterial districts.

For the evaluation of renal circulatory abnormalities by DSA, it has been suggested that 45 ml of 76% meglumine or sodium diatrizoate should be injected i.v. by mechanical injector at a rate of 30 ml per second [20]. The technique is very simple and may be carried out as an outpatient procedure.

Recently DSA with intra-arterial injection of contrast has been suggested in order to further reduce the dosage of contrast material [21]. Thus, while a concentration of 380 to 760 mg I/ml (diatrizoate meglumine) is commonly used for i.v. injection, 200 to 270 mg I/ml are employed for intra-arterial injection of 4 to 30 ml of diatrizoate meglumine at a rate of 2 to 15 ml/sec (a greater volume with reduced concentration is preferable for assuring adequate mixing) [21].

This technique will therefore reduce the risk of radiocontrast nephrotoxocity; it has another great advantage over conventional angiography, that of reducing the time required for its completion, with less discomfort for the patient.

4 Gray-Scale Ultrasonography (Echography)

Ultrasonic echography is an excellent, noninvasive procedure for visualizing kidneys and upper urinary tracts of patients with renal failure. It is also commonly used in ARF, mainly in postrenal ARF, for detecting obstruction of the urinary tract. With the recent improvement in gray-scale resolution and the availability of newer ultrasound equipment, not only strong echoes due to well-defined interfaces (e.g., hilar fat, renal capsule) but also low-level echoes of renal parenchyma may be recorded [22]. Thus, a skilled imaging technologist with serial sonograms may recognize different pathological conditions of renal parenchyma. This technique has become, therefore, particularly important in ARF, when radiocontrast procedures are not indicated (i.e., in patients at risk) or when IVP with tomography has failed to visualize the kidneys [23].

4.1 NORMAL RENAL ULTRASONOGRAM (ECHOGRAM)

The normal kidney appears as an elliptical, ring-shaped structure in longitudinal cross-sectional sonograms; in transverse sonograms, it appears more rounded. Dense echoes surrounding the kidney are due to the renal capsule; the central echo complex is primarily due to the renal sinus fat and, secondarily, to blood vessels, collecting system, and connective tissues. Between renal capsule and central echo complex, the renal parenchyma may be differentiated in cortical and medullary regions. The triangular areas of low echogenicity, with the bases oriented toward the renal capsule, are due to the medullary pyramids. The region of these sonolucent triangles is surrounded by a more echogenic cortex; the cortical echoes are numerous and homogenous, but less intense than the central echo complex. Strong echoes at the corticomedullary junction are due to arcuate arteries [22, 24].

4.2 RENAL SONOGRAM DURING OBSTRUCTION OF THE URINARY TRACT

During obstruction of the urinary tract, echo-free areas due to dilated urine-filled calyces and/or pelvis (ultrasound transmission is, in fact, improved in fluid-filled structures) are surrounded by echoes in the central part of the nephrosonogram; sometimes the urine-filled dilated renal pelvis may appear as a large echo-free area in the sonogram displacing the central echo complex [25]. Should the obstruction of the urinary tract be due to (radio-opaque or nonradio-opaque) renal calculi, they can be detected in the sonogram as echogenic foci with typical acoustic shadows obscuring deeper structures [25].

4.3 RENAL SONOGRAM IN ATN

Experimental [26] and clinical [26, 27] studies have demonstrated no changes in the nephrosonogram during ATN; this contrasts with definite sonographic findings observed during acute rejection in a transplanted kidney (see below). Thus, when ARF occurs in transplanted patients, if the sonogram does not show any change from the baseline sonogram, this negative finding points in favor of ATN [24].

4.4 RENAL SONOGRAM DURING ACUTE REJECTION IN TRANSPLANTED KIDNEY

Experimental and clinical studies in transplanted kidneys have demonstrated a series of sonographic features occurring during acute rejection: increase in renal volume, increased echogenicity of the renal cortex, enlargement of medullary pyramids, loss of the distinct corticomedullary boundary, decrease in the amplitude of the central echo complex. At least two of these features should be present for the diagnosis of acute rejection [27] (figure 9–9). The first sonographic change is enlargement of the medulla [24]; but this finding alone may be misleading since it is also observed in normal kidneys made diuretic by water load or furosemide administration (medullary pyramids have regained normal size 24 hours after furosemide) [27]. Obviously, since serial sonograms are necessary, the sonographic pattern depends on reproducibility of scans, which relies on the skills of the operator, on the stabil-

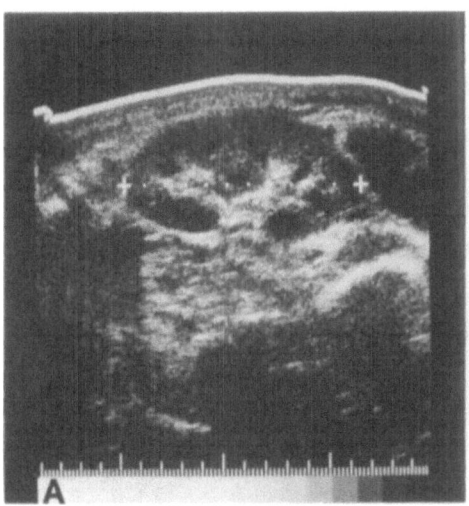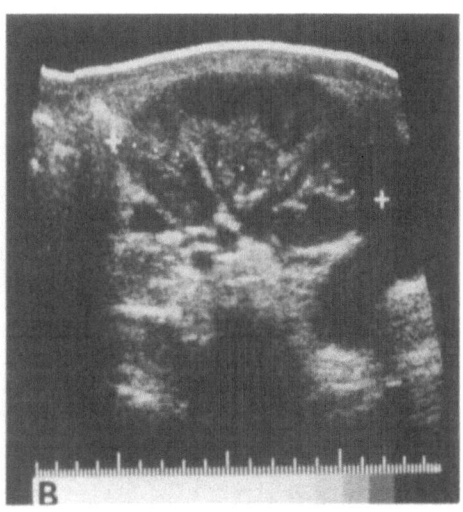

FIGURE 9–9. Renal sonogram of a patient with cadaveric renal allograft. A. Baseline longitudinal scan, showing a normal-appearing kidney. B. Longitudinal scan four weeks later during acute rejection, showing increase in renal volume, enlargement of medullary pyramids, and decrease in the amplitude of the central echo complex. (Courtesy of Dr. G. Tunisi, Second Radiology Service, Hospital of Brescia.)

ity of ultrasound instrument, and on the quality of photographic equipment [22].

4.5 RENAL SONOGRAM IN ACUTE RENAL VEIN THROMBOSIS

Experimental studies in dogs have demonstrated, after acute occlusion of one renal vein, a series of sonographic features: enlargement of the kidney, increased cortical thickness, sparsely distributed cortical echoes, indistinct corticomedullary boundary, anechoid areas in the renal parenchyma (due to hemorrhage), displacement of central echo complex, dilatation of the renal vein, and, later, renal rupture [28]. Should these sonographic findings be obtained in patients in whom renal vein thrombosis is clinically suspected, an IVP is indicated with injection of the contrast medium in the femoral vein in order to visualize the vena cava and, possibly, the renal veins [28].

5 Computerized Axial Tomography (CT)

Computerized axial tomography (CT) scanning is a useful diagnostic tool not only for evaluat-

ing a renal mass, but also for revealing the causa of nonfunctioning kidneys. It is a noninvasive, accurate, easy, and rapid procedure, independent of renal function (it may be performed in severe renal failure) and free of complication (when radiocontrast medium is not used); it is also operator- and patient-independent and a reproducible technique [22, 29]. The main disadvantages are the high cost of the equipment and exposure to ionizing radiations.

CT scanning is usually performed in the supine position, with scans obtained at 1 to 2 cm intervals; thus, at least 5 scans at 2-cm intervals are necessary for covering the whole length of the kidney.

5.1 COMPUTERIZED TOMOGRAPHY IN NORMAL KIDNEYS

The CT scan provides excellent transverse cross-sectional images of the kidneys, similar to those obtained by ultrasonography but with better resolving capability [29]. CT has a high-density resolution, allowing characterization of different tissues by their x-ray attenuation values [22]. Thus, renal parenchyma, with a relatively homogenous density, is clearly outlined by perinephric fat; it has a round shape, which becomes oval at the hilus where the vascular pedicle is clearly defined. Calyces and pelves are seen as water-density structures in patients with renal sinus and perinephric fat [29].

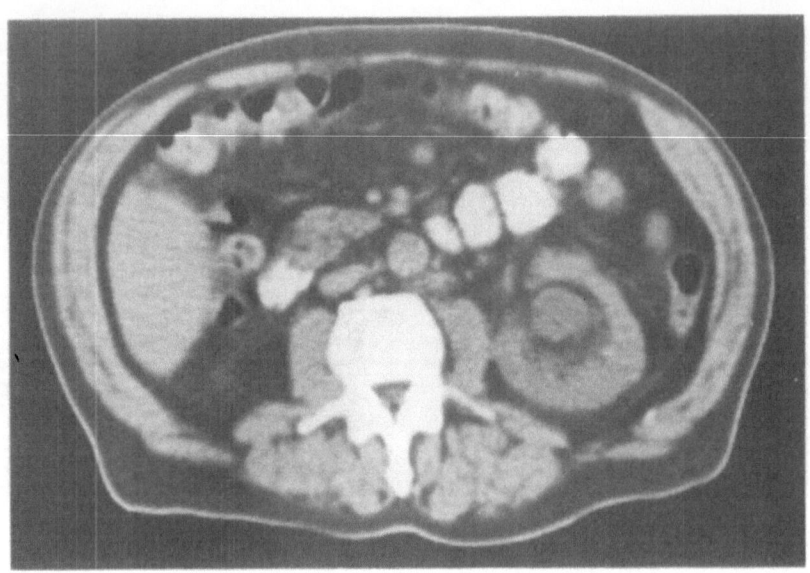

FIGURE 9–10. Postrenal ARF in a patient with a single (left) kidney. The CT scan shows an area of low attenuation within the renal shadow. An additional scan, at 1.5 cm interval, demonstrated a renal stone in the pyelocalyceal system (see figure 19–2).

Additional scans may be performed after i.v. injection of a water-soluble urographic contrast medium, such as sodium iothalamate (a bolus of 50 ml of Conray 400®, with 400 mg I/ml), which enhances visualization of the collecting systems [29]. Following i.v. injection of a contrast, the attenuation value will rise in the renal parenchyma and much more in the collecting system, allowing a sharp definition of calyces and pelves [29].

Sequential fast scanning permits differentiation between cortex and medulla. If scanning is performed during the injection of radiocontrast, the enhanced cortex is well differentiated from radiolucent pyramids not yet containing contrast; scans performed later do not permit this differentiation [22].

5.2 COMPUTERIZED TOMOGRAPHY IN ARF
CT scanning performed 24 hours after IVP in patients with oliguric ARF has been reported to reveal a persistent dense nephrogram in acute glomerulonephritis or leukemia [30].

But, undoubtedly, CT scanning is a very useful procedure to diagnose urinary tract obstruction.

5.2.1 *CT in Postrenal ARF* In an early stage of obstruction, the intrarenal part of the urinary tract may be seen, on CT scans, as areas

of low attenuation within a normal or enlarged renal shadow [22, 29, 30] (figure 9–10). In a later stage, a more severe dilatation of urine-filled pyelocalyceal system with parenchymal atrophy leads to an oval renal shape in which a thin-walled sac of water-density fluid will replace the renal parenchyma [29] (figure 9–11). A dilated ureter is commonly identified on CT scans, even without contrast, as an area of low attenuation; the level of the obstruction can be determined by serial scans [30].

In renal failure, the lesion is bilateral; it may be unilateral if there is a single kidney (figure 9–10).

CT scanning may also demonstrate the cause of obstruction. Thus, even nonradio-opaque obstructing stones of uric acid nonvisible on plain film tomograms may be easily identified on CT scans even without contrast (figure 19–2). Aortic aneurysm, retroperitoneal fibrosis, and malignancies may be seen easily on CT scanning as responsible for obstruction.

5.2.2 *CT in Transplanted Kidney* A decrease in allograft volume may be observed on CT scans, indicating chronic rejection, while a

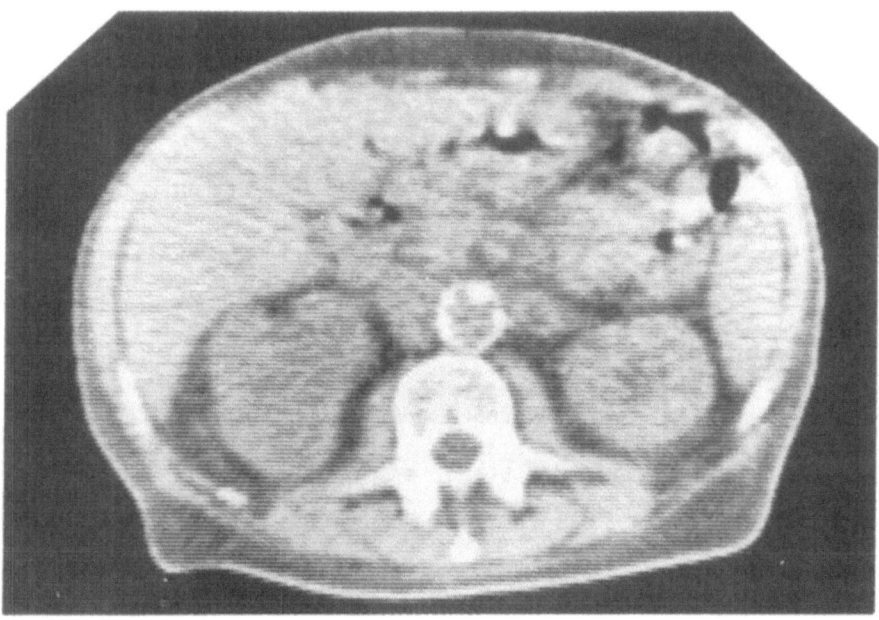

FIGURE 9–11. P.C., a 70-year-old male patient became anuric following therapy with gentamicin because of unexplained fever. The right kidney was not visible on intravenous pyelography. The CT scan demonstrated an irregular shape of the right kidney with a thin-walled sac of water-density fluid replacing the renal parenchyma.

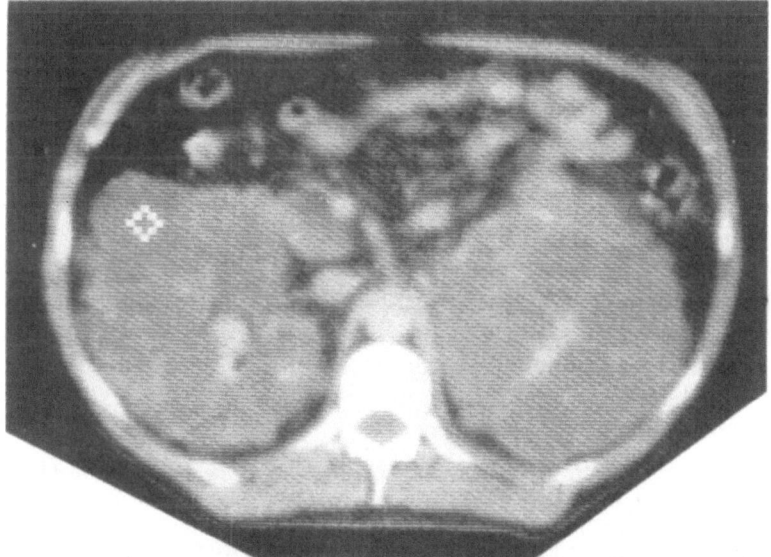

FIGURE 9–12. Postcontrast scan in polycystic kidney disease. The kidneys are enlarged with characteristic lobulated contour; the image is made by innumerable cysts of varying size, filled with water-density fluid. The collecting system is poorly defined because of reduced renal function.

218

sudden, marked increase in volume of the transplanted kidney suggests an acute rejection [29]. But CT scanning also permits the differentiation of acute rejection from other causes of ARF following transplantation; thus, hydronephrosis by ureteral obstruction, perirenal collection of blood, or urine or pus or lymphoceles may be easily identified [29].

5.3 COMPUTERIZED TOMOGRAPHY IN POLYCYSTIC KIDNEY DISEASE

Frequently, but not constantly, polycystic kidney disease is diagnosed by IVP and by renal ultrasonography. Sometimes, only CT scanning may identify this bilateral disease. The kidneys, on CT scans, appear enlarged with a characteristic lobulated contour; the image is made by innumerable cysts of varying size, filled with water-density fluid (figure 9–12). Postcontrast scans show an increased attenuation value of the remnant parenchyma and, in patients with renal failure, a poorly defined collecting system (figure 9–12).

6 Renography

Renography allows the evaluation of the arrival, uptake, and excretion of a radionuclide (usually orthoiodohippurate I^{131}, Hippuran) injected i.v. The normal renogram shows three phases. The first, the vascular phase, is the rapid rise of the curve following the i.v. injection and represents the radioactivity in blood, kidney, and other tissues under the probe. The second, the secretory phase, is the less steep rise of the curve and is due to renal handling of hippuran. The third, the excretory phase, is the descending portion of the curve depending mainly on the excretion of the radionuclide. In the opinion of some authors, renography may be useful in ARF for diagnosing acute urinary tract obstruction (post-renal ARF). If radioactivity does not leave the pelvis, in fact, the third excretory phase is no longer observed or markedly delayed [22]. It has been stated that renography is most effective for diagnosing postrenal ARF when performed within 48 hours of the onset of obstruction.

In the opinion of other authors, however, renography is a very limited usefulness in ARF because a marked delay in the excretory phase may be observed even in ATN [31].

References

1. Newhouse JH, Pfister RC. The nephrogram. Radiol Clin North Am 17: 213–226, 1979.
2. Cattell WR, McIntosh CS, Moseley F, Fry IK. Excretion urography in acute renal failure. Brit Med J 1: 275–278, 1973.
3. Mudge GH. Nephrotoxicity of urographic radiocontrast drugs. Kidney Int 18: 540–552, 1980.
4. Fry IK, Cattell WR. Radiology in the diagnosis of renal failure. Brit Med Bull 27: 148–152, 1971.
5. Sherwood T, Doyle FH, Boulton-Jones M, Joekes AM, Peters DK, Sissons P. The intravenous urogram in acute renal failure. Brit J Radiol 47: 368–372, 1974.
6. Joffre F, Durand D, Sablayrolles JL, Teisseire R, Putois J, Suc JM. Interet de l'urographie intraveineuse an cours des nécroses corticales rénales. Ann Radiol 19: 555–557, 1976.
7. Davidson AJ. Radiologic Diagnosis of Renal Parenchymal Disease. Philadelphia: WB Saunders, 1977.
8. Bowley NB. Renal opacification during intravenous urography in acute cortical necrosis (The nephrogram in cortical necrosis). Brit J Radiol 54: 524–526, 1981.
9. Deutsch V, Franke O, Drory Y, Eliahou H, Braf Z. Bilateral renal cortical necrosis with survival through the acute phase with a note on the value of selective nephroangiography. Am J Med 50: 828–834, 1971.
10. Kleinknecht D, Grunfeld J, Gomez PC, Moreau J, Garcia-Torres R. Diagnostic procedures and long-term prognosis in bilateral renal cortical necrosis. Kidney Int 4: 390–400, 1973.
11. Cattell WR. Acute renal failure. In Recent Advances in Renal Disease, Jones NF (ed). Edinburgh: Churchill Livingstone, 1975, pp. 1–47.
12. Brown CB, Glancy JJ, Fry IK, Cattell WR. High-dose excretion urography in oliguric renal failure. Lancet II: 952–955, 1970.
13. Matalon R, Eisinger RP. Successful intravenous pyelography in advanced uremia; visualization in the post-dialytic state. N Engl J Med 282: 835–837, 1970.
14. Hare WSC, McOmish D. Skinny needle pyelography: An advance in uroradiology. Med J Australia, 2: 123–125, 1981.
15. Hollenberg NK, Epstein M, Rosen SM, Basch RI, Oken DE, Merrill JP. Acute oliguric renal failure in man: Evidence for preferential renal cortical ischemia. Medicine 47: 455–474, 1968.
16. Hollenberg NK, Adams DF, Oken DE, Abrams HL, Merrill JP. Acute renal failure due to nephrotoxins: Renal hemodynamic and angiographic studies in man. N Engl J Med 282: 1329–1334, 1970.

17. Tuttle RJ, Minielly JA. The angiographic diagnosis of acute hemorrhagic renal cortical necrosis. Radiology 126: 637–638, 1978.
18. Harrington DP, Boxt LM, Murray PD. Digital subtraction angiography—Overview of technical principles. Am J Roentg 139: 781–786, 1982.
19. Ludwig JW, Verhoeven LHJ, Engels PHC. Digital video subtraction angiography (DVSA) equipment. Angiographic technique in comparison with conventional angiography in different vascular areas. Brit J Radiol 55: 545–553, 1982.
20. Hillman BJ, Ovitt TW, Capp MP, Fisher HD, Frost MM, Nudelman S. Renal digital subtraction angiography: 100 cases. Radiology 145: 643–646, 1982.
21. Crummy AB, Stieghorst MF, Turski PA, Strother CM, Lieberman RP, Sackett JF, Turnipseed WD, Detmer DE, Mistretta CA. Digital subtraction angiography: Current status and use of intra-arterial injection. Radiology 145: 303–397, 1982.
22. Barbaric ZL, Tanasescu DE, Zerhouni EA, Sanders RC. Contribution of uroradiology to the diagnosis and management of kidney disease. In Current Nephrology, Gonick HC (ed). Boston: Houghton Mifflin, 1980, vol 4, pp. 384–456.
23. Sanders RC. The place of diagnostic ultrasound in the examination of kidneys not seen on excretory urography. J Urol 114: 813–821, 1975.
24. Hricak H, Toledo-Perreyra LH, Eyler WR, Madrazo BL. Role of ultrasound in renal transplantation: A review of clinical and experimental observations. Dial Transpl 8: 818–821, 1979.
25. Andreucci VE. Chronic renal failure. In The Treatment of Renal Failure, Castro JE (ed). Lancaster: MTP Press, 1982, pp. 33–167.
26. Hricak H, Toledo-Perreyra LH, Eyler WR, Madrazo BL, Sy GS. Evaluation of acute post-transplant renal failure by ultrasound. Radiology 133: 443–447, 1979.
27. Hricak H, Cruz C, Eyler WR, Madrazo BL, Romanski R, Sandler MA. Acute post-transplant renal failure: Differential diagnosis by ultrasound. Radiology 139: 441–449, 1981.
28. Hricak H, Sandler MA, Madrazo BL, Eyler WR, Sy GS. Sonographic manifestations of acute renal vein thrombosis: An experimental study. Invest Radiol 16: 30–35, 1981.
29. Sagel SS, Stanley RJ, Levitt RG, Geisse G. Computed tomography of the kidney. Radiology 124: 359–370, 1977.
30. McClennan BL. Current approaches to the azotemic patient. Radiol Clin North Am 27: 197–211, 1979.
31. Mayo ME, Hilton PJ, Jones NF, Lloyd-Davies RW, Croft DN. [131]I hippuran renogram in acute renal failure. Brit Med J, 3: 516–517, 1971.

10. NONOLIGURIC ACUTE RENAL FAILURE

Joel A. Gordon,

Robert W. Schrier

1 Introduction

Acute renal failure (ARF) is defined as an abrupt cessation of glomerular filtration accompanied by a corresponding rise of the nitrogenous waste products, blood urea nitrogen (BUN), and creatinine [1]. Traditionally, ARF has been heralded by progressively diminishing urine output, rarely to the point of cessation of urine output (anuria), but frequently to the point of oliguria, which is arbitrarily defined as less than 400 milliliters of urine output per 24 hours [2].

The concept of nonoliguric ARF—that is, a declining glomerular filtration rate in the face of maintained or even enhanced urine output—has been rarely recognized until recently. Indeed, early reviews dealing with ARF barely mention the existence of ARF without oliguria or anuria [3, 4]. In fact, it was not until the 1960s that the entity of nonoliguric ARF was even recognized as a distant clinical entity [5, 6].

In recent years, there has been an increase in the recognition and incidence of nonoliguric forms of ARF [7, 8, 9, 10]. As noted in a recent study from our institution by Anderson and Schrier, nonoliguric forms of ARF comprised 33% of all cases seen in consultation for a rising BUN and creatinine [7].

What accounts for this dramatic rise in the recognition of nonoliguric forms of ARF? Indeed, does this dramatic rise in incidence truly reflect an increasing incidence of this variety of ARF, or have we failed to recognize this form of ARF in the past? Certainly, the modern usage of automated biochemical screening devices has made serial monitoring of plasma and serum BUN and creatinine values in patients easy and convenient for the practicing physician. In addition, the increase in usage of potent nephrotoxic aminoglycoside antibiotics, as well as potent chemotherapeutic agents such as cis-diammine dichloroplatinum, have contributed to the increasing incidence of nonoliguric forms of ARF. However, we feel that for the large part, this variety of ARF has been primarily unrecognized in the past and that more awareness of this clinical entity has contributed largely to its increased incidence.

ARF, either oliguric or nonoliguric, may present as a wide spectrum of disease. For example, the urinary volume, severity of azotemia, acidosis, and hyperkalemia may reflect the severity of the insult(s). Furthermore, various therapeutic maneuvers advocated now and in the past have been designed to "convert" oliguric to nonoliguric forms of ARF, for reasons that will be discussed later.

Moreover, ARF may occur in two phases, an oliguric phase, of variable duration and severity, followed by a polyuric or diuretic phase, which also may be of variable duration and severity. Thus, depending on when the patient is first seen, it may be difficult to classify ARF as either purely oliguric or purely nonoliguric.

V.E. Andreucci (ed.), ACUTE RENAL FAILURE.
All rights reserved. Copyright © 1984.
Martinus Nijhoff Publishing, Boston/The Hague/
Dordrecht/Lancaster.

TABLE 10-1. Etiologies of nonoliguric
acute renal failure

I. Trauma
   A. Blunt
   B. Open
   C. Head injury
   D. Burns
II. Surgery—Elective and Emergency
   A. Orthopedic
   B. Urologic
   C. Abdominal
   D. Cardiac
III. Pigment
   A. Hemoglobin
   B. Myoglobin
IV. Toxins
   A. Anesthetic agents—Methoxyflurane
   B. Radiocontrast agents
   C. Antineoplastic agents—Cis
      Disamminedichloroplatinum
   D. Antibiotic agents—Aminoglycosides and others
V. Miscellaneous
   A. Sepsis
   B. Hyperuricemia
   C. Hypercalcemia

2 Etiology

There are numerous etiologies of nonoliguric forms of ARF (table 10-1). Furthermore, each of the particular etiologies may produce either oliguric or nonoliguric forms of ARF, depending on the particular circumstance under which the insult occurs.

One of the earliest recognized causes of "high-output" ARF was traumatic injury [6, 11]. As early as 1955, Teschan et al. [11], in their review of renal insufficiency in military casualties, recognized the nonoliguric form of ARF in patients suffering from a variety of injuries sustained during combat. In fact, they pointed out that "renal insufficiency without oliguria probably occurred much more frequently than indicated here, but with absent or undiscovered oliguria and without obvious clinical uremia, such patients passed through the regular chain of evacuation." [11].

In 1964, Baxter et al. [6] reviewed the clinical course of nine patients who had high-output (nonoliguric) ARF in a civilian population suffering from both blunt and open trauma. This review emphasized the under recognition

of this variety of ARF and indicated that management of acidosis and fluid and electrolyte balance were much easier in this type of ARF as opposed to the more classical variety of oliguric ARF.

The occurrence of ARF following head trauma has been recognized for some time. In the mid-1950s, Taylor and associates [12, 13] were able to recognize that renal failure following head trauma may be either oliguric or nonoliguric, depending on the circumstances under which the trauma occurred as well as the extent of the accompanying injury.

Thermal injuries are another well-recognized cause of nonoliguric ARF. In 1956, Sevitt [14] extensively reviewed thermal injury and ARF. Of the 21 patients with extensive burns and ARF, all were considered to have the nonoliguric variety of ARF. Vertel and Knochel [5] reported nonoliguric ARF in 11 patients at the U.S. Army Surgical Research Unit. Ten of the eleven patients were victims of extensive burns, and all had nonoliguric ARF.

In addition to the traumatic causes stated above, a variety of elective and nonelective surgical procedures have been found to induce a nonoliguric form of ARF (table 10-1). In 1966, Baxter and Maynard [15] recognized that in both nontraumatic emergency surgery (usually a perforated viscus) as well as in elective surgery (abdominal), nonoliguric ARF can develop. Subsequently, other authors also noted the occurrence of high-output ARF following elective surgical procedures [16, 17].

In addition to elective orthopedic, urologic, and abdominal operations, nonoliguric ARF has been described with a surprisingly high frequency following elective cardiac surgery. Both Bhat et al. [18] and Hilberman et al. [19] found a greater than 50% incidence of nonoliguric ARF in all patients developing renal insufficiency following cardiac surgery. Furthermore, both investigators found an alarmingly high incidence of mortality (greater than 50%) in these patients with this variety of nonoliguric renal failure, a substantially higher figure than has been traditionally seen in the nonoliguric form of ARF [8]. This most likely reflects the severity of the underlying cardiac disease in these patients. Those patients whose cardiac function deteriorates after surgery are the most likely to develop ARF and fail to survive.

Pigment-induced ARF, either from hemoglobin or myoglobin, has been traditionally associated with oliguric ARF. However, nonoliguric ARF can also result from these pigment insults.

In what is probably the first clinical description of nonoliguric ARF, Shen et al. [20] described the renal complications of hemoglobinuria suffered by patients injured in the famous Coconut Grove disaster of 1942. Although the majority of the fourteen patients described by Shen had oliguria, four patients were able to re-establish urine output despite evidence of progressive azotemia. Rhabdomyolysis, accompanied by myoglobinuria, is a well-organized cause of ARF [21]. Although traditionally considered an oliguric cause of ARF, recent reports of nontraumatic rhabdomyolysis reveal that as many as 20 or 25% of these cases of ARF are of the nonoliguric variety [22, 23].

Perhaps the largest single contributor to the increasing incidence of nonoliguric forms of ARF is that of toxin-induced renal failure. As stated previously, the reason for this is twofold. First, there has been a large increase in the usage of the aminoglycoside antibiotics and antineoplastic agents such as cis-diammine dichloroplatinum. Second, the increased awareness of the nephrotoxic potential of these agents has led to increased awareness of this entity by physicians.

Prior to the introduction of these above agents, the first toxin described to be responsible for inducing a nonoliguric form of ARF was the anesthetic agent methoxyflurane. In 1966, Crandell described 16 cases of nonoliguric ARF occurring in patients who underwent elective surgical procedures [24]. The common denominator in all of these patients was methoxyflurane anesthesia. Subsequent reports occurring almost simultaneously implicated methoxyflurane anesthesia as a cause of nonoliguric ARF [25].

However, after these initial reports in the mid-1960s, there has been little mention in the literature of methyoxyflurane anesthesia as a cause of nonoliguric ARF. The reason re-mains obscure. However, the increased usage of newer and less toxic anesthetic agents and the resultant decrease usage of methoxyflurane has been largely responsible for this decline.

Acute renal failure secondary to iodinated radiocontrast agents [26] is a well-recognized complication of these pharmaceuticals and is a particularly frequent event in patients with dysproteinemia, advanced diabetes mellitus, hypertension, and pre-existing renal insufficiency [27, 28]. Although traditionally felt to be of the oliguric variety, nonoliguric ARF has been described as occurring in approximately 10% of these patients [28]. This figure of 10%, however, may overestimate the true incidence of polyuric ARF secondary to contrast agents. This is because patients who are at risk for radiocontrast induced ARF are now aggressively treated prior to and following contrast administration with maneuvers designed to expand extracellular fluid volume and promote a diuresis (furosemide, saline, mannitol). Therefore, patients identified with nonoliguric ARF secondary to contrast administration may actually represent patients with oliguric ARF whose oliguria has been reversed by these maneuvers.

In the last 10 to 15 years, the large number of antineoplastic agents available for the treatment of leukemias as well as solid tumors has dramatically increased. One agent in particular, cis-diammine dichloroplatinum (DDP), has recently gained a great deal of popularity and achieved a great deal of success in treating a variety of solid tumors. It has been particularly successful when combined with bleomycin and vinblastine in the treatment of metastatic testicular carcinomas [29]. Although a variety of toxic side effects are associated with the use of DDP, the major side effect is its nephrotoxicity [30, 31].

Recently, work from our laboratory [32] as well as work done by Safirstein et al. [33] has further clarified the nephrotoxicity and nonoliguric state induced by DDP. An early central form of diabetes insipidus (DI) followed by a later nephrogenic form of DI explains, in part, the polyuria induced by DDP. Polydipsia also contributes to the polyuria seen. The concentrating defect found by both groups of investigators was characterized by a decrease in inner medullary solute concentration. This decrease was not found to be secondary to enhanced inner medullary plasma flow, which would serve to "wash out" solutes in the inner medulla. Rather, decreased delivery of solutes, primarily urea, was found to be of particular significance in explaining this decrease in inner medullary solute concentration.

The one category of nephrotoxic agents that has probably accounted for more nonoliguric ARF over the last 10 to 15 years than any other agent is the aminoglycoside antibiotics. This conclusion is supported in two recent reviews of nonoliguric ARF in which aminoglycosides account for the largest percentage of cases of nonoliguric renal failure [7, 10].

In addition to nonoliguric ARF, the aminoglycosides are a well recognized cause of the oliguric variety of ARF. However, aminoglycosides most often cause a mild, reversible, nonoliguric form of ARF [34, 35]. The increased recognition of the nephrotoxic potential of aminoglycosides, as well as well-established dosage guidelines for patients with underlying renal insufficiency, may lead to the eventual disappearance of the severe, oliguric variety of renal failure.

In addition to the aminoglycosides, the cephalosporins, either alone or in combination with the aminoglycosides, have been shown to induce nonoliguric ARF [36].

Finally, there have been a number of miscellaneous causes of nonoliguric ARF. Among these are sepsis and metabolic disorders such as hypercalcemia and hyperuricemia.

3 Pathophysiology

The exact pathophysiologic mechanisms responsible for both oliguric as well as nonoliguric ARF have not been entirely elucidated. In fact, over the last 20 years, the majority of the research has been devoted to discovering the mechanisms responsible for the oliguric form of ARF, with little attention paid to the milder, polyuric form.

As stated by Stein et al. in their excellent review of the pathophysiology of ARF: "Last, investigators should begin to evaluate models

that are characterized by a polyuric form of ARF. This area has been surprisingly neglected in the past." {37}. A number of studies performed over the last several years have attempted to elucidate the mechanisms responsible for this particular form of ARF. Some of these will be discussed below.

Our understanding of the pathophysiology of oliguric ARF has become quite sophisticated over the last 30 years. Vascular and tubular phenomena, as well as alterations in glomerular capillary permeability, have become focal points for the study and understanding of the pathogenesis of oliguric ARF {38}.

Are the same factors potentially responsible for the nonoliguric form of ARF? Furthermore, are there additional factors that are unique to this particular variety of renal failure? Finally, pathophysiologically, what determines whether a particular insult (toxic, ischemic) leads to oliguric or nonoliguric acute renal failure? These questions are not yet answered, but we will attempt to formulate a hypothesis on the pathophysiology of nonoliguric ARF.

In table 10–2 are listed the factors commonly believed to be responsible for (oliguric) ARF. We will examine each of these categories individually and discuss the role each may play in the pathophysiology of nonoliguric ARF. Finally, to conclude the discussion on pathophysiology, we will introduce the concept of "nephron heterogeneity" as being particularly important in the pathophysiology of this form of ARF.

Vascular phenomena have been recognized to be involved in the initiation of many forms of ARF. Indeed, the term *vasomotor nephropathy*

TABLE 10–2. Factors responsible for oliguric acute renal failure

---

I. Vascular Factors
   A. Decreased renal blood flow
   B. Increased renal vascular resistance
II. Glomerular Factors
   A. Decrease in ultrafiltration coefficient (K_f)
      i. Changes in effective capillary surface area
      ii. Changes in hydraulic conductivity
III. Tubular Factors
   A. Intratubular obstruction
   B. Passive backleak of filtrate

---

evolved from the suggestion that afferent arteriolar vasoconstriction accompanied by increased renal vascular resistance was primarily responsible for the oliguric state following both nephrotoxic and ischemic insults [39, 40]. It is clear, however, that normalization of renal blood flow does not reverse established ARF [37].

Nonoliguric ARF has been described following renal ischemia in both experimental animals and man [41–44]. In three recent clinical reports by Myers and Hilberman [19, 43, 44], a virtually 100% nonoliguric form of ARF was described following elective cardiac surgery. The pathogenetic factor common to all of these patients was a prolonged but temporary decrease in renal blood flow induced by poor cardiac performance. These investigators found, however, that in addition to the initiation of nonoliguric ARF by an ischemic insult, tubular "backleak" of glomerular filtrate appeared to be involved in the maintenance phase of the ARF (see below). In addition, these investigators postulated that the usage of "protective" agents, such as mannitol, furosemide, and dopamine may have attenuated the ischemic insult and potentially converted an oliguric form to a nonoliguric form of ARF. The mechanism(s) operating here to convert oliguric to nonoliguric acute renal failure postcardiac surgery, however, remains speculative. It may be that prevention of severe renal vasoconstriction and improvement of renal blood flow during the initiation phase, as well as enhancement of solute and water excretion and prevention of cellular swelling and tubular obstruction during the maintenance phase, may have facilitated this conversion.

In summary, based on both experimental and clinical studies, there is good evidence to support vascular factors as being pathophysiologically important in the initiation phase of nonoliguric ARF. However, as is the case with oliguric ARF, there is little evidence to support the role of reduced renal blood flow during the maintenance phase.

The glomerular factor that may be altered and account for the decrease in glomerular filtration rate characteristic of ARF is a change in the ultrafiltration coefficient (K_f). This decrease in K_f may be due to alterations in effective capillary surface area or alterations in hydraulic conductivity.

In two recent experimental models of ARF a fall in K_f has been demonstrated. Blantz [45], in a model of nephrotoxic ARF in the rat following uranyl nitrate administration, found a decrease in K_f that was similar to the decrease in K_f found by Bayliss et al. [46] in a model of nephrotoxic ARF following gentamicin administration. It is interesting to note that in both of these models of nephrotoxin-induced ARF, a comparable decrease in K_f occurred although polyuria was observed during the ARF. Thus, despite a declining GFR and K_f following these two insults, urine flow rate remained preserved.

From these studies, we conclude that while a decline in K_f may indeed be substantial enough to lower GFR, it may not be sufficient enough to diminish urine flow rate. On the other hand, a particular insult to the kidney significant enough to profoundly decrease K_f may lead to a more severe reduction in GFR and actually diminish urine flow rate. Thus, it may be that, depending on the severity of a particular insult, the degree of change in K_f and subsequent change in GFR may dictate whether oliguria or polyuria is present.

In addtion to glomerular and vascular factors, tubular factors have been felt for some time to be playing a substantial role in the pathophysiology of ARF. The two factors most often implicated in the pathogenesis of ARF are tubular backleak and intratubular obstruction. As early as 1942, Bywaters [47] suggested that tubular obstruction was the major pathogenetic factor responsible for the oliguria seen in ARF following crush injuries. Let us first examine the role of tubular obstruction in the pathogenesis of nonoliguric ARF.

From the experimental laboratory, we have learned that tubular obstruction may play a prominent role in some forms of ischemic and toxin-induced oliguric ARF [48, 49]. However, it is not known whether tubular obstruction may play a role in nonoliguric ARF. Partial tubular obstruction, whether from cellular necrosis or swelling, sloughing of debris, or cast formation, could be associated with polyuria if the volume of filtrate in the patient with nonoliguric ARF is relatively greater than in the patient with oliguric renal failure.

Relative amounts of tubular backleak could also be an important determinant of the ultimate urine volume seen in patients following a variety of ischemic or toxic insults. As alluded to earlier, Myers et al. [19, 43, 44], found "tubular backleak of filtrate" to be playing a substantial pathogenic role in their patients with ischemia-induced nonoliguric ARF following elective cardiac surgery. In spite of substantial "tubular backleak" found by these investigators, these patients were all nonoliguric, thereby suggesting that other renal mechanisms must be operating in patients with nonoliguric ARF to account for their maintenance of urine output in the presence of a fall in glomerular filtration rate. What are some of the factors that may be operating in the nonoliguric state? Table 10–3 summarizes these factors. We will now discuss each of these in some detail.

First a diminution in tubular handling of sodium may account for the preservation of urine flow in spite of a decrease in glomerular filtration rate. An ischemic or toxic insult may cause significant cellular injury and diminish normal sodium transport by tubular epithelium. For example, if a diminution in tubular reabsorption of sodium occurs in the proximal tubule and thick portion of the ascending limb of Henle, sodium delivery to the distal nephron may overwhelm distal tubular capacity in reclaiming the sodium; hence, a natriuresis would occur. This would be characterized by an elevated fractional excretion of sodium (FE_{Na}) as well as a renal failure index (RFI) of greater than 2, values typically found in both oliguric and nonoliguric ARF [50] (see chapter 7). Hence, clinical evidence exists that patients with both oliguric and nonoliguric ARF have a marked abnormality in tubular sodium reabsorption. However, it is not known whether this tubular defect is more severe in the nonoliguric state and hence contributes to the preservation of urine flow characteristic of this form of ARF.

Abnormalities in tubular water handling by damaged tubular epithelia may also contribute to the polyuria seen in nonoliguric ARF. Clinical observations in patients with nonoliguric ARF frequently reveal signs and symptoms of volume deletion. These patients frequently complain of being thirsty. Physical examination reveals orthostatic hypotension, tachycardia, dry mucous membranes, and tenting of the skin. Laboratory evidence reveals abnormalities in sodium and water conservation, including an inappropriately low urinary osmolality and a urine-plasma osmolality ratio of approximately 1, all indicative of a defect in renal concentrating ability. Studies have been carried out in several laboratories to identify the mechanisms responsible for this defect in urinary concentrating capacity. Indeed, studies from our own laboratory have confirmed a nephrogenic origin of the defect in water conservation in both an ischemic and nephrotoxic model of nonoliguric ARF {32, 41]. As alluded to earlier, a major defect in interstitial tonicity was found to contribute to the concentrating defect found in nonoliguric ARF induced by cisplatin {32, 33]. This decrease in interstitial tonicity was found to be primarily due to a decrease in solute reabsorption from the water impermeable portion of the distal nephron rather than to an increase in inner medullary plasma flow. Thus, defects in the tubular reabsorption of water may also contribute to the polyuria in the nonoliguric form of ARF.

Finally, and perhaps the newest and most intriguing hypothesis regarding the unique pathogenesis of nonoliguric ARF, is the concept of "nephron heterogeneity" in this form of renal insufficiency [51]. By changing the anesthetic agent used to induce ischemic ARF in experimental animals, Finn et al. [51] produced either an oliguric or nonoliguric form of ARF. What was most intriguing about these differences was the marked discrepancy in nephron populations between the oliguric and nonoliguric animals. In the animals with oli-

TABLE 10–3. Factors important in the nonoliguric form of acute renal failure

I. Altered tubular sodium reabsorption
II. Altered water transport and conservation
III. Nephron heterogeneity

guric renal failure, the kidneys were composed of a homogenous population of nephrons, all with tubular disarray and casts. In contrast, the kidneys from the animals with nonoliguric renal failure were composed of a heterogeneous population of nephrons. While two-thirds of the nephrons exhibited tubular damage and casts, approximately one-third of the nephrons were completely normal, with patent tubules, no casts, and brisk tubular fluid flow. This fascinating finding may be the biggest clue yet as to what is responsible for the polyuria in nonoliguric renal failure. Could it be that there is a subset of nephrons that are not damaged by an ischemic or toxic insult; these nephrons continue to maintain filtration and urine flow in nonoliguric renal failure? Further investigation into this intriguing hypothesis in the future should help answer this question.

In summary, many of the same mechanisms found to be important in oliguric ARF appear to be operating in nonoliguric ARF. It may be the nature, severity, and inherent conditions of a particular insult (toxic or ischemic) that dictate whether the oliguric or nonoliguric variety of ARF becomes clinically apparent.

4 Clinical Features of Nonoliguric Acute Renal Failure

Patients with ARF, whether oliguric or nonoliguric, require hospitalization not only for making the proper etiologic diagnosis but for initiating appropriate therapeutic measures. However, the clinical features encountered in these two groups of patients are generally quite different.

Patients with these two varieties of acute renal failure often have different presenting symptoms. This difference relates to little or no urine output versus normal or enhanced urine output. Patients with oliguric ARF are often hypertensive and tachypneic, with signs of volume overload, including rales and/or peripheral edema. Substantial weight gain has occurred during the illness.

The patient with nonoliguric renal failure may show signs of extra-cellular fluid volume depletion, including orthostatic hypotension, poor skin turgor, and dry mucous membranes.

TABLE 10–4. Biochemical abnormalities encountered in oliguric and nonoliguric acute renal failure

	Oliguric patients (n = 38)	Nonoliguric patients (n = 54)	p Value
Mean maximum BUN (mg/dl)	114 ± 5	95 ± 5	<0.02
Mean maximum serum creat (mg/dl)	9 ± 0.5	6 ± 0.3	<0.001
BUN/Cr >50/5 mg/dl (days)	18 ± 2	8 ± 0.8	<0.001
Metabolic acidosis	45%	20%	<0.025

Source: Adopted from Anderson RJ et al., Non-oliguric acute renal failure, NEJM 296: 1134, 1977, with permission.

Furthermore, when weights are known, weight loss is often discovered over the preceding few days. It should be emphasized, however, that excessive fluid intake can also lead to fluid overload in patients with nonoliguric ARF.

The severity of the renal failure encountered in these two groups of patients ultimately depends on the degree of impairment of the GFR as well as the degree of impairment of urinary flow. Based on these two assumptions, the physician would logically and correctly assume that patients with nonoliguric ARF have a milder degree of renal failure. Patients with nonoliguric renal failure have enhanced renal elimination of water, fewer electrolyte abnormalities, less accumulation of nitrogenous wastes, and milder metabolic acidosis [7–10]. A comparison of some of these biochemical abnormalities encountered in patients with these two forms of ARF is shown in table 10–4.

If patients with nonoliguric ARF have a milder degree of renal failure, it might be expected that they may also have significantly less morbidity and mortality. Indeed, patients with nonoliguric ARF require substantially fewer dialyses, experience fewer complications, and as a group, have a significantly lower mortality rate than those with oliguric ARF [52]. In table 10–5 are summarized some of these differences that are evident between these two groups of patients.

TABLE 10–5. Morbidity and mortality in oliguric and nonoliguric acute renal failure

	Oliguric patients (n = 38)	Nonoliguric patients (n = 54)	p Value
Hospitalization (days)	31 ± 3	22 ± 2	<0.01
Dialysis required (percentage)	84	28	<0.001
Complications (percentage) septicemia	42	20	<0.05
Gastrointestinal hemorrhage	39	19	<0.05
Neurologic abnormalities	50	30	<0.05
Mortality (percentage)	50	26	<0.05

Adapted from Anderson RJ et al., Non-oliguric Acute Renal Failure, NEJM 296: 1134, 1977, with permission.

5 Treatment

The therapy of ARF can be classified by treatment undertaken during the three phases of ARF: the initiation phase, the maintenance phase, and the recovery phase.

Treatment undertaken during the initiation phase primarily consists of maneuvers designed to enhance urine flow and simultaneously improve glomerular filtration rate. This is done because, as discussed earlier, there is evidence that the nonoliguric state in patients with ARF is accompanied by milder renal failure and significantly less morbidiy and mortality [7, 52]. Whether such conversion is associated with a similar lower mortality rate of patients as with spontaneous nonoliguric renal failure is not known.

The agents that have been primarily involved in this conversion from the oliguric to nonoliguric state include the potent "loop" diuretics, ethacrynic acid and furosemide, as well as the well-known polymeric sugar, mannitol [53]. Is there any evidence, based on controlled or uncontrolled clinical studies that these agents work, and, if so, does this conversion from oliguria to polyuria result in an improvement in morbidity and mortality?

First, there is some evidence that the administration of potent diuretic agents (furosemide) to patients with oliguric ARF leads to a sustained diuresis and lower mortality. Anderson et al. [7], in an uncontrolled study, found that

18 of 40 patients were converted by furosemide from an oliguric to a nonoliguric state. However, in a retrospective analysis, Minuth, Terrell, and Suki failed to demonstrate a predictable and beneficial response to parenteral furosemide in patients suffering from oliguric ARF [54]. In the only controlled trial to date examining the role of furosemide in oliguria, Kleinknecht [55] found that furosemide did not modify or change the oliguric phase of ARF in the 33 randomly selected patients who received the medication.

Even though there is little conclusive evidence that agents such as furosemide or ethacrynic acid reverses the oliguria in a significant number of patients who are treated, the question remains whether the conversion of oliguira to polyuria found in some patients improves morbidity and enhances survival. The data regarding this issue remain unsettled and controversial. As stated previously, Anderson et al. [7] in their study of nonoliguric ARF found that patients with oliguric ARF who were converted to nonoliguric renal failure following furosemide therapy had a milder and less severe course than those who failed to respond to furosemide. Minuth et al. in their retrospective analysis of ARF, found that patients who responded to furosemide had degrees of metabolic complications similar to those patients who do not resond. The only improvement they could demonstrate was the diminished need for dialytic therapy in those patients who responded to furosemide therapy [54].

In summary, therefore, treatment during the initiation phase of (oliguric) ARF with agents such as furosemide and mannitol to enhance urine flow rate, improve GFR, and reverse the renal insufficiency remains to be proven in controlled therapeutic trials. However, there does appear to be a subset of patients who if treated early during the initiation phase of oliguric ARF with parenteral furosemide or mannitol may respond with polyuria, a milder form of renal failure, and an improvement in survival.

During the maintenance of the established phase of ARF, the goals of therapy in the nonoliguric variety are similar to those found in the oliguric variety, with few special exceptions.

First, the prevention and treatment of hemorrhage and infectious complications, the leading causes of death in all forms of ARF, are identical in both varieties of ARF. Second, attempts are made in nonoliguric renal failure to maintain an adequate level of nutrition. Since patients with nonoliguric renal failure are not often as sick as those with oliguria, oral feedings are often carried out in an appropriate fashion, depending on specific caloric and mineral needs. If patients with nonoliguric renal failure are unable to eat, parenteral alimentation or hyperalimentation with concentrated amino acid and gluose solutions is frequently undertaken. In fact, since many of these patients have urine volumes greater than 1000 ml/day, administration of large volumes of intravenous and/or oral fluids is often done with little risk of circulatory overload and pulmonary congestion, complications frequently encountered in oliguric patients.

Finally, with regard to uremic complications and symptoms, the management of nonoliguric patients is identical with that undertaken in patients with oliguric renal failure. If patients with nonoliguric ARF have uremic symptoms such as nausea, vomiting, diarrhea, pruritus, anorexia, confusion, or signs such as asterixis, stupor or coma, dialysis should be initiated. The choice of which mode of dialysis is initiated, whether it be hemodialysis or peritoneal dialysis, must be individualized. However, patients with nonoliguric ARF are often not as catabolic, acidotic, hyperkalemic, or encephalopathic as their oliguric counterparts; thus, they often require less intense dialytic therapy. Therefore, the nephrologist can often choose peritoneal dialysis as the mode of therapy and avoid the infectious and vascular complications associated with the use of arteriovenous shunts in hemodialysis.

The specific management of electrolyte problems encountered in nonoliguric ARF deserves special mention. First, as mentioned earlier, because of the maintenance of urine flow, less severe restriction of sodium and water intake can be implemented in patients with nonoliguric ARF. Therefore, oral intake and parenteral administration of fluids can be liberalized in these patients. Second, the incidence of hyperkalemia found in patients with nonoliguric and oliguric ARF is comparable [8]. Therefore, dietary and parenteral potassium restriction, as well as therapeutic measures to lower serum potassium, are identical in both forms of ARF.

Finally, there does appear to be one unique electrolyte abnormality encountered in nonoliguric renal failure that is markedly different from that found in the oliguric form of ARF. Hypomagnesemia, as opposed to hypermagnesemia, is encountered in two particular varieties of nonoliguric ARF. Schilsky and Anderson [56] described hypomagnesemia in greater than 50% (23 out of 44) of patients receiving cis-diammine dichloroplatinum as a chemotherapeutic agent in treating a variety of solid tumors. As mentioned earlier, cisplatin is an agent with significant and predictable nephrotoxicity, and it specifically induces the nonoliguric variety of ARF [30–33]. With the increasing usage of cisplatin in treating solid tumors, the incidence of nonoliguric ARF is certain to rise, and clinicians should be aware of the renal magnesium wasting that it causes and the subsequent, often severe, symptomatic hypomagnesemia.

Hypocalcemia may accompany the hypomagnesemia and lead to signs such as muscular twitching and irritability, a positive Chvostek sign, and frank tetany. Correction of the magnesium depletion will often restore serum calcium values to normal, and resolution of the signs and symptoms accompanying hypocalcemia.

The second circumstance in which severe renal magnesium wasting is encountered when an agent known to cause a nonoliguric variety of ARF has been used was described by Bar and his colleagues in 1975 following high-dose gentamicin therapy [57]. Again, in a similar fashion to cisplatin therapy, severe renal magnesium wasting, hypomagnesemia, and symptomatic hypocalcemia was found in two patients following high-dose aminoglycoside (gentamicin) therapy. Curiously enough, in these two patients, in spite of the high-dose gentamicin therapy and the tubular defects encountered, there was no evidence of renal insufficiency. Therefore, the simultaneous occurrence of nonoliguric ARF and renal magnesium wasting has yet to be described following gentamicin therapy. However, clinicians should be aware that both complications can result from gentamicin therapy.

Finally, treatment during the recovery phase from nonoliguric ARF differs from oliguric ARF only in the sense that treatment has been the same thoughout the entire course of nonoliguric renal failure. The recovery phase of oliguric ARF is often synonymous with the "diuretic" phase. This is the time when urine output is re-established, and the patient's GFR begins to return toward normal. Liberalization of sodium, potassium, and water restriction can now be instituted.

During the recovery phase in nonoliguric renal failure, there is rapid restoration of GFR toward normal, correction of tubular defects, and hence more physiologic handling of monovalent (sodium and potassium) and divalent (magnesium, calcium) cations as well as monovalent and divalent anions. The internal milieu in which enzymes function and physiologic processes occur is rapidly returned to normal, and the homeostasis of fluid and electrolytes is again regulated to the kidney.

6 Summary and Conclusion

Nonoliguric acute renal failure is a common form of ARF, which, prior to the use of potent nephrotoxic antibiotic and antineoplastic agents, was frequently unrecognized. It is characterized by the maintenance of urine output despite a compromise and decline in glomerular filtration rate. Although caused by a diverse group of etiologic agents, both ischemic as well as nephrotoxic insults can lead to the nonoliguric state. The renal failure encountered in the nonoliguric variety is usually mild, with less azotemia, fewer metabolic complications and an improved survival rate when compared to its oliguric counterpart. Treatment of nonoliguric ARF differs little from that of its oliguric counterpart, with the exception of less rigid fluid and electrolyte restriction as well as special attention to problems with divalent cations such as magnesium and calcium. With proper recognition and management of this

syndrome, perhaps there will be a substantial improvement in the alarmingly high mortality and morbidity rate encountered in all forms of ARF.

References

1. Levinsky NL, Alexander EA, Venkatachalam M. Acute renal failure. In The Kidney, Brenner BM, Rector FC Jr (eds). Philadelphia: WB Saunders, 1981, pp. 1181–1236.
2. Harrington JT, Cohen JJ. Acute Oliguria. N Engl J Med 292: 89–91, 1975.
3. Swann RC, Merrill JP. The clinical course of acute renal failure. Medicine 32: 215–293, 1953.
4. Strauss MB. Acute renal insufficiency due to lower nephron nephrosis. N Engl J Med 239: 693, 1948.
5. Vertel RM, Knochel JP. Nonoliguric acute renal failure. JAMA 200: 118–122, 1967.
6. Baxter CR, Zelditz WD, Shires GT. High output acute renal failure complicating traumatic injury. J Trauma 4: 567–580, 1964.
7. Anderson RJ, Linas SL, Berns AS, Henrich WL, Miller TR, Gabow PA, Schrier RW. Non-oliguric acute renal failure. N Engl J Med 296: 1134–1137, 1977.
8. Anderson RJ, Schrier RW. Clinical spectrum of oliguric and non-oliguric acute renal failure. In Acute Renal Failure, Brenner BM, Stein JH (eds). New York: Churchill Livingstone, 1980, pp. 1–16.
9. Myers C, Roxe BM, Hano JE. The clinical course of non-oliguric acute renal failure. Cardiov Med 4: 699–672, 1977.
10. Danovitch G, Carvounis C, Weinstein E, Levenson S. Nonoliguric acute renal failure. Isr J Med Sci 15: 5–8, 1979.
11. Teschan P, Post RS, Smith LH, Abernathy RS, Davis JH. Post-traumatic renal insufficiency in military casualties: I. Clinical characteristics. Am J Med 18: 172–186, 1955.
12. Taylor WH, Reid JVO. Acute uremic renal failure and head injury and surgical operation. J Clin Pathol 9: 184, 1956.
13. Taylor WH. Management of acute renal failure following surgical operation and head injury. Lancet 2: 703–707, 1957.
14. Sevitt S. Distal tubular necrosis with little or no oliguria. J Clin Pathol 9: 12–30, 1956.
15. Baxter CR, Maynard DR. Prevention and recognition of surgical renal complications. Clin Anesthesia 3: 322–333, 1968.
16. Gant NF et al. Non-oliguric renal failure—Report of a case. Obst Gynec 34: 675–679, 1969.
17. Ireland GW, Cass AS. The recognition and management of acute high output renal failure. J Urol 108: 40–43, 1972.

18. Bhat JG, Gluck MC, Lowenstein J, Baldwin DS. Renal failure after open-heart surgery. Ann Intern Med 84: 677–682, 1976.

19. Hilberman M, Myers BD, Carrie BJ, Derby G, Jamison RL, Stinson EB. Acute renal failure following cardiac surgery. J Thorac Cardiovas Surg 77: 880–888, 1979.

20. Shen SC, Ham TH, Fleming EM. Studies on the destruction of red blood cells. III: Mechanisms and complications of hemoglobinuria in patients with thermal burns: Spherocytosis and increased osmotic fragility of red blood cells. N Engl J Med 229: 701–713, 1943.

21. Knochel JP. Rhabdomyolysis and myoglobinuria. Seminars in Nephrology 1: 75–86, 1981.

22. Grossman RA, Hamilton RW, Morse BD, Penn AS, Goldberg M. Non-traumatic rhabdomyolysis and acute renal failure. N Engl J Med 291: 807–811, 1974.

23. Koffler A, Friedler RM, Massry SG. Acute renal failure due to non-traumatic rhabdomyolysis. Ann Intern Med 85: 23–28, 1976.

24. Crandell WB, Pappas SG, Macdonald A. Nephrotoxicity associated with methyoxyflurane anesthesia. Anesthesiology 27: 591–608, 1966.

25. Pezzi PJ, Frosbese AS, Greenberg SR. Methoxyflurane and renal toxicity. Lancet 1: 823, 1966.

26. Van Zee BE, Hay WE, Talley TE, Jaenike JR. Renal injury associated with intravenous pyelography in non-diabetic and diabetic patients. Ann Intern Med 89: 51–54, 1978.

27. Porter GA, Bennett WM. Nephrotoxin-induced acute renal failure. In Acute Renal Failure, Brenner BM, Stein JH (eds). New York: Churchill Livingstone, 1980, pp. 123–162.

28. Ansari Z, Baldwin D. Acute renal failure due to radiocontrast agents. Nephron 17: 28–40, 1976.

29. Einhorn LH, Williams SD. The role of cisplatinum in solid tumor therapy. N Engl J Med 300: 289–291, 1979.

30. Madias NE, Harrington JT. Platinum nephrotoxicity. Am J Med 65: 307–314, 1978.

31. Blackley JD, Hill JB. Renal and electrolyte disturbances associated with cis-platin. Ann Intern Med 95: 628–632, 1981.

32. Gordon JA, Anderson RJ, Peterson LK. Water metabolism after cis-platinum in the rat. Am J Physiol 243: F36–43, 1982.

33. Safirstein R, et al. Cis platin nephrotoxicity in rats: Defect in papillary hypertonicity. Am J Physiol 241: F175–F185, 1981.

34. Gray N, Buzzeo L, Salaki J, Eisenger RP. Gentamicin associated acute renal failure. Arch Intern Med 136: 1101–1104, 1976.

35. Cronin RJ. Aminoglycoside nephrotoxicity: Pathogenesis and prevention. Clin Nephrol 11: 251–256, 1979.

36. Fung-Herrera CB, Mulvaney WP. Cephalexin nephrotoxicity: Reversible nonoliguric acute renal failure and hepatotoxicity associated with cephalexin therapy. JAMA 229: 318–319, 1974.

37. Stein J, Lifschitz M, Barnes L. Current concepts on the pathophysiology of acute renal failure. Am J Physiol 234: F171–F181, 1978.

38. Finn WF, Arendshorst WJ, Gottschalk CW. Pathogenesis of oliguria in acute renal failure. Circ Res 36: 675–681, 1975.

39. Oken DE. Modern concepts of the role of nephrotoxic agents in the pathogenesis of acute renal failure. Prog Biochem Pharmacol 7: 1–29, 1971.

40. Oken DE. Nosologic considerations in the nomenclature of acute renal failure. Nephron 8: 505–510, 1971.

41. Anderson RJ, Gordon JA, Peterson LK, Gross P, Ellis M. The renal concentration defect following non-oliguric acute renal failure in the rat. Kidney Int 21: 583–591, 1982.

42. Cronin RE, Erickson AM, DeTorrente A, McDonald KM, Schrier RW. Norephinephrine-induced acute renal failure; a reversible ischemic model of acute renal failure. Kidney Int 14: 187–190, 1978.

43. Myers BD, Chui F, Hilberman M, Michaels AS. Trans-tubular leakage of glomerular filtrate in human acute renal failure. Am J Physiol 237: F319–F325, 1979.

44. Myers BD, Carrie BJ, Yee RR, Hilberman M, Michael AS. Pathophysiology of hemodynamically mediated acute renal failure in man. Kidney Int 18: 594–604, 1980.

45. Blantz RC. Mechanisms of acute renal failure after uranyl nitrate. J Clin Invest 55: 621–635, 1975.

46. Bayliss C, Rennke H, Brenner BM. Mechanisms of the defect in glomerular ultrafiltration associated with gentamicin administration. Kidney Int 12: 344–353, 1977.

47. Bywaters EGL, Dible JH. The renal lesion in traumatic anuria. J Path & Bact 54: 111–120, 1942.

48. Arendhorst W, Finn WF, Gottschalk CW. Pathogenesis of acute renal failure following renal ischemia in the rat. Circ Res 37: 558–568, 1975.

49. Cronin RE, DeTorrente A, Miller PM, Bulger RE, Burke JJ, Schrier RW. Pathogenic mechanisms in early norepinephrine-induced acute renal failure: Functional and histological correlates of protection. Kidney Int 14: 115–125, 1978.

50. Miller TR, Anderson RT, Linas SL, Henrich WL, Berns AS, Gabow PA, Schrier RW. Urinary diagnostic indices in acute renal failure. Ann Intern Med 89: 47–50, 1978.

51. Finn WF. Nephron heterogeneity in polyuric acute renal failure. J Lab Clin Med 98: 21–30, 1981.

52. McMurray SD, et al. Prevailing patterns and predictor variables in patients with acute tubular necrosis. Arch Intern Med 138: 950–955, 1978.

53. Ng RCK, Suki WN. Treatment of acute renal failure. In Acute Renal Failure, Brenner BM, Stein JH (eds). New York: Churchill Livingstone, 1980, pp. 229–275.

54. Minuth AW, Terrell JB, Suki WW. Acute renal failure: A study of the course and prognosis of 104 patients and of the role of furosemide. Am J Med Sci 271: 317–324, 1976.
55. Kleinknecht D, Ganevae D, Gonzalez-Duque LA, Fermanian J. Furosemide in acute oliguric renal failure: A controlled trial. Nephron 17: 51–58, 1976.
56. Shilsky RL, Anderson T. Hypomagnesemia and renal magnesium wasting in patients receiving cisplatin. Ann Intern Med 90: 929–931, 1979.
57. Bar RS, Wilson HE, Mazzaferri EL. Hypomagnesemic hypocalcemia secondary to renal magnesium wasting: A possible consequence of high-dose gentamicin therapy. Ann Intern Med 82: 646–649, 1975.

11. HEPATORENAL SYNDROME

Solomon Papper

1 Introduction

The hepatorenal syndrome is a specific form of acute renal failure occurring in patients with parenchymal liver disease of diverse etiology.

In addition to a consideration of clinical features and treatment, this chapter also deals specifically with areas of confusion, controversy, and uncertainty. These areas include the term *hepatorenal syndrome* and its definition, criteria for the diagnosis of the syndrome, and the pathogenesis.

2 History and the Term *Hepatorenal Syndrome*

In 1863, Austin Flint [1] recorded the fact that patients with cirrhosis and hydroperitoneum might develop severe oliguria and die. The term *hepatorenal syndrome* (HRS) was introduced 50 years ago to designate unexplained renal failure following biliary tract surgery [2]. Although in retrospect no one can state with certainty the precise nature of the renal failure described in these early studies, it has since become known that biliary tract obstruction predisposes to acute tubular necrosis. Subsequently, the label HRS was applied so generally and loosely to virtually all associations of renal and hepatic disturbances that the term becomes meaningless, vague, and misleading

Portions of this chapter are taken from Papper S, "The Hepatorenal Syndrome," in *The Kidney in Liver Disease* (2nd ed.), Murray Epstein (ed.) (Elsevier Science Publishing Co., Inc., 1983). Reprinted by permission of the publisher and editor, copyright 1983 by Elsevier North Holland, Inc.

V.E. Andreucci (ed.), ACUTE RENAL FAILURE.
All rights reserved. Copyright © 1984.
Martinus Nijhoff Publishing, Boston/The Hague/
Dordrecht/Lancaster.

clinically. With that background, it is not surprising that in the 1940s experts were generally skeptical that there was any particular variety of renal failure that occurred in liver disease that could not be ascribed to other known causes.

In the 1950s, however, the existence of an unexplained renal failure in cirrhosis with quite specific clinical and renal functional characteristics was documented. In 1956, Hecker and Sherlock [3] reported nine patients with terminal liver failure. In those patients, who also had renal failure, the authors noted the absence of proteinuria, a low urinary concentration of sodium, and a poor response to therapy. In 1958 and 1959, my colleagues and I reported 22 patients with cirrhosis and renal failure and included clinical observations on the spectrum of the severity of liver disease with renal failure, as well as detailed studies of renal function [4, 5]. At that time, evidence was also presented to "suggest that we might well search primarily for factors adversely affecting the renal circulation . . . rather than renal parenchymal disease" [4]. However, our attempts to improve the renal circulation with saline, blood, and dextran were without benefit. In 1962, Vesin [6] confirmed these findings and suggested the term *functional renal failure*. In the early 1960s, many groups throughout the world added considerable data to confirm the existence of HRS and its functional nature [7]. In 1965, Shear et al. [8] demonstrated that acute tubular necrosis (ATN) may also supervene.

Despite efforts to apply other names to this specific hepatic-renal relationship, such as "renal failure of cirrhosis," "hemodynamic renal failure," "functional renal failure," "cirrhotic

234

nephropathy," "hepatic nephropathy" and others, the apparently more appealing term *hepatorenal syndrome* has been most commonly used and has persisted. Whether or not this is a regrettable term for what is quite a specific variety of renal failure, there is no real advantage in continuing the debate. And I shall refer to this one condition as the hepatorenal syndrome.

There is probably still need to define and describe specifically this renal failure of liver disease that is not due to the usual known causes of renal functional impairment. Even as recently as 1978, a symposium mostly of European experts gathered "to attain one limited goal: an internationally acceptable definition of the Hepato-Renal syndrome, together with the establishment of its diagnostic criteria" [9]. And in 1980, an editorial in *Lancet* entitled "Hepatorenal Syndrome or Hepatic Nephropathy?" also made a plea for the more specific use of the term HRS or for substituting another term [10]. In both the European symposium's conclusion and in *Lancet,* the conclusions for the definition and diagnostic criteria of HRS are largely consistent with those we and others have proposed and published in the past [3–8, 11, 12] and more recently [13–16].

3 Definition of HRS

The hepatorenal syndrome may be defined as incompletely explained renal failure occurring in patients with parenchymal liver disease in the absence of clinical, laboratory, or anatomic evidence of other known causes of renal failure. Early in its course, its renal functional characteristics are indistinguishable from prerenal azotemia except that it is not responsive or at best only transiently responsive to volume expansion. Hence, we include a test for adequacy of effective circulating volume in section 8 on diagnostic criteria. In some patients, with time, there is a transition into acute tubular necrosis (ATN).

The hepatorenal syndrome is potentially reversible. In some instances, it reverses spontaneously with improvement of liver function. How often spontaneous reversal occurs is not known; while in most series (including our own) this appears to be a very uncommon outcome, other careful observers give figures of 10 to 20% spontaneous remission. Reversal of renal failure occurs with change in the hepatic environment. Thus, the kidney from a patient with HRS may be used successfully as a donor for transplantation in a patient with a normal liver [17]. Conversely, the kidney in a patient with HRS recovers function if the patient undergoes successful liver transplantation [18].

The relative frequency of different types of liver disease, including cirrhosis associated with HRS, depends on geographic and other incompletely understood circumstances. In the United States, we deal mostly with the alcoholic type—that is, Laënnec's cirrhosis—while some of our colleagues in other parts of the world have greater experience with postnecrotic, idiopathic, or primary biliary cirrhosis. There is also evidence that HRS may complicate other varieties of liver disease, e.g., viral hepatitis, fulminant hepatic failure, fatty liver of pregnancy, primary and secondary malignancy of the liver, and even hepatic resection. (It is also possible that HRS may rarely follow biliary tract obstruction and biliary tract surgery where ATN is far more common.) Although the pathophysiology may be similar in the renal failure of these diverse causes of liver disease, it is perhaps premature to assume that pathogenesis of the renal dysfunction is identical in all instances.

Another aspect of definition might well include the major differential diagnosis, that is, conditions other than the one designated as HRS, but which also are characterized by both hepatic and renal disturbances (see table 11–1). The list is large. However, there are five main categories of clinical conditions that may be confused with the hepatorenal syndrome. First, there are the circumstances in which hepatic and renal dysfunction result from simultaneous injury to both organs, sometimes referred to as the "pseudo-hepatorenal" syndrome. These are outlined in table 11–2. Second, immune complex glomerulonephritis may develop in the course of hepatitis B disease. Third, some patients with acute liver disease develop disseminated intravascular coagulation (DIC), which may damage the kidney. Fourth, patients with

TABLE 11-1. Conditions (other than HRS) with both hepatic and renal involvement

1. Simultaneous hepatic and renal injury ("pseudo-hepatorenal" syndrome—see table 11–2).
2. Immune complex glomerulonephritis secondary to hepatitis B disease.
3. Renal injury secondary to disseminated intravascular coagulation in patients with severe liver injury.
4. Acute tubular necrosis secondary to obstructive jaundice.
5. Prerenal azotemia in patients with liver disease.

TABLE 11-2. "Pseudo-hepatorenal" syndromes

1. Generalized Disorders
   Infections (sepsis, hepatitis B, leptospirosis, yellow fever, Reye's syndrome)
   Circulatory (shock, heart failure)
   Genetic (polycystic disease, sickle-cell anemia)
   Collagen-vascular (systemic lupus erythematosus, polyarteritis nodosa)
   Unknown nature (toxemias of pregnancy, amyloidosis, sarcoidosis, hyperthermia)
2. Toxins
   Carbon tetrachloride, paracetamol (acetaminophen), Amanita phalloides poisoning, methoxyflurane, halothane, tetracycline, copper, chromium, streptomycin, sulfonamides, iproniazid
3. Neoplasms
   Metastatic, renal cell carcinoma

Source: Adapted from Conn HO [11]. (Courtesy of the Williams & Wilkins Co. and the author).

TABLE 11-3. Renal failure in cirrhosis (200 patients)

Associated (precipitating?) events	No. of patients
Mild gastrointestinal bleeding[a]	76
Abdominal paracentesis	11
Induced diuresis	10
Severe or progressive jaundice	80[b]
No apparent associated event	49

[a] Guaiac positive stool only.
[b] Twenty-six of these patients also had other associated events and are therefore reported in other categories (16, guaiac positive stool; 8, induced diuresis; 2, paracentesis).

obstructive jaundice have a poorly understood predilection to the development of ATN. And fifth, "prerenal" azotemia is a likely occurrence in patients who are actively forming ascites, especially if their intake of solute and fluids is meager and there are associated losses of the body fluids due to vomiting, diarrhea, and forced diuresis. "Prerenal" azotemia is difficult if not impossible to distinguish from early HRS except by the response to expansion of extracellular fluid volume and may actually predispose to HRS, as is considered later in this chapter.

It is difficult to know the incidence and prevalence of HRS in the broad spectrum of patients with liver disease. However, HRS is probably not uncommon in patients with terminal cirrhosis: incidence figures of 44% and 84% are given in some studies [8].

4 Clinical Features

My colleagues and I have studied more than 200 patients with alcoholic cirrhosis and HRS. I shall draw heavily on this personal experience in conjunction with the studies of others.

a. Although oliguria is the hallmark of HRS, it may occur in the nonoliguric form. We have had only 12 patients out of 200 without oliguria.
b. HRS may develop in the course of liver disease without any apparent precipitating event (see table 11–3). We and others have observed its occurrence following abdominal paracentesis, even when as little as three liters of fluid are removed or after fluid loss due to forced diuresis. We have also seen renal failure in patients with slight blood loss manifested only by guaiac-positive stool, in the absence of gross gastrointestinal hemorrhage, and without decrease in hematocrit or clinical shock.
c. Renal failure may develop with great rapidity. Patients may develop HRS in a matter of months, weeks, or even 24 to 48 hours after normal renal function has been documented.
d. In our group of patients, ascites was generally present, but varied considerably in degree. Most of our patients had 3 to 4 + ascites.
e. Jaundice ranges from severe to minimal and from progressive to declining. While most of the reported patients with HRS have evidence of severe hepatocellular disease, there are many in whom the liver disease is less advanced.

f. In 181 of 200 patients, there was a modest reduction in blood pressure from previous values. For example, a blood pressure of 120/80 mm Hg in the past might now be in the order of 110/65. It has been documented in a number of instances that this reduction in blood pressure may occur after renal failure already exists.

g. Hepatic encephalopathy was present in 161 of 200 patients.

h. This condition usually develops in the hospital, therefore raising the question of whether events in the hospital might precipitate the syndrome. Obviously, forced diuresis is an example of a hospital event that might precipitate HRS, but there may well be others presently undefined, but conceivably of great importance. (Perhaps one should consider not only positive hospital circumstances but also omissions, such as alcohol.)

5 Clinical Course

There are no apparent features that identify patients with cirrhosis who will ultimately develop renal failure.

The development of renal failure in the course of Laënnec's cirrhosis is of grave prognostic significance. Only two patients in our entire group had a spontaneous recovery. On the other hand, spontaneous recovery is well documented. Reynolds [19] reported 13% spontaneous recovery in a series of 62 patients. Gordon and Anderson estimate that "perhaps as many as 20–30% of patients will obtain peak serum creatinine values of 2–5 mg/dl (177–442 μmol/l) which later decline" [20]. Although the exact figures may depend on a number of factors, including severity at the time the diagnosis is made, spontaneous recovery occurs in a minority of instances. The carefully documented recoveries have appeared to follow a dramatic and rapid improvement in the condition of the liver.

In many instances, the course is rapid, with the development of terminal liver failure in a week or two. In other patients, the course progresses over several weeks or a month or two with patients who feel poorly and have mild mental obtundation and who die of terminal liver failure, gastrointestinal bleeding, or infection. In a retrospective study, gastrointestinal bleeding was the most common cause of death [21].

In many patients, it is difficult to attribute the poor outcome of HRS directly to renal failure when GFR is of the order of 15 to 20% of normal. (Blood urea nitrogen [BUN] and serum creatinine concentrations may underestimate the degree of renal functional impairment in patients with liver disease because of impaired urea synthesis in the case of BUN and decreased muscle mass in interpreting serum creatinine.) It seems likely that renal failure may be a reflection or a part of a broader lethal event and that in most instances it is not in itself the most important determinant of how long the patient will survive. On the other hand, we have had patients with more severe renal failure and serum creatinine concentrations of 1.15 to 1.24 mmol/l (13 to 24 mg/dl). As is true of most series, we have not seen many patients with a truly uremic death.

6 Renal Function

a. The urine is generally acid and may contain small amounts of protein. Hyaline and granular casts as well as microscopic hematuria are commonly observed.

b. Urinary concentration is variable, but one common pattern is a scanty, quite concentrated urine (perhaps two to three times the concentration of plasma) early in the course of renal failure. There is often a subsequent gradual decrease in urinary concentration toward that of plasma, while the patient remains oliguric. Some patients die while their urine is still concentrated, and others have urinary osmolalities only slightly above that of plasma at the time the diagnosis is made. In some patients with HRS, oliguria does not occur.

c. In our series, with the exception of an occasional patient with a urinary sodium concentration (U_{Na}) of 20 to 30 mmol/l, U_{Na} is less than 10 mmol/l, including those patients who do not have oliguria. In many instances, U_{Na} is only 1 to 2 mmol/l. Gordon and Anderson report U_{Na} as 14 ± 3 in HRS [20]. There is an occasional patient whose course begins with a very low urinary sodium concentration that increases to levels approaching 40 mmol/l. Such a phenomenon raises the question of "transition" into acute tubular necrosis.

d. Diluting ability is difficult to study and interpret in patients who are so ill. The secretion of antidiuretic hormone (ADH) may be stimulated for reasons totally unrelated to the presence of liver disease, for example, pain, discomfort, drugs, etc. However, under carefully controlled circumstances, with the aforementioned limitations, none of the patients can elaborate a dilute urine. The serum sodium concentration is usually but not always reduced. It has been shown that early in the course of renal failure, the serum sodium concentration may be normal, declining as a consequence of administered water in excess of that excreted [7].

e. Hall and Ricanati [22] have shown that patients with HRS have normal renal tubular handling of beta-2-microglobulin (β_2M). Urinary β_2M is generally increased in primary tubular disorders with or without concomitant liver disease.

f. As already mentioned, the levels of serum creatinine do not generally reach those seen in terminal stages of primary renal disease—but on occasion they do. Along with the striking decrease in glomerular filtration rate (GFR) and renal plasma flow (RPF), the filtration fraction is either normal or low. Because of the only modest reduction in arterial pressure, the calculated renal vascular resistance is greatly elevated.

g. There is potent vasoconstriction in the outer segments of the renal cortex with preservation of blood flow to the deeper cortical and medullary segments [23]. Patients also exhibit a very striking arterial instability during contrast fluororadiography [23]. However, the entire arterial tree fills normally when injected postmortem. The corticomedullary shift of blood with afferent vasoconstriction is not a finding unique to the hepatorenal syndrome, but occurs in other states as well—e.g., heart failure. However the great renal vascular instability seems to be characteristic of this group of patients. Vascular instability has also been observed in a few severely decompensated cirrhotic patients without renal failure [24].

7 Pathology

In our series, the kidney was either perfectly normal or had some minimal changes but without any evidence of an identifiable primary renal disease.

Through the years, renal lesions have been described in cirrhosis. The reports of glomerular lesions have included "cirrhotic glomerulosclerosis" [25]. This lesion is seen in postnecrotic and biliary cirrhosis as well as in alcoholic liver disease, and pathologists continue to debate whether it is even specific for chronic liver disease. In addition, mesangial thickening, basement membrane thickening, proliferative glomerulonephritis, and immunoglobulin deposits have been noted. The observations describe a deposition of osmophilic granules, proteinaceous material, and irregular black particles, mainly in the mesangium. There have also been findings of a thick glomerular basement membrane and some fusion and focal destruction of foot processes. Other investigators have found gamma globulin glomerular fixation by immunofluorescence microscopy of renal biopsies. These have been identified as IgA, IgG, IgM, or C_3. These deposits have been primarily in the mesangium and the capillary wall. The glomerular findings often do not correlate with proteinuria or elevation in serum creatinine concentration, rendering their clinical significance uncertain. In one study, control subjects without liver disease had glomerular sclerosis and deposits. Although immune disease is possible, it seems more likely that the deposits result from precipitation in glomeruli of either aggregated immunoglobulins or circulating immune complexes.

Tubular lesions have also been described. "Biliary or cholemic nephrosis" has no functional significance because azotemia can exist without the lesion, and the latter may be observed in the presence of normal renal function.

Other apparently minor tubular alterations have been observed. As already mentioned, ATN has also been described [8]. In our experience, ATN is rare although others have noted it more frequently, particularly in fulminant hepatic failure rather than in cirrhosis [26].

With the exception of acute tubular necrosis, when it is present, the etiologic, functional, and clinical significance of the other anatomic findings is far from evident: the lesion of glomerular sclerosis does not correlate with the presence or absence of proteinuria or azotemia, and, histologically, the appearance of the kidney in cirrhosis may vary from normal to the observation of a number of glomerular and tubular abnormalities. Therefore, the observed lesions do not seem critical to the initiation of the hepatorenal syndrome. Furthermore, the lesions may or may not be specific to cirrhosis, and if they are, the mechanism of their development is not known.

Tubular necrosis has been described in some patients with cirrhosis and renal failure. It is unlikely that ATN accounts for the initial renal failure in any appreciable number of patients. We recognize that one may have a course consistent with tubular necrosis at a time when examination of the kidney with light microscopy fails to reveal any abnormality; nonetheless, the functional changes seen in the majority of patients with the hepatorenal syndrome constitutes strong evidence against such an initiating mechanism. As will be discussed later (see section 9 on pathogenesis), we regard ATN as most likely an occasional consequence of the functional circulatory abnormalities of HRS.

8 Diagnostic Criteria

Although the HRS is a specific syndrome, there are intrinsic difficulties in firmly establishing the diagnosis in particular patients. First there is no specific test for HRS. Second, the diagnosis includes negative criteria, that is, the absence of other known causes of renal failure. Invoking negative criteria is always intellectually disquieting and tends to place the diagnosis in individual patients in some doubt. Finally, the renal functional changes early in the course of HRS are indistinguishable from prerenal azotemia. However, in our world as clinicians, many specific conditions offer difficulty in diagnosis for similar reasons. In HRS as in these other states, the diagnosis is made as a composite that includes the clinical setting in which the renal failure develops, positive and negative clinical features, the renal functional changes, the course, and the response to certain measures, notably volume expansion. These diagnostic criteria may be summarized as follows.

8.1 CLINICAL

a Presence of liver disease.
b. Absence of primary renal disease or known causes of renal failure.
c. Acute or subacute onset of renal functional impairment that is usually progressive over a matter of days or weeks.
d. No sustained improvement with cautious expansion of the vascular space (to achieve a central venous pressure of greater than 8 cm water).

TABLE 11–4. Renal functional changes in the hepatorenal syndrome

	Early*	Late (days to weeks)	Progression to ATN
GFR	Low	Low	Low
Urine sodium concentration	<10–20 mmol/l	<10–20 mmol/l	>40 mmol/l
FE_{Na}	<1	<1	>2
Urine Concentration U/Posm	>1 (concentrated)	>1 to 1 (concentrated to isoosmotic)	1 (isoosmotic)

*Early HRS is functionally indistinguishable from "prerenal azotemia." However, HRS does not have sustained response to expansion of vascular volume.

8.2 RENAL FUNCTION

The early renal functional changes (see table 11–4) are indistinguishable from "prerenal azotemia," except that in HRS there is not a sustained response to expansion of vascular volume. The urine sodium concentration is less than 10 to 20 mmol/l, the fractional excretion of sodium (FE_{Na}) is less than 1, and the urine is concentrated (table 11–4).

Later in the course, although U_{Na} and FE_{Na} remain low, the urinary concentration decreases toward isoosmotic levels (table 11–4).

9 Pathogenesis

Despite intense investigation, the etiology of the renal failure of cirrhosis is not known. One of the major obstacles is the lack of an appropriate comparable animal model. From the rapidity of onset of HRS in cirrhosis, the possible pathogenetic mechanisms are confined to those producing acute or subacute renal failure rather than a chronic disease. Among the acute and subacute renal diseases, we find no evidence for glomerulonephritis, vasculitis, or interstitial nephritis. There is no question that ATN occurs in some patients with HRS. The lesion has been seen histologically, and urinary lysozyme concentrations have been elevated in some patients [27]. But ATN is probably not common for the following reasons. The renal functional characteristics of HRS—i.e., maintained concentrating ability early in the course, very low urinary sodium concentration, and high urinary-osmolar/plasma-osmolar ratio—constitute strong evidence against ATN. In our own series, we have seen it twice; in both instances, the urine changed late in the course from the above characteristics to isoosmotic and urinary sodium concentrations above 60 mmol/l. The likelihood of "transitional" forms—i.e., progression from the functional underperfused kidney to indications of tubular necrosis—has already been proposed. These are characterized by the development of isoosmotic urine and increases in urinary sodium concentration from less than 10 to 20 mmol/l to the 30 to 50 mmol/l range. It is probable that these transitional forms and frank ATN, when they occur, are the consequence of the severely altered renal circulation in a vulnerable patient, rather than of the initiating mechanism.

The role of bilirubin itself has been considered. However, there is no evidence that bilirubin directly damages the kidney except in the Gunn rat [28]. There is evidence that under certain conditions—for example, obstructive jaundice—bilirubin or bile acids make the kidney more sensitive to other influences, such as ischemia. (This subject is carefully reviewed by Better and Berl [29].) As will be considered later, jaundiced serum may contain material other than bilirubin that increases vascular responsiveness to vasoconstrictor stimuli. In HRS, there is poor correlation with the degree of jaundice; in fact, some of our patients had only minimal jaundice, and in several others, bilirubin concentrations were declining at the time HRS developed.

There is no substantive evidence in man that hyponatremia causes renal functional impairment; in any case, there is good evidence that hyponatremia develops after renal failure in oliguric patients who continue to receive water. The presence of a concentrated urine early in the disease course, along with the absence of the characteristic vacuolization of the proximal tubules, allows us to dismiss the possibility of hypokalemic nephropathy.

As stated earlier, in 1958, we presented evidence to "suggest that we might well search primarily for factors adversely affecting the renal circulation . . . rather than renal parenchymal disease" [4]. The largest body of evidence still supports a circulatory mechanism for the production of HRS (table 11–5). In summary form, this evidence includes the following observations: Renal failure may develop with great rapidity. Early in HRS, the combination of reduced GFR, concentrated urine, and very low urinary sodium concentration is characteristic of a diminution in effective renal perfusion. Although we exclude all patients with gross clinical shock from our own series, a slight decrease in blood pressure was the rule. There is good evidence that the mild reduction in blood pressure was not the cause of the renal failure, but rather that the change in blood pressure was further evidence of an altered circulation. The onset of renal failure following

TABLE 11-5. Evidence for circulatory pathogenesis of hepatorenal syndrome (HRS)

CLINICAL
1. HRS may develop rapidly.
2. HRS may follow reduction in circulating volume.

RENAL FUNCTION
1. Early: low GFR; low U_{Na}; concentrated urine.
2. Afferent vasoconstriction.
3. Expansion of volume may cause transient improvement.
4. Vasoactive drugs may cause transient improvement.
5. Relative cortical ischemia.
6. Unstable renal arterial circulation.

EXTRARENAL CIRCULATION
1. Blood pressure modestly reduced.
2. Vasodilatation and shunting.
3. Cardiac output may be high.
4. Hepatic and cerebral blood flow may be low.
5. Splanchnic pooling.

MORPHOLOGY
1. Normal or nondiagnostic.

REVERSIBILITY IN NORMAL HEPATIC ENVIRONMENT
1. HRS kidney functions as transplanted donor organ.
2. Liver transplantation in HRS results in renal recovery.

clinical circumstances that serve to cause some reduction in effective circulating volume— e.g., mild occult gastrointestinal bleeding, paracentesis, forced diuresis—all lend support to the importance of circulatory derangement. The administration of saline, ascitic fluid, blood plasma, or dextran has been shown to cause a transient increase in urine volume and the presence of a more dilute urine [4]. The administration of the pressor amine metaraminol is often followed by increased GFR, an increase in urine flow, and the elaboration of a more dilute urine [30]. We have already indicated that the histologic appearance of the kidney is not diagnostic, is often normal, and, in that negative sense, is consistent with decreased renal perfusion. The relative cortical ischemia and grossly unstable renal arterial tree also constitute evidence of intrarenal circulatory changes. The HRS kidney is capable of normal renal function if its environment is changed to include a normal liver. This has been accomplished by using successfully the HRS kidney as a donor for renal transplantation in a noncirrhotic patient [17] and by the return of renal

function when the patient with HRS successfully receives a liver transplant [18].

10 The Circulation

The mechanism of the altered renal circulation in HRS is not known. Because it may be important to consider all circulatory changes in cirrhosis in order to understand those in the kidney, a brief summary of the extrarenal as well as the renal circulatory disturbances seems appropriate (see table 11–6).

Although the earlier studies reported elevated cardiac output (as is commonly the case in cirrhosis without HRS) it was found subsequently that cardiac output may be normal or reduced [30, 31]. Blood pressure is modestly reduced [4], and measured plasma volume is increased, normal, or reduced [32]. Patients also have decreased cerebral and hepatic blood flow [3, 33]. In patients with elevated cardiac output, there is peripheral vasodilatation and arteriovenous shunting in several organ systems [31]. The renal circulatory changes, in addition to reduced GFR and RBF [4, 7], include intense afferent vasoconstriction [24], relative cortical ischemia [24], and an unstable arterial circulation [24].

Some evidence has been presented that pa-

TABLE 11-6. Circulatory changes in patients with hepatorenal syndrome (HRS)

EXTRARENAL CIRCULATION
1. Cardiac output may be high, normal, or low.
2. Blood pressure is modestly reduced.
3. Plasma volume may be increased, normal, or decreased.
4. There is reduced cerebral and hepatic blood flow.
5. In those patients with elevated cardiac output, there are peripheral vasodilatation, arteriovenous shunting of blood in muscles, lung, and possibly in the kidney and liver.

RENAL CIRCULATION
1. Renal blood flow and glomerular filtration are reduced.
2. There is vasoconstriction involving the branches of the main renal artery, the interlobar arteries, as well as the smaller arteries (i.e., there is afferent vasoconstriction).
3. Relative cortical ischemia is present.
4. The renal arterial circulation is unstable.

tients with HRS might comprise two groups according to circulatory changes. One group may have decreased plasma volume, reduced cardiac output, and increased renal vascular resistance and transient renal response to volume expansion. Another group may have normal or increased plasma volume, increased cardiac output, increased renal vascular resistance, and no response to volume expansion [34]. More observations are needed to consider this grouping of findings. We doubt this separation is so precise because we have noted response to volume expansion in some patients with high cardiac output.

It is evident that these are very broad circulatory derangements in HRS. It suggests two possible pathogenetic generalizations: (a) that a single cause is operating differently on the various circulatory beds or (b) that there may not be a single explanation to account for these alterations in the circulation.

At the present time, one cannot describe a precise mechanism of the circulatory basis for HRS. Two general hypothetical approaches have evolved: (a) the abnormal renal circulation may be viewed as the physiologic response to alterations in extrarenal circulation resulting in "prerenal azotemia," and (b) it is conceivable that a humoral or neurohumoral agent produced by or inadequately inactivated by the diseased liver or bypassing the liver via portal-systemic shunts may be primarily responsible for the renal circulatory abnormalities. It is possible that both mechanisms interact in the pathogenesis of HRS. As these two possibilities are now considered, it is important to keep in mind that there may not be a single "cause." Thus, there is considerable evidence that insults leading to renal ischemia stimulate many factors that increase renal vascular resistance [20].

10.1 PHYSIOLOGIC RESPONSE

It is conceivable that the renal afferent vasoconstriction that characterizes HRS may be due, at least in part, to alterations in the extrarenal distribution of blood. A body of evidence regarding cirrhosis indicates that despite the presence of an increased total extracellular volume, the kidney perceives the volume as reduced. That is, there is a reduction in "effective" (as distinguished from "total") extracellular fluid volume; in other words, there is prerenal azotemia [35]. (There is also alternative evidence consistent with the view that extracellular volume [ECV] is expanded due to primary sodium retention and that the enlarged ECV "overflows" into the peritoneal cavity where the dynamics are conducive to ascites [35].) If there is, in fact, a reduction in effective circulating volume, it may be due to splanchnic pooling as a consequence of portal hypertension as well as to a diversion of systemic blood into arteriovenous shunts in skin, muscle, and other organs. It is also known that patients with advanced liver disease may have a reduction in cerebral and hepatic blood flow. Therefore, it is conceivable that many patients with cirrhosis may have a high cardiac output, with blood coursing preferentially into shunted areas—for example, the skin and muscle—and depriving the kidney, as well as other viscera, of blood.

Evidence in animals and man indicates that the opening of an arteriovenous fistula results in a decrease in effective circulation and renal afferent vasoconstriction. While this relatively simple mechanism, which we have sometimes referred to as the "diversion theory," cannot be dismissed entirely, there is evidence that this mechanism is not the sole explanation. Some patients with cirrhosis and renal failure have normal or even reduced cardiac output. Because cardiac output is determined by many factors, a normal output in and of itself would not negate the possible impact of a reduced effective extracellular fluid volume without increased cardiac output in the pathogenesis of afferent vasoconstriction.

A large body of physiologic evidence indicates that the kidney responds by vasoconstriction to a reduction in effective circulating volume. However, the response in HRS to expansion of intravascular volume results in inconsistent and only transient improvement in renal function [4, 34, 36]. Furthermore, it is apparent that the renal fraction of the cardiac output is reduced markedly, irrespective of the magnitude of the cardiac output [30]. Finally, it is difficult to explain in this way the very abrupt onset of HRS in some patients. One would have to postulate that there had been a small but critical decrement in the already contracted effective extracellular fluid volume, or that there had been an inapparent change in the distribution of body fluids, or that the kidney's response to the long-standing diminished extracellular fluid volume had been altered.

If the kidney perceives a decrease in effective volume, no matter what its cause, the consequent renal afferent vasoconstriction might be mediated via increased renal sympathetic tone or increased renin activity.

The evidence for increased sympathetic tone is not supported at this time: patients with HRS do not have increased excretion of urinary catecholamines, metanephrine, and 5-hydroxyindoleacetic acid, and 5-hydoxytrypamine levels in blood and urine are not elevated [37]. Phentolamine (Regitine) injected into the renal artery failed to modify renal hemodynamics in cirrhotic patients with renal cortical ischemia, although it is possible that systemic hypotension secondary to the phentolamine might have influenced the result [24]. On the other hand, transient increases in renal plasma flow with minor changes in GFR were induced by the simultaneous systemic injections of albumin to prevent hypotension and of the alpha-adrenergic blocking agent phenoxybenzamine (Dibenzyline) [38].

The role of the renin-angiotensin system is considered in more detail later under possible humoral mechanisms in the pathogenesis of HRS.

It may well be that the kidney in HRS is responding physiologically to a reduction in effective circulating volume secondary to altered extrarenal circulation; that is, "prerenal" azotemia is produced. However, there are sufficient data to question this as the sole mechanism.

10.2 HUMORAL AGENT(S)

The possibility of a humoral mechanism was mentioned in 1893 by Pavlow, who described "nephritis" following diversion of portal blood into systemic circulation [39]. He postulated that the renal disorder was due to intestinal toxins. This possibility has attracted considerable attention ever since the elegant work of

Shorr and co-workers describing the influence on renal function of vasoactive materials of hepatic origin [40]. It is conceivable that one or more substances, inadequately destroyed by the diseased liver or produced by it or bypassing it, are capable of producing both peripheral vasodilatation and, independently, vasoconstriction in other circulatory beds such as the kidney.

A humoral agent is consistent with the few observations of spontaneous recovery accompanying rapid improvement in liver function, as well as with the response to renal and liver transplantation already suggested. The role of a humoral agent is also consistent with observations in some patients in whom there is an apparent discrepancy between the degree of liver functional impairment as judged by the usual tests of liver function and the presence of HRS. For example, some patients with very little jaundice develop renal failure, and still other patients develop HRS while liver function appears to be recovering. There are also alterations in renal function in patients with liver metastases, thereby supporting the thesis that substances may be produced by a damaged liver independent of the usual evidence of hepatic tissue destruction or jaundice, and yet may have the capacity to produce HRS [41]. Thus, one might postulate that the release of the humoral agent is a consequence not of general hepatocellular insult per se, but rather of some other aspect of hepatic abnormality. At the present time, there is insufficient evidence for the proof of the role of a humoral substance, but it remains a distinct possibility.

Some of the humoral agents under consideration are vasodilator material, jaundiced serum, false neurotransmitters, endotoxins, the renin-angiotensin system, prostaglandin deficiency, vasoactive intestinal polypeptide, and the kallikrein-kinin system.

10.2.1 Vasodilator Material (VDM) VDM was described in the 1930s by Shorr et al. to inhibit the vasoconstrictor actions of epinephrine on the rat mesappendix [40]. This material, subsequently identified as ferritin, has its highest serum levels in the presence of hepatitis. It seems unlikely that it plays a significant role as a humoral agent in HRS.

10.2.2 Jaundiced Serum The relation of jaundice or some constituent of jaundiced serum to renal function in general and to HRS specifically is not defined [29]. As already stated, HRS may develop while jaundice is actually decreasing, or renal failure may occur in the presence of very minimal jaundice. However, some other material that accumulates in jaundiced blood may conceivably sensitize the renal circulation of a cirrhotic patient to other vasoconstrictor influences [42]. This has been suggested for patients and animals with obstructive jaundice. For example, experiments performed in the rat with only unconjugated hyperbilirubinemia showed no difference in the incidence of ischemia-induced renal impairment between animals with and those without bile duct ligation (without conjugated bilirubin) [43], while Wistar rats with bile duct ligation and conjugated hyperbilirubinemia exhibited a very high incidence of renal failure [44]. These observations suggested that the high levels of conjugated bilirubin or bile acids render the kidney more susceptible to ischemia. Other studies in baboons with obstructive jaundice may also be relevant. Perfusion of the rabbit isolated kidney with plasma obtained from jaundiced baboons evokes an increased pressor response to norepinephrine. Whether or not this is a nonspecific finding is not clear. Other studies indicate relative cortical ischemia and increased sensitivity to norepinephrine during xenon-clearance studies in the jaundiced primates [13]. Hence, the vascular response to norepinephrine may be potentiated by something in the plasma of baboons with obstructive jaundice. Perfusion with betalipoproteins from the serum of jaundiced baboons also resulted in enhanced vasoconstriction. Many observations indicating greater predilection for the development of ATN in people with obstructive jaundice suggest that the renal circulation is vulnerable in the presence of obstructive jaundice [29]. The relevance of these observations to HRS, where there is generally some degree of intrahepatic obstruction but the liver disease is primarily parenchymal, is unknown.

10.2.3 False Neurotransmitters Mashford et al. [45] administered tyramine and norepi-

nephrine to patients with cirrhosis. While normotensive, nonazotemic cirrhotics had a "normal" blood pressure response, patients with HRS had a diminished blood pressure response. On this background of possible depleted stores of epinephrine, Fischer and Baldessarini [46] have speculated that potently vasoactive amines such as norepinephrine and dopamine are replaced in HRS by relatively inactive amines, i.e., "false" neurotransmitters such as octopamine and phenylethanolamine. The latter amines are postulated to derive from bacteria in the gut that are shunted into the systemic circulation. The proponents of this theory view it as consistent with the transient beneficial effects on renal function observed following administration of the sympathomimetic amine metaraminol, with the latter drug functioning as a substitute transmitter. On the other hand, intravenous infusions of dopamine do not substantially change filtration rate or urine flow, although there is an increase in renal plasma flow. The evidence supporting the false transmitter thesis, in my judgment, is neither confirmed nor established. Since the α-adrenergic activity of the kidney is vasoconstrictor, a false transmitter might be expected to cause less rather than more vasoconstriction as characterizes HRS.

10.2.4 Endotoxins Endotoxins, the lipopolysaccharide constituents of the cell wall of certain bacteria, are potent renal vasoconstrictors [47]. It has been postulated that endotoxins derived from intestinal bacteria may reach the systemic circulation in large amounts in cirrhosis and cause HRS. Indeed, investigators have shown a correlation between the level of endotoxins in the blood and renal failure in cirrhosis [48]. But more recent observations question such a relationship [49, 50]. The Limulus tests for endotoxin have variations, and their individual accuracy is controversial. A correlation with renal failure in cirrhosis may reflect retention of endotoxins rather than a causal relation of endotoxins to HRS. Endotoxemia is appealing as a possible humoral agent not only because it may cause renal vasoconstriction, but also because it may produce vasodilatation in other circulatory beds and offers the possibility of therapeutic value. Over 20 years ago,

Dr. Wesley Spink indicated personally to the author the likeness of HRS to "slow endotoxin shock." Nonetheless, endotoxemia is far from established as playing a role in the pathogenesis of HRS.

10.2.5 Renin-Angiotensin System The renin-angiotensin system has found its way into consideration in the pathogenesis of the hepatorenal syndrome. It is known that plasma renin activity is increased in the hepatorenal syndrome, it is also known that plasma concentration of renin substrate normally produced by the liver and kidney is decreased in most patients with cirrhosis of the liver. There is experimental evidence that high renin levels within the kidney may produce afferent renal vasoconstriction through unknown mechanisms. The persistence of high renin levels in cirrhosis has at least two theoretical explanations. First, there may be the perception by the kidney of a reduction in effective extracellular volume, which stimulates renin release. Second, the thesis has been presented that the reduction in substrate results in reduced angiotensin levels, that the normal inhibitory feedback mechanism is therefore impaired, and that renin secretion continues [51]. In fact, Berkowitz et al. have postulated that reduced renin substrate is the primary cause of renal vasoconstriction in HRS [51]. The levels of angiotensin II that are generated in the face of low substrate and high renin levels are debated. If angiotensin II is elevated as some believe it is, rather than reduced, there is reason to ask whether increased angiotensin II can cause the vasoconstriction observed in HRS. There is evidence that angiotensin does not cause constriction of the interlobular and arcuate arteries; vasoconstriction of these vessels is present in HRS [52]. It is certainly possible that the increased plasma renin levels are not the cause of the renal ischemia, but are rather the consequence of renal ischemia. This interpretation of the data is consistent with the observation that dopamine-induced increases in renal blood flow in cirrhosis are accompanied by decreased plasma renin activity. Furthermore, salarasin, an antagonist of endogenous angiotensin II, failed to improve renal function in three patients with HRS [53].

The studies of Schroeder et al. [54] are of considerable interest. They studied patients with HRS before and after peritoneovenous or portacaval shunt. In the patients who survived the surgery, the previously elevated plasma renin activities became normal and the reduced levels of renin substrate increased. Before surgery, saralasin produced hypotension and increased renin levels and was without effect postoperatively. Renal function improved significantly postoperatively. Plasma volume and cardiac output also rose although they were not low preoperatively. Schroeder et al. believed their data were most consistent with a surgically induced expansion of "effective" plasma volume and secondary improvement in renal function and suppression of renin. The data are perhaps most consistent with hyperreninemia and reduced substrate as consequences rather than causes of the renal vasoconstriction.

However, there is no final answer on the role of the renin-angiotensin system in HRS either as a physiologic response to volume contraction or in the context of a humoral agent.

10.2.6 Prostaglandins The role of prostaglandins in HRS is unknown although some interesting data are developing. Some studies suggest increased PGE levels in cirrhosis [55, 56]. Boyer, Zia, and Reynolds [57] reported that indomethacin, an effective inhibitor of prostaglandin synthetase, causes a decrease in glomerular filtration rate and renal plasma flow in patients with cirrhosis and ascites. Zipser et al. [55] also noted that inhibition of prostaglandin synthetase with indomethacin and ibuprofen was followed by a 57% reduction in creatinine clearance in patients with cirrhosis. These observations suggest that a failure in prostaglandin synthesis or release may be a factor in the causation of HRS. While exogenous prostaglandins have not proved beneficial to date, the relevance of such an experimental design in evaluating the role of a local tissue hormone has been challenged. More studies on enhancing endogenous prostaglandins might be of greater interest.

10.2.7 Vasoactive Intestinal Polypeptide Said et al. [58] isolated from the small bowel a vasoactive intestinal polypeptide (VIP) that produced some of the common hemodynamic changes of cirrhosis when injected into experimental animals: peripheral vasodilatation, increased cardiac output, pulmonary shunting, and hyperventilation. Hunt et al. [59] have confirmed the earlier work of Said's group indicating that VIP blood levels are often elevated in cirrhosis. However, VIP levels are elevated in renal failure in the absence of cirrhosis, adding to the difficulty in studying any causal relationship between HRS and VIP. The unconfirmed studies of Espinel et al. [60] (presented in abstract form), in which varying doses of VIP were injected into conscious rats and renal function studied, are interesting. At lower doses, VIP caused an increase in GFR and RPF, as well as sodium excretion, reminiscent of the supernormal hemodynamics sometimes seen in cirrhosis. At larger doses of VIP, there was a substantial reduction in renal hemodynamics and sodium excretion. These are intriguing data, but even if confirmed, they do not prove that VIP is relevant to the genesis of HRS.

10.2.8 Kallikrein-Kinin System Bradykinin levels are reduced in cirrhosis, perhaps due to liver dysfunction. Wong et al. [61] have noted that functional plasma prekallikrein is reduced even further in patients with HRS. Plasma bradykinin was also reduced. Wong's group speculates that perhaps the kinin deficiency induces a decrease in vasodilator activity. If one administers large amounts of bradykinin intravenously in normal subjects, there is a rise in RPF, possibly mediated by increased release of certain prostaglandins. Whether or not bradykinin deficiency can play a role in the genesis of HRS cannot be stated.

10.2.9 Tubuloglomerular Feedback Because of the close anatomic proximity of the macula densa to the juxtaglomerular apparatus, Thurau and Schnermann [62] investigated a functional relationship between the two. They found that increasing the sodium load in the macula densa resulted in a decrease in glomerular filtration. This "tubuloglomerular feedback" mechanism seemed capable of serving homeostatic purposes (see chapter 1). The question has also been raised about its possible role in the pathogene-

sis of various forms of acute renal failure. Wunderlich et al. [63] have shown that treated sera from patients with liver dysfunction and acute renal failure perfused through Henle's loop enhance the tubuloglomerular feedback system in rats, thus resulting in greater reductions in GFR than serum from a normal subject or from patients with prerenal azotemia. Although this requires more investigation, it is consistent with a "humoral" material capable of adversely altering renal function.

Figure 11–1 presents an entirely conjectural outline of how a humoral agent might fit into the scheme of things. It also indicates how a humoral agent and a decrease in effective volume secondary both to alterations in extrarenal distribution of blood and to reduced intake and excess loss of fluid and solute might operate together to influence the evolution of HRS. In addition, figure 11–1 attempts to demonstrate the similarity and differences of HRS and renal hypoperfusion ("prerenal" azotemia) without the hepatorenal syndrome. The scheme also suggests how decreased effective plasma volume might not only simulate but also aggravate and perhaps precipitate the hepatorenal syndrome. Finally, the figure depicts the possible relationship of HRS to the development of ATN in patients with liver disease with or without HRS.

In summary, the data suggest that renal failure in cirrhosis is due to a circulatory mechanism characterized by afferent renal vasoconstriction, relative cortical ischemia, and an unstable renal arterial circulation. Although the precise nature of the circulatory disturbance is not evident, one must consider three possibilities: (a) that the observed renal circulatory disturbances are a physiologic response to altered extrarenal distribution of blood; (b) that there may be a humoral agent(s) capable of producing both extrarenal alterations in blood distribution and intrarenal circulatory modifications; and (c) that it is possible that both of these mechanisms are operative.

11 Treatment

Treatment may be divided into three categories: prevention, initial phase therapy, and treatment when HRS is fully established.

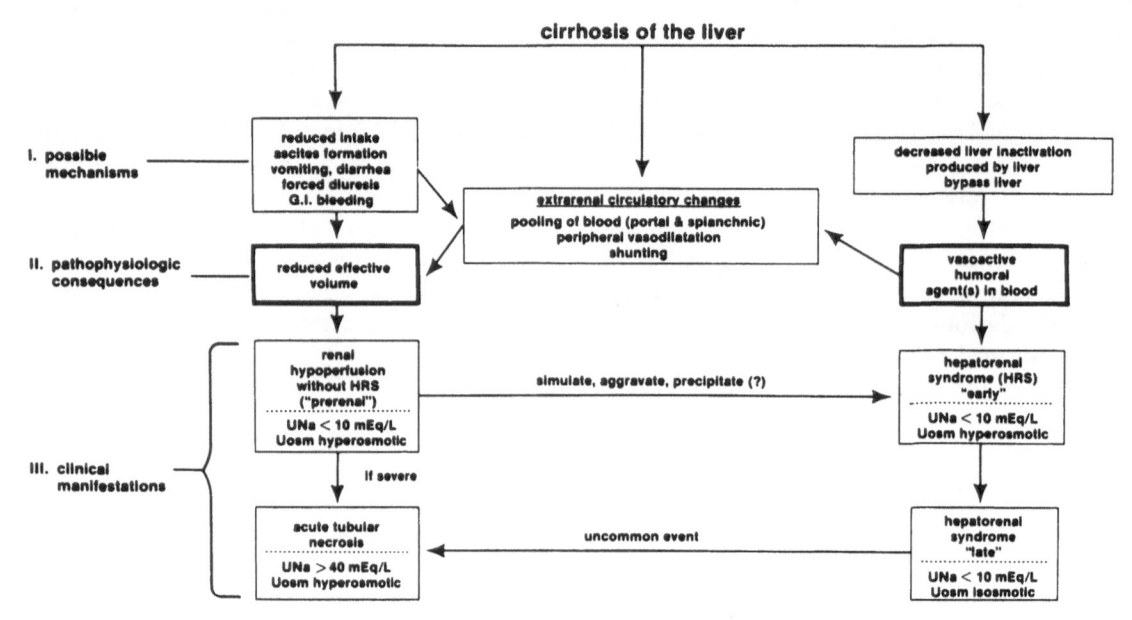

FIGURE 11–1. A conjectural formulation of the interrelationships of hypoperfusion and a humoral agent in the genesis of hepatorenal syndrome (HRS)

11.1 PREVENTION

In the absence of known causes, it is difficult to know with certainty how to prevent the development of HRS. A few points are reasonable:

a. Many data indicate reduced effective circulating volume in cirrhosis. Therefore, one should avoid any further reduction in volume that might reduce renal perfusion. For example, paracentesis beyond diagnostic and therapeutic requirements should be avoided. Diuretics should be used in a manner that results in a slow and gradual diuresis of no more than 0.5 kg daily, rather than as aggressive, forced diuresis.

b. Because of data suggesting that certain nonsteroidal anti-inflammatory agents may lower GRF in unstable cirrhosis, these drugs should be avoided.

c. Nephrotoxic drugs and radiographic contrast materials may theoretically be more dangerous in the face of kidneys prone to underperfusion. Their use, therefore, may require the most stringent indications.

11.2 INITIAL PHASE THERAPY

a. The first step is to be certain that one is not dealing exclusively or significantly with reversible volume depletion, which may be present despite edema and ascites. There are many ways to accomplish this. We prefer normal saline until the central venous pressure is 8 to 10 cm water. If an increase in GFR and diuresis occur, volume is maintained at the effective level. Colloid solutions may be used in place of normal saline but offer no known advantage as far as the observed transient response to volume expansion is concerned. Such expansion must be undertaken with special caution because excessive expansion may not only worsen ascites and edema, but increase portal pressure and the risk of variceal bleeding.

b. Consider the possibility of other causes of renal failure—especially treatable ones, such as obstruction, infection, nephrotoxic agents, heart failure, and unrelated primary renal disease aggravated by the presence of liver disease.

c. If dialysis has any role, it may be that of allowing time for a full assessment in an unclear clinical situation. In that event, a single dialysis should suffice [64].

11.3 TREATMENT OF ESTABLISHED HRS

When HRS is clearly established, treatment is very unsatisfactory. The following approaches may be summarized [11–16]:

a. The ideal approach is to improve liver function; sadly, this is seldom possible. Liver transplantation remains experimental although results have improved substantially in recent years.

b. The expansion of volume beyond repair of deficits with blood, plasma, albumin, dextran, and saline has not been useful.

c. Vasoactive drugs are without sustained benefit. Although low-dose dopamine is commonly used, its general usefulness is not established.

d. Corticosteroids are now undergoing controlled study and should not presently be used because of potential risk pending the results of the study [20].

e. Abdominal paracentesis with or without reinfusion of ascitic fluid has not proved beneficial [65].

f. Treatment with conventional intermittent hemodialysis and peritoneal dialysis has not been effective [66, 67]. Further testing is needed employing the membranes that remove larger molecules and with hemoperfusion. There is one optimistic report employing hemodialysis and charcoal hemoperfusion in one patient [68].

g. Fresh plasma to replenish renin substrate has failed to result in improvement [51]. Exchange transfusions are not useful. I know of no published experience with plasmaphoresis.

h. Polymyxin B, an antibiotic with anti-endotoxin effect, has been alleged to result in improvement in renal function in some instances [69]. However, the polymyxins are quite nephrotoxic. I do not believe this is currently acceptable therapy.

i. The parenteral administration of prostaglandin A_1 and the intrarenal use of prostaglandin E_1 were not effective for patients with severe renal failure [56, 70].

j. There have been isolated reports of recovery from HRS following portasystemic anastomosis [11, 71]. Schroeder's group describes the results in five carefully studied patients [54]. Three died within one to eight weeks postoperatively, while two patients are well two and ten years after the surgery. On the other hand, portacaval anastomosis has been reported to initiate renal failure [72] or to be of no value therapeutically [73]. If portasystemic anastomosis is useful in HRS, the mechanism of its efficacy is not known. It may be due to improving the effective circulation by decompressing the splanchnic pool or to some other mechanism. Even if valuable for individual patients, it would be important to have means of selecting those who might tolerate the surgery and benefit from it. For most of our patients, the risk would be prohibitive.

k. The peritoneal jugular-venous shunt (PVS) has received much attention as effective therapy for HRS [74–76]. In evaluating the results of PVS, it is especially important to distinguish between HRS and prerenal azotemia with a test of expanding effective volume as described earlier. Unfortunately, this has not regularly been done in the reported studies. One would not be surprised to find improvement in renal function in pure prerenal azotemia following continuous transfer of ascitic fluid into the circulation. Schroeder et al. have treated five patients with PVS [54]. In two patients, the shunt clotted; in one a second PVS was placed while the other was treated with a mesocaval shunt. Of the four patients who were left with a PVS in place, one died in ten weeks and the other three remained improved three months to one and one-half years after the surgery. Further evidence for the possible effectiveness of the procedure is to be found in those instances of initial improvement after PVS followed by deterioration when the shunt clotted, and when improvement occurred again after a second effective shunt was placed [54, 77]. There is need for a systematic investigative approach to the possible role of PVS in the treatment of established HRS, as defined in the text under 8 *section on diagnostic criteria* [78]. We are currently engaged in such a study. As in any other experimental treat-

248

ment, all advantages and disadvantages must be assessed. Complications of PVS include clotting, infection, volume overload, and intravascular coagulation. If PVS proves effective, the mechanism remains unclear; it might be due to the re-establishment of effective circulating volume or by infusing some physiologically important material contained in the ascitic fluid. Until appropriate studies are completed, PVS should not be assumed to be of proved usefulness in the treatment of HRS.

The best approach for the clinician at present is not to equate renal functional impairment in cirrhosis with the development of HRS in any individual patient. Rather, we should search for treatable causes of decreased renal function.

12   Summary

A specific variety of renal failure may develop in the course of patients with parenchymal liver disease of diverse etiology. I refer only to this renal failure as the hepatorenal syndrome. It occurs in the absence of other causes of renal failure and early on has the renal functional characteristics of an hypoperfused kidney, including a concentrated urine and low urine sodium concentration. However, HRS does not respond to expansion of effective volume as prerenal azotemia does. If the renal changes are progressive, there are defined alterations in renal function, including a concentrated urine becoming isoosmotic while urine sodium concentration remains low. Acute tubular necrosis is an uncommon consequence of HRS.

While the development of renal failure in general bears a poor prognosis, spontaneous recovery can occur. The data suggest that, for the most part, patients die "in" rather than "of" renal failure. The latter seems to be only part of a broader, more fundamental disturbance. While the evidence supports an impairment of effective renal perfusion, the precise pathogenetic factor or factors in generating impaired renal circulation are not known. Treatment is currently unsatisfactory although the peritoneal jugular-venous shunt warrants and is receiving detailed investigation. Emphasis in individual

patients is presently best placed on searching for more treatable causes of renal functional impairment in individual patients.

References

1. Flint A. Clinical report on hydro-peritoneum, based on an analysis of forty-six cases. Am J Med Sci 45: 306–339, 1863.
2. Helwig FC, Schutz CB. A liver kidney syndrome. Clinical, pathological and experimental studies. Surg Gynecol Obstet 55: 570–580, 1932.
3. Hecker R, Sherlock S. Electrolyte and circulatory changes in terminal liver failure. Lancet 2: 1121–1125, 1956.
4. Papper S. The role of the kidney in Laënnec's cirrhosis of the liver. Medicine (Baltimore) 37: 299–316, 1958.
5. Papper S, Belsky JL, Bleifer KH. Renal failure in Laënnec's cirrhosis of the liver: I. Description of clinical and laboratory features. Ann Intern Med 51: 759–773, 1959.
6. Vesin P. Late functional renal failure in cirrhosis with ascites: Pathophysiology, diagnosis and treatment. In Aktuelle Probleme der Hepatologie, Martini GA, Sherlock S (eds). Stuttgart: Georg Thieme Verlag, 1962, pp. 98–109.
7. Baldus WP, Feichter RN, Summerskill WHJ, Hunt JC, Wakim KG. The kidney in cirrhosis: II. Disorders of renal function. Ann Intern Med 60: 366–377, 1964.
8. Shear L, Kleinerman J, Gabuzda GJ. Renal failure in patients with cirrhosis of the liver: I. Clinical and pathologic characteristics. Am J Med 39: 184–198, 1965.
9. Bartoli E, Chiandussi L (eds). Hepato-Renal Syndrome. Padova, Italy: Piccin Medical Books, 1979.
10. Editorial. Hepatorenal syndome or hepatic nephropathy? Lancet 1(8172): 801–803, 1980.
11. Conn HO. A rational approach to the hepatorenal syndrome. Gastroenterology 65: 321–340, 1973.
12. Papper S. Renal failure in cirrhosis (the hepatorenal syndrome). In the Kidney in Liver Disease, Epstein M (ed). New York: Elsevier-North Holland, 1978, pp. 91–112.
13. Epstein M (ed). The Kidney in Liver Disease. New York: Elsevier-North Holland, 1978.
14. Vaamonde CA, Papper S. The kidney in liver disease. In Strauss and Welt's Diseases of the Kidney (3rd ed), Earley LE, Gottschalk CW (eds). Boston: Little, Brown, and Company, 1979, pp. 1289–1317.
15. Papper S. Hepatorenal syndrome. Contri Nephrol 23: 55–74, 1980.
16. Papper S. Hepatorenal syndrome. In The Liver in Kidney Disease (2nd ed), Epstein M (ed). New York: Elsevier Science Publishing Co., Inc., 1983 pp. 87–106.
17. Koppel MH, Coburn JW, Mims MM, Goldstein

H, Boyle JD, Rubini ME. Transplantation of cadaveric kidneys from patients with hepatorenal syndrome. Evidence for the functional nature of renal failure in advanced liver disease. N Engl J Med 280: 1367–1371, 1969.

18. Iwatsuki S, Popovtzer MM, Corman JL, Ishikawa M, Putnam CW, Katz FH, Starzl TE. Recovery from "hepatorenal syndrome" after orthotopic liver transplantation. N Engl J Med 289: 1155–1159, 1973.

19. Reynolds TB. The hepatorenal syndrome. In The Liver and Its Diseases, Schaffner F, Sherlock S, Leevy CM (eds). New York: Intercontinental Medical Book Corp, 1974, pp. 307–313.

20. Gordon JA, Anderson RJ. Hepatorenal syndrome. Seminars in Nephrology 1(1): 37–41, 1981.

21. Arras S, Faedda R, Satta A, Saggia G, Olmeo N, Bartoli E. Retrospective analysis of the incidence of the hepato-renal syndrome in patients with liver disease. In Hepato-Renal Syndrome, Bartoli E, Chiandussi L (eds). Padova, Italy: Piccin Medical Books, 1979, pp. 427–451.

22. Hall PW III, Ricanati ES. Renal handling of beta-2-microglobulin in renal disorders: With special reference to hepatorenal syndrome. Nephron 27(2): 62–66, 1981.

23. Epstein M, Berk DP, Hollenberg NK, Adams DF, Chalmers TC, Abrams HL, Merrill JP. Renal failure in the patient with cirrhosis. The role of active vasoconstriction. Am J Med 49: 175–185, 1970.

24. Epstein M, Schneider N, Befeler B. Relationship of systemic and intrarenal hemodynamics in cirrhosis. J Lab Clin Med 89: 1175–1187, 1977.

25. Berger J, Yaneva H, Nabana B. Glomerular changes in patients with cirrhosis of the liver. In Advances in Nephrology, vol. 7, Hamburger J, Crosnier J, Grunfeld J-P, Maxwell MH (eds). Chicago: Year Book Medical Publishers, 1977, pp. 3–14.

26. Wilkinson SP, Williams R. Defining "hepatorenal syndrome." In Hepato-Renal Syndrome, Bartoli E, Chiandussi L (eds). Padova, Italy: Piccin Medical Books, 1979, pp. 21–34.

27. Wilkinson SP, Portmann B, Hurst D, Williams R. Pathogenesis of renal failure in cirrhosis and fulminant hepatic failure. Postgrad Med J 51: 503–505, 1975.

28. Odell GB, Natzschka JC, Storey GNB. Bilirubin nephropathy in the Gunn strain of rat. Am J Physiol 212: 931–938, 1967.

29. Better OS, Berl T. Jaundice and the kidney. In The Kidney in Systemic Disease (2nd ed), Suki WN, Eknoyan G (eds). New York: John Wiley, 1981, pp. 521–537.

30. Lancestremere RG, Klingler EL Jr, Frisch E, Papper S. Simultaneous determination of cardiac output and renal function in patients with Laënnec's cirrhosis during the administration of the pressor amine, metaraminol. J Lab Clin Med 61: 820–825, 1963.

31. Murray JF, Dawson AM, Sherlock S. Circulatory changes in chronic liver disease. Am J Med 24: 358–367, 1958.

32. Lieberman FL, Reynolds TB. Plasma volume in cirrhosis of the liver: Its relation to portal hypertension, ascites, and renal failure. J Clin Invest 46: 1297–1208, 1967.

33. Fazekas JF, Tictin HE, Ehrmantrant WR, Alman RW. Cerebral metabolism in hepatic insufficiency. Am J Med 21: 843–849, 1956.

34. Tristani FE, Cohn JN. Systemic and renal hemodynamics in oliguric hepatic failure: Effect of volume expansion. J Clin Invest 46: 1894–1906, 1967.

35. Epstein M. Renal sodium handling in cirrhosis: A reappraisal. Nephron 23: 211–217, 1979.

36. Reynolds TB, Lieberman FL, Redeker AG. Functional renal failure with cirrhosis: The effect of plasma expansion therapy. Medicine (Baltimore) 46: 191–196, 1967.

37. Barnado DE, Summerskill WHJ, Strong CG, Baldus WP. Renal function, renin activity and endogenous vasoactive substances in cirrhosis. Am J Dig Dis 15: 419–425, 1970.

38. Baldus WP. Etiology and management of renal failure in cirrhosis and portal hypertension. Ann NY Acad Sci 170: 267–278, 1969.

39. Lancet Paris Correspondent. The antitoxin functions of the liver. Lancet 2: 1092–1093, 1893.

40. Shorr E. Hepatorenal vasotropic factors in experimental cirrhosis. In Transactions of the 6th Conference on Liver Injury, May 1–2, 1947. New York: Josiah Macy Foundation, 1947, pp. 33–39.

41. Kew MC, Limbrick CA, Varma RR, Williams HS, Sherlock S. Renal blood flow in malignant disease of the liver. Gut 13: 421–426, 1972.

42. Bloom D, McCalden TA, Rosendorff C. Effects of jaundiced plasma on vascular sensitivity to noradrenalin. Kidney Int 8: 149–157, 1975.

43. Baum M, Stirling GA, Dawson JL. Further study into obstructive jaundice and ischemic renal damage. Br Med J 2: 229–231, 1969.

44. Dawson JL. Jaundice and anorexic renal damage: Protective effect of mannitol. Br Med J 1: 810–811, 1964.

45. Mashford ML, Mahon WA, Chalmers TC. Studies of the cardiovascular system in the hypotension of liver failure. N Engl J Med 267: 1071–1074, 1962.

46. Fischer JE, Baldessarini RJ. False neurotransmitters and hepatic failure. Lancet 2: 75–80, 1971.

47. Gillenwater JY, Dooley ES, Frohlich ED. Effects of endotoxin on renal function and hemodynamics. Am J Physiol 205: 293–297, 1963.

48. Clemente C, Rodes J, Bosch J, Arroyo V, Mas A, Teres J. Functional renal failure in cirrhosis. A possible role for endotoxin? Digestion (abstract) 12: 295, 1975.

49. Gatta A, Milani L, Merkel C, Amodio P, Caregaro L, Zuin R (letter to editor). Lancet 2(8237): 101–102, 1981.

50. Fulenwider, JT, Sibley C, Stein SF, Evatt B, Nordlinger BM, Ivey GL. Endotoxemia in cirrhosis; an

observation not substantiated. Gastroenterology 78: 1001–1004, 1980.

51. Berkowitz HD, Miller LD, Rosato E. Renin substrate depletion in the hepatorenal syndrome. N Engl J Med 290: 461, 1974.

52. Elkin M, Meng CH. The effects of angiotensin on renal vascularity in dogs. Am J Roentgenol 98: 927–934, 1966.

53. Arroyo V, Bosch J, Rodes J. The renin-angiotensin system in cirrhosis. In Hepato-Renal Syndrome, Bartoli E, Chiandussi L (eds). Padova, Italy: Piccin Medical Books, 1979, pp. 201–227.

54. Schroeder ET, Anderson GH Jr, Smulyan H. Effects of portacaval or peritoneovenous shunt on renin in the hepatorenal syndrome. Kidney Int 15: 54–61, 1979.

55. Zipser RD, Hoefs JC, Speckart PF, Zia PK, Horton R. Prostaglandins: Modulators of renal function and pressor resistance in chronic liver disease. J Clin Endocrinol Metab 48: 895–900, 1979.

56. Zusman RM, Axelrod L, Tolkoff-Rubin N. The treatment of the hepatorenal syndrome with intrarenal administration of prostaglandin E_1. Prostaglandins 13: 819–830, 1977.

57. Boyer TD, Zia P, Reynolds TB. Effect of indomethacin and prostaglandin A_1 on renal function plasma renin activity in alcoholic liver disease. Gastroenterology 77: 215–222, 1979.

58. Said SI, Mutt V. Polypeptide with broad biological activity: Isolation from small intestine. Science 169: 1217–1218, 1970.

59. Hunt S, Vaamonde CA, Rattassi T, Berian G, Said SI, Papper S. Circulating levels of vasoactive intestinal polypeptide in liver disease. Arch Intern Med 139: 994–996, 1979.

60. Espinel CH, Said SI, Maklouf GM. Different effects of the peptide homologues, VIP (vasoactive intestinal polypeptide) and glucagon on renal transport and hemodynamics (abstract). Clin Res 24: 36A, 1976.

61. Wong PY, Talamo RC, Williams GH. Kallikrein-kinin and renin-angiotensin systems in functional renal failure of cirrhosis of the liver. Gastroenterol 73: 1114–1118, 1977.

62. Thurau K, Schnermann J. Die Natriumkonzentration an den Macula densa-Zellen als regulierender Faktor fur das Glomerulumfiltrat. Klin Wochenschr 43: 410–413, 1965.

63. Wunderlich PF, Brunner FP, Davis JM, Haberle, DA, Tholen H, Thiel G. Feedback activation in rat nephrons by sera from patients with acute renal failure. Kidney Int 17: 497–506, 1980.

64. Perez GO, Oster JR. A critical review of the role of

dialysis in the treatment of liver disease. In The Kidney in Liver Disease, Epstein M (ed). New York: Elsevier-North Holland, 1978, pp. 325–336.

65. Levy VG, Opolon P, Pauleau N, Caroli J. Treatment of ascites by reinfusion of concentrated peritoneal fluid—review of 318 procedures in 210 patients. Postgrad Med J 51: 564–566, 1975.

66. Wilkinson SP, Weston MJ, Parsons V, Williams R. Dialysis in the treatment of renal failure in patients with liver disease. Clin Nephrol 8: 287–292, 1977.

67. Ring-Larsen H, Clausen E, Ranek L. Peritoneal dialysis in hyponatremia due to liver failure. Scand J Gastroenterol 8: 33–40, 1973.

68. Krumlovsky FA, del Greco F, Niederman M. Prolonged hemoperfusion and hemodialysis in management of hepatic failure and hepatorenal syndrome. Trans Am Soc Artif Intern Organs 24: 235–238, 1978.

69. Wilkinson SP. Endotoxins and liver disease. Scand J Gastroenterol 12: 385–386, 1977.

70. Arieff AI, Chidsey CA. Renal function in cirrhosis and the effects of prostaglandin A_1. Am J Med 56: 695–703, 1974.

71. Schroeder ET, Numann PJ, Chamberlain BE. Functional renal failure in cirrhosis. Recovery after protocaval shunt. Ann Intern Med 72: 923–928, 1970.

72. Garrett JG, Voorhees AB Jr, Sommers SC. Renal failure following portasystemic shunt in patients with cirrhosis of the liver. Ann Surg 172: 218–225, 1970.

73. Ring-Larsen H, Hesse B, Stigsby B. Effect of portal systemic anastomosis on renal hemodynamics in cirrhosis. Gut 17: 856–860, 1976.

74. Grosberg SJ, Wapnick S. A retrospective comparison on functional renal failure in cirrhosis treated by conventional therapy or the peritoneovenous shunt (LeVeen). Am J Med Sci 276: 287–291, 1978.

75. Plodson TR, Panish RM. Hepatorenal syndrome: Recovery after peritoneovenous shunt. Arch Intern Med 137; 1248–1249, 1977.

76. Berkowitz, HD, Mullen JL, Miller LD, Rosato EF. Improved renal function and inhibition of renin and aldosterone secretion following peritoneovenous (LeVeen) shunt. Surgery 84: 120–126, 1978.

77. Witte MH, Witte CL, Jacobs S, Kut R. Peritoneovenous (LeVeen) shunt: Control of renin-aldosterone system in cirrhotic ascites. JAMA 239: 31–33, 1978.

78. Epstein M. The peritoneovenous shunt in the management of ascites and the hepatorenal syndrome. Gastroenterol 82: 790–799, 1982.

12. MYOGLOBINURIA AND ACUTE RENAL FAILURE

Vittorio E. Andreucci

1 Rhabdomyolysis and Myoglobinuria

Rhabdomyolisis is muscle cell lysis (as hemolysis is lysis of red blood cells) with liberation of cell content into the circulation. As hemolysis liberates hemoglobin, rhabdomyolysis liberates myoglobin. The occurrence of myoglobinuria indicates extensive destruction of striated muscle, that is, the damage of at least 200 grams of normal muscles [1]. That is why myoglobinuria is not prominent after myocardial infarction.

The occurrence of rhabdomyolysis has been supposed to be a rare phenomenon. This is not so. It is a frequent clinical event, but many times it is not recognized because muscular symptoms are slight or absent and/or urine containing myoglobin is so diluted that its color is not different from normal concentrated urine [2]. Furthermore, urinary excretion of myoglobin may be minimal by the time patients reach the hospital. Thus, it may come about that rhabdomyolysis-induced ARF is regarded as ATN of undetermined etiology or even as ARF secondary to glomerulonephritis or to acute interstitial nephritis occurring as a hypersensitivity reaction to antibiotics. Sometimes the condition is recognized by the incidental discovery of elevated serum levels of muscle enzymes. The inconstancy of myoglobinuria in patients with rhabdomyolysis suggests the use of "rhabdomyolysis" rather than "myoglobinuria" to define the syndrome that follows muscle injury.

2 Consequences of Muscle Damage

Rhabdomyolysis allows escape of cell contents into the extracellular fluid: myoglobin; enzymes such as creatine phosphokinase (CPK), glutamic oxoloacetic transaminase (GOT), lactic dehydrogenase (LDH), aldolase; electrolytes such as potassium and phosphate; nucleoproteins and their metabolites and unidentified organic acid(s) [3].

2.1 MYOGLOBIN

Myoglobin is a heme pigment composed of a folded polypeptide (protein) portion, globin, and a prosthetic group, heme, which contains an atom of iron. It is a muscle protein (mol wt 17,800 daltons) that is located in the soluble phase of the sarcoplasma of striated skeletal and cardiac muscles, near the sarcolemma but not bound to it [4, 5]. It is synthesized by muscle ribosomes [6]. Myoglobin normally constitutes 1 to 2% of the wet weight of skeletal muscle, but it may reach 3.5% of the wet weight in highly trained subjects [7].

Only 0.3 mg of myoglobin is released daily from muscles under normal conditions [8]. Normal serum concentrations of myoglobin average 33 ng/ml [9] and do not normally exceed 50 ng/ml [8, 10]. In patients with CRF (serum creatinine greater than 265 μmol/l, 3 mg/dl), serum myoglobin levels have been reported to average 466 ng/ml [9]. In uremic patients on maintenance hemodialysis, mean values of 170 ng/ml [8] and 343 ng/ml [9] have been reported.

For a long time, myoglobin has been regarded as a store for oxygen; it seems, however, that it plays a key role in the transport of oxygen into and within muscle cells through

252

its property of reversibly binding molecular oxygen [2, 11]. The weakness that follows myoglobinuria may therefore be accounted for, at least in part, by the loss of this function [2].

Myoglobin is liberated into the bloodstream by any illness that results in rhabdomyolysis, as hemoglobin is liberated by hemolysis. But while hemolysis is followed by a pink, red, or brownish staining of serum, rhabdomyolysis does not stain the serum. The serum is not stained because hemoglobin is bound to a specific serum protein, haptoglobin, and is excreted into the urine only when the binding haptoglobin is saturated; this occurs when hemoglobin concentration exceeds 100 mg/dl [7]. Thus, when hemolysis is mild, the serum is pink while the urine retains its clear yellow color; when hemolysis is massive, both serum and urine are stained. Following rhabdomyolysis, the myoglobin released from muscle cells is readily filtered and appears in the urine (its clearance is 75% that of creatinine). According to Kagen [11] this occurs despite a myoglobin-binding capacity by human serum (apparently due to either an alpha-2 or a beta globulin) of 23 mg/dl; but at serum levels below this maximum-binding capacity, free and bound myoglobin coexist, so that free myoglobin is readily filtered. Thus, stained urine with unstained serum argues in favor of rhabdomyolysis [7]. In order to detect a high value of serum myoglobin (a serum concentration of 5.6 mg/dl has been reported in rhabdomyolysis-induced ARF) [10], blood samples should be obtained soon after the muscle damage since both urinary excretion of the pigment and its metabolism to bilirubin will normalize serum levels within one to six hours [3]. Quantitative myoglobin assays are usually not suitable for clinical use so that serum myoglobin cannot be measured in clinical practice. As we will discuss later in this chapter, however, serum concentrations of enzymes will readily allow the diagnosis of rhabdomyolysis. On the other hand, it has been demonstrated that serum myoglobin levels can be predicted from serum concentrations of creatine phosphokinase (CPK), glutamic oxaloacetic transaminase (GOT), or lactic dehydrogenase (LDH) [12].

It has been stated that the renal threshold for

myoglobin is as low as 0.3 mg/dl of plasma [2]; according to others, it is as high as 10 mg/dl [13]. The latter value is too high. Apparently, the correct renal threshold is 0.5 to 1.5 mg/dl [3, 11, 12].

Because of the rapid clearance of myoglobin from plasma, serum levels may be normal by the time the patient is hospitalized; on the other hand, the urine appears grossly stained when its myoglobin concentration is greater than 100 mg/dl [3, 7]. When hospitalization occurs a long time after muscle damage, myoglobinuria may not be detected even by orthotolidine dipstick [3] (a method as sensitive as immunodiffusion or immunoelectrophoresis in detecting myoglobin in urine) [7, 14]. In a recent series of 87 episodes of rhabdomyolysis in 77 patients, a negative orthotolidine dipstick test for myoglobin was found in 26% of patients [3].

2.2 CREATINE PHOSPHOKINASE (CPK)

Creatine phosphokinase (CPK) is an enzyme that transfers a high-energy phosphate moiety from phosphocreatine to adenosine diphosphate (ADP) to form adenosine triphosphate (ATP). Thus, it catalyzes, in striated and cardiac muscles, the following reaction

$$ADP + \text{phosphocreatine} \underset{}{\overset{CPK}{\rightleftharpoons}} ATP + \text{creatine}.$$

This reaction is very important for the continuous chemical regeneration of ATP, which is the immediate energy source for muscular contraction and probably also for sarcolemma integrity [2].

Actually, three isoenzymes of CPK have been identified: CPK–BB (brain type, or CPK–I), CPK–MB (intermediate type, or CPK–II), and CPK–MM (muscle type, or CPK–III) [15]. CPK–I and CPK–II are not present in serum; the isoenzyme CPK–MM, which is normally present in serum (normal values up to 125 mU-ml), is responsible for the normal muscle metabolism [16].

Serum CPK (isoenzyme CPK–MM) is increased in conditions of muscle damage. Elevated levels (233.6 mU/ml) have been observed in uremic patients on maintenance hemodialysis (242.3 mU/ml) or peritoneal dialysis (85.2 mU/ml) and have been attributed to uremic myopathy [16].

Following rhabdomyolysis, CPK is released by damaged muscle cells into the extracellular fluid. Serum CPK reaches a peak within 24 hours after muscle injury; then it declines with an approximate half-life of 48 hours [3]. Persistently high levels of CPK indicate continuous muscle injury.

It has been stated that serum CPK is the most sensitive marker of muscle damage, and it may be used (even if there is no myoglobinuria) as the single diagnostic criterion for rhabdomyolysis, when its serum level is at least five times greater than normal and in the absence of cardiac or brain injury [3]. In contrast with the behavior of myoglobin, serum levels of CPK remain high for many days because of its slow clearance; it has been observed that the decline of serum CPK concentration is about 39% of the previous day's value per day [3].

2.3 GLUTAMIC OXALOACETIC TRANSAMINASE (GOT)

Glutamic oxaloacetic transaminase (GOT) is an enzyme that catalyzes the reversible reaction by which oxaloacetate and glutamate interact to form alpha ketoglutarate and aspartate. GOT is in greatest concentration in myocardium and, in decreasing order of concentration, in liver, skeletal muscle, brain, kidney, and other organs.

Serum levels of GOT increase significantly not only after myocardial infarction and hepatocellular necrosis but also following rhabdomyolysis.

2.4 LACTIC DEHYDROGENASE (LDH)

Lactic dehydrogenase (LDH) is a glycolytic enzyme that catalyzes the reversible reaction of pyruvate to lactate in the presence of diphosphopyridine nucleotide (DPN):

$$\text{piruvic acic} + \text{DPNH} + \text{H}^+ \underset{\longleftarrow}{\overset{\text{LDH}}{\rightleftharpoons}} \text{lactic acid} + \text{DPN}$$

LDH is ubiquitous, but it is mainly represented in the cells of myocardium, muscles, liver, and kidney. Its serum concentration,

therefore, is significantly increased in any condition of cell necrosis, mainly myocardial infarction, muscular dystrophy, dermatomyositis, crush syndrome, and hepatic and renal diseases.

2.5 ALDOLASE

Aldolase is a glycolytic enzyme that is present in the serum of normal subjects. Usually the serum levels of aldolase increase in the same conditions in which increase of serum LDH occurs. But aldolase is a more sensitive indicator of muscle damage.

2.6 CREATINE AND CREATININE

Creatine is an amino acid that may be either ingested (exogenous creatinine) or synthesized in the liver from glycine, arginine and methionine and then delivered to the skeletal muscles, which contain most (90 to 98%) of total body creatine. Normal serum concentration of creatine is 15 to 46 μmol/l (0.2–0.6 mg/dl). It plays a key role in the biochemical adaptation of skeletal muscles to provide energy for contraction. As mentioned above, creatine represents a substrate for CPK; with ATP it yields ADP and phosphocreatine; the latter is then available to phosphorylate ADP in order to supply the ATP necessary for muscle contraction. Skeletal muscles contain about 400 mg of creatine per 100 grams of muscle, more than half in the form of phosphocreatine [17].

Creatinuria is normally modest; less than 760 μmol (100 mg) of creatine are usually excreted with urine in 24 hours. Urinary excretion of creatine is increased in hypercatabolic states (fever, hyperthyroidism, starvation, etc.). In patients with rhabdomyolysis, creatine is released in great amounts from damaged muscles and its excretion increases significantly; thus, elevated creatinuria has been observed in normal subjects after intense physical training [18].

A constant percentage (1.5 to 2%) of creatine-phosphocreatine is converted daily into creatinine (the anhydride of creatine) by a nonenzymatic mechanism that is increased by acid pH [19, 20]. Muscle concentration of creatinine is low.

The urinary excretion of creatinine is much greater than that of creatine, ranging from 176 to 265 μmol/kg b.w./day (20 to 30 mg/kg b.w./day) in men and from 88 to 220 μmol/kg b.w./day (10 to 25 mg/kg b.w./day) in women. Normal subjects fed with creatine expand their creatine pool and therefore increase their creatinine excretion in the urine [21]. For this reason, creatinine is influenced by diet as well as by lean body mass [20]. Furthermore, since cooking converts creatine into creatinine, an increase in cooked meat eaten rapidly increases creatinine excretion [20]. In patients with rhabdomyolysis, the urinary excretion of creatinine is also increased soon after the muscle injury [18].

Data from the literature on serum concentration of creatine in patients with renal disease are conflicting. High serum levels have been found in uremic patients [22]. Apparently, as renal function declines, the extrarenal clearance of creatinine increases both by recycling creatinine to creatine and by degrading creatinine to products other than creatine [20]. As demonstrated by Jones and Burnett [23], creatinine is subject to enteric cycling like urea and uric acid; it is secreted into the gastrointestinal tract and metabolized by gut microflora. Creatinine may be converted to either N-methylhydantoin or to creatine; N-methylhydantoin is formed by desimidation of creatinine by creatinine desimidase, and creatine is formed enzymatically by hydration of creatinine by creatinine hydrolase; creatine is further metabolized to urea and sarcosine by the creatine amidinohydrolase [24].

Serum concentrations of creatine and creatinine are greatly increased in patients with ARF secondary to rhabdomyolysis, apparently, much more than usually expected in ARF. We have observed high values of serum creatine with serum creatine–creatinine ratio markedly elevated in patients with posttraumatic ARF and extensive muscle injury [25] (see below). It has been stated that a disproportionately faster rise of serum creatinine (greater than 221 μmol/l/day, 2.5 mg/dl/day) [26] than of BUN is typical of rhabdomyolysis and is indicative of muscle damage [27]. Values of BUN of 18.57 mmol/l (52 mg/dl) or 15 mmol/l (42 mg/dl) with simultaneous values of serum creatinine of 1,202 μmol/l (13.6 mg/dl) and 928 μmol/l

(10.5 mg/dl) with BUN-to-serum-creatinine ratios (BUN/S_{Cr} in mg/dl) of 3.8 and 4, respectively, are striking [27, 28]. BUN/S_{Cr} is approximately 10 in normal subjects and in patients with renal failure (unless uremic patients are on a low-protein diet). According to Knochel [28], these low values of BUN/S_{Cr} are limited to the first 24 hours after muscle injury, normalizing after the second day. There were patients, however, who exhibited a low BUN/S_{Cr} much longer, up to the fourth day [27]. Apparently, part of this markedly elevated serum creatinine derives from creatine released from injured muscle cells and spontaneously dehydrated to creatinine [7]. However, this unexpected behavior of BUN/S_{Cr} has been denied on the basis of clinical [3] and experimental studies [29]. Probably, the contention is due to the lack of constancy of low values of BUN/S_{Cr}; thus, Koffler et al. [26] have observed it in only 7 out of 21 patients with ARF due to nontraumatic rhabdomyolysis.

2.7 POTASSIUM

Since potassium concentration within muscle cells is extremely high (an average of 156 mmol/kg H_2O) [30] as compared to the concentration of the cation in extracellular fluid (and serum), hyperkalemia is expected to occur after rhabdomyolysis. On reviewing the literature, however, Gabow et al. [3] have observed an incidence of hyperkalemia (i.e., serum potassium greater than 5.5 mmol/l) of only 43%; furthermore, only 7 (6 of whom had ARF) of their 77 patients exhibited a serum potassium greater than 5.5 mmol/l. Severe hyperkalemia appears to occur quite frequently in rhabdomyolysis associated with oliguric ARF, particularly in the presence of metabolic acidosis [3, 25, 26].

2.8 PHOSPHORUS

Phosphate concentration in muscle cells is also high (an average of 95 mmol/kg H_2O) [30] as compared to extracellular fluid (and serum). Thus, hyperphosphatemia is expected to occur following extensive skeletal muscle breakdown. When renal function is preserved, however, serum phosphate levels are normal. Hyperphosphatemia is frequently observed in rhabdomyolysis associated with ARF [26]; under such circumstances, serum phosphorus concentration has been found directly correlated with serum anion gap and inversely with serum bicarbonate; this finding suggests that hyperphosphatemia is partly due to phosphorus released from hydrolyzed ATP, which is liberated by damaged muscle cells with some unidentified organic acid(s) responsible for the increase in anion gap [3] (see below).

Hyperphosphatemia may cause calcification of damaged muscles leading to hypocalcemia [31] (see below).

2.9 URIC ACID

The release of great amounts of nucleoproteins and their metabolites after muscle cell destruction can provide adequate substrate to increase urate production in the liver. This mechanism clearly accounts for the marked hyperuricemia observed after rhabdomyolysis. Reduced tubular secretion of uric acid (because of increased production of other organic acids that compete with uric acid for the secretory site in the kidney) may also contribute to hyperuricemia; this may be the case in lactic acidosis following exercise or after ingestion of alcohol; even low doses of aspirin or i.v. infusion of sodium lactate may further increase serum uric acid levels by inhibiting uric acid secretion (see chapter 2, section 13). Obviously, when rhabdomyolysis is followed by ARF, hyperuricemia will become more marked [3, 26]; values as high as 2.97 mmol/l (50 mg/dl) have been observed.

Severe hyperuricemia seems more frequent in cases secondary to unaccustomed strenuous muscular exertion or heat exhaustion [10, 18, 28], to illicit drug (phencyclidine) abuse [32], and to repeated grand mal fits [33]. Apparently, the increased production of uric acid from precursors that have been released by damaged skeletal muscles is associated, in these cases, with reduced renal excretion of uric acid because of the lactic acidosis that follows exertion and epileptic fits.

3 Causes of Rhabdomyolysis

Rhabdomyolysis may be hereditary or sporadic. The hereditary forms of rhabdomyolysis include glycogen diseases with phosphorylase deficiency (McArdle's disease) or with phosphofructokinase deficiency (Tarni's disease), and a disorder of muscle lipid metabolism with a lack of carnitine palmityl transferase [2, 28].

The causes of sporadic rhabdomyolysis include:

a. Exertion. Severe physical exertion in untrained but normal individuals [27, 34] or even in trained subjects, such as marathon runners [35, 36]; generalized or unilateral convulsions (status epilepticus) [37]; agitated delirium [2]; seizures induced by therapeutic or accidental high-voltage electric shock [10, 38].

b. Crush. Compression of muscles by fallen weights with crushing and tearing (wars, earthquakes, auto accidents, etc.) [2, 25, 39–41]; muscle compression by body in deeply comatose individuals: when a position is maintained for hours or days, the compression of muscles and their arterial supply by the body weight may cause ischemic muscle necrosis because of an increase in intramuscular pressures of 26 to 240 mm Hg [42] as may occur in drug abuse (alcohol, heroin, barbiturate) or in carbon monoxide intoxication [2, 42–44].

c. Ischemia. Arterial occlusion by embolus or thrombosis [45]; open-heart surgery or dissecting aneurysm of the aorta [46]; prolonged operation in knee-chest position [47]; compartmental syndrome [48] (i.e., any condition in which the swelling of a muscle within a tight fascial compartment, by causing arterial compression and occlusion, will create a self-perpetuating edema-ischemia cycle, which will result in rhabdomyolysis), such as anterior tibial syndrome [49], or the crush syndrome itself (in which ischemia plays an important pathogenetic role).

d. Metabolic depression or toxicity. Drugs, such as barbiturates or narcotics [2], phenothiazines, haloperidol and tricyclic antidepressants causing neuroleptic malignant syndrome [50], heroin [51, 52], phencyclidine [32]; hypothermia [53]; heat injury [10, 18, 54]; carbon monoxide intoxication [2]; alcoholism [3, 26]; sea snakebite poisoning [55]; allergy to seafood

[13]; potassium depletion [18, 56–59]; ingestion of licorice (with glycyrrhizic acid which has a mineralcorticoid-like action) [60]; administration of carbenoxolone (which also contains glycyrrhizic acid) to treat gastric ulcer [61–63] or amphotericin B [64] (which may act through potassium depletion).

e. Progressive muscle disease and infections affecting muscles. Muscular dystrophy, myotonia congenita, dermatomyositis, and polymyositis [65]; infections such as gangrene, Rocky Mountain spotted fever, Legionnaire's disease [7], or even influenza infection [66, 67].

f. Cause unknown. In some patients, rhabdomyolysis occurs in the absence of any known cause.

Some authors prefer a differentiation between "exertional" and "nonexertional" rhabdomyolysis, basing this classification on relation to strenuous exercise. Others have defined "nontraumatic rhabdomyolysis" as those forms occurring in the absence of overt muscle damage. Actually, quite frequently many factors may contribute to rhabdomyolysis. Thus, in the crush syndrome, while the direct trauma to muscle with crushing and tearing plays a key role in generating muscle damage, other factors may be very important in maintaining and potentiating muscle injury; thus, a compartmental syndrome resulting from the initial insult, by compressing the major arteries, may cause ischemic injury to the muscle; shock and hypotension may further contribute in reducing muscle nutrition. In cases of drug abuse (e.g., alcohol, heroin, barbiturate) or in carbon monoxide intoxication, the metabolic depression effect of drugs or toxins may be combined with a prolonged deep coma in which compression of muscles and their arterial supply will create a crush syndrome.

Physical exertion is more likely to cause rhabdomyolysis in the presence of potassium [59] and/or phosphate depletion [68] through relative muscle ischemia (see below).

4 Pathogenesis of Rhabdomyolysis

Because the frequent occurrence of myoglobinuria in patients with phosphorylase or phosfruktokinase deficiency, Rowland and Penn [2] suggested a common mechanism in the pathogenesis of rhabdomyolysis: the depletion of ATP in muscle cells. When glycogen cannot be utilized (because of hereditary deficit, metabolic depression, strenuous exhausting exercise, etc.) other mechanisms of ATP synthesis are activated, mainly the oxidation of fatty acids in mitochondria. Should these alternative mechanisms be insufficient, cellular ATP would fall. In a similar fashion, ATP production in muscle mitochondria may be severely impaired in other conditions that are usual causes of rhabdomyolysis, such as ischemia, direct trauma, increased pressure on muscular fibers, hypothermia, depressant drugs, carbon monoxide intoxication [2]. Even the rhabdomyolysis that follows potassium depletion (with serum potassium levels as low as 1.4 mmol/l) [57] has been attributed to relative muscle ischemia during even a little muscle exercise [59]. During exercise, the integrity of muscles is preserved by the capacity of blood flow to muscles to increase or to match the metabolic demand. Local changes in pH, or increase in osmolality or in phosphate or potassium concentrations have been implicated as local mediators [59]. Should potassium ion play a main role in causing local hyperemia during muscular exercise [69], potassium depletion would be responsible for an insufficient release of the ion during exercise with a secondary insufficient increase in muscle blood flow; the resulting relative ischemia may cause rhabdomyolysis [11, 59].

Thus, many clinical conditions could cause ARF through potassium depletion: diuretics, licorice ingestion [60], renal tubular acidosis [57], diarrhea or nasogastric drainage [59], carbenoxalone sodium administration [61], amphotericin B [64], heat stroke [58]. The fact that rhabdomyolysis in potassium-deficient states is unusual may be due to the limited muscular activity of those patients who exhibit generalized weakness and paralysis [57].

As mentioned above, phosphate concentration also may be important to regulate muscle perfusion to metabolic demand. Thus, phosphate depletion has been shown to cause rhabdomyolysis [68, 70]; a fall in serum phosphorus level to less than 0.32 mmol/l (1 mg/dl) for one to two days was, in fact, followed by a sharp increase in serum CPK to about 10,000 U/l [71].

ATP is the immediate energy source that drives the active sodium-potassium exchange and sarcolemmal calcium efflux [72]; it is necessary to maintain the integrity of sarcolemma (the muscle cell membrane) [2]. ATP deficiency in muscle cells may cause cytoplasmic sodium and calcium accumulation, severe cellular injury, and myoglobin release, that is, the typical features of rhabdomyolysis.

Optimal sarcoplasmic concentration of ionized calcium is critical for normal muscle function; thus, any impairment in the regulation of sarcoplasmic calcium may cause cell injury [72]. It has been demonstrated that experimental agents that permit accumulation of calcium in muscle cells produce ultrastructural damage characteristic of early rhabdomyolysis; rhabdomyolysis is prevented by the simultaneous administration of verapamil (which prevents calcium accumulation in the cytoplasm) [73]. It has been therefore suggested that when sarcoplasmic calcium is severely elevated, some dormant enzymes that can cause autodestruction are activated [72]. Recently, a calcium-activated neutral protease has been identified in muscle cells, which may cause myofibril dissolution with lesions very similar to those observed in rhabdomyolysis [72, 74]. This neutral protease normally operates in slowly decomposing myofibrillar proteins so that synthetic processes can rebuild them; when calcium concentration in muscle cell protoplasm is elevated, the activity of neutral protease is greatly increased, leading to cell destruction [7].

Other mechanisms may cause accumulation of calcium in muscle cells. Thus, low levels of $1,25(OH)_2D$, which have been observed in patients with rhabdomyolysis-induced ARF [75] may allow high sarcoplasmic concentration of calcium ions [72].

5 Clinical Outcome of Rhabdomyolysis

5.1 SYMPTOMS

In many cases of rhabdomyolysis, the patient is weak, unable to walk, with nausea, vomiting, and severe myalgia, which increases with movement. The muscles may be edematous and tender, frequently with edema and hemorrhagic discoloration of the overlying skin. In severe rhabdomyolysis, tendon reflexes may be absent. If the diaphragm is involved, respiratory failure may occur. There may be fever and, frequently, ARF.

The swelling, tenderness, and edema of the limbs, the myalgia, and extreme weakness are all presumably accounted for by the muscle necrosis secondary to ischemic or toxic injury [2].

5.2 LABORATORY FEATURES

5.2.1 Urinalysis Myoglobin is the first component of urine we should look for when there is a diagnostic suspicion of rhabdomyolysis.

In case of pigmenturia, the differential diagnosis involves porphyria, myoglobinuria, and hemoglobinuria. Porphyria is ruled out by negative benzidine and orthotolidine tests in the urine, which are positive for both other conditions. In hemoglobinuria, the serum is pink (because of the hemoglobin bound to serum haptoglobin) and serum enzymes are normal. In myoglobinuria, the serum is unstained, serum enzymes are greatly elevated, and the urine usually contains no or just a few red blood cells per high-power field on microscopic examination of a centrifuged specimen. For urine to be visibly stained, myoglobin concentration should be at least 100 mg/dl [7]. Thus, a dipstick based on orthotolidine reaction is sufficient in most cases, particularly when history and physical examination argue in favor of rhabdomyolysis. Associated hematuria, however, does not allow the diagnosis of myoglobinuria by the orthotolidine dipstick test. And hematuria is not infrequent; it was present in 32% of 87 episodes of rhabdomyolysis in a recent review [3].

The sensitivity of the orthotolidine dipstick test is very high, ranging from 0.01 to 0.1 mg/dl [7]. Other specific but expensive tests include: hemoagglutination test, immunodiffusion techniques, and immunoelectrophoresis and radioimmunoassay techniques, the latter being the only one more sensitive than the orthotolidine dipstick [76].

Because of the rapid clearance of myoglobin

from plasma, urine myoglobin may not be detected by the time of hospitalization; the absence of myoglobin, therefore, does not exclude the diagnosis of rhabdomyolysis; thus, the orthotolidine dipstick test was found negative in 18% of 87 episodes of rhabdomyolysis [3].

Proteinuria is very frequent; an incidence of 67% has been reported in a single study, but an incidence of 90% resulted from a review of the literature [3]. It is usually a mild proteinuria, only rarely exceeding 3g/24 hours.

5.2.2 Serum Chemistry As mentioned above, serum levels of CPK, GOT, LDH, and aldolase are increased. The rise of serum CPK, in particular, is by itself of diagnostic value when it reaches five times the normal serum level. Hyperkalemia, hyperphosphatemia, and metabolic acidosis usually occur when ARF is present (see below). Severe hyperuricemia is frequent.

Marked hypoalbuminemia may occur in the first days following extensive rhabdomyolysis because of loss of serum albumin due to capillary damage; under such circumstances the i.v. infusion of albumin may increase the edema [7]. In the posttraumatic form of rhabdomyolysis, both hypercatabolism and protein loss through the wound may make the fall in serum albumin even more marked [25] (table 12–1).

Finally, it should be mentioned that leukocytosis (around 20,000/mm^3) has been observed as a frequent feature of rhabdomyolysis and is unrelated to infections [10, 32].

6 Rhabdomyolysis-Induced ARF

In a recent prospective study, 25% of the cases of ARF were reported as associated with nontraumatic rhabdomyolysis [77]. But myoglobinuria is not always associated with ARF. In a recent report, ARF was observed in 33% of patients with rhabdomyolysis, and the presence of myoglobinuria at the time of hospitalization did not predict the development of ARF [3].

In order to identify those patients with rhabdomyolysis who will develop ARF, Gabow et al. [3] have recently suggested a predictive formula:

$$R = 0.7 [K] + 1.1 [Cr] + 0.6 [Alb] - 6.6,$$

where the serum concentration of potassium [K] in mmol/l, creatinine [Cr] in md/dl, and albumin [Alb] in g/dl would predict the risk of ARF in patients with rhabdomyolysis; an R value less than 0.1 indicates a low risk of ARF, while an R value equal to or greater than 0.1 indicates a high risk of ARF; according to the authors, this formula yields a high incidence of false positives but a low incidence of false negatives. It therefore appears important to start immediately those measures (such as saline infusion, mannitol, furosemide) that may prevent ARF (see below).

6.1 PATHOGENESIS

Glycerol-induced ARF is the experimental model that most closely resembles human ARF associated with rhabdomyolysis (see chapter 1, section 5). It is therefore possible that the same factors responsible for the initiation and maintenance of glycerol-induced ARF are involved in the pathophysiology of rhabdomyolysis-induced ARF.

6.1.1 Plasma Volume Contraction and Impairment in Renal Perfusion It is well known that ARF does not necessarily follow single episodes of myoglobinuria, as hemoglobinuria does not invariably lead to ARF after incompatible blood transfusion. Similarly, the i.v. infusion of either myoglobin or hemoglobin does not impair renal function when urine flow is adequate [7]. On the other hand, a severe bout of exercise in a hospital patient induced myoglobinuria and oliguric ARF lasting 14 days [13]. Similarly, exhausting exercise performed in a hot climate with severe dehydration from massive sweating has been reported to be followed by myoglobinuric ARF [18]. It is therefore reasonable to conclude that the occurrence of ARF after muscle injury is not directly related to the amount of myoglobin released from damaged muscles, but is dependent on the combination of predisposing factors such as dehydration, hypotension, and/or shock. The occurrence of severe hypotension and even shock is not uncommon following a traumatic event. Also, in nontraumatic but extensive rhabdomyolysis, even in the absence of frank dehydration or ECV depletion, the associated capillary leak of fluid and circulating albumin into the injured muscle bed may cause plasma volume contraction and the consequent impairment in renal perfusion, in a fashion quite similar to that observed in glycerol-induced ARF in experimental animals (see chapter 1, section 5). That this occurs is demonstrated by the observation that as much as 10 liters of normal saline in the first 12 to 24 hours after injury may be necessary in patients with extensive rhabdomyolysis who were not obviously dehydrated in order to stabilize their blood pressure [7]. External fluid losses, such as vomiting, severe sweating, etc., may further reduce the circulatory volume and greatly favor ARF.

6.1.2 Reduction in K_f A reduction in glomerular capillary ultrafiltration coefficient (K_f) may occur in rhabdomyolysis-induced ARF, but it has not been demonstrated. Reduction in K_f may be secondary to high plasma levels of arginin vasopressin, which have been found in glycerol-induced ARF [78] (see chapter 1, section 5).

6.1.3 Tubular Obstruction Obstructing casts have been observed many times in histologic preparations of renal specimens obtained by renal biopsy or at autopsy of patients with rhabdomyolysis-induced ARF. Widespread tubular obstruction may be responsible for the maintenance of ARF (see chapter 1). Tubular obstruction in ARF associated with rhabdomyolysis may occur by three mechanisms: (a) myoglobin precipitation, (b) toxic epithelial damage with luminal accumulation of cell debris, and (c) deposition of uric acid crystals.

The experimental injection of myoglobin into rabbits has been demonstrated to cause ARF when urine was acid; no impairment of renal function occurred when urine pH was neutral or alkaline [79]. It has therefore been suggested that, in salt-depleted patients with a low urine pH, when myoglobinuria is associated with highly concentrated urine, myoglobin precipitates, causing tubular obstruction.

Some evidence has been provided in favor of a toxic role of heme, which may cause a metabolic injury to tubular epithelium. In vitro studies using kidney slices have demonstrated

that while intact molecules of myoglobin and hemoglobin do not impair tubular transport, free heme does [80].

As mentioned above, muscle injury is frequently followed by marked hyperuricemia. The resulting increase in urinary excretion of uric acid may cause tubular obstruction by uric acid crystals. This mechanism has been postulated as particularly important in cases of rhabdomyolysis-induced ARF secondary to unaccustomed strenuous muscular exertion or heat exhaustion [18] and to epileptic fits [33, 81]. Metabolic acidosis, constantly present in these conditions, predisposes (through the acid urine) to uric acid crystalluria and precipitation of uric acid crystals in the distal tubules and collecting ducts (see chapter 2, section 13). (For this reason, serum uric acid should be monitored and dehydration avoided in patients with repeated epileptic fits) [81].

6.2 CLINICAL OUTCOME

The clinical outcome of nontraumatic rhabdomyolysis-induced ARF is similar to that of other forms of ATN, with the addition of symptoms and laboratory features typical of rhabdomyolysis (see section 5 in this chapter). However, because of the hypercatabolic state due to muscle cell damage, biochemical abnormalities are exaggerated: marked hyperkalemia, hyperuricemia, and hyperphosphatemia are, as a rule, associated with severe metabolic acidosis; under such conditions serum anion gap is markedly elevated, significantly higher than the anion gap of other forms of ARF, suggesting a release of unidentified organic acid(s) from damaged muscle cells [3]. Patients frequently have fever, tachycardia, and leukocytosis even in the absence of infections. Hypocalcemia is very frequent in the oliguric phase, usually followed by hypercalcemia in the diuretic recovery phase. Serum calcium derangement, however, deserves a more detailed analysis (see below). Disseminated intravascular coagulation (DIC) (see chapter 6) is common in major rhabdomyolysis [7]. In these cases, fibrin degradation products (FDP) will be found in serum and urine, in association with thrombocytopenia, hypofibrinogenemia, and prolonged prothrombin time [25].

6.3 SERUM CALCIUM DERANGEMENT

6.3.1 Hypocalcemia Marked hypocalcemia (with serum calcium levels as low as 0.88 mmol/l, 3.5 mg/dl) is an almost constant biochemical feature of the oliguric phase of ARF associated with rhabdomyolysis. It has been observed that the degree of hypocalcemia is strictly related to the severity of hyperphosphatemia, which, in turn, is dependent on the extent of muscle injury [82]. The excessive breakdown of skeletal muscles causes phosphate release; the hyperphosphatemia due to this and phosphate retention (secondary to the fall in renal function) will cause calcium salt deposition in damaged skeletal muscles; traumatized muscles avidly accumulate calcium, especially in conditions of renal failure [31, 83]. Plasma levels of 25-hydroxycholecalciferol (25OH D) in these hypocalcemic patients have been found either low [84] or in the low-normal range [75]. Llach et al. [75] have recently observed very low plasma levels of $1,25(OH)_2D$ (about half of the normal level) associated with marked hypocalcemia, hyperphosphatemia, and increased serum immunoreactive parathyroid hormone (PTH). Since serum phosphate plays a very important role in $1,25(OH)_2D$ synthesis [85], it has been suggested that hyperphosphatemia is the main factor in depressing $1,25(OH)_2D$ production by the malfunctioning kidney [79] and that the low levels of $1,25(OH)_2D$ may cause hypocalcemia through depressed intestinal calcium absorption and skeletal resistance to the calcemic action of PTH [72, 75, 86, 87]; despite the high levels of PTH, therefore, serum calcium remains low. Important roles in depressing $1,25(OH)_2D$ synthesis may also be played by metabolic acidosis (usually severe in rhabdomyolysis-induced ARF) and by insulin resistance, which is characteristic of uremia [72].

In a recent report, the hypocalcemia observed in rhabdomyolysis-induced ARF was not different, either in frequency or in severity, to that observed in ARF without rhabdomyolysis, and 56% of hypocalcemic patients with rhabdomyolysis-induced ARF had normal serum phosphorus [3].

The administration of calcium salts in rhab-domyolysis-induced ARF may result in only a transient correction of hypocalcemia [82]. On the basis of this observation and the possibility that cellular injury is potentiated by elevation of serum calcium (which may favor calcium accumulation in muscle cells), calcium salts should be given only to patients with life-threatening hyperkalemia [7, 72].

6.3.2 Hypercalcemia As hypocalcemia is characteristic of the oliguric phase, hypercalcemia is a typical feature of the diuretic phase of rhabdomyolysis-induced ARF. According to Feinstein et al. [88], in as many as 36 out of 48 patients with hypercalcemia, the ARF was clearly associated with rhabdomyolysis; in the remaining 12 patients, rhabdomyolysis had probably occurred even if not demonstrated.

Hypercalcemia usually occurs during the early stage of the diuretic phase [14, 26, 52, 88–93]. It was more frequently noted during the third to eleventh day of the diuretic phase [26, 89–91, 93]; but it has been observed, in a few cases, 14 [88], 35 [94], and even 55 days [88] after the onset of the diuresis. Its duration varied from 1 to 35 days with a mean of 13 days [88]. On a few occasions only has hypercalcemia been reported in the oliguric period of ARF [95–97].

The pathogenesis of the hypercalcemia during the diuretic phase of rhabdomyolysis-induced ARF is still a matter of debate. Resolution of soft-tissue calcification (i.e., remobilization of calcium salts sequestered in damaged muscles) has been postulated as the main mechanism [14, 26, 96]. Akmal et al. [31] have supported this hypothesis by demonstrating deposition of calcium in the injured muscles during the oliguric phase and disappearance of calcium from muscles during healing. The recovery of the transport system in muscle cells with resumption of renal function may be followed by the release of accumulated calcium from skeletal muscle tissue in sufficient quantity to cause hypercalcemia [72].

Increase in calcium resorption from bone and increase in gut calcium absorption have also been suggested as possible mechanisms [72, 75].

Feinstein et al. [97] have reported high blood levels of $25OH D_3$ in a patient who developed hypercalcemia during the oliguric phase of rhabdomyolysis-induced ARF. Similarly, high blood levels of 25OH D_3 have been associated with hypercalcemia occurring in the diuretic phase; the blood level of 25OH D_3 was normalized when the patient became normocalcemic [88]. It has therefore been suggested that rhabdomyolysis may release vitamin D (which is stored in muscles) from injured muscles into the circulation, thus accounting for the high blood levels of 25OH D_3 and for the consequent hypercalcemia [88].

Llach et al. [75] have recently reported that in patients with rhabdomyolysis-induced ARF, the serum levels of 1,25 $(OH)_2D$, which were very low in the oliguric phase, became elevated in the polyuric phase in association with elevated PTH levels; meanwhile, the high values of serum phosphorus observed in the oliguric phase were normalized in the polyuric phase. This observation has suggested a normalization of vitamin D metabolism by the kidney and a resumption of bone responsiveness to PTH; if this is true, hypercalcemia may have resulted from gut calcium absorption and from bone and soft-tissue resorption [75].

Although hyperparathyroidism does not seem to play an important role in the genesis of hypercalcemia [26, 52, 91, 93, 96], it has been stated that high blood levels of PTH may contribute to hypercalcemia [88].

On the basis of recent studies on the metabolism of immobilized bone and on bone histology, Zabetakis et al. [92] have recently suggested that the hypercalcemia occurring in ARF is not dissimilar from immobilization hypercalcemia. Apparently, immobilized bone has two phases of metabolic activity: the first phase, lasting for six to ten days, is characterized by a decrease in pCO_2 and an increase in blood flow, pH, pO_2, and bone deposition; the second phase is characterized by vascular congestion, a decrease in pH and pO_2, and an increase in bone resorption [92]. Patients with rhabdomyolysis-induced ARF exhibit a prolonged decrease in activity because of severe weakness and myalgia, which increases with movement. It is therefore not surprising that patients with this form of ARF usually exhibit hypercalcemia, which may be accounted for by

increased bone resorption. The occurrence of hypercalcemia in the diuretic phase of ARF is not specifically related to the entity of urine output, but is due to the temporal coincidence of the diuretic phase of ARF with the second phase of immobilized bone metabolism [92]. This hypothesis may well account for the possible occurrence of hypercalcemia during the oliguric phase of ARF, as observed by some authors, when either oliguria lasts longer or bone resorption occurs earlier than usual. In this context, the greater incidence of hypercalcemia in young patients seems to be related to the higher rates of bone turnover [92].

This suggested pathogenetic mechanism for hypercalcemia is corroborated by the case reported by Miach et al. [94]. In this patient with ARF secondary to severe trauma (motor car accident), hypercalcemia (up to 3.75 mmol/l, 15 mg/dl) lasted as long as five months. The patient was compelled to undergo almost complete immobilization for six months because of the need for assisted ventilation, traction for fractured pelvis, septic episodes, and circulatory instability. Metastatic calcification occurred in the liver and skin during the first month after the accident when the serum calcium-phosphate (in mg/100 ml) product was greater than 80. Serum immunoreactive PTH was undetectable, bone biopsy did not suggest hyperparathyroidism, and subtotal parathyroidectomy was unsuccessful in lowering serum calcium; even the administration of calcitonin did not significantly modify hypercalcemia. While mobilization of calcium and phosphate from soft tissues may have contributed to increased serum levels of calcium in this patient, increased bone resorption during the prolonged immobility undoubtedly must have played a primary role; the final normalization of serum calcium during rehabilitation was attributed both to the reincorporation of calcium in bone and to continuous urinary excretion of calcium [94].

All these observations appear to support strongly the extreme heterogeneity and the multifactorial nature of the mechanisms underlying hypercalcemia, occurring in rhabdomyolysis-induced ARF [88].

Acute severe hypercalcemia may cause hypertension with a sharp increase in systolic and diastolic blood pressure, especially when renal function is impaired. This was, for instance, observed by Feinstein et al. [88] in a 17-year-old patient who was normotensive at the end of the oliguric phase, became hypertensive (180/120 mm Hg) when hypercalcemia (peak serum calcium of 3.9 mmol/l, 15.6 mg/dl) occurred 14 days after the onset of diuresis, and returned to normotension (140/90 mmHg) after the disappearance of hypercalcemia.

Hypercalcemia may be very hazardous when it occurs associated with hyperphosphatemia; an elevated serum calcium-phosphorus product may cause metastatic calcification in vital organs, such as lungs and heart, and cause life-threatening cardiopulmonary insufficiency [88, 96, 97]. This is frequent when hypercalcemia develops during the oliguric phase of ARF; but soft-tissue calcification has also been observed in the diuretic phase [88]. Calcium deposition in the kidneys may prolong the duration of ARF, thus delaying the recovery phase [96].

The possibility of delayed hypercalcemia following ARF should warn physicians to include determination of serum calcium and phosphorus in the follow-up after ARF.

6.4 PREVENTION

In patients with extensive rhabdomyolysis ATN, may be prevented by massive fluid administration and maintenance of normal circulation; massive infusion (up to 10 liters) of normal saline (0.9 g/dl, 154 mmol/l NaCl) may be necessary in the first 12 to 24 hours to maintain a normal blood pressure [7]. But even when dehydration and salt depletion are not present, great amounts of fluid must be given (a) because of the capillary leak into the damaged muscles and (b) to maintain a high urine output through ECV expansion. This massive infusion, although necessary, may increase the edema in injured muscles and even cause compartmental compression syndrome.

In addition to volume expansion, mannitol and/or furosemide may be helpful in maintaining a high urine flow to dilute myoglobin and other toxic products [7, 98].

The i.v. infusion of sodium bicarbonate has been suggested as a preventive measure by some authors [98] but denied by others [7];

the rationale for its use is that alkalinization of urine would solubilize myoglobin.

Compartmental compression syndrome may require fasciotomy to relieve pressure, thereby preventing a secondary wave of ischemic muscle necrosis due to vascular compression [7]. In my opinion, fasciotomy should be performed only when peripheral pulses are impaired.

6.5 SPECIFIC TREATMENT

Since it is widely accepted that myoglobin is chiefly responsible for renal shutdown in ARF associated with rhabdomyolysis, the prompt removal of myoglobin from the bloodstream is regarded as an important aim in the treatment of this condition. This may be obtained sometimes by parenteral fluid administration, but often dialytic therapy is necessary.

The following protocol may be used [98]:

a. Volume depletion should be immediately corrected by adequate intravenous solutions, which may possibly include sodium bicarbonate solution.

b. Then as early as possible, a solution with 25 g (137 mmol) of mannitol and 100 mmol of sodium bicarbonate in one liter of 5 g/dl (278 mmol/1) dextrose in water should be infused intravenously at a rate of 250 ml/hour for four hours.

The use of sodium bicarbonate may help in solubilizing not only myoglobin but also uric acid, (which is possibly involved in the pathogenesis of rhabdomyolysis-induced ARF.)

c. Patients exhibiting a diuretic response should be given supplemental infusions of normal saline to replace adequately urinary electrolyte and water loss until serum creatinine starts to fall and there is no evidence of myoglobinuria.

d. Nonresponders to mannitol-sodium bicarbonate infusion may be given furosemide 200–250 mg i.v. over 10 to 15 minutes. If a diuretic response occurs, saline infusion should replace urinary losses.

e. Nonresponders should start dialysis therapy.

When choosing the type of dialysis, we might take into account the possibility of myoglobin removal. Because of its molecular weight (17,800), myoglobin is removed by peritoneal dialysis. It is not dialyzed through cuprophane membrane [25]. Good results were to be expected with polyacrilonitrile membranes (RP610 and RP6 by Hospal), which have a cutoff greater than 20,000 Daltons. However, when crushed patients with ARF were dialyzed with RP610 dialyzers, they did not do any better when compared with other crushed patients dialyzed with cuprophane dialyzers [25]. This observation is supported by the demonstration that plasma concentration of myoglobin, in patients with ARF associated with rhabdomyolysis (due to heat stroke or to electrical injury by high-voltage current), did not fall in a significant fashion when the patients were dialyzed with RP–6 dialyzers; the fall was no different from that obtained when hemodialysis was carried out with AM–10 dialyzers (i.e., cuprophane capillary dialyzers) [10].

There is evidence that plasma exchange is quite successful in removing significant amounts of myoglobin; as many as 31.2 mg of myoglobin have been removed in a three-liter plasma exchange session [10].

It should be stressed that while hypocalcemia does not require therapy, severe hypercalcemia must be treated and possibly prevented. An important preventive measure is early mobilization of patients with rhabdomyolysis-induced ARF [92]. In diuretic patients, massive i.v. infusion of saline solution and the use of furosemide are very efficient means for inhibiting tubular reabsorption of calcium and thereby increasing calcium excretion. In the oliguric phase of ARF or in any condition in which conservative treatment is not adequate to normalize serum calcium, hemodialysis with calcium-free dialysate becomes necessary.

7 Illicit Drug Abuse and Rhabdomyolysis

Because of the increasing frequency of illicit drug abuse, I would like to focus the attention of physicians on the possibility of rhabdomyolysis in illicit drug intoxication.

The description of rhabdomyolysis-induced ARF in addicts is relatively recent. It was first reported in heroin intoxication [51]. Heroin addiction may cause either a glomerulonephritis with or without the nephrotic syndrome [99] or rhabdomyolysis [26, 51, 52]. In recent years, rhabdomyolysis-induced ARF has been more frequently reported in phencyclidine abusers [32, 100–102].

Phencyclidine is a dissociative anesthetic no longer utilized as an anesthetic agent but now used as a street drug. Among users, it is usually called a "peace pill," "angel dust," "crystal," "hog"; it is smoked (alone or mixed with marijuana), ingested, inhaled, or even injected parenterally [32]. Phencyclidine has been found to be an ingredient in 184 out of 237 illicit drugs [103]. Its abuse is frequent in the United States. In two years (1978–1979), 1,000 addicts with phencyclidine intoxication were admitted to the University of Southern California Medical Center: 25 of them had rhabdomyolysis (2.5%), 17 of which (1.7%) had either a functional (prerenal ARF) or organic ARF (ATN) [32].

Rhabdomyolysis has also been observed after poisoning by strychnine, which is sometimes used for cutting cocaine [104]. This observation stresses that not only illicit drug use but also substances used for cutting them may cause rhabdomyolysis.

The pathogenetic mechanism of rhabdomyolysis in illicit drug intoxication is still undefined. Increased muscle activity (muscle spasm, seizures) and heightened isometric tension, comatose state, severe hyperthermia, and direct muscle injury by the drug have all been postulated as possible causes of rhabdomyolysis [26, 32]. On many occasions, rhabdomyolysis has been observed without coma, thus ruling out (at least in these cases) muscle compression as a possible cause [3, 26, 51].

Clinical features, prevention, and treatment of rhabdomyolysis-induced ARF are not dissimilar from those described for other forms of nontraumatic rhabdomyolysis-induced ARF (see section 6 of this chapter).

8 Posttraumatic ARF

We may define posttraumatic ARF as that form of renal shutdown that follows a traumatic event or occurs in association with complications of the traumatic event (such as hemorrhage, ECV depletion, sepsis, antibiotic nephrotoxicity, etc.), with the injury itself being the main determinant of ARF [25, 40]. It has been stated that myoglobinuria is the pathogenetic factor of ARF that follows crush injuries. Undoubtedly, rhabdomyolysis, with release of myoglobin and other cellular components, will greatly contribute to renal damage. The important role of muscle injury is demonstrated by the clinical observation that this form of ARF is more frequent and severe in subjects with large muscle mass, who would release greater amounts of myoglobin and other cell components into the circulation [7]. However, the posttraumatic ARF as defined above cannot be regarded as the simple consequence of myoglobinuria. Many factors may contribute to the pathogenesis of renal impairment: hemorrhage, ECV depletion, and shock, with resulting renal ischemia and other complications, such as infections, antibiotic nephrotoxicity, and blood transfusion reaction, which may worsen the clinical outcome of the renal shutdown.

The first description of ARF following traumatic injury to skeletal muscles was that of Bywaters and Beall [39] after the London bombing during the World War II. Because of the association of ARF with extensive crushing injuries in the muscles of various parts of the body (particularly the limbs), posttraumatic ARF has also been called "crush syndrome."

Most information on posttraumatic ARF derives from military experience. But the same syndrome may be observed in other catastrophic events involving civilians or in isolated cases of severe trauma (e.g., vehicular accidents, crushing injuries of any type, gunshots). With better knowledge of the pathogenetic mechanism, the incidence of posttraumatic ARF has dramatically decreased in recent years. Thus, among American military casualties during World War II, one in every 20 casualties developed ARF; during the Korean War, the incidence fell to one in every 800; during the Vietnam War it further fell to one in every 1,800 casualties [105].

We have recently reported our own clinical experience following the earthquake in southern Italy on 23 November 1980 [25] (table 12–1). On the basis of my personal experience

and of data obtained from the literature, I will now review the peculiar features of posttraumatic ARF, since I am confident that it will be of some help to physicians in improving the management of this severe form of ARF.

8.1 GENERAL CONSIDERATIONS

When first observed, an injured patient with acute deterioration in renal function may have experienced one or more of the following phenomena: (a) a prolonged period of hypotension, (b) mismatched blood transfusions (as emergency treatment of massive blood loss), (c) extensive muscle damage; (d) extensive third-degree burns, (e) internal organ injury, (f) wound infections and systemic sepsis, (g) severe salt depletion and/or dehydration, (h) excessive i.v. infusions of salt-free solutions in the emergency attempt to restore intravascular volume.

The patient should be immediately evaluated for fluid-volume status; the most urgent laboratory determinations must include serum electrolytes, potassium, and bicarbonate in particular.

The time interval between injury and the occurrence of ATN is variable, depending on preexistent renal function, duration of hypotension, extent of muscle damage, and so forth. In our series, two children who were admitted to our unit 48 hours after injury, were in shock, dehydrated, anuric, without blood pressure; despite the long interval after injury, they exhibited prerenal ARF, which was reversed by appropriate reconstitution of intravascular volume and normalization of blood pressure [25].

8.2 ACCELERATED CATABOLISM

As in all similar patients with posttraumatic ARF, accelerated catabolism was a rule in our series of 12 casualties. Stress of wounding and surgery (in some of them), fever, infections, immobility imposed by wounds, and starvation, all contributed to accelerate tissue catabolism with the consequent release of urea and potassium. Multiple blood transfusions may have increased serum levels of potassium. Metabolic acidosis further contributed to the life-threatening hyperkalemia usually observed when patients were first admitted to our observation, 36 to 48 hours after the earthquake

TABLE 12–1. Posttraumatic ARF in 12 casualties after the earthquake in southern Italy on 23 November 1980

Patients	Sex	Age (years)	Occurrence of ARF (days from injury)	Duration of oliguria (days)	Recovery of renal function (days from injury)	Serum CPK IU/L	Serum GOT IU/L	Serum creatine (A) mg/dl	Serum creatinine (B) mg/dl	$\frac{A}{B}$	Plasma urea mg/dl	Serum K^+ mmol/L	Serum protein g/dl[a]	Type of dialysis[b]
1. M.C.	M	22	2	12	29	111,000	990	7.4	6.6	1.12	280	7.9	4.34	PD—H
2. M.R.	M	46	2	18	41	21,000	224	7.3	7.5	0.97	296	6.0	5.00	PD—H
3. C.L.	F	33	2	12	24	42,000	600	5.8	4.7	1.23	139	6.3	5.90 (4.20)	PD—H
4. C.M.P.	F	16	1	34	53	82,000	1,340	11.6	4.3	2.70	150	7.0	5.00 (4.10)	PD—H
5. L.D.	M	46	2	35	90	16,000	131	4.2	5.1	0.82	212	7.1	5.80 (5.00)	PD—H
6. F.M.	M	9	1	1	2	29,100	220	—	1.7	—	75	5.5	—	Prerenal ARF
7. Fi.P.	F	11	1	1	1	14,000	—	—	0.9	—	85	5.9	5.80 (5.50)	Prerenal ARF
8. Fa.P.	M	32	2	24	exitus[c]	132,000	1,750	—	3.0	—	150	5.5	5.50 (4.00)	PD—H
9. P.G.	M	37	2	6	exitus[d]	34,000	450	11.6	7.3	1.59	205	6.1	5.80 (4.40)	H
10. D.V.R.	M	22	1	3	exitus[d]	85,500	1,040	—	4.6	—	101	8.2	5.70	H
11. D.F.E.	F	46	1	3	exitus[d]	45,000	800	—	4.8	—	135	8.2	4.30	PD
12. A.M.	F	45	2	6	exitus[d]	44,000	600	—	4.3	—	107	4.1	3.20	PD

[a] In parenthesis, the lowest observed value despite massive administration of albumin.
[b] PD = peritoneal dialysis; H = hemodialysis.
[c] The patient died from an intracerebral hemorrhage.
[d] The patient died because of irreversible shock and/or acute respiratory distress syndrome.

[25]. The very high levels of plasma urea and the persistent hyperkalemia (table 12–1) despite conservative therapy forced us to perform early and intensive dialysis. But even in those cases without these urgent needs, early and frequent dialyses were performed; our purpose, in fact, was to prevent uremic symptoms and allow patients to be fed in order to compensate tissue wasting. Marked wasting of both subcutaneous fat and muscles, in fact, occurred, as mirrored by the marked hypoalbuminemia and by severe weight loss, despite massive i.v. infusions of proteins, glucose, and even lipids: a 46-year-old man, 79 Kg b.w. on admission, was finally discharged completely healed, having lost 26 Kg in 39 days. Vigorous efforts were made from the beginning to obtain in all patients an adequate calorie intake both by feeding (whenever possible) and by parenteral nutrition. In most cases, however, our attempts were only partially successful.

Undoubtedly, a great contribution to the low serum concentration of protein resulted from the protein loss through infected surgical wounds (because of fasciotomies and/or amputations) and through the peritoneum during peritoneal dialysis [25].

8.3 TYPE OF DIALYSIS

After the catastrophic earthquake of November 1980 in southern Italy, we expected to receive in our unit many patients with posttraumatic ARF. In order to avoid overwhelming our limited hemodialysis facilities, we decided to treat all patients by peritoneal dialysis (which does not limit the number of patients under treatment), reserving hemodialysis for those patients for whom peritoneal dialysis was not satisfactory. Since only 12 patients arrived under our observation, peritoneally dialyzed patients could be transferred to hemodialysis after a few days. Thus, two patients were treated conservatively (they had prerenal ARF, which was readily reversed despite myoglobinuria and was associated with severe dehydration, salt depletion and shock); two were treated only by extracorporeal hemodialysis; eight were initially managed by continuous (up to eight days) peritoneal dialysis, but six of them were then transferred to hemodialysis while the other two

died on peritoneal dialysis [25] (table 12–1).

The main reasons for transferring patients from continuous peritoneal dialysis to hemodialysis were (a) a tendency to peritoneal infection due to contamination from infected wounds; (b) marked hypoproteinemia despite massive i.v. infusions of proteins (up to 120 g/day of albumin in form of 20 g/dl albumin and plasma); (c) difficulty in controlling fluid retention despite the use of hypertonic solutions and continuous treatment (up to eight consecutive days). Undoubtedly, the increased rate of formation of water of oxydation by the catabolized tissues greatly contributed to the occurrence of generalized edema despite fluid restriction; only by using ultrafiltration hemodialysis associated with massive i.v. infusion of proteins was a dry body weight obtained. In two patients, a few sessions of hemodialysis were combined with the continuous peritoneal dialysis, both to remove fluid and to decrease plasma urea and serum potassium.

8.4 MYOGLOBIN REMOVAL

Unfortunately, in our patients with posttraumatic ARF, myoglobin could not be measured by radial immunodiffusion technique in urine and peritoneal dialysate samples until one week after the earthquake. Five days after the onset of ARF, myoglobinuria was detected in only one patient, a 16-year-old girl with an infected fasciotomy wound on the left leg, who underwent amputation two days later; a continuous muscle injury was therefore still present five days after the onset of ARF. In this patient, severe oliguria lasted 35 days and renal function was completely normalized 53 days after the earthquake [25].

After the first 24 hours of peritoneal dialysis, myoglobin was detected in samples of peritoneal dialysate in three patients, with concentrations of 0.22, 0.51, and 0.61 mg/dl [25].

8.5 COMPLICATIONS

In our series of 12 patients, complications included a bleeding diathesis related to coagulation defect (one case), severe gastrointestinal hemorrhage secondary to stress ulcer (one case), respiratory insufficiency with severe hypoxemia (four cases), irreversible shock (one case), and infections (six cases).

Infection was the most frequent complication with Pseudomonas aeruginosa as the predominant organism in urine, blood, wound, and peritoneal dialysate cultures. Infections of wounds (fasciotomy or amputation) were usually the source for systemic infections [25].

8.6 SUGGESTIONS FOR MANAGEMENT

a. After severe trauma, the patient should be resuscitated as soon as possible and then rapidly transported to sophisticated treatment facilities that should include the artificial kidney.

b. Emergency therapy may include blood transfusion, i.v. infusion of plasma, 20 g/dl human albumin, plasma expanders, isotonic saline, and, in anuric patients, sodium bicarbonate solution (to treat hyperkalemia), in addition to the commonly used dextrose solution. Massive infusion of normal saline may be necessary to maintain normal blood pressure and circulation and to prevent or reverse prerenal ARF.

c. Fasciotomy should be performed in markedly swollen limbs of crushed patients when peripheral pulses are impaired. Fasciotomy should be avoided when peripheral pulses are intact because of the risk of wound infection.

d. Serum electrolyte (particularly potassium), serum creatinine, plasma urea, and hematocrit should be obtained immediately after trauma and then repeated daily with serum uric acid, protein, CPK, GOT, LDH, aldolase, calcium, and phosphorus. Serum potassium should preferably be repeated twice a day.

e. Intensive dialysis should be performed as early as possible to correct hyperkalemia (after the conservative emergency therapy) and high plasma levels of urea due to accelerated catabolism; to prevent uremic symptoms; to facilitate adequate nutrition and wound healing. In my opinion, daily hemodialysis is preferable. Advantages of peritoneal dialysis include the lack of need for special facilities, the possibility of treating many patients simultaneously (this is important in the event of a catastrophe), the lack of need for vascular access, and efficacy in dialyzing myoglobin. Disadvantages of perito-

neal dialysis include protein loss with dialysate; inadequacy in removing fluid, potassium, and urea; and the high incidence of peritonitis [25].

f. Massive i.v. infusions of 25g/dl human albumin are necessary to correct the low serum levels of albumin due to accelerated catabolism, protein loss through exposed wounds, protein loss by peritoneal dialysis.

g. Efforts should be made to provide adequate calorie intake both by parenteral nutrition and by feeding.

h. All measures should be used to prevent and treat infections. Frequent débridement of devitalized tissue in exposed wounds may help in preventing infection. Urine, blood, wound, and peritoneal dialysate cultures should be performed daily. Antibiotic therapy should be started on evidence of culturally proven infection on the basis of sensitivity results. If antibiotic therapy has to be instituted before identification of the responsible microorganism, agents effective against Gram-negative, Gram-positive, and anerobic organisms should be used. An aminoglycoside will be the agent of first choice for Gram-negative coverage, bearing in mind the need to reduce dosage (see chapter 3). Doxycycline is a very useful agent for covering Gram-positive and anaerobic microorganisms; it is not nephrotoxic, it does not produce catabolic effects (as other tetracyclines do), and it does not accumulate in conditions of reduced renal function so that it not require reduction in dosage [41, 106].

Tests for viral infections should be performed in severely ill patients with unexplained fever.

References

1. Berenbaum MC, Birch CA, Moreland JD. Paroxysmal myoglobinuria. Lancet 1: 892–895, 1953.
2. Rowland LP, Penn AS. Myoglobinuria. Med Clin North Am 56: 1233–1256, 1972.
3. Gabow PA, Kaehny WD, Kelleher SP. The spectrum of rhabdomyolysis. Medicine 61: 141–152, 1982.
4. Kagen LJ, Christian CL. Immunologic measurements of myoglobin in human adult and fetal skeletal muscle. Am J Physiol 211: 656–660, 1966.

5. Kagen LJ, Gurewich R. Localization of myoglobin in human skeletal muscle using fluorescent antibody technique. J Histochem Cytochem 15: 436–441, 1967.

6. Kagen LJ, Linder S. Biosynthesis of myoglobin by muscle polysomes. Biochim Biophys Acta 195: 522–530, 1969.

7. Knochel JP: Rhabdomyolysis and myoglobinuria. Ann Rev Med 33: 435–443, 1982.

8. Hallgren R, Karlsson FA, Roxin LE, Venge P. Myoglobin turnover: Influence of renal and extrarenal factors. J Lab Clin Med 91: 246–254, 1978.

9. Hart PM, Feinfeld DA, Briscoe AM, Nurse HM, Hotchkiss JL, Thomson GE. The effect of renal failure and hemodialysis on serum and urine myoglobin. Clin Nephrol 18: 141–143, 1982.

10. Kuroda M, Katsuki K, Uehara H, Kita T, Asaka S, Miyazaki R, Akiyama T, Tofuku Y, Takeda R. Successful treatment of fulminating complications associated with extensive rhabdomyolysis by plasma exchange. Artif Organs 5: 372–378, 1981.

11. Kagen LJ. Myoglobin: Biochemical, Physiological and Clinical Aspects. New York: Columbia University Press, 1973.

12. Olerud JE, Homer LD, Carroll HW. Serum myoglobin levels predicted from serum enzyme values. N Engl J Med 293: 483–485, 1975.

13. de Wardener. The Kidney. Edinburgh: Churchill Livingstone. 1973.

14. Grossman RA, Hamilton RW, Morse BM, Penn AS, Goldberg M. Nontraumatic rhabdomyolysis and acute renal failure. N Engl J Med 291: 807–811, 1974.

15. Van Der Veen KJ, Willibrands AF. Isoenzymes of creatine phosphokinase in tissue extracts and in normal and pathological sera. Clin Chim Acta 12: 312–316, 1966.

16. Soffer O, Fellner SK, Rush RL. Creatine phosphokinase in long-term dialysis patients. Arch Intern Med 141: 181–183, 1981.

17. Fitch CD, Lucy DD, Bornhofen JH, Dalrymple GV. Creatine metabolism in skeletal muscle. II. Creatine kinetics in man. Neurology 18: 32–42, 1968.

18. Knochel JP, Dotin LN, Hamburger RJ. Heat stress, exercise and muscle injury: Effects on urate metabolism and renal function. Ann Intern Med 81: 321–328, 1974.

19. Crim MC, Calloway DH, Margen S. Creatine metabolism in men: Urinary creatine and creatinine excretions with creatine feeding. J Nutr 105: 428–438, 1975.

20. Mitch WE, Collier VU, Walser M. Creatinine metabolism in chronic renal failure. Clin Sci 58: 327–335, 1980.

21. Crim MC, Calloway DH, Margen S. Creatine metabolism in men: Creatine pool size and turnover in relation to creatine intake. J Nutr 106: 471–481, 1976.

22. Lazdins O, Dawson JK. Concentration of guani-dines in normal human plasma. Clin Exp Pharmacol Physiol 5: 75–80, 1978.

23. Jones JD, Burnett PC. Creatinine metabolism in humans with decreased renal function: Creatinine deficit. Clin Chem 20: 1204–1212, 1974.

24. Jones JD, Burnett PC. Creatinine metabolism and toxicity. Kidney Int 7: S294–S298, 1975.

25. Andreucci VE, Dal Canton A, Usberti M, Federico S, Calderaro V, Cianciaruso B, Russo D, Balletta M, Sabbatini M, Capuano A. Posttraumatic acute renal failure: Clinical experience after the earthquake in southern Italy. In Acute Renal Failure, Seybold D, Gessler U (eds). Basel: Karger, 1982, pp. 219–239.

26. Koffler A, Friedler RM, Massry SG. Acute renal failure due to nontraumatic rhabdomyolysis. Ann Intern Med 85: 23–28, 1976.

27. Hamilton RW, Gardner LB, Penn AS, Goldberg M. Acute tubular necrosis caused by exercise-induced myoglobinuria. Ann Intern Med 77–82, 1972.

28. Knochel JP: Renal injury in muscle disease. In The Kidney in Systemic Disease, Suki WN, Eknoyan G (eds). New York: John Wiley, 1976, pp. 129–140.

29. Swenson RS, Pellascio ML, Spreiter SC. Evidence that creatinine generation is not increased in experimental rhabdomyolysis acute renal failure. Abstracts Am Soc Nephrol, 12th Meeting, Boston, 1979, p 7A.

30. Hays RM. Dynamics of body water and electrolytes. In Clinical disorders of fluid and electrolyte metabolism, Maxwell MH, Kleeman CR (eds). New York: McGraw-Hill, 1980 (3rd ed), pp 1–36.

31. Akmal M, Goldstein DA, Telfer N, Wilkinson E, Massry SG. Resolution of muscle calcification in rhabdomyolysis and acute renal failure. Ann Intern Med 89: 928–930, 1978.

32. Akmal M, Valdin JR, McCarron MM, Massry SG. Rhabdomyolysis with and without acute renal failure in patients with phencyclidine intoxication. Am J Nephrol 1: 91–96, 1981.

33. Warren DJ, Leitch AG, Leggett RJ. Hyperuricemic acute renal failure after epileptic seisures. Lancet 2: 385–387, 1975.

34. Smith RF. Exertional rhabdomyolysis in naval officer candidates. Ann Intern Med 121: 313–319, 1968.

35. Schiff HB, MacSearraigh ETM, Kallmeyer JC. Myoglobinuria, rhabdomyolysis and marathon running. Quart J Med 47: 463–472, 1978.

36. MacSearraigh ETM, Kallmeyer JC, Schiff HB. Acute renal failure in marathon runners. Nephron 24: 236–240, 1979.

37. Diamond I, Aquino TI. Myoglobinuria following unilateral status epilepticus and ipsilateral rhabdomyolysis. N Engl J Med 272: 834–837, 1965.

38. Selzer ML, Reinhart MJ, Deeney JM. Acute renal failure following EST. Ann J Psychiat 120: 602–603, 1963.

39. Bywaters EGL, Beall D: Crush injuries with im-

pairment of renal function. Brit Med J 1: 427–432, 1941.

40. Whelton A, Donadio JV Jr. Post-traumatic acute renal failure in Vietnam. A comparison with the Korean War experience. Johns Hopkins Med J 124: 95–105, 1969.

41. Whelton A. Post-traumatic acute renal failure. Bull N Y Acad Med 55: 150–162, 1979.

42. Owen CA, Mubarak SJ, Hargens AR, Rutherford L, Garetto LP, Akeson WH. Intramural pressures with limb compression. Clarification of the pathogenesis of drug-induced muscle-compartment syndrome. N Engl J Med 300: 1169, 1979.

43. Schreiber SN, Liebowitz MR, Bernstein LH, Srinivasan K. Limb compression and renal impairment (crush syndrome) complicating narcotic overdose. N Engl J Med 284: 368–369, 1971.

44. Penn AS, Rowland LP, Fraser DW. Drugs, coma, and myoglobinuria. Arch Neurol 26: 336–343, 1972.

45. Haimovici H. Arterial embolism, myoglobinuria and renal tubular necrosis. Arch Surg 100: 639–645, 1970.

46. Kagen LJ. Immunologic detection of myoglobinuria after cardiac surgery. Ann Intern Med 67: 1183–1189, 1967.

47. Gordon BS, Newman W. Lower nephron syndrome following prolonged knee-chest position. J Bone Joint Surg 35A: 764–768, 1953.

48. Mubarak S, Owen CA. Compartmental syndrome and its relation to the crush syndrome: A spectrum of disease. Clin Orthop 113: 81–89, 1975.

49. Getzen LC, Carr JE. Etiology of anterior tibial compartment syndrome. Surg Gynec Obstet 125: 347–350, 1967.

50. Eiser AR, Neff MS, Slifkin RF. Acute myoglobinuric renal failure. A consequence of the neuroleptic malignant syndrome. Arch Intern Med 142: 601–603, 1982.

51. Richter RW, Challenor YB, Pearson J, Kagen LJ, Hamilton LL, Ramsey WH. Acute myoglobinuria associated with heroin addiction. JAMA 216:1172–1176, 1971.

52. Robinson SF, Woods AH. Heroin induced rhabdomyolysis and acute renal failure. A case report. Ariz Med 31: 246–251, 1974.

53. Marshall RJ, McCanghey WTE. Hypothermic myxedema coma with muscle damage and acute renal tubular necrosis. Lancet 2: 754–757, 1956.

54. Vertel RM, Knochel JP. Acute renal failure due to heat injury Am J Med 43: 435–451, 1967.

55. Reid HA. Myoglobinuria and sea snake-bite poisoning. Brit Med J 1: 1284–1289, 1961.

56. Heitzman EJ, Patterson JF, Stanley MM. Myoglobinuria and hypokalemia in regional enteritis. Arch Intern Med 110: 117–124, 1962.

57. Campion DS, Arias JM, Carter NW. Rhabdomyolysis and myoglobinuria. Association with hypokalemia of renal tubular acidosis. JAMA 220: 967–969, 1972.

58. Knochel JP, Schlein EM. On the mechanism of rhabdomyolysis in potassium depletion. J Clin Invest 51: 1750–1758, 1972.

59. Nadel SM, Jackson JW, Ploth DW. Hypokalemic rhabdomyolysis and acute renal failure. Occurrence following total parenteral nutrition. JAMA 241: 2294–2296, 1979.

60. Gross EG, Dexter JD, Roth RG. Hypokalemic myopathy with myoglobinuria associated with licorice ingestion. N Engl J Med 274: 602–606, 1966.

61. Mohamed SD, Chapman RS, Crooks J. Hypokalemia, flaccid quadriparesis and myoglobinuria with carbenoxolone (biogastrone). Brit Med J 1: 1581–1582, 1966.

62. Mitchell ABS. Duagastrone-induced hypokalemic nephropathy and myopathy with myoglobinuria. Postgrad Med J 47: 807–813, 1971.

63. Barnes PC, Leonard JHC. Hypokalemic myopathy and myoglobinuria due to carbenoxolone sodium. Postgrad Med J 47: 813–815, 1971.

64. Drutz DJ, Fan JH, Tai TY. Hypokalemic rhabdomyolysis and myoglobinuria following amphotericin B therapy. JAMA 211: 824–826, 1970.

65. Pirovino M, Neff MS, Sharon E. Myoglobinuria and acute renal failure with acute polymyositis. N Y State J Med 79: 764–767, 1979.

66. Simon NM, Rovner RN, Berlin BS. Acute myoglobinuria associated with type A2 (Hong Kong) influenza. JAMA 212: 1704–1705, 1970.

67. Minow RA, Gorbach S, Johnson BL, Dornfeld L. Myoglobinuria associated with influenza A infection. Ann Intern Med 80: 359–361, 1974.

68. Fitzgerald F. Clinical hypophosphatemia. Ann Rev Med 29: 177–189, 1978.

69. Kjellmer I. The potassium ion as a vasodilator during muscular exercise. Acta Physiol Scand 63: 460–468, 1963.

70. Knochel JP, Barcenas C, Cotton JR, Fuller TJ, Haller R, Carter NW. Hypophosphatemia and rhabdomyolysis. J Clin Invest 62: 1240–1246, 1978.

71. Knochel JP. The pathophysiology and clinical characteristic of severe hypophosphatemia. Arch Intern Med 137: 203, 1977.

72. Knochel JP. Serum calcium derangements in rhabdomyolysis. N Engl J Med 305: 161–163, 1981.

73. Publicover SJ, Duncan CJ, Smith JL. The use of A23187 to demonstrate the role of intracellular calcium in causing ultrastructural damage in mammalian muscle. J Neuropathol Exp Neurol 37: 544–557, 1978.

74. Reddy MK, Etlinger JD, Rabinowitz M, Fischman DA, Zak R. Removal of Z-lines and α-actinin from isolated myofibrils by a calcium-activated neutral protease. J Biol Chem 250: 4278–4284, 1975.

75. Llach F, Felsenfeld AJ, Haussler MR. The pathophysiology of altered calcium metabolism in rhabdomyolysis-induced acute renal failure. N Engl J Med 305: 117–123, 1981.

76. Adams EC. Differentiation of myoglobin and he-

moglobin in biological fluids. Ann Clin Lab Sci 10: 493–499, 1980.

77. Anderson RJ, Linas SL, Berns AS, Henrich WL, Miller TR, Gabow PA, Schrier RW. Nonoliguric acute renal failure. N Engl J Med 296: 1134–1138, 1977.

78. Hofbauer KG, Forgiarini P, Imbs F, Wood JM. Effects of a competitive vasopressin antagonist in glycerol-induced acute renal failure in rats. In Acute Renal Failure, Eliahou HE (ed). London: John Libbey, 1982, pp. 194–198.

79. Perri GC, Gorini P. Uremia in the rabbit after injection of crystalline myoglobin. Brit J Exp Pathol 33: 440–444, 1953.

80. Braun SR, Weiss FR, Keller AI, Ciccone JR, Preuss HG. Evaluation of the renal toxicity of heme proteins and their derivatives: A role in the genesis of acute tubular necrosis. J Exp Med 131: 443–460, 1970.

81. Editorial. Acute renal failure, hyperuricemia and myoglobinuria. Brit Med J 1: 1233–1234, 1979.

82. Meroney WH, Herndon RF. The management of acute renal insufficiency. JAMA 155: 877–883, 1954.

83. Meroney WH, Arney GK, Segar WE, Balch HH. The acute calcification of traumatized muscle, with particular reference to acute post-traumatic renal insufficiency. J Clin Invest 36: 825–832, 1956.

84. Pietrek J, Kokot F, Kuska J. Serum 25-hydroxyvitamin D and parathyroid hormone in patients with acute renal failure. Kidney Int 13: 178–185, 1978.

85. Gray RW, Wilz DR, Caldas AE, Lemann JJr. The importance of phosphate in regulating plasma 1,25 (OH)$_2$ vitamin D levels in humans: Studies in healthy subjects in calcium-stone formers and in patients with primary hyperparathyroidism. J Clin Endocrinol Metab 45: 299–306, 1977.

86. Massry SG, Arieff AI, Coburn JW, Palmieri G, Kleeman CR. Divalent ion metabolism in patients with acute renal failure: Studies on the mechanism of hypocalcemia. Kidney Int 5: 437–445, 1974.

87. Massry SG, Stein R, Garty J, Arieff AI, Coburn JW, Norman AW, Friedler RM. Skeletal resistance to the calcemic action of parathyroid hormone in uremia: Role of 1,25(OH)$_2$D$_3$. Kidney Int 9: 467–474, 1976.

88. Feinstein EI, Akmal M, Telfer N, Massry SG. Delayed hypercalcemia with acute renal failure associated with nontraumatic rhabdomyolysis. Arch Intern Med 141: 753–755, 1981.

89. Tavill AS, Evanson JM, Baker SB, Hewitt V. Idiopathic paroxysmal myoglobinuria with acute renal failure and hypercalcemia. N Engl J Med 271: 283–287, 1964.

90. Segal AT, Miller M, Moses AM. Hypercalcemia during the diuretic phase of acute renal failure. Ann Intern Med 68: 1066–1068, 1968.

91. Leonard CD, Eichner ER. Acute renal failure and

transient hypercalcemia in idiopathic rhabdomyolysis. JAMA 211: 1539–1540, 1970.

92. Zabetakis PM, Singh R, Michelis MF, Murdaugh HV. Acute renal failure. Bone immobilization as cause of hypercalcemia. NY State J Med 79: 1887–1891, 1979.

93. Weinstein RS, Hudson JB. Parathyroid hormone and 25-hydroxycholecalciferol levels in hypercalcemia of acute renal failure. Arch Intern Med 140: 410–411, 1980.

94. Miach PJ, Dawborn JK, Douglas MC, Jerums G, Xipell JM. Prolonged hypercalcemia following acute renal failure. Clin Nephrol 4: 32–36, 1975.

95. Butikofer E, Molleyres J. Akute ischamische Muskelnekrosen, reversible Muskelverkalkungen und sekundare Hypercalcemia bei akuter Anurie. Schweiz Med Woch 98: 961–965, 1968.

96. de Torrente A, Berl T, Cohn PD, Kawamoto E, Hertz P, Schrier RW. Hypercalcemia of acute renal failure: Clinical significance and pathogenesis. Am J Med, 61: 119–123, 1976.

97. Feinstein EI, Akmal M, Goldstein DA, Telfer N, Massry SG. Hypercalcemia and acute widespread calcifications during the oliguric phase of acute renal failure due to rhabdomyolysis. Mineral Electrolyte Metab 2: 193–199, 1979.

98. Eneas JF, Schoenfeld PY, Humphreys MH. The effect of infusion of mannitol-sodium bicarbonate on the clinical course of myoglobinuria. Arch Intern Med 139: 801–805, 1979.

99. Llach F, Descoeudres C, Massry SG. Heroin-associated nephropathy Clinical and histological studies in 19 patients. Clin Nephrol 11: 7–11, 1979.

100. Cogen FC, Rigg G, Simmons JL, Domino EF. Phencyclidine-associated acute rhabdomyolysis. Ann Intern Med 88: 210–212, 1978.

101. Barton CH, Sterling ML, Vaziri ND. Rhabdomyolysis and acute renal failure associated with phencyclidine intoxication. Arch Intern Med 140: 568–569, 1980.

102. Patel R, Das M, Patazzolo M, Ansari A, Balasubramariam S. Myoglobinuric acute renal failure in phencyclidine overdose. Report of observations in eight cases. Ann Emerg Med 9: 549–553, 1980.

103. Hart JB, McChesney JD, Grief M. Composition of illicit drugs and the use of drug analysis and abuse abatement. J Psychedelic Drugs 5: 83–88, 1972.

104. Boyd RE, Brennan PT, Deng JF, Rochester DF, Spyker DA. Strychnine poisoning. Recovery from profound lactic acidosis, hyperthermia and rhabdomyolysis. Am J Med 74: 507–512, 1983.

105. Bichet OD, Burke TJ, Schrier RW. Prevention and pathogenesis of acute renal failure. Clin Exper Dial Apheresis 5: 127–141, 1981.

106. Whelton A, Schach Von Witenau M, Twomey TM, Gordon Walker W, Bianchine JR. Doxycycline pharmacokinetics in the absence of renal function. Kidney Int 5: 365–371, 1974.

13 ACUTE RENAL FAILURE IN GLOMERULAR DISEASE

J. Stewart Cameron

Acute renal failure (ARF) can occur in glomerular disease from a variety of circumstances. These are in brief:

a. *A result of glomerular inflammation:* The infiltration of the glomerulus with polymorphonuclear leucocytes, monocytes, and proliferation of local cells may be so intense that glomerular filtration is seriously and acutely compromised. This may be the result of predominantly endocapillary proliferation and infiltration or of predominantly extracapillary proliferation and infiltration with the formation of "crescents" of cells around the glomerulus. Some of the latter group may also show arteritic lesions.
b. *A result of ill understood hemodynamic events:* In severe nephrotic syndromes, ARF may appear. On occasion, this is clearly related to hypotension, sometimes accompanied by septicemia, but in other nephrotics the reasons are obscure; in some, antiprostaglandin agents may be implicated.
c. *A result of interstitial nephritis:* Drug-induced interstitial nephritis, particularly from the use of diuretics, may occur in nephrotic patients.
d. *A result of major vascular thrombosis:* In nephrotic patients, ARF may follow acute renal venous thrombosis.
e. *A result of microvascular thrombosis:* In some glomerulonephritides, capillary thrombi may be a feature and can be widespread in some patients with ARF. Clearly, this relates to both disseminated intravascular coagulation on the one hand, and hemolytic-uremic syndrome on the other.

V.E. Andreucci (ed.). ACUTE RENAL FAILURE.
All rights reserved. Copyright © 1984.
Martinus Nijhoff Publishing. Boston/The Hague/
Dordrecht/Lancaster.

This chapter is principally concerned with (a) and (b) above; (c) is dealt with in chapter 2, (d) in chapter 14, and (e) in chapter 16, although some mention is made of this topic in this chapter. The diagnosis of different stages of ARF is discussed in chapters 7 and 8, although, again, some mention of characteristic clinical and urinary findings is made in this chapter.

1 Acute Renal Failure in Glomerulonephritis

1.1 DIAGNOSIS

The diagnosis of acute renal failure from glomerulonephritis can be very straightforward, but on occasion is very difficult. Once acute tubular necrosis (ATN) and oliguria are established, there may be little to distinguish glomerulonephritis from ATN since both are characterized by hematuria; granular casts, including on occasion red cell casts; proteinuria of several grams per liter; normal-sized or large kidneys on x-ray; scan or ultrasound; and oliguria. The urinary sodium, however, usually remains low in acute forms of glomerulonephritis [1–3], while osmolality is high [4], and may be used to distinguish ATN from acute glomerulonephritis, especially if the FE_{Na} is calculated [3] (see chapter 7). Two circumstances, however, may obscure the usefulness of this measurement: the prior use of diuretics to induce a diuresis or a concomitant ATN as part of the acute glomerulonephritis. In problem patients, the diagnosis will depend on suspicion, and particularly on the history. A prior infection, a prodrome of myalgia, fever, or clinical and chemical evidence of a nephrotic state will make one suspicious, especially if

272

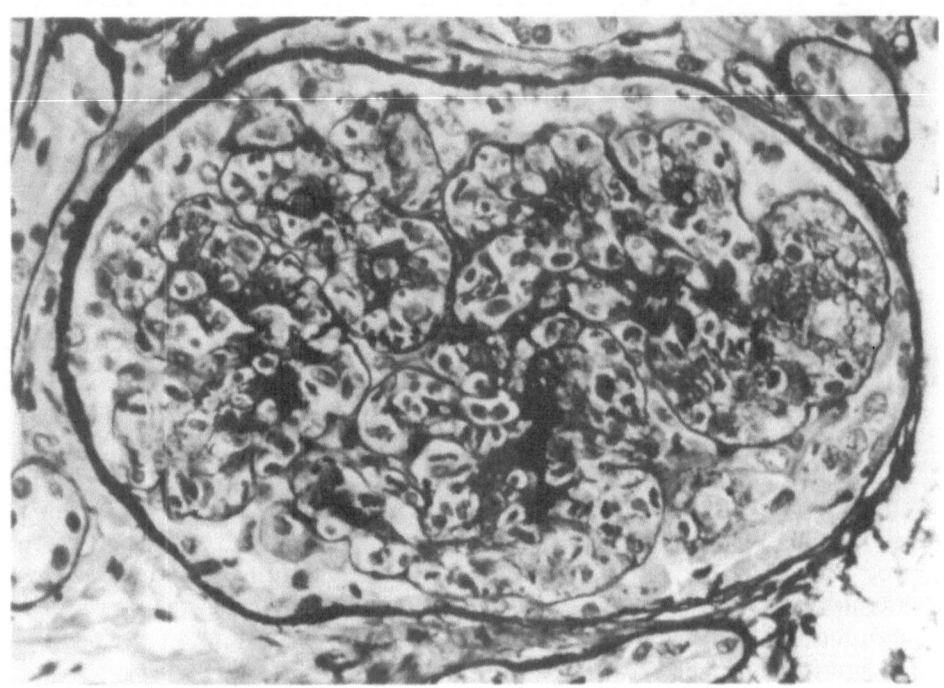

FIGURE 13–1. An acute endocapillary glomerulonephritis, from the patient whose clinical course is shown in figure 13–3. The glomerular tuft is swollen and congested with polymorphonuclear leucocytes, monocytes, and proliferated endocapillary cells. There is also mild extracapillary prominence, but no true crescent formation. Tubules showed vacuolation and necrosis (not shown here). After seven days' oliguria, a diuresis was obtained without specific treatment. Biopsy taken on the second day of oliguria. (Silver methenamine counterstained with hematoxylin and eosin, ×450.)

there are no obvious circumstances that might lead to ATN. Finally, however, the diagnosis can be made only by renal biopsy, and the decision when to perform this may not be easy [5]. In general, if there is a suspicion of a glomerular cause for the ARF, it is better to perform the biopsy early rather than late since prognosis differs so much among the various subgroups and since treatment may be indicated for some varieties (see below).

1.2 ACUTE RENAL FAILURE IN ENDOCAPILLARY GLOMERULONEPHRITIS

A mild reversible oliguria is usual in classical postinfectious glomerulonephritis with purely endocapillary glomerulonephritis on renal biopsy (figure 13–1). This is usually accompanied by a mild rise in the blood urea and plasma creatinine [6], but in almost all patients this falls short of a requirement for dialysis. On occasion, however, the oliguria is severe and prolonged, the uremia advances, and dialysis is necessary [2, 7]; usually the patient is supposed to have crescentic glomerulonephritis (see below) on clinical grounds, but on biopsy only an endocapillary glomerulonephritis or a nephritis with only a minority of glomeruli affected by small crescents is found. Often, the

acute endocapillary glomerulonephritis follows an infection including streptococcal disease. In this case, the infection may be in the throat or skin, but may be elsewhere such as a deep abscess on a heart valve or on an infected jugulo-atrial shunt or other intravascular prosthesis [8]. The ASOT or other streptococcal antibodies may be high in some cases, and hypocomplementemia is common, but not invariable, and becomes less common after the first few days of illness. The glomerular inflammation and infiltration is presumed to have a basis in glomerular localization of the immune complexes (usually present in abundance in the circulation) within the glomeruli, but in situ immune complex formation of separately deposited antigens and antibodies may play a role in acute glomerulonephritis, as it does in mem-

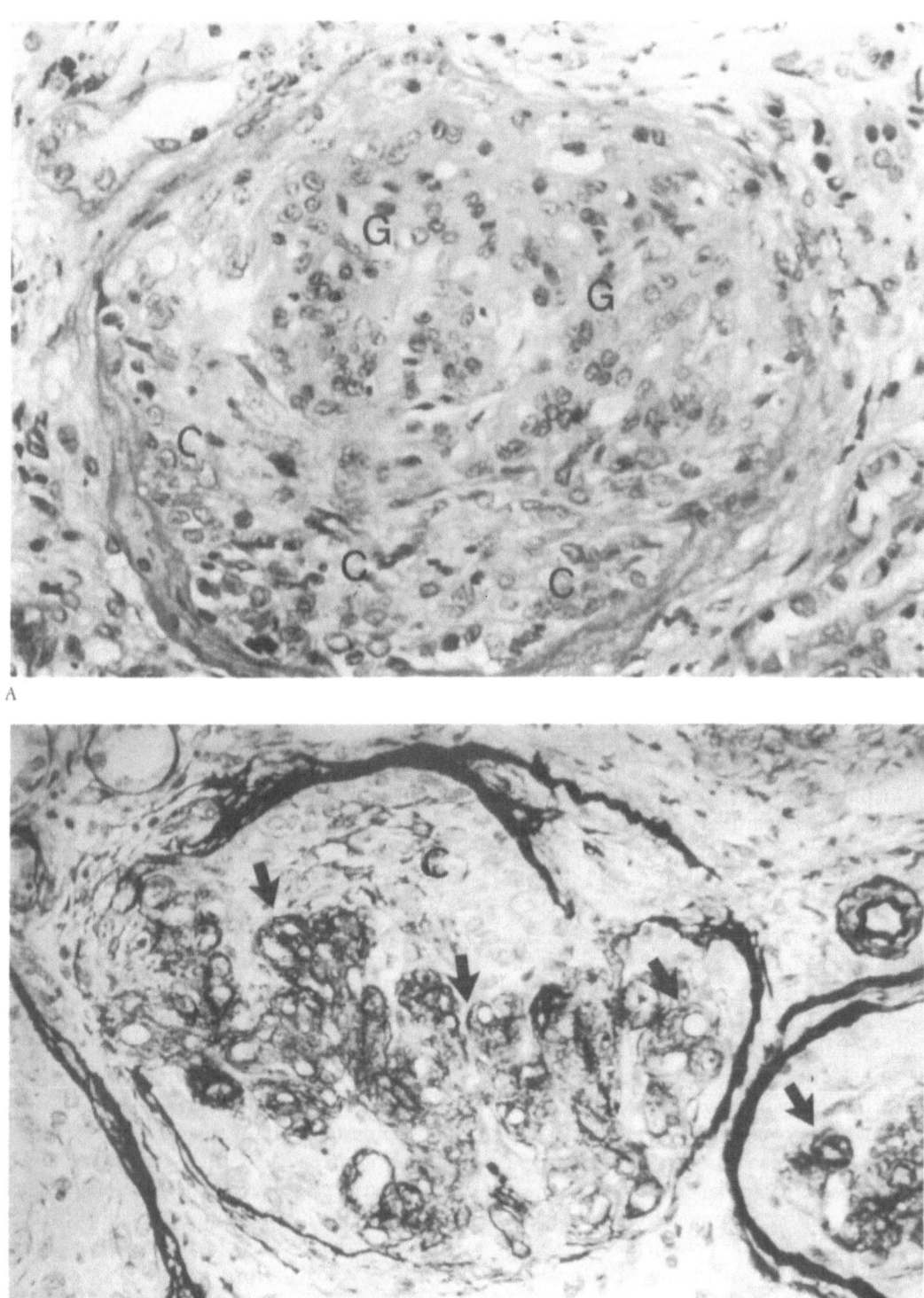

FIGURE 13–2. Mesangiocapillary glomerulonephritis (MCGN) **A.** In addition to endocapillary proliferation within the glomerular tuft (G, top right) there is increase in mesangial matrix and a large crescent C, bottom left). Peripheral capillary walls (not well seen in this hematoxylin and eosin-stained preparation) are thickened. The patient had rapidly progressive renal failure (×450). **B.** A silver-methenamine preparation from another patient with crescentic MCGN. The crescent (C) surrounds the glomerular tuft, in which the peripheral capillary walls show the typical "double contour" appearance of MCGN (arrows) (×450).

274

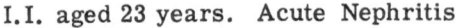

I.I. aged 23 years. Acute Nephritis

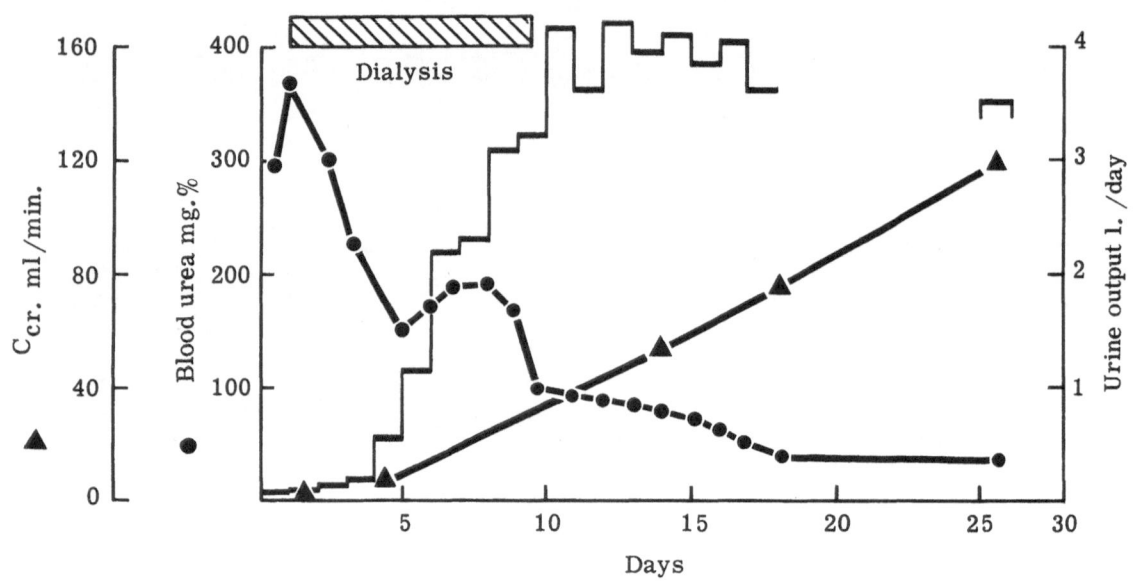

FIGURE 13–3. The clinical course of a young man with poststreptococcal glomerulonephritis, whose biopsy is shown in figure 13–1. Acute hematuria and oliguria followed 11 days after a sore throat; his ASOT was 800 units, and C3, 34%, normal. He presented with oliguria and required peritoneal dialysis for 10 days. At 7 days, his blood pressure rose suddenly to 190/130 and he had a fit. As the diuresis appeared, proteinuria rose to 5.5 G/24h, but was only 0.2 G/24h by day 26. He has remained completely well, without proteinuria and with normal renal function and blood pressure, for the last 15 years.

branous nephropathy, especially in the formation of the extra capillary deposits usually called "humps." Occasional small crescents are common, involving fewer than 50% of the glomeruli [6].

In other postinfectious glomerulonephritis with acute renal failure (for example, shunt nephritis and subacute bacterial endocarditis) [8, 9], the glomerular appearance may be one of mesangiocapillary glomerulonephritis (figure 13–2 A and B) or, less commonly, a focal segmental proliferative glomerulonephritis. In the series of severe postinfectious nephritides with ARF described by Beaufils et al. [8], four patients had mesangiocapillary patterns, complicated by 20 to 60% of glomeruli with crescents in three, while three other patients had focal segmental proliferative glomerulonephritis. Two of the former were oligoanuric at presentation. Only two patients of 11 had simple endocapillary glomerulonephritis.

In occasional patients with uncomplicated acute postinfectious nephritis, the oliguria is severe, prolonged, and the uremia severe enough to require dialysis. This may be aggravated by uncontrolled or ill-advised fluid administration, leading to exaggerated circulatory

overload, hypertension, and pulmonary edema. How the oliguria comes about is not clear, but the glomerular tuft in biopsy specimens is usually ischemic with occluded capillary loops. In some patients, the more prolonged oliguria is associated with appearances of acute tubular necrosis in the tubules, which may account for the acute renal failure in some. In others, the tubulointerstitial infiltrate normally present, together with immune complexes in the TBM, is much more prominent, and the suspicion of tubulo-interstitial component is present. Very rarely, anti-TBM antibodies are present, and linear deposition of IgG is found along the tubular basement membranes [10].

Complete recovery is the rule in patients with endocapillary glomerulonephritis and

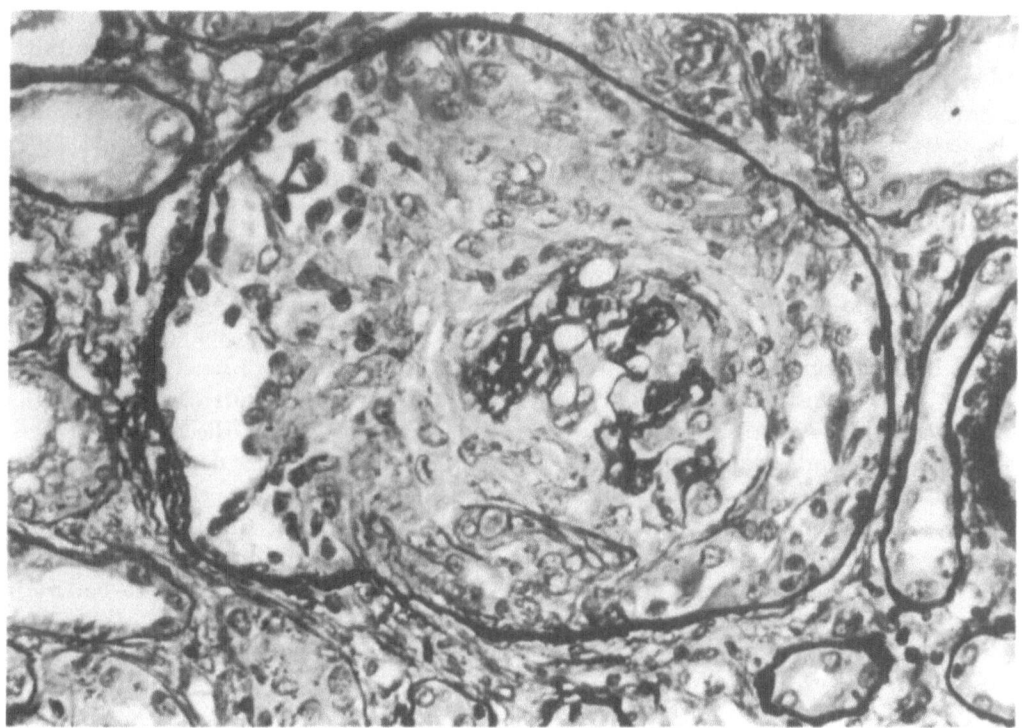

FIGURE 13–4. A crescentic glomerulonephritis. The glomerulus has been cut tangentially, through the crescent, which almost obliterates Bowman's space. The glomerulus itself is collapsed and shows no obvious pathology. Contrast this with the swollen and proliferated glomerulus in figure 13–2 in which crescents complicate a mesangiocapillary glomerulonephritis. (Silver methenamine counterstained with hematoxylin and eosin, ×450.)

ARF (figure 13–3), unless persistent infection within the circulation is a feature [8], or the histological picture changes to one of extracapillary proliferation [11]. The duration of oliguria is often brief, lasting at most two or three days. Dialysis is rarely required, especially now that powerful loop-acting diuretics are available. In most patients with oliguria from acute glomerulonephritis, a large dose of frusemide (e.g., 250 mg to 1G), or equivalent agent such as bumetanide, will induce a diuresis and obviate the need for dialysis. It may also relieve the hypertension, which may be severe, with diastolic pressures of 130 mm Hg or higher; an important differential diagnostic point is that these very pressures are not accompanied by retinopathy or papilloedema. Hypertension may need treatment in its own right, as may the fits that can follow. Valium

is best for these, since it is predominantly excreted via the liver.

There is no evidence that oral corticosteroids affect the oliguria of acute endocapillary glomerulonephritis; reports of the use of intravenous methylprednisolone in this rare situation are lacking, although a number of patients with advancing renal failure and minor numbers of crescents have been plasmapheresed [12] or given anticoagulants [13]. The results do not allow any conclusion to be drawn since numbers are small, the population is heterogenous, and treatments have differed.

A final form of acute renal failure is the peculiar recurrent resolving renal failure in children with IgA nephropathy and otherwise benign course. This was described by Talwalkar et al. [14], and we have seen one similar case.

1.3 ACUTE RENAL FAILURE IN EXTRACAPILLARY (CRESCENTIC) GLOMERULONEPHRITIS
This is a good deal more common than acute endocapillary glomerulonephritis, although still rare. It must be emphasized from the outset that this group of patients is neither patho-

logically nor clinically homogeneous [14,15]. Only the supposition that the presence of large numbers of crescents (see figure 13–4) is the main determinant of prognosis, overriding that of the underlying or associated glomerulopathy, justifies considering them together. Here, we have to consider those patients who present in ARF with oliguria or anuria, rather than the more common patients with a history of a nephrotic syndrome and a documented decline in renal function over weeks or months.

In considering this group of patients, it is important to define terms. First, *crescent* is used in various ways by various writers to mean anything from a mere capsular adhesion through a small segmental crescent to a large occluding lesion. Here, it is employed to mean *major* crescents only, with a layer of cells at least two or three cells thick or more occupying at least half the circumference of the glomerulus in the plane of section. Of course, geometry of the cut will determine to some extent what the size of any crescent appears to be, but with large numbers of glomeruli this random effect will cancel out. Such considerations are especially important if the number of glomeruli affected by "crescents" is taken to be important. Two studies have shown the extent of individual crescents and the percentage of glomeruli affected to be highly correlated [13, 17], although an exception is Henoch-Schönlein purpura, in which a high percentage—on occasions, 100% of glomeruli—may be affected by small segmental crescents [18].

The glomerular tuft in predominantly crescentic glomerulonephritis is frequently collapsed, especially if it is not the site of obvious endocapillary disease; interpretation of the glomerular changes under these circumstances is difficult. There is often intense interstitial cellular infiltrate near or around affected glomeruli, with plasma cells, monocytes, and polymorphonuclear leucocytes. Bowman's capsule may be ruptured. Some crescents are almost entirely cellular, but in time they become fibrocellular, with synthesis of new basement membranelike material within the crescent, and eventual sclerosis.

The nature and genesis of crescents have been the subject of much debate. Current thoughts on their pathogenesis are summarized in figure 13–5 A and B. Breaks in the basement membrane are seen in most forms of crescentic glomerulonephritis [19], but may be found without crescent formation. Fibrin is found with great regularity in crescents [17, 19], the more so in cellular crescents presumed to be in an early state of evolution, less so in fibrocellular crescents. Factor VIII is absent, however [20], suggesting that the fibrin is generated by a pathway not involving this factor since it is normally present in thromboses. In this context, the report of crescentic glomerulonephritis following the bite of Russell viper is of interest [21]. Evidence from work in rabbits suggests very strongly that the presence of fibrin in the blood and then in the extracapillary space is essential to the formation of crescents [22], and this is likely to be true in humans also.

The nature of the cells forming the crescent is a controversial issue. To begin with, it was assumed that they were formed from proliferation of epithelial cells of the glomerulus and/or cells lining Bowman's capsule. Recent studies, including specific stains, transplantation [23], and glomerular culture techniques [24], suggest that in both animal and human crescents the predominant cell is the macrophage, together with some polymorphonuclear leucocytes. Platelets and platelet-related antigens are absent [25].

The natural history of crescents is not clear, but it is evident from studies in both humans and animals that not only unaffected glomeruli may survive intact. Presumably, organized crescents do not resolve whereas cellular crescents may. This point, if true, could be of importance in considering whether to treat patients with crescentic glomerulonephritis.

Extensive crescent formation may be found in almost every form of glomerulonephritis (table 13–1) both primary, or in a setting of a systemic disease or vasculitis. Examination of the glomerulus, or of the patient, may give clues immediately as to which form is present, but the glomeruli may be so destroyed as to make this difficult. Examination by immunofluorescence is crucial [15, 16] since it may give an immediate clue to the nature of the condi-

Breaks in glomerular capillary wall

Fibrin exudation into extracapillary
space

Monocytes invade ± local proliferation

CRESCENT FORMATION

A

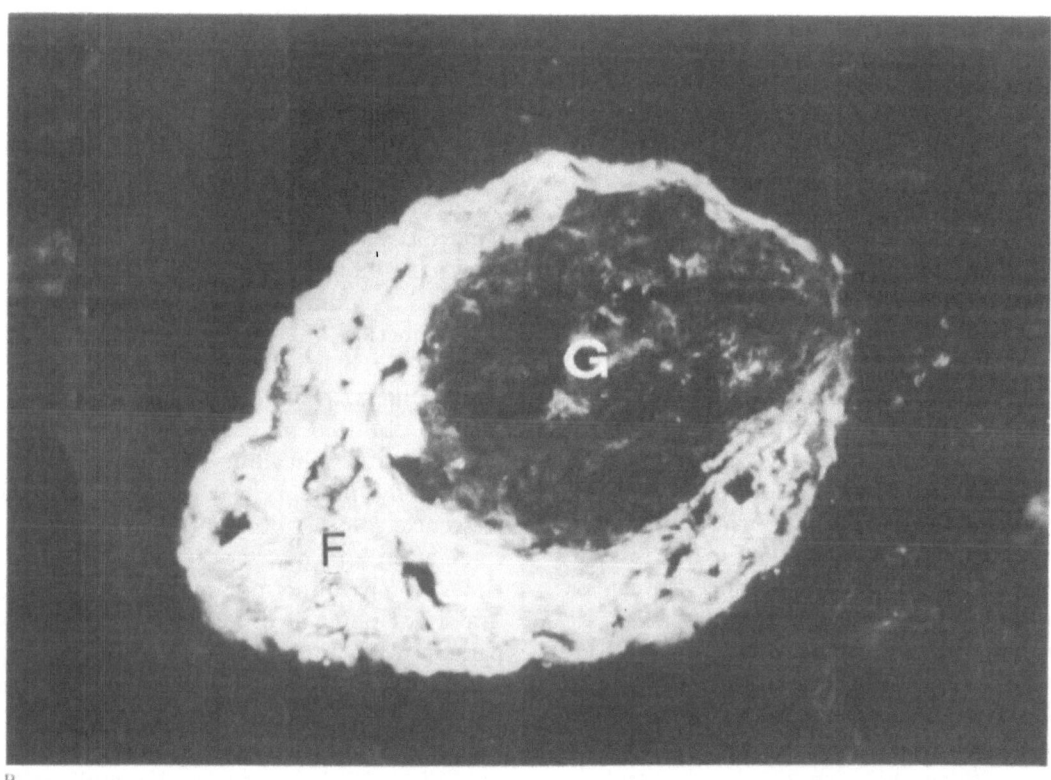

B

FIGURE 13–5. **A.** The genesis of crescents, according to current theories. This is a summary of both animal experiments and observations on human disease (see text.) **B.** Immunofluorescent preparation showing fibrin (F) in a crescent surrounding a glomerulus (G).

tion. The finding of linear IgG (occasionally linear IgA) [35] indicates anti-GBM disease, which may present without lung involvement or present with lung involvement that is not evident to ordinary clinical examination. Conversely, a "Goodpasture-like" syndrome of nephritis and lung involvement may be seen in rare instances in Henoch-Schönlein purpura, SLE, poststreptococcal glomerulonephritis, and, of course, commonly in forms of polyarteritis [36].

278

TABLE 13–1. Classification of oliguric
glomerulonephritis [14, 15]

Classification	Reference
APPARENTLY PRIMARY	
Common	
"idiopathic" crescentic glomerulonephritis	27
endocapillary glomerulonephritis + crescents	13
mesangiocapillary glomerulonephritis (types I or II) + crescents	28
focal segmental glomerulonephritis + crescents	—
anti-GBM nephritis with crescents	8
Uncommon	
IgA nephropathy + crescents	29
membranous nephropathy + crescents	30
SECONDARY	
Common	
Henoch-Schönlein purpura	18
microscopic polyarteritis nodosa	31
Wegener's granuloma	31
Uncommon	
systemic lupus erythematosus	32
Behçet's syndrome	33
essential mixed cryoglobulinemia	34
infections	
streptococcal	13
shunt nephritis	9
deep abscesses	8
subacute bacterial endocarditis	9
neoplasia	17

In some patients, a focal segmental necrotizing glomerulonephritis or a crushed but apparently normal glomerulus is seen, with immunofluorescence studies negative, except perhaps for fibrin [15, 16, 27]. A number of such patients have evident polyarteritis, other later develop signs of polyarteritis, or it is evident outside the kidney at postmortem examination. What, then, of similar patients with no evidence of polyarteritis? Some have called these patients "idiopathic" crescentic glomerulonephritis [27], while others have not observed such patients at all in their series [37]. In our own studies (Neild et al, in preparation), we have patients in all the categories mentioned, including "idiopathic" glomerulonephritis, although they are in a minority. At the moment, it seems best to keep an open mind on this subject since, at a practical level, patients with apparently idiopathic, "nonimmunologic" crescentic glomerulonephritis are found.

Small crescents frequently complicate an otherwise straightforward endocapillary exudative glomerulonephritis [6], whether or not an antecedent infection is identifiable, but rather rarely the crescents may be extensive and, even more rarely, the patient presents anuric. Crescents affecting some glomeruli are equally common in mesangiocapillary glomerulonephritis of either type [28], but more than 60% of glomeruli were affected in only 8 of 104 patients in our own series [38] (5/69 type I and 3/35 type II). Only occasional patients with extensive crescents complicating either membranous nephropathy [30] or IgA nephropathy [29] have been described.

1.3.1 Clinical Presentation [13, 15, 17, 37]
Crescentic glomerulonephritis is rare in childhood and almost unknown in infancy. It seems to become more common with age and in the elderly, accompanied or unaccompanied by arteritis, and is one of the more frequent forms of glomerulonephritis [39]. The clinical presentation varies, from a disease with an evolution over months involving fever, myalgia, a nephrotic syndrome with a steady decline in renal function, to the sudden onset of oligoanuria "out of the blue." The signs of a systemic illness, such as Henoch-Schönlein purpura in children or polyarteritis or Wegener's granulomatosis in adults may be evident; SLE very rarely presents with rapidly progressive crescentic glomerulonephritis [32]—only six cases of 119 in our series, although rapid declines in renal function are more often seen. An important point in differential diagnosis is that patients with anti-GBM disease, if there is not severe lung purpura, are often extremely well, without the prodrome of myalgia, fever, and malaise associated frequently with polyarteritis or "idiopathic" crescentic glomerulonephritis. Acute postinfectious nephritis may present with a variable number of crescents, and in these patients the complement levels may be depressed; they are low also (especially C4) in active cryoglobulinemia with nephritis and in subacute bacterial endocarditis with nephritis. In other forms of crescentic glomerulonephritis, including polyarteritis, concentrations of all complement components are usually normal. Antinuclear factors may be present in

TABLE 13–2. Summary of treated and untreated patients with crescentic glomerulonephritis (>50% of glomeruli with crescents)[a]

Total No. of patients	No. not treated	No. judged to have improved	Total no. treated[b]	No. judged to have improved
328	115	13 (11.3%)	213	90 (42%)

[a]World literature, 1964–1980. Excluding patients with anti-GBM disease, known or suspected vasculitis, SLE, or Henoch-Schönlein purpura. Includes unpublished Guy's daya (Neild et al., in preparation) on 39 patients.
[b]Prednisone alone, 3; prednisone + azathioprine or cyclophosphamide, 36; prednisone + i.v. methylprednisone, 10; combined 27. In a total of 14 patients described in references, [17] and [27], it is not clear what each patient received.

both essential cryoglobulinemia [34] and in polyarteritis, but dsDNA binding is normal. In patients with "essential cryoglobulinemia" and with polyarteritis, tests for hepatitis B antigen may be positive although this is variable according to geographical area; for example, we have never found a positive test in either condition. An important test is a search for anti-GBM antibodies since there may be no pulmonary involvement even in fulminating crescentic anti-GBM disease.

The distinction of rapidly progressive glomerulonephritis from other forms of renal failure or from other forms of glomerulonephritis can be made only by renal biopsy [5], which plays a crucial role in the management of the patients (see chapter 8).

1.3.2 Outcome The natural prognosis of crescentic glomerulonephritis is a very confused issue because it is not a homogenous group of patients to begin with and, even within homogenous subgroups, patients of differing severity have been compared. Here, it is worth considering principally patients with more than 50 or 60% of glomeruli affected by crescents, since oligo-anuria is rarely seen with disease less severe than this. In this group as a whole (but excluding anti-GBM disease, polyarteritis, and other arteritides), analysis of the available literature shows that only about 11% of such patients recover or retain useful renal function without any specific treatment at all (table 13–2); other published analyses have given somewhat higher figures but have included patients with less than 50 to 60% of glomeruli affected by crescents. The effect of oligo-anuria requiring dialysis is adverse in all series, but it is very difficult to find patients who have been treated with dialysis and supportive treatment alone! Including patients treated in a variety of fashions, analysis of six recent series of patients shows a recovery of renal function in 18 out of 78 patients (23%) who presented in oligo-anuria (table 13–3); Bolton and Couser's more selective analysis [44] suggests that only 7% of such patients show recovery irrespective of treatment. The proportion of patients with oligo-anuria at presentation, not surprisingly, increases with increasing proportion of glomeruli affected by crescents (table 13–4).

Some histological features may give a clue to likely prognosis. As just mentioned, patients presenting with oligo-anuria and glomerulonephritis usually show a high proportion of crescents. Overall (including nonoliguric and oliguric patients), prognosis is weakly correlated with the number of crescents present in the glomeruli (table 13–5). However, tubulo-inter-

TABLE 13–3. Reported recovery of renal function after presentation of crescentic nephritis with oligo-anuria

Author	Reference	No. of patients		Histology			
		TOTAL	RECOVERY	ANTIGBM	POST STREP.	ENDOCAPILLARY	IDIOPATHIC CRESCENTIC GN
Leonard et al. (1976)	[40]	20	2	0	2	0	0
Sonsino et al. (1972)	[41]	26	5	0	2	2	1
Beirne et al. (1977)	[42]	22	4	1	0	1	2
Morrin et al. (1978)	[43]	17	6	0	0	2	4
Stilmant et al. (1979)	[27]	4	1	0	0	0	1
		78	18 (23%)	1	4	5	8

Note: All patients treated with various regimens of corticosteroids ± cytotoxic agents.

TABLE 13–4. Frequency of an oligo-anuric presentation in crescentic glomerulonephritis*

% Crescents	% of patients with oligo-anuria
60–70	0
70–80	40
80–90	44
90–100	72
100	92

*Excluding anti-GBM, polyarteritis, SLE, and Henoch-Schönlein purpura.
Source: Data of Sonsino et al. [41] and Cameron [45].

stitial damage is also a valuable guide to prognosis. In our own series of patients with 60% crescents, 14 out of 26 patients with low indices of tubulo-interstitial damage showed recovery of renal function, while only 5 out of 13 with high scores did so (Neild et al, in preparation). These features, together with a high degree of fibrocellularity and sclerosis within the crescents, and the degree of glomerulosclerosis, may suggest a poor outcome. Conversely, cellular crescents and an absence of glomerulosclerosis, fibrocellular crescents, and tubulo-interstitial damage suggests disease that may remit spontaneously or respond to treatment.

Finally, within the whole group of patients with extensive crescents, different subgroups may have different prognoses. Those forms of glomerulonephritis following infection, which show "humps" on electron microscopy or endocapillary deposits with endocapillary proliferation, may do better in most series [41, 45] than those that show no deposits, with or without evident associated arteritis. In general, also, patients with obvious proliferation in the

glomeruli, even if a history of infection is absent, are thought to do better than those with "idiopathic" crescentic glomerulonephritis with a normal or nearly normal glomerular tuft [41, 45]. However, I have analyzed elsewhere [46] the data supporting the thesis that patients with disease of equivalent severity and post-streptococcal crescentic glomerulonephritis do no better than other crescentic nephritis. In Beaufils' series [8] of four patients with infections and extensive crescent formation alone, two died oliguric and two regained renal function but remained in chronic renal failure. In our eight patients with mesangiocapillary glomerulonephritis complicated by more than 60% of glomeruli with occluding crescents [38] two presented with oliguria and neither regained function; of the remaining six with less aggressive disease clinically, only two still have renal function. Thus, although the prognosis of mesangiocapillary and endocapillary glomerulonephritis complicated by crescents may be somewhat better than that found in those with "idiopathic" crescentic glomerulonephritis, it is still very poor, especially when oligo-anuria is present.

The finding of anti-GBM antibodies together with oligo-anuria requiring dialysis indicates a very poor prognosis for renal function. In 1973, Wilson and Dixon [47] reported only 3 patients of 32 with any form of Goodpasture's syndrome surviving without dialysis or transplantation, and more recently Beirne et al.[42] mentioned only 3 of 17 patients retaining or regaining renal function. Those few patients who have shown recovery of renal function have often not had extensive crescent formation round their glomeruli. Even with

TABLE 13–5. Effect of number of glomeruli with crescents on recovery or retention of renal function in crescentic nephritis

	Percentage of glomeruli with crescents				
	100%	90–99%	80–89%	70–79%	60–69%
No. of patients	66	43	36	35	20
No. "improved"	10	14	18	20	11
% improved	15%	32%	50%	56%	55%

Note: Review of world literature, 1964–1980, including Guy's published (44) and unpublished data. Patients treated with a variety of agents, including prednisone, ± cytotoxic agents, i.v. methylprednisolone, and combined immunosuppression and anticoagulation.

aggressive treatment, recovery of renal function in oliguric anti-GBM disease is rare (see below). There are no data giving any idea of the outlook for untreated polyarteritis with extensive crescents and oligo-anuria. But since this represents the worst group from among all polyarteritic patients, and the untreated survival was only of the order of 12% after five years for all forms of polyarteritis together [48], we can assume with some security that survival—far less recovery of renal function—is very rare since of itself the presence of oligo-anuria is an indicator of poor prognosis (table 13–5), with or without treatment. The question arises immediately of how justified aggressive therapy may be in the situation of glomerulonephritis with extensive crescents and oligo-anuria, in any of its various subgroups.

1.3.3 · Treatment of Oligo-Anuric Crescentic Glomerulonephritis

1.3.3.1 GOODPASTURE'S SYNDROME AND ANTI/GBM NE-PHRITIS. The prognosis for renal function in oligo-anuric Goodpasture's syndrome requiring dialysis is negligible [42, 47], as noted above. Is this very poor prognosis improved by treatment?

Since the data just quoted were taken from patients treated principally with prednis(ol)one alone, or together with cytotoxic agents, it is evident that these agents make little or no impact.

Although most of the evidence favoring the use of anticoagulants in the treatment of glomerulonephritis was obtained with models of anti-GBM nephritis [22], very little use of anticoagulation alone or together with immunosuppression has been made in the human disease. We have treated two anuric patients with the combination without any effect, and the risk of precipitating or worsening pulmonary hemorrhage perhaps accounts for the lack of reports in the literature. Note that in table 13–6, nine patients received anticoagulation as well as plasmapheresis.

There are almost as few reports of the use of intravenous doses of methylprednisolone in anti-GBM nephritis. Bolton [49] gave a preliminary report on eight patients so treated without evident benefit, all patients being oligo-anuric and requiring dialysis. The abstract of Bruns and colleagues [50] is a little more encouraging. Some workers, however, have reported resolution of pulmonary hemorrhage after the use of i.v. methylprednisolone

TABLE 13–6. Effect of plasmapheresis on survival with renal function in Goodpasture's syndrome

	Ref	Beginning treatment with renal function[b]		Beginning of treatment oligo-anuric		Immunosuppression used[d]
		TREATED	MAINTAINED OR IMPROVED FUNCTION	TREATED	FUNCTION RETURNED	
Lockwood & Peters 1980	[53]	18	12	10	0	P+C+A
Johnson et al. 1978	[54]	3	3	1	0	P+C
Walker et al. 1977	[55]	4	2	0	0	P+C+A
Swainson et al. 1978	[56]	1	0	2	0	P+C
Erikson et al. 1979	[57]	4	3	2	0	P+C
Munk & Skamene 1979	[58]	1	1	1	0	P,nil
McKenzie et al. 1979	[12]	3	3	1	0	P+C
Asaba et al.[c] 1980	[59]	1	1	1	0	P+A
Cameron et al 1981	(unp)	0	0	2	0	P+C+A
		35	25 (71%)	20	0 (0%)	

[a]NB. Single case reports not included (see text). Most, but not all, patients have extensive crescentic glomerulonephritis.
[b]P_{creat} < 1000 μmol/l (11.3 mg/dl)/,GFR > 5 ml/min plus urine output and no requirement for dialysis.
[c]Using a plasma membrane filter.
[d]P = prednis(ol)one; A = azathioprine; C = cyclophosphamide. Walker used prednisone and azathioprine in one patient, prednisone and cyclophosphamide in three. In addition, two of Lockwood's, both of Asaba's, and all of Walker's patients received anticoagulant treatment in addition (heparin/warfarin plus dipyridamole).

[51], and we must regard the question of whether methylprednisolone achieves any benefit in anti-GBM nephritis as an open one.

Most interest has centered recently on the use of plasmapheresis or plasma exchange in patients with anti-GBM disease. This has almost always been combined with immunosuppression—often intense immunosuppression—because of the supposed risks of antibody "rebound" following removal of circulating antibody by plasma exchange [52]. Whether any possible benefit arises directly from removal and suppression of injurious antibody is not clear. Obviously, also, removal of humoral mediators of injury could be important, but in experimental animals, complement seems to be most important in the brief, reversible heterologous phase of anti-GBM antibody fixation, and not in the autologous phase, although here fibrinogen is of central importance [22].

In the largest series of plasmapheresed patients suffering from anti-GBM disease, that treated at the Hammersmith Hospital in London [53], the immunosuppression used has been azathioprine 1 mg/kg/24h, cyclophosphamide 3 mg/kg/24h, plus a variable dosage of prednisolone orally. Various replacement fluids have been used, depending on availability, and daily 4-1 exchanges performed for 7 to 10 days.

In considering the published results of such treatment in a rare disease, it is probably better to ignore all single case reports since single case reports of failure are unlikely and make their way into the literature, whereas "success" is more frequently publicized: table 13–6 gives an analysis of a published series of two or more patients up to the end of 1981. It is immediately noticeable that despite encouraging results in patients with rapidly aggressive glomerulonephritis short of renal failure, there has been uniform failure to benefit patients with oligo-anuria.

A preliminary communication of more recent results from the Hammersmith group [60] confirms this impression; of 21 oligo-anuric patients with anti-GBM disease treated with plasmapheresis and immunosuppression, none recovered renal function and 11 died.

Thus, it seems that treatment with immunosuppression and plasmapheresis confers no benefit, so far as renal function is concerned, on patients with the oligo-anuric form of anti-GBM nephritis, and is not worth pursuing since the complications (principally infections) are by no means negligible. The main indication for using this form of treatment in oligo-anuric patients then is for severe pulmonary disease, if present. Of 23 treated patients reported in the literature who had varying degrees of pulmonary involvement (life-threatening in some patients), only a single patient among those described by McKenzie and colleagues [12] appeared to have gained no benefit. A further consideration is the persistence of anti-GBM antibody in the circulation: this is brief in patients plasmapheresed [53], usually detectable for only a few months at most, whereas antibody may persist for years in patients left untreated. This may influence subsequent transplantation attempts.

1.3.3.2 PRESUMED IDIOPATHIC IMMUNE COMPLEX CRESCENTIC GLOMERULONEPHRITIS. This is a rare and heterogenous group of patients, principally involving endocapillary proliferative glomerulonephritis, many postinfectious or mesangiocapillary in pattern. One can also include under this heading the more dubious group of "idiopathic" crescentic glomerulonephritis since it is not possible in all published series to distinguish exactly what the authors have described.

Usually, in oligo-anuric patients, more than 60% of glomeruli are affected by crescents, but occasional patients with 50 to 60% of glomeruli showing crescents present in this fashion [2, 7, 12, 13]. In some of these patients, the remaining glomeruli do not show the expected intense proliferation and infiltration, and the mechanism of the oliguria is obscure. Thus, the boundary between "crescentic" or endocapillary glomerulonephritis with anuria is not an absolute one.

Analysis of the literature up to 1970 shows about 100 patients who were in the main treated with prednisone, with or without cytotoxic agents. The results of these analyses have been published [44, 61] and show that about one-quarter of patients with more than 60% of glomeruli affected by crescents managed in this fashion showed retention or recovery of renal function. Of those with oligo-anuria, 10% or less showed recovery of function. It is doubtful if these figures differ from the figure of 11% spontaneous recovery for all cases given no treatment (table 13–2) who mostly had some renal function at presentation.

Despite the fact that animal work using anticoagulants has been almost exclusively on the model of anti-GBM nephritis [62], and the doses of heparin or warfarin used were lethal in many animals, clinically it has been in presumed immune complex glomerulonephritis that anticoagulants have been used, almost always in association with some form of immunosuppression.

In our own series, eight patients in the immune complex group who were oligo-anuric were treated, and two out of four with idiopathic immune complex crescentic nephritis recovered renal function and retained it. In Arandt's small controlled trial [13] in poststreptococcal glomerulonephritis with extensive crescent formation, two patients in the test group and one in the control group required dialysis; all recovered renal function, and there was no overall difference between test and control groups. When it has been employed, this form of treatment has been used almost always in patients with a rapid decline in renal function rather than those requiring dialysis [13, 62–65] and so, again, data are insufficient to draw firm conclusions.

In 1976, Cole [66] and colleagues first reported the use of very large doses of methyl-prednisolone intravenously for severe forms of glomerulonephritis, after others had used it to treat transplant rejection [67] and systemic lupus erythematosus [68]. Table 13–7 summarizes these and subsequent reports. As in other situations, the presumed "response" of patients with oligo-anuria to treatment is poorer (8 of 17, 47%) than those without (19 of 21, 90%). The simplicity, brevity, and relative lack of toxicity of this treatment (usually involving the injection of 1 G of methylprednisolone daily for 3 consecutive days) has made it popular, and these apparently impressive results when compared with historical controls have made this almost the standard treatment for immune complex rapidly progressive glomerulonephritis. Bolton and colleagues have since given a brief report [70] on a controlled comparison, which appears to be consistent with the preliminary results in table 13–7.

Unlike the fairly clear role for plasmapheresis in anti-GBM nephritis outlined above, there are no clear answers as to whether plasmapheresis is better than other approaches, including no treatment. Also, how plasma exchange might work in patients with immune complex disease is even less clear than in the case of anti-GBM nephritis. As well as the possibility of depletion of mediator of injury, removal of immune complexes from the circulation may have various effects. It is still possible that these complexes represent the pathogenic

TABLE 13–7. Treatment of patients with glomerulonephritis without vasculitis and >60% crescents with i.v. methylprednisolone: summary of the literature

	Ref.	Total	(Of whom oligo-anuric)	Response*		
Cole et al. 1976	[66]	2	(0)	2	(–)	
O'Neill et al. 1979	[69]	10	(7)	4	(2)	1 G daily for 7 days
Bolton 1981	[70]	10	(7)	9	(6)	30 mg/kg, 3 doses
Oredugba et al. 1979	[71]	5	(0)	5	(–)	1 G daily for 5 days
Bruns et al. 1980	[50]	9	(3)	7	(–)	30 mg/kg 4–11 doses
	Totals	36	(17)	27 (75%)	(8) (47%)	

*Figures in parentheses give no. of patients with oligo-anuria who "responded."
Notes: 1. No. of pulses of 1 G methylprednisolone given: 3–11 G.
2. Initial plasma creatinines: 450–1610 μmol/l (5.1–18.2 mg/dl).
3. Final plasma creatinines (6–36 months follow-up): 80–283 μmol/l (0.9–3.2 mg/dl). (One patient died of cryptococcal meningitis with a plasma creatinine of 80 μml/l (0.9 mg/dl).)
4. Bolton 1981 [70] includes 5 patients described in Bolton and Couser 1979 [44].
5. Note that patients with less than 60% of glomeruli involved by crescents have been excluded, as have patients with anti-GBM disease.

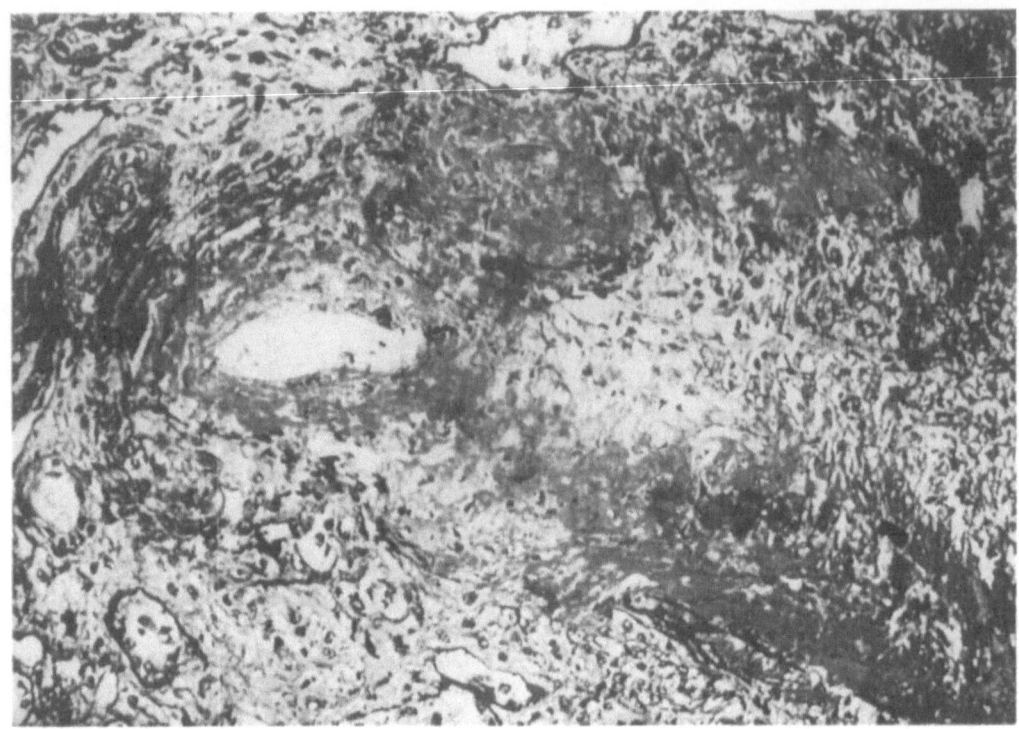

FIGURE 13–6. Acute arteritis within the kidney. The wall of an artery is focally replaced with necrotic material which stains as fibrin surrounded by inflammatory cells. Only about one-third of patients with microscopic polyarteritis and glomerulonephritis show vasculitis in renal biopsy specimens. (Martius scarlet-blue counterstained with silver, ×250.)

agents, although this now seems less likely. If circulating complexes truly represent those complexes localizing in the kidney, then removal and antibody suppresion might arrest progress of the disease. In addition, the effect of circulating complexes in blocking the reticuloendothelial system, thus permitting more toxic complexes to persist, has been advocated [53]. Finally, if soluble immune complexes regulate the immune response in part, then their removal might "reset" the system, either in a beneficial fashion, or to the patient's detriment.

Thus, patients with presumed immune complex glomerulonephritis treated by plasma exchange are inevitably more mixed population than those with anti-GBM disease. In a number of reports [12, 50, 72–75], all or most of the patients had vasculitis, Henoch-Schönlein purpura, or systemic lupus as well as severe glomerulonephritis. The patients with presumed immune complex disease not associated with vasculitis are in the minority, although encouraging results have been published in a total of 31 patients (21 "improved") whose disease was treated at a point short of renal failure (plasma creatinines 100–800 μmol/l, 1–9 mg/dl), there are almost no accounts of oligoanuric patients with idiopathic glomerulonephritis treated by plasma exchange who also required dialysis. Of a total of four patients [60, 74], none recovered renal function. Thus, the value of plasma exchange in oliguric patients in this group remains unstudied, although clearly there may be a role in patients, with or without crescentic glomerulnephritis, who have advancing renal failure.

1.3.3.3 CRESCENTIC NEPHRITIS AS PART OF VASCULITIS. The microscopic form of polyarteritis (figure 13–6) is frequently complicated by a focal segmental necrotising glomerulonephritis (figure 13–7 A and B and extensive crescent formation is often seen [2], even in the presence of mostly normal glomeruli [31]. Thus, crescentic glomerulonephritis with vasculitis is more common than immune complex glomerulonephritis without vascular involvement.

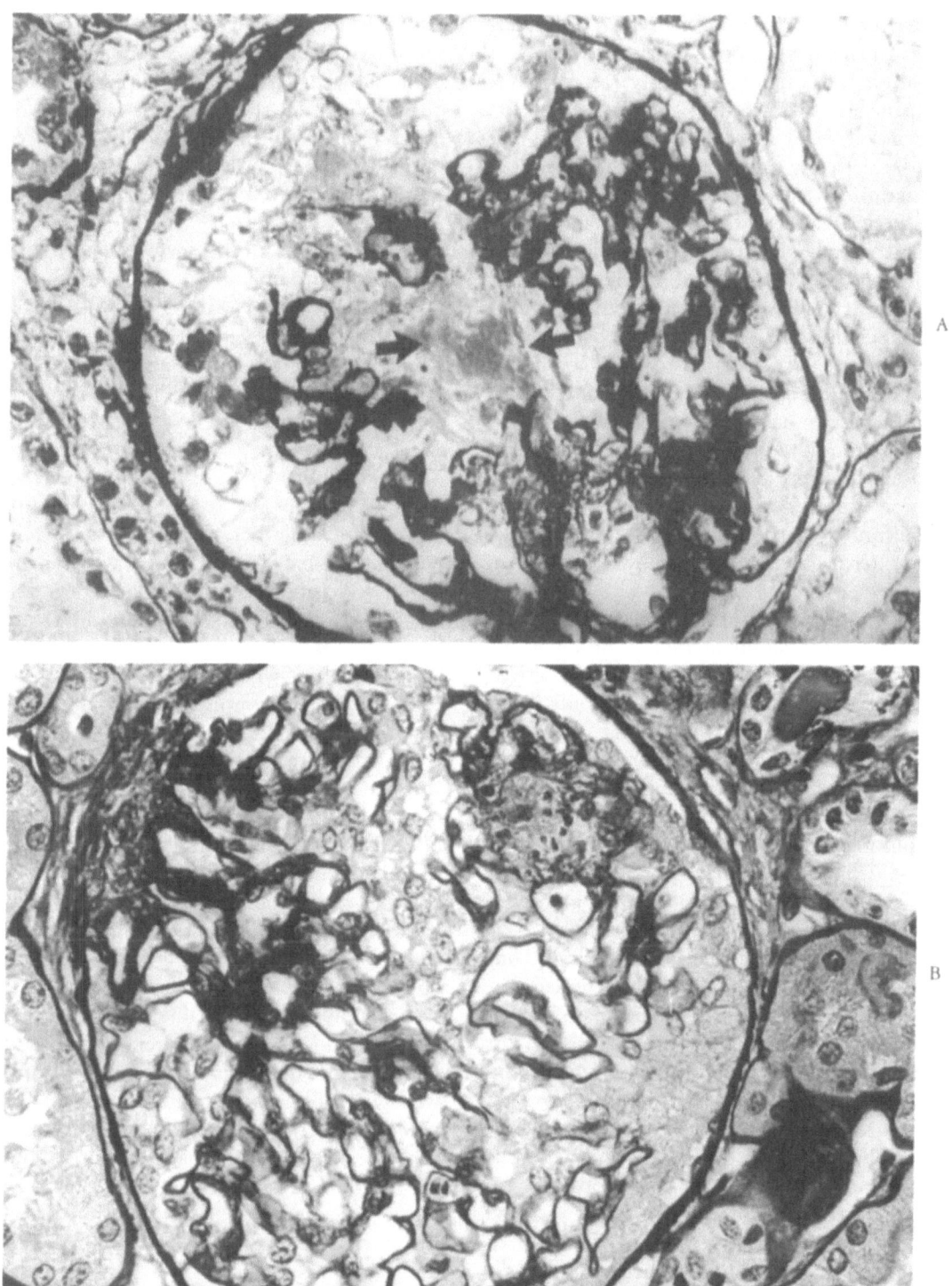

FIGURE 13–7. **A.** Focal segmental necrotizing glomerulonephritis in a setting of polyarteritis. This is the microscopic form of the disease in which the glomerular capillaries are commonly affected, in contrast to the "classical" form of the disease in which major arteries are the principal seat of disease. The necrotic area contains fibrin (arrows). Such lesions may be found with and without crescents. (Methenamine silver counterstained with haematoxylin and eosin, ×450.) **B.** A milder lesion showing nuclear debris and small surrounding crescents from a patient with SLE. (Silver methenamine counterstained with hematoxylin and eosin, ×500.)

The overall prognosis of untreated polyarteritis is in general very poor, both in Wegener's granuloma and microscopic polyarteritis, five-year survivals of 12 to 15% being the rule irrespective of renal involvement [48]. This has been dramatically improved by the introduction first of corticosteroids, which raised overall five-year survival rates to 50 to 60% and finally cytotoxic agents, which have given survivals of up to 80% at five years [48]. Therefore, any treatment of severe renal improvement in the vasculitides must be seen against a background of treatment with corticosteroids, cytotoxic agents being used at least in the acute phase, and probably in the long-term for many patients. Although cyclophosphamide has received most attention [76], results with azathioprine are as good; perhaps it is better to use the former in the acute disease and the latter long-term in view of its lower long-term toxicity.

Surprisingly, there are few accounts in the literature giving details of more than a few patients with polyarteritis and glomerulonephritis [2]. In our own series of 55 such patients (Serra et al., in preparation), including three patients with biopsy-proven Wegener's granuloma and two cases of relapsing polychondritis, 21 patients were oligo-anuric at presentation with plasma creatinines of 600 to 2,000 μmol/l (6.8–22.6 mg/dl) and required dialysis. Of these 21, 13 had more than 60% of glomeruli involved by crescents; of the remainder, two showed intense endocapillary proliferation, one showed capillary thrombi, and the remainder, lesser degrees of crescent formation. Thus, as in idiopathic glomerulonephritis, although the majority of patients with oligo-anuria show extensive crescent formation, this is not present in all. Of the 21 patients, only one, whose biopsy showed only the mildest mesangial changes and whose oliguria was of obscure origin, recovered renal function. Another patient with 90% crescents recovered renal function after two years on dialysis. Furthermore, only two other patients survived on dialysis, the remainder dying on dialysis of complication of their disease, of treatment, or both. Five patients were given no treatment other than dialysis because of age, or other disease, while six were treated with methylprednisolone and seven with anticoagulants (three with both); none showed a diuresis. The adverse effect of oliguria itself is shown by the fact that of nine other patients with 60 to 100% of glomeruli affects by crescents who did not have oligo-anuria (plasma creatinines 132 and 290–430 μmol/l 1.5 and 3.3–4.9 mg/dl), seven are now alive with their own kidneys, two with normal renal function.

Only four other patients with polyarteritis and oligo-anuric crescentic glomerulonephritis who were treated with pulse methylprednisolone have been reported [70, 77]; three of Bolton's [70] patients were able to come off dialysis, but Neild's [77] oligo-anuric patient did not. Thus, the advantages of methylprednisolone do not seem to be great, taking all these data together. Friedman and Kincaid-Smith [78] had better results with anticoagulation and immunosuppression. They treated a total of eight patients with vasculitis, crescentic nephritis, and oliguria, two with steroids at one (both of whom failed to regain function) and six with combined treatment, four of whom regained function.

Plasmapheresis has been used in a number of similar patients, especially at Hammersmith Hospital [60, 72]; many of these patients have been called "Wegener's granuloma" in published accounts, but these reports are unclear on the criteria on which this diagnosis was based. In the majority, the diagnosis was made from the combination of arteritis and lung involvement and might be included as microscopic polyarteritis in other series. Nevertheless, the most recent brief report [60] from the Hammersmith group mentions 24 patients who were oligo-anuric at presentation, all of whom had either microscopic polyarteritis [7] or Wegener's granuloma [18] and a mean of 77% glomeruli affected by crescents. Of these, 14 (58%) recovered renal function after plasmapheresis, after up to 28 days of treatment on dialysis; subsequently, one patient developed end-stage renal failure. Nine patients (33%) had plasma creatinines of 200 to 400 μmol/l 2.3–4.5 mg/dl at last follow-up, six who recovered function having died, three of infection. On the basis of three results, intensive daily 4-1 plasma exchanges with background immunosuppression using prednisone and cytotoxic agents appear to offer a better prognosis for patients with arteritis and severe crescentic glomerulonephritis with anuria than either anticoagulation or methylprednisolone.

1.3.4 Systemic Lupus Erythematosus (SLE)

Severe oliguric glomerulonephritis with or without extensive crescent formation is very rare in SLE [32], despite the fact that severe nephritis is quite common, and decline in renal function may be rapid. Only occasional cases are reported [32, 79–81] in series totaling more than 1,000 patients with lupus nephritis. In our own series [82], six patients presented with more than 60% of glomeruli affected by crescents and another patients developed crescents later. Only this patient and two others were oligo-anuric. Some patients without crescents develop acute renal failure, in association with arteritis or glomerular thrombosis [83].

Pateints with severe proliferative glomerulonephritis are almost always treated using oral prednisone, and in many units with cytotoxic agents as well. The appearance of acute oliguria may be in a setting of such treatment in the past.

Following the use of intravenous methylprednisolone for acute transplant rejection [67], this treatment has been tried in patients with severe lupus nephritis [68, 80–82, 84, 85], usually in the form of 1 G intravenously on three consecutive days. Patients with a recent deterioration in function and without glomerulosclerosis have shown encouraging responses, but only six of the reported cases were oligo-anuric and required dialysis [80, 81], of whom four responded with return of renal function. Thus, high-dose intravenous methylprednisolone seems worth a trial even in oligo-anuric lupus nephritis with crescents.

Plasmapheresis has also been applied to the treatment of SLE nephritis [12, 86–88], but all the patients treated have had mild to moderate impairment of renal function only. The role of this treatment in severe lupus nephritis with oliguria has not been evaluated.

Ponticelli and colleagues [83] pointed to the importance of glomerular thrombi in acute renal failure in SLE and reported favorably on treatment with anticoagulants in four cases, all of whom regained function. We have also used combined anticoagulation and immunosuppression in a total of eight patients with severe lupus nephritis, three of whom required dialysis. However, none of the three oliguric patients retained renal function.

1.3.5 Henoch-Schönlein purpura

Severe oliguric renal failure is even more rare in Henoch-Schönlein purpura nephritis [30]. In a series of now over 200 patients, we have seen acute oligo-anuric renal failure and severe crescentic glomerulonephritis in only two patients, who both failed to respond to combined immunosuppression and anticoagulation. Usually, glomerulonephritis with extensive crescent formation in a setting of Henoch-Schönlein purpura presents as a progressive renal failure over months or years, and even this outcome is rare [89]. There seem to be no data on the use of methylprednisolone in this situation, although McKenzie [12] and Kaufmann and Houwert [90] report three cases treated with plasmapheresis.

1.3.6 Essential Cryoglobulinemia

Occasionally, monoclonal cryoimmunoglobulinemia [91] and rather more commonly mixed cryoglobulinemia [34, 91, 92] may present with ARF, whether an underlying disease can be identified or not ("essential mixed cryoglobulinemia"). In many instances, the acute renal failure reverses with immunosuppression [34], especially intravenous methylprednisolone; the use of plasma exchange would seem to have particular advantages, especially when large amounts of cryoglobulin and immune complexes are present in the circulation McKenzie et al. [93] report on a case of severe progressive nephritis, short of oliguria, treated by plasmapheresis and immunosuppression.

1.3.7 Conclusions

It is evident that aggressive treatment of oliguric forms of glomerulonephritis associated with severe crescent formation has not been evaluated fully in any instance. Nor, if one examines the data critically, is it clear what advantages such aggressive treatment may have over supportive treatment, including dialysis. Perhaps the clearest indication from these uncontrolled data is that survival can be improved in Goodpasture's syndrome, especially with pulmonary involvement, by plasmapheresis, and that perhaps this treatment also improves the prognosis for oliguric crescentic nephritis in polyarteritis. Even less certain are the results of intravenous methylprednisolone in nonsystemic crescentic glomerulonephritis; it would appear that once oliguria has become established, reversal is unlikely whatever treatment is given although about one in five cases of recovery has been reported.

An important factor of immunosuppressive treatments is that the side effects, especially infections, may be worse than the disease [94]. This is particularly so with plasmapheresis combined with high doses of cytotoxic agents and steroids [94, 95]. In balancing the decision of whether and when to employ such treatments, this will remain an important consideration.

2 Acute Renal Failure in Nephrotic Patients with Minor Glomerular Abnormalities

Fifteen years ago, Wrong and colleagues [96, 97] pointed out that patients with minor or minimal change lesions in their glomeruli, but a severe nephrotic syndrome, could go into acute renal failure. In their patients, oliguria was prolonged and dialysis necessary, but in most a diuresis was obtained one to four months later. They also noted a similar state in patients with severe amyloidosis and profuse proteinuria. Subsequently, a number of other authors have reported acute oliguria and uremia requiring dialysis in nephrotic patients with minimal change lesions [98–107], the prognosis varying from immediate return of renal function with volume replacement and diuretics through brief or prolonged periods of oliguria to apparently permanent renal failure.

2.1 CLINICAL DIAGNOSIS
Almost all patients reported in the literature have been adults, usually over 50 or 60 years of age; one of our own patients with a minimal

change nephrotic syndrome who went into ARF was 82 (figure 13–8). There is only one report of ARF in children with minimal lesions and a nephrotic syndrome [108] which describes two boys of eight and twelve who required dialysis for acute reversible renal failure. We have seen three cases of acute reversible renal failure in nephrotic children with minimal change: one, aged 2½, precipitated by pneumococcal septicemia and peritonitis another from extreme prolonged hypotension, which also resulted in aortic thrombosis and loss of both legs. A fourth child died anuric despite peritoneal dialysis. The more common situation in children and young adults is a patient who may be uremic and oliguric, but whose urine output responds promptly to volume replacement with intravenous albumin together with diuretics. An inquiry of three units, who between them have seen more than 2,000 nephrotic children, revealed no further unpublished cases; therefore, established ARF must be accounted very rare in nephrotic children (RHR White, I Greifer, M Broyer, personal communications 1982).

Obviously, it is very important to distinguish between a minimal change lesion with immediately reversible oliguria, the same situation but with established ARF, and the patients with a proliferative glomerulonephritis, usually crescentic. Renal vein thrombosis [109] and acute interstitial nephritis [110] also need exclusion. In the early stages of acute oliguria in minimal change nephrotics, the urine is highly concentrated (U/P osmolality $>1.3:1$), almost devoid of sodium (<5 mmol/l), and usually does not contain red cells; the latter is, of course, not true in patients with focal glomerulosclerosis. If casts are present, they are usually only of the hyaline variety. Once tubular necrosis has become established, however, and oliguria resistant to volume replacement and diuretics is present, the urine will be that of ATN with a higher sodium concentration (20–60 mmol/l), abundant granular casts, and red cells. Red cell casts, however, are usually absent. Finally, in acute glomerulonephritis, the urine may show low sodium but with abundant red cells, red cells and other casts, and proteinuria.

Thus, the urine findings are particularly

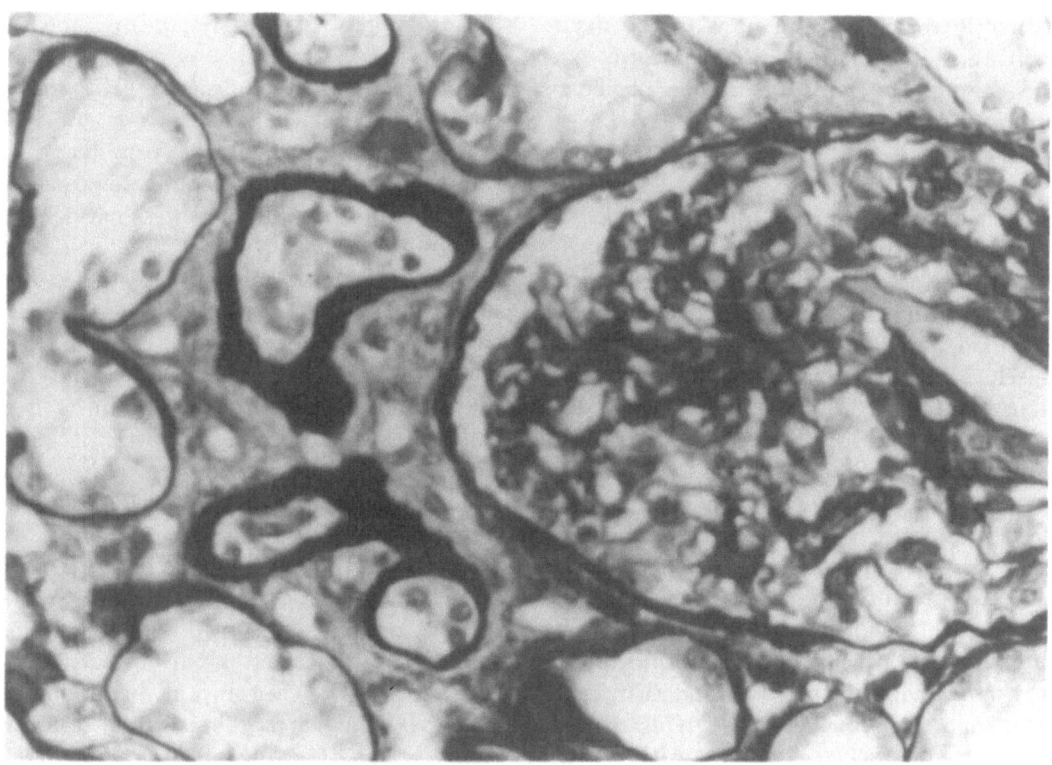

FIGURE 13–8. Renal biopsy in an 82-year-old man with a nephrotic syndrome and acute renal failure. The glomerulus is essentially normal (allowing for age), but tubules show extensive vacuolation and necrosis. Intravenous albumin (which failed to achieve a diuresis) put him into pulmonary edema. He died later still on dialysis. (Silver methenamine counterstained with hematoxylin and eosin, ×250.)

helpful if the urinary findings suggest a minimal change lesion with reversible oliguria; any other finding may have to be sorted out by judicious administration of fluids, colloid, and diuretics, and by renal biopsy. The history of a nephrotic syndrome will obviously by of great value, and renal vein thrombosis may need to be excluded by ultrasonography or venography (see below, however, on the toxicity of contrast agents in nephrotic patients.)

Recently, several reports have appeared of nephrotic patients whose renal failure followed ingestion of prostaglandin synthetase inhibitors [111–116], such as indomethacin [113, 114] or fenoprofen [115, 116]. In some, the changes were slow, in others acute. These drugs are known to cause an acute reversible drop in glomerular filtration rate [117] and may also give rise to an interstitial nephritis, which was

noted in some of the reported cases, in nonnephrotic as well as those with a nephrotic syndrome. Obviously, a search should be made in the history for other factors that might relate to renal failure, including other nephrotoxic drugs and agents (see chapter 2), other reasons for acute renal hypoperfusion or toxic pigmenturia.

2.2 RENAL BIOPSY APPEARANCES

Renal biopsies in nephrotic patients with acute renal failure do not show the usual distribution of glomerular histological patterns: although occasional patients with mesangiocapillary glomerulonephritis, membranous nephropathy, or amyloidosis have been recorded, the great majority show minimal changes, mild mesangial increase, or focal segmental glomerulosclerosis. The tubules and interstitium may be normal, allowing for age, but extensive tubular necrosis with or without regenerative changes may be seen. A few patients may show extensive interstitial infiltrates [99]; if this is so, the possibility of drug sensitization should be considered (see chapter 2). But this is not always present, and a recent report suggests that this may relate directly to the pathogenesis of the disorder, in that minimal change nephrotic syndrome may arise from a disorder of T-cell function [116].

2.3 PATHOGENESIS

At first, such cases were all thought to result from acute and prolonged hypovolemia [118], perhaps aggravated by other hypotensive events such as bleeding, anesthesia, and surgery, or septicemia, by whatever mechanisms lead to post-ischaemic ATN in nonnephrotic patients without preexisting hypovolemia [119] (see chapter 2). In our own series of 12 nephrotic patients with ARF, such factors were important in three patients. Thus, the spectrum of "prerenal" uremia, established ARF, and irreversible renal failure is seen in both nephrotic and nonnephrotic patients. However, it has become clear that the pathognesis of edema in the nephrotic patient [120] is more complicated than previously supposed and that hypovolemia and consequent renal hypoperfusion cannot account for all cases of ARF in nephrotics.

First, hypovolemia is present only in some nephrotic patients [121], others having normal or even expanded plasma volumes. This may have importance in the use of intravenous albumin in the management of the nephrotic patient in ARF (see below). Most hypovolemic patients with high renin levels are those with minimal change lesions or minor changes [122]. In the untreated nephrotic patient, plasma volume appears to return to around normal levels, at the price of a grossly expanded interstitial volume, visible as edema. Second, a number of nephrotic patients with minimal change lesions are hypertensive [98, 121] rather than hypotensive, even when hypovolemic; this may arise from, or relate to, high renin levels. Finally, although most patients with an active minimal change nephrotic syndrome show depressed glomerular filtration rates or creatinine clearances, in the few in whom plasma flow has been measured at the same time this was normal, or less prominently depressed, so that the filtration fraction was decreased [112, 121] rather than increased as might be supposed. If only some cases of ARF in nephrotic patients arise from acute renal hypoperfusion, what is responsible for the remaining cases?

Lowenstein and colleagues [104] have suggested that renal edema causes a rise in interstitial pressure in nephrotic patients that could result in tubular collapse. Measurements of intrarenal interstitial pressures have not been made in nephrotic patients as yet, although the kidneys are well known to be large in X-ray or ultrasonography in such patients. A possible role for altered glomerular permeability has been discussed; in minimal change children [123] and adults [124], permeability to molecules of low molecular weight is decreased. In contrast to the increased permeability to molecules of higher molecular weight and in rats rendered hypoalbuminemic, the ultrafiltration coefficient fell, with no increase in the GFR (which would be expected from the fall in plasma oncotic pressure) [125]. Further experiments by the same group in rats made nephrotic with puromycin aminonucleoside showed a fall in capillary ultrafiltration coefficient [126]. The morphological alterations in podocyte foot process structure in both experimental animals and human patients with nephrotic syndromes may provide the morphological correlate of this observation. At the moment, although we cannot be sure of what is going on in the majority of nephrotics in ARF, a change in ultrafiltration coefficient seems the most attractive explanation.

In some patients, other factors involved in acute or tubular damage may be involved, including large doses of contrast media [127] nephrotoxic drugs other than prostaglandin synthetase inhibitors, septicemia, jaundice, myoglobinuria, etc. (see chapters 2, 11, and 12). In our own series, three patients had episodes of ARF following injections of large doses of meglimine ditrozoate for renal venography, using the technique of venous phase arteriography. Thus, the contrast was delivered directly into the renal artery, and it is now clear that this technique carries considerable risk. Another patient had septicemia and another a major secondary hemorrhage from a surgical renal biopsy.

2.4 CLINICAL MANAGEMENT

Two immediate goals (apart from dealing with

uremia per se) are first to distinguish between a nephrotic syndrome arising from proliferative glomerulonephritis, and one the result of minimal or minor changes alone; and second, to determine the reversibility of the lesion. As discussed above, a finding of highly concentrated urine with a very low sodium concentration, when coupled with a urine devoid of red cells and granular casts, strongly suggests a nephrotic syndrome arising from a minimal change lesion, which is at least potentially reversible. However, a urine with a higher sodium concentration, isoosmolar with plasma, and containing red cells and granular casts can arise either in a patient with severe glomerulonephritis or from a minimal change nephrotic syndrome with superadded ATN. Under these circumstances, only a renal biopsy can distinguish between the two possibilities. A history of a nephrotic syndrome is in itself a favor of ATN in a nephrotic patient with minimal change since a nephrotic syndrome is unusual as a prodrome to an oligo-anuric crescentic glomerulonephritis.

To determine the reversibility of the oliguric state, and avert established ARF administration of powerful diuretics, intravenous albumin solutions, or both are often used. Both have dangers. If the patient is critically hypovolemic and a response to the diuretic is obtained, the hypovolemia may be worsened and ARF rendered irreversible. If albumin is given indiscriminately and no diuresis is obtained, the sudden expansion of a normally filled or overfilled circulation may lead to acute pulmonary edema. Thus, both agents should be given together, under careful and continuous observation of the hourly urinary output and the cardiovascular status; in patients with normally filled or overfilled jugular veins, albumin should be avoided. A central venous pressure line assists when the neck veins cannot be seen easily. Up to 1 G or more of frusemide may be needed to obtain a diuresis.

The use of more powerful renal vasodilators, such as dopamine in low dosage (1–2 μg/kg/min) or oral captopril, is attractive, but no reports of their use in this situation have yet appeared.

If no response is obtained to the restoration of a depleted circulating volume (if present) and diuretics in large dosage, then further administration of diuretics can lead to toxicity. Likewise, if a bladder catheter has been used in the initial stages to determine the hourly urine output, it may now be removed. Management now centers on the management of a state of uremia that may last days, weeks, or months [97, 99], sometimes complicated by continued losses of large amounts of albumin in the urine.

The combination of a nephrotic state and uremia is dangerous, and the danger may be further increased by giving corticosteroids and/or immunosuppressants with the aim of putting the minimal change lesion into remission. Probably, the continued risks of proteinuria—and its massive increase when a diuresis is obtained—are less than adding immunosuppression to hypoproteinemia and uremia, but this can be judged only for the inidividual patient. It is usual for proteinuria to remain in the nephrotic range despite oliguria severe enough to require dialysis.

2.5 PROGNOSIS

As indicated, this state is serious, and since many of the patients are over 60, death from complications is seen. However, in some patients, renal function does not return [99, 104, 106], for reasons as obscure as the nature of the whole condition. There do not appear to be any clues as to which patients have irreversible renal failure, and the prolonged oliguria in some patients (mean 43 days in Wrong's series) [96, 97] means that dialysis must be pursued in any case.

References

1. Swann RC, Merrill JP. The clinical course of acute renal failure. Medicine 32: 215–292, 1953.
2. Harrison CV, Loughridge LW, Milne MD. Acute oliguric renal failure in acute glomerulonephritis and polyarteritis nodosa. Quart J Med 33: 39–55, 1964.
3. Espinel CH, Gregory AW. Differential diagnosis of acute renal failure. Clin Nephrol 13: 73–77, 1980.
4. Hilton PJ, Jones NF, Barraclough MA, Lloyd-Davies RW. Urinary osmolality in acute renal failure due to glomerulonephritis. Lancet 2: 655–656, 1969.
5. Wilson DM, Turner DR, Cameron JS, Ogg CS, Brown CB, Chantler C. Value of renal biopsy in

acute intrinsic renal failure. Brit Med J 2: 459–461, 1976.

6. Lewy JE, Salinal-Madrigal L, Herdson PB, Pirani CL, Metcoff J. Clinicopathological correlations in acute post-streptococcal glomerulonephritis. Medicine 50: 453–501, 1971.

7. Nakamoto S, Dunea G, Koloff WJ, McCormack LJ. Treament of oliguric glomerulonephritis with dialysis and steroids. Ann Int Med 63: 359–368, 1965.

8. Beaufils M, Morel-Maroger L, Sraer J-D, Kanfer A, Kourilsky O, Richet G. Acute renal failure of glomerular origin during visceral abcesses. N Engl J Med 295: 185–189, 1976.

9. Kim Y, Michael AF. Chronic bacteremia and nephritis. Ann Rev Med 29: 319–325, 1978.

10. Morel-Maroger L, Kourilsky O, Mignon F, Richet G. Antitubular basement membrane antibodies in rapidly progressive post-streptococcal glomerulonephritis: Report of a case. Clin Immunol Immunopathol 2: 185–194, 1974.

11. Gill DG, Turner DR, Chantler C, Cameron JS. The progression of acute proliferative post-streptococcal glomerulonephritis to severe epithelial crescent formation. Clin Nephrol 8: 449–452, 1977.

12. McKenzie PF, Taylor AE, Woodroffe AJ, Seymour AE, Chan Y-L, Clarkson AR. Plasmapheresis in glomerulonephritis. Clin Nephrol 12: 97–108, 1979.

13. Roy S, Murphy WM, Arant BS. Poststreptococcal crescentic glomerulonephritis in children: Comparison of quintuple therapy versus supportive care. J Peditr 98: 403–410, 1981.

14. Talwalkar YB, Price WH, Musgrave JE. Recurrent resolving renal failure in IgA nephropathy. J Pediatr 92: 596–597, 1978.

15. Glassock RJ. A clinical and immunopathologic dissection of rapidly progressive glomerulonephritis. Nephron 22: 253, 1978.

16. Spargo BH, Ordoñez NG, Ringus JC. The differential diagnosis of crescentic glomerulonephritis. The pathology of specific lesions with prognostic implications. Hum Pathol 8: 187–204, 1977.

17. Whitworth JA, Morel-Maroger L, Mignon F, Richet G. The significance of extracapillary proliferation. Clinicopathological review of 60 patients. Nephron 16: 1–19, 1976b.

18. Levy M, Broyer M, Habib R. Pathology and immunopathology of Schönlein-Henoch nephritis. In Progress in Glomerulonephritis, Kincaid-Smith P, D'Apice AJF, Atkins RC (eds). New York: John Wiley, 1979, pp. 261–282.

19. Stejskal J, Pirani CL, Okada M, Mandelanakis N, Pollak VE. Discontinuities (gaps) of the glomerular capillary wall and basement membrane in renal diseases. Lab Invest 28: 149–169, 1973.

20. Hoyer JR, Michael AF, Hoyer LW. Immunofluorescent localization of antihemophilic factor antigen and fibrinogen in human renal disease. J Clin Invest 53: 1375–1384, 1974.

21. Sitprija V, Boonpucknavig V. Extracapillary proliferative glomerulonephritis in Russell's viper bite. Br Med J 1: 1417, 1980.

22. Naish P, Penn GB, Evans DJ, Peters DK. The effects of defibrination on nephrotoxic nephritis in the rabbit. Clin Sci 42: 643–646, 1972.

23. Cattell V, Jameson SW. The origin of glomerular crescents in experimental nephrotoxic serum nephritis in man. Lab Invest 39: 584–590, 1978.

24. Atkins RC, Holdsworth SR, Glasgow EF, Matthews FG. The macrophage in human rapidly progressive glomerulonephritis. Lancet: 830–832, 1976.

25. Miller K, Dresner IG, Michael AF. Localization of platelet antigens in human kidney disease. Kidney Int 18: 472–479, 1980.

26. Morita T, Suzuki Y, Churg J. Structure and development of the glomerular crescent. Amer J Pathol 72: 349–360, 1973.

27. Stilmant MM, Bolton WK,, Sturgill BC, Schmitt GW, Couser WG. Crescentic glomerulonephritis without immune deposits: Clinicopathologic features. Kidney Int 15: 184–195, 1979.

28. Habib R, Kleinknecht C, Gubler M-C, Levy M. Idiopathic membranoroliferative glomerulonephritis in children. Report of 105 cases. Clin Nephrol 1: 193–214, 1973.

29. Martini A, Magrini U, Scelsi M, Capelli V, Barberis L. Chronic mesangioproliferative IgA glomerulonephritis complicated by a rapidly progressive course in a 14-year-old boy. Nephron 29: 164–166, 1981.

30. Moorthy AV, Zimmerman SW, Burkholder PM, Harrington AR. Association of crescentic glomerulonephritis with membranous glomerulopathy: Report of three cases. Clin Nephrol 6: 319–325, 1976.

31. Heptinstall RH. Pathology of the Kidney. Boston: Little, Brown, 1974 (2nd ed), pp. 601–622.

32. Baldwin DS, Lowenstein J, Rothfield NF, Gallo G, McCluskey RT. The clinical course of the proliferative and membranous forms of lupus nephritis. Ann Int Med 73: 929–942, 1970.

33. Olsson PJ, Gaffney E, Alexander RW, Mars DR, Fuller TJ. Proliferative glomerulonephritis with crescent formation in Behçet's syndrome. Arch Int Med 140: 713–714, 1980.

34. Tarantino A, de Vechi A, Montagnino G, Imbasciati E, Mihatsch MJ, Zollinger HU, di Belgiojoso GB, Busnach G, Ponticelli C. Renal disease in essential mixed cryoglobulinemia. Long-term follow-up of 44 cases. Quart J Med 45: 1–30, 1981.

35. Border WA, Baehler RW, Bhathena D, Glassock RJ. IgA anti-basement membrane nephritis with pulmonary hemorrhage. Ann Int Med 91: 21–25, 1979.

36. Matthay RA, Bromberg SI, Putman CE. Pulmonary-renal syndromes—A review. Yale J Biol Med 53: 497–523, 1980.

37. Cohen AH, Border WA, Shankel E, Glassock RJ.

Crescentic glomerulonephritis: Immune vs nonimmune mechanisms. Am J Nephrol 1: 78–83, 1981.

38. Cameron JS, Turner DR, Heaton J, Williams DG, Ogg CS, Chantler C, Haycock GB, Hicks J. Idiopathic mesangiocapillary glomerulonephritis: Comparison of types I and II in children and adults, and long-term prognosis. Am J Med 1982.

39. Moorthy AV, Zimmerman SW. Renal disease in the elderly: Clinicopathologic analysis of renal disease in 115 elderly patients. Clin Nephrol 15: 223–229, 1980.

40. Leonard CD, Nagle RB, Striker GE, Cutler RE, Scribner BH. Acute glomerulonephritis with prolonged oliguria. Ann Int Med 73: 703–711, 1976.

41. Sonsino E, Nabarra B, Kazatchkine M, Hinglais N, Kreis N. Extracapillary proliferative glomerulonephritis. So-called malignant glomerulonephritis. Adv Nephrol 2: 121, 163, 1972.

42. Beirne GJ, Wagnild JP, Zimmerman SW, Machon PD, Burkholder PM. Idiopathic crescentic glomerulonephritis. Medicine 56: 349–381, 1977.

43. Morrin PAF, Hinglais N, Nabarra B, Kreis H. Rapidly progressive glomerulonephritis. A clinical and pathological study. Am J Med 65: 446–460, 1978.

44. Bolton WK, Couser WG. Intravenous methylprednisolone therapy of acute crescentic rapidly progressive glomerulonephritis. Am J Med 66: 594–502, 1979.

45. Cameron JS. The treatment of severe glomerulonephritis with combined immunosuppression and anticoagulation. In Proceedings of the 6th International Congress of Nephrology, Montreal, 1978. Basel: Karger, 1978, pp. 419–424.

46. Cameron JS. The natural history of glomerulonephritis. In Renal Disease, Black DAK, Jones NF (eds). Oxford: Blackwell Scientific Publications, 1979 (4th ed), pp. 329–382.

47. Wilson CB, Dixon FJ. Antiglomerular basement membrane antibody-induced glomerulonephritis. Kidney Int 3: 74–89, 1973.

48. Leib ES, Restivo C, Paulus HE. Immunosuppressive and corticosteroid therapy of polyarteritis nodosa. Am J Med 67: 941–947, 1979.

49. Bolton WK. Pulse methylprednisolone therapy (Rx) of idiopathic aute crescentic rapidly progressive glomerulonephritis (AC-RPGN). Abstracts, American Society of Nephrology, 1980, p. 13A.

50. Bruns FJ, Fraley DS, Alder S, Segel DP. Megadose methylprednisolone versus plasmapheresis in treatment of rapidly progressive glomerulonephritis (RPGN). Abstracts, 13th Annual Meeting American Society of Nephrology, 1980, p. 14A.

51. de Torrente A, Popvtzer MM, Guggenheim SJ, Schrier RW. Serious pulmonary hemorrhage, glomerulonephritis and massive steroid therapy. Ann Int Med 83: 218–219, 1975.

52. Balow JE. The role of immunosuppressive drugs in plasmapheresis therapy. In Proceedings of the 8th International Congress of Nephology, Athens, 1981. Basel: Karger, 1981, pp. 674–680.

53. Lockwood CM, Peters KD. Plasma exchange in glomerulonephritis and related vaculitides. Ann Rev Med 31: 167–179, 1980.

54. Johnson JP, Whitman W, Briggs WA, Wilson CB. Plasmapheresis and immunosuppressive agents in antibasement membrane antibody-induced Goodpasture's syndrome. Am J Med 64: 354–359, 1978.

55. Walker RG, D'Apice AJF, Becker GJ, Kincaid-Smith P, Craswell PWT. Plasmapheresis in Goodpasture's syndrome with renal failure. Med J Aust 1: 875–879, 1977.

56. Swainson CP, Robson JS, Urbaniak SJ, Keller AJ, Kay AB. Treatment of Goodpasture's disease by plasma exchange and immunosuppression. Clin Exp Immunol 32: 233–242, 1978.

57. Erikson SB, Kurtz SB, Donadio JV, Holley KE, Wilson CB, Pineda AA. Use of combined plasmapheresis and immunosuppression in the treatment of Goodpasture's syndrome. Mayo Clin Proc 54: 714–720, 1979.

58. Munk ZM, Skamene E. Goodpasture's syndrome—Effects of plasmapheresis. Clin Exp Immunol 36: 244–249, 1979.

59. Asaba H, Rekola S, Bergstrand A, Wasserman H, Bergstrom J. Clinical trial of plasma exchange with a membrane filter in treatment of crescentic glomerulonephritis. Clin Nephrol 14: 60–65, 1980.

60. Hind CRK, Lockwood CM, Evans DJ, Rees AJ. The prognosis after immunosuppression of patients with crescentic nephritis requiring dialysis. Quart J Med, 1982 (in press) (abstract).

61. Brown CB, Turner DR, Cameron JS, Ogg CS, Chantler C, Gill D. Combined immunosuppression and anticoagulation in rapidly progressive glomerulonephritis. Lancet 2: 1166–1172, 1974.

62. Cameron JS. The treatment of glomerulonephritis with inhibitors of coagulation. In Glomerulonephritis, Kluthe R, Vogt A, Batsford S (eds). New York: Wiley, 1977, pp. 154–164.

63. Nakamoto Y, Dohi K, Fujioka M, Kida H, Hattori N, Takeuchi J. Combined anticoagulant and immunosuppressive treatment in rapidly progressive glomerulonephritis (RPGN). A long-term follow-up study. Jap J Med 18: 210–217, 1979.

64. Arieff A, Pinggera W. Rapidly progressive glomerulonephritis treated with anticogulants. Archs Int Med 129:77–84, 1972.

65. Kincaid-Smith P. The treatment of chronic mesangiocapillary (membranoproliferative) glomerulonephritis with impaired renal function. Med J Aust 2: 587–592, 1972.

66. Cole BR, Brocklebank JT, Kienstra RA, Kissane JM, Robson AM. "Pulse" methylprednisolone therapy in the treatment of severe glomerulonephritis. J Pediatr 88: 307–314, 1976.

67. Bell PRF, Briggs JD, Calman KC, Paton AM, Wood RFM, Macpherson SG, Kyle K. Reversal of

acute clinical and experimental organ rejection using large doses of intravenous prednisolone. Lancet 1: 876–880, 1971.

68. Cathcart ES, Idelson BA, Scheinberg MA, Couser WG. Beneficial effects of methylprednisolone "pulse" therapy in diffuse proliferative lupus nephritis. Lancet 1: 163–166, 1974.

69. O'Neill WM, Etheridge WB, Bloomer A. High-dose corticosteroids. Their use in treating idiopathic rapidly progressive glomerulonephritis. Arch Int Med 139: 514–518, 1979.

70. Bolton K. Pulse methylprednisolone therapy of rapidly progressive glomerulonephritis. In Controversies in Nephrology, 2, Schreiner G, Winchester JF (eds). New York: Plenum Press, 1982 (in press).

71. Oredugba O, Mazumdar DC, Meyer JS, Lubowitz H. Pulse methylprednisone therapy in idiopathic, rapidly progressive glomerulonephritis. Ann Int Med 92: 504–506, 1980.

72. Lockwood CM, Rees AJ, Pinching AJ, Bussell B, Sweny P, Uff J, Peters DK. Plasma exchange and immunosuppression in the treatment of fulminating immune-complex crescentic nephritis. Lancet 1: 63–67, 1977.

73. Harmer D, Finn R, Goldsmith HG, Bone JM, Forbes AW. Plasmapheresis in fulminating crescentic nephritis. Lancet 1: 679, 1979 (letter).

74. Russ GR, D'Apice AJF. Plasma exchange and immunosuppression in crescentic glomerulonephritis. In Proceedings of the 8th International Congress of Nephrology, Athens, 1981. Basel: Karger, 1981, pp. 667–673.

75. Becker GJ, D'Apice AJF, Walker RG, Kincaid-Smith P. Plasmapheresis in the treatment of glomerulonephritis. Med J Aust 2: 693–697, 1977.

76. Fauci As, Katz P, Haynes BF, Wolff SM. Cyclophosphamide therapy of severe systemic necrotizing vasculitis. N Engl J Med 301: 235–238, 1979.

77. Neild GH, Lee HA. Methylprednisolone pulse therapy in the treatment of polyarteritis nodosa. Postgrad Med J 53: 382–387, 1977.

78. Friedman A, Kincaid-Smith P. Arteritis with impaired renal function. In Glomerulonephritis, Kincaid-Smith P, Mathew TH, Becker EL (eds). New York: Wiley, 1973, pp. 1047–1056.

79. Sinniah R, Feng PH. Lupus nephritis: Correlation with light, electron microscopic and immunofluorescent findings and renal function. Clin Nephrol 6: 340–351, 1976.

80. Kimberlly RP, Lockshin MD, Sherman RL, McDougal JS, Inman RD, Christian CC. High-dose intravenous methylprednisolone pulse therapy in systemic lupus erythematosus. Am J Med 70: 817–824, 1981.

81. Dosa S, Cairns SA, Lawler W, Mallick NP, Slotki IN. The treatment of lupus nephritis by mehylprednisolone pulse therapy. Postgrad Med J 54: 628–632, 1978.

82. Adu D, Cameron JS. Lupus nephritis. In Clinics in Rheumatic Diseases, vol 8, no 1, Hughes GRF (ed), Chapter 11, 1982.

83. Ponticelli C, Imbasciati E, Brancaccio D, Tarantino A, Rivolta E. Acute renal failure in systemic lupus erythematosus. Br Med M 3: 716–719, 1974.

84. Ponticelli C, Zucchelli P, Banti G, Cagnoli L, Scalia P, Pasquali S, Imbasciati E. Treatment of diffuse proliferative lupus nephritis by intravenous high-dose methylprednisolone. Quart J Med 51: 16–24, 1982.

85. Fessel J. Megadose corticosteroid therapy in systemic lupus erythematosus. J Rheumatol 7: 486–500, 1980.

86. Jones JV, Vernier RL, Cumming RH, Bacon PA, Evers J, Fraser ID, Tothanley J, Tribe CR, Davis P, Hughes GRV. Evidence for a therapeutic effect of plasmapheresis in patients with systemic lupus erythematosus Quart J Med 48: 555–576, 1979.

87. Parry HF, Nineham LJ, Moran CJ, Hay FC, Snaith ML, Morrow WJM, Richards JDM, Roitt IM, Goldstone AH. Plasma exchange in systemic lupus erythematosus. Ann Rheum Dis 40: 224–228, 1981.

88. Clark WF, Lindsay RM, Ulan RA, Cordy PE, Linton AL. Chronic plasma exchange therapy in SLE nephritis. Clin Nephrol 16: 20–23, 1981.

89. Counahan R, Winterborn MH, White RHR, Heaton JM, Meadow SR, Bluett NH, Swetschin H, Cameron JS, Chantler C. Prognosis of Henoch-Schönlein nephritis in children. Br Med J 2: 11–14, 1977.

90. Kaufmann RH, Houwert DA. Plasmapheresis in rapidly progressive Henoch-Schönlein glomerulonephritis and the effect on circulating IgA immune complexes. Clin Nephrol 16: 155–160, 1981.

91. Ponticelli C, Imbasciati E, Tarantino A, Pietrogrande M. Acute anuric glomerulonephritis in monoclonal cryoglobulinemia. Br Med J 2: 948–949, 1977.

92. Morel-Maroger L, Verroust P. Glomerular lesions in dysproteinemias. Kidney Int 5: 249–252, 1974.

93. McKenzie RG, Anarekar SN, Dawborn JK, Evans SM, Ham K, McPherson G, Riglar AG, Xipell JM. Glomerulonephritis secondary to mixed polyclonal cryoglobulinemia: Response to immunosuppression and plasmapheresis. Aust NZ J Med 11: 529–533, 1981.

94. Cohen J, Pinching AJ, Rees AJ, Peters DK. Infection and immunosuppresion. A study of the infective complications of 75 patients with immunologically mediated disease. Quart J Med 51: 1–15, 1982.

95. Wing EJ, Bruns FJ, Fraley DS, Segel DP. Infectious complications with plasmapheresis in rapidly progressive glomerulonephritis. JAMA 244: 2423–2426, 1980.

96. Chamberlain MJ, Pringle A, Wrong OM. Oliguric renal failure in the nephrotic syndrome. Quart J Med 35: 215–235, 1966.

97. Conolly ME, Wrong OM, Jones OM. Reversible

renal failure in idiopathic nephrotic syndrome with minimal glomerular changes. Lancet 1: 665–668, 1968.

98. Cameron JS, Turner DR, Ogg CS, Sharpstone P, Brown CB. The nephrotic syndrome in adults with "minimal change" glomerular lesions. Quart J Med 43: 461–488, 1974.

99. Raij L, Keane WF, Leonard A, Shapiro FL. Irreversible acute renal failure in idiopathic nephrotic syndrome. Am J Med 61: 207–214, 1976.

100. Holdsworth DR, Stephenson P, Dowling JP, Atkins RC. Reversible acute renal failure in the nephrotic syndrome with minimal glomerular pathology. Med J Aust 2: 532–533, 1977.

101. Stephens VJ, Yates APB, Lechler RI, Baker LRI. Reversible uremia in normotensive nephrotic syndrome. Br Med J 3: 705–706, 1979.

102. Case records of the Massachusetts General Hospital. Case No 28, 1978: discussants: Rose BD, Colvin RB. N Engl J Med 299: 136–145, 1978.

103. Hulter HN, Bonner EL Jr. Lipoid nephrosis appearing as acute oliguric renal failure. Arch Int Med 140: 403–405, 1980.

104. Lowenstein J, Schacht RG, Baldwin DS. Renal failure in minimal change nephrotic syndrome. Am J Med 70: 227–233, 1981.

105. Esparza AR, Kahn SI, Garella S, Abuelo JG. Spectrum of acute renal failure in nephrotic syndrome with minimal (or minor) glomerular lesions: Role of hemodynamic factors. Lab Invest 45:510–521, 1981.

106. Imbasciati E, Ponticelli C, Case N, Altieri P, Bolasco F, Mihatsch MJ, Zollinger HU. Acute renal failure in idiopathic nephrotic syndrome. Nephron 28: 186–191, 1981.

107. Case Records of the Massachusetts General Hospital. Case 4—1982: discussant: Barnard D. N Engl J Med 306: 221–231, 1982.

108. Steele BT, Bacheyie GS, Baumal R, Rance CPh. Acute renal failure of short duration in minimal lesion nephrotic syndrome of childhood. Int J Ped Nephrol 3: 59–62, 1982.

109. Llach F, Papper S, Massry SG. The clinical spectrum of renal vein thrombosis: Acute and chronic. Am J Med 69: 819–827, 1980.

110. Lyons H, Pinn VW, Cortell S, Cohen JJ, Harrington JT. Allergic interstitial nephritis causing reversible renal failure in four patients with idiopathic nephrotic syndrome. N Engl J Med 288: 124–218, 1973.

111. Brezin JH, Katz SM, Schwartz AB, Chinitz JL: Reversible renal failure and nephrotic syndrome associated with non-steroidal anti-inflammatory drugs. N Engl J Med 301: 1271–1273, 1979.

112. Rennke HG, Roos PC, Wall SG. Drug-induced interstitial nephritis with heavy glomerular proteinuria. N Engl J Med 302: 691–692, 1980 (letter).

113. Kleinknecht C, Broyer M, Gubler M-C, Palcoux J-B. Irreversible renal failure after indomethacin in steroid-resistant nephrosis. N Engl J Med 302: 691, 1980 (letter).

114. Baumelou A, Agrafiotis A, Jacobs C, Legrain M. Acute renal insufficiency during indomethacin treatment: Six cases. In Prostaglandin Synthetase Inhibitors: New Clinical Applications. New York: AR Liss, 1980, pp. 293–302.

115. Curt GA, Kaldany A, Whitley LG, Crosson AW, Rolla A, Merino MJ, D'Elia JA. Reversible rapidly progressive renal failure with nephrotic syndrome due to fenoprofen calcium. Ann Int Med 92: 72–73, 1980.

116. Finkelstein A, Fraley DS, Stachura I, Feldman HA, Gandy DR, Bourke E. Fenoprofen nephropathy—Lipoid nephrosis and interstitial nephritis—a possible lymphocyte T disorder. Am J Med 72: 81–87, 1982.

117. Arisz L, Donker AJM, Brentjens JRH, van der Hem GK. The effect of indomethacin on proteinuria and kidney function in the nephrotic syndrome. Acta Med Scand 199: 121–125, 1976.

118. Yamauchi H, Hopper J. Hypovolemic shock and hypotension as a complication in the nephrotic syndrome. Report of ten cases. Ann Int Med 60: 242–254, 1964.

119. Levinsky NG. Pathophysiology of acute renal failure. N Engl J Med 296: 1453–1458, 1977.

120. Bernard DB, Alexander EA. Edema formation in the nephrotic syndrome: Pathophysiologic mechanisms. Cardiovasc Med 4: 605–626, 1979.

121. Mees EJF, Roos JC, Boer P, Yoe OH, Simatupang TA. Observations on edema formation in the nephrotic syndrome in adults with minimal lesions. Am J Med 67: 378–384, 1979.

122. Meltzer JI, Keim HJ, Laragh JH, Sealey JE, Jan K-M, Chien S. Nephrotic syndrome: Vasoconstriction and hypervolemic types indicated by renin-sodium profiling. Ann Int Med 91: 688–696, 1979.

123. Robson AM, Giangiacomo J, Kienstra RA, Naqvi ST, Inglefinger JR. Normal glomerular permeability and its modification by minimal change nephrotic syndrome. J Clin Invest 54: 1190–1199, 1974.

124. Carrie BJ, Salyer WR, Myers BD. Minimal change nephropathy: An electrochemical disorder of the glomerular membrane. Am J Med 70: 262–268, 1981.

125. Baylis C, Ichikawa I, Willis WT, Wilson CB, Brenner BM. Dynamics of glomerular ultrafiltration. IX. Effects of plasma protein concentration. Am J Physiol 232: F58–F71, 1977.

126. Bohrer MP, Baylis C, Robertson CR, Brenner BM. Mechanisms of the puromycin-induced defects in the transglomerular passage of water and macromolecules. J Clin Invest 60: 152–161, 1977.

127. Mudge GH. Nephrotoxicity of urographic radiocontrast drugs. Kidney Int 18: 540–552, 1980.

14. VASCULAR NEPHROPATHIES AND ACUTE RENAL FAILURE IN ADULTS

Jean-Daniel Sraer,

Gabriel Richet

Approximately 5% of all cases of acute renal failure (ARF) are related to renovascular diseases [1–3]. This estimate is drawn from the results of renal biopsies performed when the clinical diagnosis of acute tubular necrosis (ATN) was uncertain. If anything, these statistics therefore underestimate the true frequency.

1 Characteristics of Acute Renal Failure in Renovascular Diseases

Acute renal failure in renovascular diseases is hallmarked by one or several features that should lead to immediate diagnosis and urgent etiopathogenic treatment.

1.1 HISTORY

Although it is often not apparent in the medical history, the kidney may have been injured in the past, even if renal function is normal. A long-standing history of hypertension is also common [4].

1.2 ONSET

The onset of renal failure is less abrupt than in ATN, and the initial phase can last from a few days to several weeks [5].

The help of the nephrological group of Hopital Tenon is deeply aknowledged, specially that of L. Morel-Maroger renal pathologist, F. Mignon, A. Meyrier, A. Kanfer, M. Beaufils and L. Moulonguet Doleris, the physicians in charge of most of the cases upon which this study relies.

V.E. Andreucci (ed.). ACUTE RENAL FAILURE.
All rights reserved. Copyright © 1984.
Martinus Nijhoff Publishing. Boston/The Hague/
Dordrecht/Lancaster.

1.3 CLINICAL FEATURES

In addition to the manifestations of renal failure, the following clinical features can occur:

a. Hypertension is almost always present. It is generally severe, is usually associated with organic complications, and is preceded by a period of benign essential hypertension [4]. Malignant hypertension can occur before, a few days after, or at the same time as the onset of acute uremia.

b. Other clinical features are arthralgia, myalgia with or without amyotrophy, various central and peripheral neurological signs (the latter commonly presenting as mononeuritis), vascular purpura, and other cutaneous lesions and jaundice. This list cannot pretend to be exhaustive because of the frequent associations with multiple visceral lesions.

1.4 LABORATORY FINDINGS

a. Anemia is a constant feature. The combination of microangiopathic hemolytic anemia and evidence of intravascular coagulation is particularly significant.

b. Abnormal immunological processes can sometimes be detected; these vary according to the etiology of the renovascular disease. They include cryoglobulinemia, Latex and Waaler Rose agglutination, circulating immune complexes, hypocomplementemia, positive Coombs test, and hepatitis B antigens and antibodies.

c. The most constant element of the urinary syndrome is gross or microscopic hematuria. Proteinuria is often abundant, up to 10 to 15 g per liter, but the 24-hour excretion rate is low, due to oligo-anuria.

1.5 RADIOLOGICAL FEATURES

Splanchnic angiography can reveal aneurysms, dead tree, and stationary wave aspects [5].

Renal arteriography can complete this picture, showing distal ischemia in favor of cortical ischemia, which is sometimes total.

1.6 HISTOPATHOLOGY

The histopathological alterations vary according to the vascular syndrome. Arterial lesions are often less severe than arteriolar lesions. The abnormalities include intimal thickening, thrombosis, and fibrinoid necrosis with or without perivascular granulomata. The glomerular lesions vary according to the type of renovascular disease: ischemic retraction of the flocculus; microectasia of the glomerular capillaries; heterogeneous intraluminal deposits that can alter the capillary's permeability, so-called hyaline subendothelial deposits; thrombosis; endo- or extracapillary proliferation. The tubulo-interstitial lesions are nonspecific. Immunofluorescent microscopy easily detects fibrinogen and sometimes deposited immunoglobulins and complement. In some syndromes, there are extrarenal lesions, granulomata, or acute angiitic vascular lesions in the blood vessels of the skin, skeletal muscles, and the pituitary.

Among all the features discussed above, microangiopathic hemolytic anemia is clinically the most indicative of the vascular origin of acute renal failure. It explains the emphasis that must be placed on the hemolytic uremic syndrome. The only exceptions are the lesions of necrotizing angiitis, which are not usually accompanied by microangiopathic hemolysis. In fact, acute renal failure in angiitis is accompanied by a glomerular syndrome and manifestations of cutaneous or visceral arterial thrombosis and rupture.

2 Hemolytic Uremic Syndromes (HUS) of the Adult

These syndromes can occur independently from or in association with a pre-existing vascular disease.

2.1 THE CLINICAL IMPORTANCE OF MICROANGIOPATHIC HEMOLYTIC ANEMIA

This anemia often goes unnoticed as the lowered hemoglobin may be only transitory. It is the presence of this particular anemia that leads to the question of performing sophisticated investigations such as renal biopsy or renal arteriography. They are indeed the two most rewarding investigations, but both have potential hazards. Hemolytic anemia should be excluded at the onset of every case of ARF.

The anemia is often severe with low or absent plasma haptoglobin levels, brisk reticulocytosis (over 100,000/ml), and bone marrow erythroid hyperplasia. The red blood cells are fragmented, forming schizocytes. The Coombs test is negative. The serum bilirubin level is slightly elevated (25–34 μmol/l, 1.5–2.0 mg/dl).

However, it must not be overlooked that microangiopathic hemolytic anemia can exist in the absence of renal lesions, for example, in association with adenocarcinomata [6], toxemia of pregnancy [7, 8], Kasabach-Merrit syndrome [9], and disseminated intravascular coagulation [10].

2.2 HEMOLYTIC UREMIC SYNDROMES IN THE ADULT WITHOUT ANY KNOWN VASCULAR DISEASE

2.2.1 History. In 1955, Gasser [11] described the coincidence of hemolytic anemia, thrombocytopenia, and ARF with cortical necrosis in a child. A little later, Habib [12] defined the clinical and pathological entity of the hemolytic uremic syndrome (HUS) with thrombotic microangiopathy, frequently reversible in children. The first adult cases were recognized from 1966 onward by Waddell and Matz [13], Dunea et al. [14], and Mery et al. [15]. Since then, many cases, both primary and secondary to vascular disease, have been reported. In the primary forms, the clinical and histopathological features are similar to those observed in the child.

2.2.2 Clinical, Biochemical, and Radiological Description

a. The premonitory phase is rarely absent. The symptoms are fatigue, even exhaustion, weight loss, fever, and various gastrointestinal complaints that can lead to laparotomy. In a series of 35 patients, this phase lasted from 7 to 60 days [2]. Two patients underwent laparotomy, which did not reveal any surgical abnormality.

b. The renal failure appears abruptly and is marked by the characteristic features of acute uremia. Oligo-anuria is common. The most significant additional sign is hypertension, which can occur either just before, just after, or at the same time as the acute renal failure. In the majority of cases, this hypertension is malignant with diastolic blood pressure exceeding 120 mm Hg. The clinical picture can include left ventricular failure, acute pulmonary edema, hypertensive encephalopathy with signs of inflammatory hypertensive retinopathy (hemorrhages, papilledema, and sometimes retinal detachment). Central neurological manifestations, such as convulsions, stupor, confusion, and coma, may occur even after the hypertension has been controlled. Arthralgia and purpura are frequent. Muscular wasting is virtually constant despite all efforts to avoid denutrition [16]. Hemorrhage, sometimes gastrointestinal but more often uterine, can occur. The biological features of microangiopathic hemolytic anemia are always distinct.

c. Arteriography of the aorta and its branches shows renal cortical ischemia, irregular arteries almost completely interrupted at the corticomedullary junction, and sometimes intrarenal or intrasplenic microaneurisms. Lastly, it can show "stationary wave" images, similar to those obtained in the splanchnic vessels of the rat after infusion of angiotensin II [17].

2.2.3 *Clinical Course* The outcome can be fatal due to visceral hemorrhage, cerebral or pulmonary edema, uncontrollable hypertension, or even cachexia. Renal failure is often irreversible and dialysis and/or transplantation are required. However, cases of complete recovery of renal function after weeks or months of oligo-anuria have been reported. The patient's age, the etiology of the hemolytic uremic syndrome, more important still the precocity and the efficacy of the treatment, and the extent of the arteriolar (and secondarily the glomerular) lesions are the major factors governing both mortality rates and renal recovery [18].

2.2.4 *Histopathology* Transcutaenous renal biopsy has revealed the initial renal lesions involved and their evolution. This procedure does carry risks because of the frequency of hemostatic disorders, vascular lesions, and hypertension in these patients. Rupture of the kidney occurred in three of our patients 25 to 32 days after biopsy. The number of minor perirenal hematomas is undoubtedly far higher [2].

a. On light microscopy, the initial lesions are similar to those found in the child (figure 14–1). The glomerular capillary walls are initially thickened by large deposits projecting between the glomerular basement membrane and the swollen endothelium. These "clear deposits" are eosinophilic, heterogeneous. With silver staining, the capillary lumen is reduced or even obstructed by a fibrillar network. Capillary thrombi caused by an amalgamation of eosinophilic material and red blood cell aggregates are frequent. Some capillary loops are filled with red cells and distended. There is no cellular proliferation. The lesions differ from one glomerulus to the next. This unequal injury persists at a later stage. Some lobules are sclerosed. In some places, the clear deposits persist. Sometimes, glomerular ischemia causes folding and retraction of the capillary walls. Some loops are filled with a homogenous, eosinophilic, nonfibrillar substance that is purple on PAS staining and that entirely obstructs the capillary lumen. This probably reflects the transformation of a fibrino-cruoric thrombus. Arterioles may be normal initially. More often they are damaged. At first, the lesions are patchy involving some arteriolar segments, sparing others. They consist in so-called fibrinoid necrosis of the vascular wall, likely to be due to red cells and plasma passing the endothelial lining and infiltrating the muscular bed. Within the lumen, thrombi, including platelets, are seen here and there. The intima is abnormal: swelling of the endothelial cells projecting into the lumen, edema contributing to lumen narrowing, and local detachment of the endothelial sheet. Later lesions become organized, leading to obstruction of the arteriolar lumen by an onion skin proliferation of smooth muscle cells and fibroblasts. This concentric endarteriolitis, although more extensive than

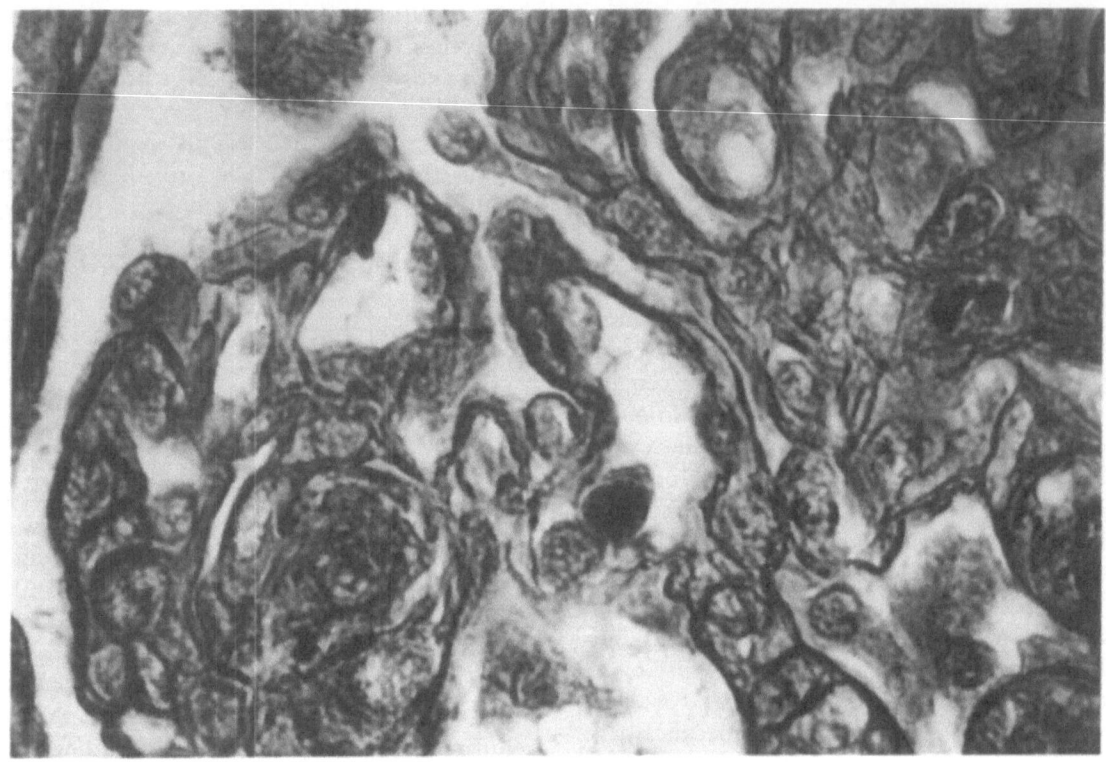

FIGURE 14-1. Glomerular lesions in the hemolytic-uremic syndrome. (×400)

the early lesions, is still irregularly distributed within the kidney. In larger arteries, there is rarely proliferative endarteritis. The internal elastic lamina is intact. There is no parallel between the degree of glomerular and arterial injury: a damaged glomerulus can be irrigated by a healthy afferent arteriole and vice versa. Tubular atrophy and necrosis is frequent. The tubules often contain hyaline or red blood cell casts. There are signs of interstitial involvement: edema, fibrosis, and in some cases, inflammatory cells [19–22].

b. Electron microscopy better analyzes the glomerular abnormalities. Cytoplasmic hyperplasia of the capillary endothelial cell is responsible for luminal narrowing. This cytoplasm contains a voluminous ergastoplasm and a fine peripheral laminar network that can be recognized at a low magnification. Multiple inclusions containing red blood cell and platelet debris suggest intense phagocytic activity. Glomerular basement membrane lesions are limited to the area between the lamina densa and the endothelial cytoplasm. This zone is far wider than the normal lamina rara interna and

contains a deposit that is as opaque as the lamina densa in some places and appears lighter but cloudy in the spaces in between. The capillary lumen is full of a proteinaceous substance containing red blood cells and platelets that have sometimes agglutinated; in places, this substance extends through the endothelium to reach the lamina densa. There is a striking resemblance between this intracapillary substance and the clear deposit seen with light microscopy [19, 23].

c. Immunofluorescent microscopy is of great value because of the rapidity with which it provides results. It is an emergency investigation. Large fibrin deposits are visible in the glomerular tuft and on the arteriolar lesions. Neither complement nor immunoglobulins are deposited. The discovery of fibrin immediately differentiates the renal lesions from those of ATN or extracapillary glomerulonephritis [18, 20].

There seem to be three distinct histopathological groups in the HUS of the adult. The

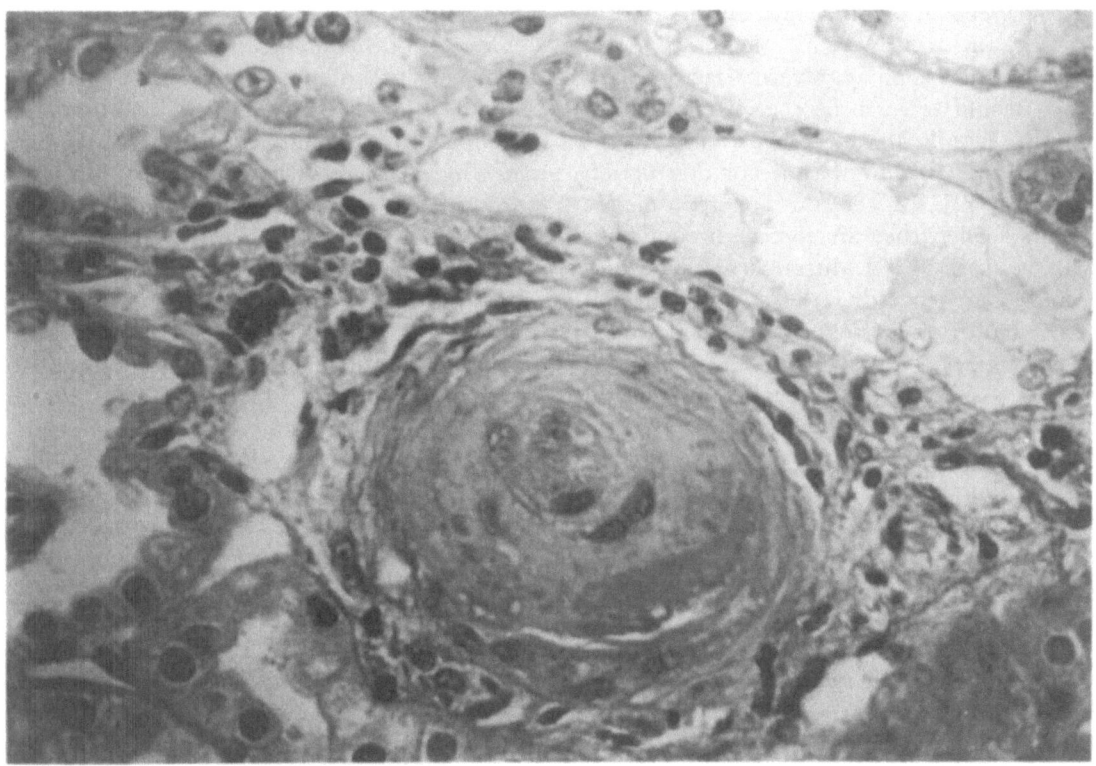

FIGURE 14–2. "Onion-skin" arteriole. (×400)

first group is characterized by exclusively or predominantly glomerular lesions. Any existing arteriolar lesions are discrete, limited to narrow zones of necrosis or tumefaction of the endothelium. These lesions can be reversible, and hopefully there follows at least partial recovery of renal function. Some glomerular sclerosis and arteriolar obstruction have been observed in the course of the disease in this group, but renal integrity is not compromised. The distinctive feature of the second group is a diffuse proliferation of the arteriolar endothelium. These vessels are often obstructed ("onion-skin arterioles") (figure 14–2). This lesion is frequently associated with fibrinoid necrosis. Most of the glomeruli are ischemic; the remaining few have clear subendothelial deposits and fibrillar matting. In most cases, a severe high renin hypertension makes an early appearance. Renal failure is generally permanent. A third group combines the two types described above. This association of arteriolar and glomerular lesions is especially frequent when the renal biopsy is carried out late in clinical course, when acute renal failure is prolonged. Renal prognosis is again poor. At the present date, it is unknown whether these three groups should be classified as separate anatomical entities or whether all the lesions are due to the same initial insult injuring either glomerular or arteriolar endothelial cells, or both. Indeed, if it were possible to prove in some patients that the arteriolar lesions existed in their own right, independent from hypertension, before the appearance of glomerular alterations, these cases would be no different from those labeled malignant nephroangiosclerosis. This theory, which was proposed by Bohle, is of fundamental importance [24–27]. The endothelial lesion is considered by some as primary and therefore critical [27].

2.2.5 Pathophysiology The pathophysiology is far from clear. There is definitely a relationship between the arteriolar fibrin deposits and hemolysis. The work of Symmers [28], Monroe and Strauss [29], Brain et al. [6], and Gavras et al. [30] showed that the schizocytosis is mechanical, the red blood cells being injured when they encounter the intraluminal fibrin deposits in the arterioles and glomeruli. Arterial hypertension is an aggravating factor. Schizocytosis would seem to be the initial phase of hemolysis. Plasma from these patients engenders neither RBC deformation nor destruction in vitro [31, 32]. On the contrary, red cells are fragmented when they are forced through a fibrin network [33–35]. Intravascular coagulation could be then either the cause of the hemolysis, due to fibrin deposits and endothelial lesions it creates, or the consequence of hemolysis, due to intraglomerular thromboplastin liberation [36–44]. Great emphasis has recently been placed on platelet aggregation along the glomerular and arteriolar endothelial cells. A theory suggests that the plasma of patients with the HUS contains factors that inhibit the endothelium's physiological reaction to increased platelet Thromboxane A_2 synthesis [45–50]. In fact, inhibition of vascular prostacyclin synthesis has been demonstrated in three patients. After treatment by plasma exchange, endothelial prostacyclin synthesis returned to normal. The suppression of prostacyclin formation seems to be related to complex humoral mechanisms involving oxidating and antioxidating factors. Direct damage to the endothelium of small renal vessels and glomeruli is another initiating mechanism to be taken into consideration. Endothelial injury could be caused by local modifications in the renal microcirculation, due to vasoactive hormone release during a shock syndrome [51, 52]. The same endothelial lesions have been demonstrated in endotoxic shock and in immune complex deposits. These initial endothelial lesions induce local coagulation with platelet aggregation and, secondarily, hemolysis by RBC fragmentation. The RBC membranes appear to bring about disseminated intravascular coagulation by release of a thromboplastin-like substance. For some reason, the injured endothelium is no longer capable of secreting plasminogen-activating enzymes [53], which are usually abundant and fast-acting in the glomerulus. This we have proved in the rat—in which the induction of disseminated intravascular coagulation is immediately followed by release of these enzymes—with disappearance

of the intracapillary thrombi sixty minutes after the thrombin infusion is stopped [54, 55]. In human pathology, renal intravascular coagulation has been proved both by immunohistochemical and biological methods, the latter showing an increase in platelet and fibrinogen turnover [56]. The cause of the endothelial lesions is not well understood. Perhaps they are due to immunological phenomena, but immunoglobulin and complement deposits are rare on renal biopsy. However, in thrombotic microangiopathy in the adult, it has been possible to detect brief hypocomplementemia, circulating complement fragments, and circulating immune complexes [57–61]. Coagulation could be induced locally by complement activation. Mechanical phenomena would then be responsible for fibrin deposits and microangiopathic hemolytic anemia. Platelet adhesion could explain the thrombocytopenia.

2.2.6 *Treatment* If a cause, such as infection or oral hormonal contraceptives, is discovered, appropriate therapeutic measures should be taken, even though their efficacy cannot be ascertained once the pathological process has begun. These specific measures are discussed in the chapter dealing with different clinical forms. However, the major therapeutic decisions, apart from those destined to control the manifestations of renal failure, are directed by the specific symptoms and the presumed pathophysiology of this syndrome.

2.2.6.1 SYMPTOMATIC THERAPEUTIC MEASURES. Treatment of hypertension: Malignant hypertension is a medical emergency that requires urgent therapy aimed at reducing arterial blood pressure to normal levels (systolic < 150 mm Hg, diastolic < 90 mm Hg) within a few hours. Antihypertensive vasodilators such as diazoxide and parenteral dihydralazine must be used. Precautions should be taken to avoid compromising the blood supply to the major organs due to vasodilatation, by maintaining a sufficient blood volume. In our experience, an intravenous bolus of diazoxide results in fast return to normal blood pressure, whenever intramuscular dihydralazine is ineffective. We rarely use intravenous nitroprusside because of renal failure and the risk, however small it may be, of cyanide poisoning. At this highly acute stage of the disease, both oral Captopril and Minoxidil are effective and can be administrated. Some consider Captopril, at a minimal dose of 75 mg, to be the treatment of choice. Whichever vasodilator is chosen, it must be used in conjunction with a beta-adrenergic receptor-blocking agent that, among other actions, reduces renin output by already ischemic kidneys. Clonidine can be used intramuscularly but not intravenously because of its agonist effect on alpha receptors. In general, after an initial phase of three to four days when parenteral therapy is essential, blood pressure can be controled by oral administration of beta blockers and vasodilators, complemented, if necessary, by depletion of extracellular fluid by ultrafiltration during dialysis.

Anticoagulant therapy: Heparin therapy, followed up by vitamin K antagonists, has been proposed for the past 15 years [18, 62–72]. A precise evaluation of its use is impossible. Nevertheless, we continue to use anticoagulant therapy because we have been impressed by the occurrence of relapses when these drugs were withdrawn. However, we only resort to anticoagulants when renal biopsy shows little or no arterial injury, as they are of no avail once the arteriolar lesions are organized and have caused glomerular ischemia. Streptokinase was proposed but then abandoned because of hemorrhagic complications.

Inhibitors of platelet aggregation, such as dipyridamole, have not yet been proved efficient when used alone [71, 73].

2.2.6.2 PHYSIOPATHOLOGICAL THERAPY. Physiopathological therapy is aimed at suppression of platelet Thromboxane elaboration or neutralization of its harmful effects by stimulation of endothelial cell prostacyclins. Other forms of therapy, including immunosuppressive agents, corticosteroids [5, 74], prostacyclins [75], fresh plasma transfusions, and plasma exchanges [76–79], have also been employed, but the successful reports of treatment in individual patients are ambiguous and often unconvincing; moreover, no controlled studies are available. We have twice observed complete recovery with symptomatic therapeutic measures alone. In view of the uncertainty surrounding

treatment of this syndrome, certain authors now adopt a purely symptomatic, supportive, therapeutic attitude.

Symptomatic or physiopathological therapy must be closely supervised, as complications from long-term use of these drugs are particularly frequent in patients with renal failure. Strict, prolonged compliance to the treatment is essential since recovery of renal function sufficient to forego dialysis often occurs after several weeks, or even months, of oligo-anuria. This favorable evolution has become more frequent since efficient vasodilators such as Captopril and Minoxidil, used in association with beta blockers, have been available. For these reasons, the dosage of the drugs used must be carefully adapted to obtain near normal blood pressure and blood volume and satisfactory hemostasis.

If uremia is irreversible, survival is maintained by dialysis. Hypertension is the main therapeutic problem. Because of the wide range of antihypertensive agents now available, refractory hypertension has become exceptional and there is hardly ever need for bilateral nephrectomy, which was frequently employed 10 years ago. Renal transplantation is not contraindicated. In our own experience of seven patients, six have evolved favorably, with no recurrence in the transplant and no acute vascular rejection; one of our patients was transplanted over 10 years ago [5, 80].

2.2.7 *Etiological Variants of Hemolytic Uremic Syndromes in Patients Without Any Known Vascular Disease*

a. There is often an infectious cause involved: Typhoid fever [81], E. Coli septicemia [82, 83], pseudomonas [84], some neuraminidase-producing pneumococci [85], shigella [86, 87]. Viral infection is often invoked [82, 88–90]. In addition to these well-documented cases, there is a remarkable frequency of intense signs of infection in the premonitory phase; moreover, some cases of familial HUS have been reported, which cannot be due exclusively to genetic factors [89]. A HUS was diagnosed in two children of different parents living in the same home in connection with a familial viral infection due to the Asiatic influenza virus 2 [90, 91].

b. Hemolytic uremic syndrome in pregnancy: After exclusion of all cases appearing as complications of septic abortion [82, 91], placental retention, and retroplacental hematoma [92–94], pregnancy is a cause of the HUS in its own right [6, 62, 63, 95, 96]. The syndrome can occur as early as the fifth month of pregnancy [97]. However, in most cases, it occurs in the days or weeks following an uncomplicated delivery and an apparently normal pregnancy. The longest interval recorded is 10 months [5]. The features of the HUS are the same as those described above. The premonitory phase is short, often marked by uterine hemorrhages. Blood pressure frequently rises a few days after the onset of anuria. In our series of seven cases, the renal lesions healed completely in two women, but the remaining five survived, thanks only to dialysis and transplantation. These patients' renal prognosis is therefore always severe. In some other series, mortality is higher than in ours.

c. Hemolytic uremic syndrome and oral contraceptives: The frequency of this syndrome during hormonal contraceptive treatment is low, but not negligible (98–100). Three important facts must be taken into consideration: the interval between the start of oral contraception and the onset of the disease is anything from a few weeks to ten years; there is no connection between the HUS and hypertension, which can also occur occasionally during contraceptive treatment; high doses of oestrogens, and not progesterones, are responsible for the syndrome. A good illustration is provided by the case of a HUS occurring five months after a pregnancy, on oral contraceptives; three years later, a renal transplant was carried out; the HUS recurred ten months after substitution of pure progestatives by estroprogestatives [101, 102].

d. Hemolytic uremic syndrome and multisystem diseases. This association is rare, with one reported case of lupus [103], one of our patients with rheumatoid arthritis [104], one case of familial glomerulitis [105], and

some cases after mitomycin treatment [106].

e. Hemolytic uremic syndrome and hyperacute rejection of transplant are frequently associated.

2.2.8 Relationship Between Hemolytic Uremic Syndrome and Thrombotic Thrombocytopenic Purpura

These two syndromes have much in common. Classically, they differ by the higher frequency of brain damage and the lower frequency of kidney damage in thrombotic thrombocytopenic purpura. In fact, this clinical distinction is not so clear-cut as it appears. However, renal histology may differentiate the two syndromes. Although fibrinoid thrombi are present in both cases, the glomerular lesions observed in thrombotic thrombocytopenic purpura, such as the thickened capillary walls without clear deposits and the discrete endocapillary proliferation, are absent in the HUS. These arguments are not definitive [107, 108].

2.2.9 Relationship Between Hemolytic Uremic Syndrome and Cortical Necrosis.

The first cases of HUS described by Gasser [11] in the child involved cortical necrosis. Renal arteriography performed early in both syndromes shows ischemia. But ischemia and cortical necrosis are not identical although early in the course of the disease, radiological appearance are the same. However, a recent study showed that the HUS was present in only two out of 38 cases of cortical necrosis [93, 109]. The evolution is different: definitive anuria probably occurs in the HUS because the distal lesions affect all the arterioles, whereas cortical necrosis results from the juxtaposition of ischemic zones, separated by areas of intact parenchyma, enough to provide satisfactory renal function.

2.3 HEMOLYTIC UREMIC SYNDROME IN PATIENTS WITH VASCULAR DISEASE

2.3.1 Hemolytic Uremic Syndrome in Malignant Hypertension

2.3.1.1 CLINICAL FEATURES. Malignant hypertension is a clinical syndrome first described by Volhard and Fahr in 1914 [110]. Uremia due to ARF is part of this syndrome. More recently [28–30], it appeared that, although clinically discrete, microangiopathic hemolytic anemia is constant, always biochemically detectable, even if the onset of malignant hypertension is very progressive. The hemolytic uremic syndrome is associated with the other clinical features of malignant hypertension. The ocular and neurological signs are most severe [5]. Hypertensive retinopathy is constant, with soft exudates, hemorrhages, and retinal detachment. Papilledema is found in approximately 75% of cases [111, 112]. The manifestations of hypertensive encephalopathy are thirst, severe headache, vomiting, confusion, stupor, even coma. In some cases, generalized or localized convulsions can occur, imitating a tumoral syndrome [111, 113]. Hypertensive encephalopathy results from either multiple cerebral arteriolar thrombi or from plasmatic exudates through cerebral arteriolar walls; successive arteriolar segments are alternately dilated then constricted [113–117]. The rapid, considerable weight loss of these patients is equally impressive [76, 111]. This, in combination with muscular wasting, is a major clinical feature we have frequently observed. The patient's degree of hydration varies according to time elapsed since onset of renal failure, intensity of gastrointestinal losses, whether the patient continues to eat and drink, and the treatment given. This must be estimated rapidly, and if the extracellular volume is depleted, it must be corrected simultaneously or even before commencing antihypertensive treatment, as there is a danger of hypotensive shock when vasodilators are used in dehydrated patients. Most patients have elevated peripheral plasma renin activity levels and increased aldosterone production, even when normally hydrated [118]; this in turn lowers kalemia and raises bicarbonate levels. This secondary hyperaldosteronism is a consequence of increased juxtaglomerular cell activity in reply to renal ischemia. This activity persists even when renal failure is far advanced.

2.3.1.2 EVOLUTION. The evolution of HUS in malignant hypertension is always extremely severe. Mortality is high, due to cerebral hemorrhage, cardiac infarction, hemorrhagic pancreatitis, or rapidly progressing cachexia due to poor mesenteric blood flow, as shown by splanchnic arteriography [119]. However, survival rates have improved with the advent of new antihypertensive agents that are essentially vasodilators, in particular Captopril, used in conjunction with beta blockers and that decrease renin secretion; systematic prevention and treatment of the extracellular dehydration that often occurs have also improved prognosis [120–122]. Although therapy is far from guaranteeing prevention of renal destruction, it does permit survival and maintains blood flow to the major organs. Contrary to what was considered as established fact, belated improvement of renal function can occur, even after two or three years of dialysis [123, 124]. Such cases are rare, but usually come about when blood pressure has been perfectly controlled. Bilateral nephrectomy, advocated a few years ago when hypertension was difficult to control, is no longer considered. No undue complications are encountered on chronic dialysis or transplantation. We have not observed any case of recurrence in our transplanted patients.

2.3.1.3 THE HEMOLYTIC UREMIC SYNDROME OF PRIMARY AND OF SECONDARY MALIGNANT HYPERTENSION. They are not entirely identical.

a. HUS in secondary malignant hypertension is by far the more frequent. It complicates a hypertensive vascular disease, that was first detected anytime from one to 20 previously [5, 125–127]. About 1% of patients with permanent hypertension will develop the malignant phase. Men are slightly more commonly affected than women (60% compared to 40%). The average age at diagnosis is 40 to 50 years [128]. Malignant hypertension more often occurs in the course of essential hypertension, but can also complicate secondary hypertension, which has usually appeared recently. The premonitory signs are rise in diastolic pressure levels above 120 mm Hg, inefficacy of treatment, and symptoms such as headache, vertigo, visual disturbances, and weight loss. After onset, the feature of malignant hypertension are those described above.

b. HUS in primary malignant hypertension was actually the one described by Volhard and Fahr [110], then Schurmann and MacMahon [129]. In the past few years, Bohle et at. [25, 26] have carried out impressive clinical and anatomical studies on this syndrome, which they have called primitive malignant nephroangio-

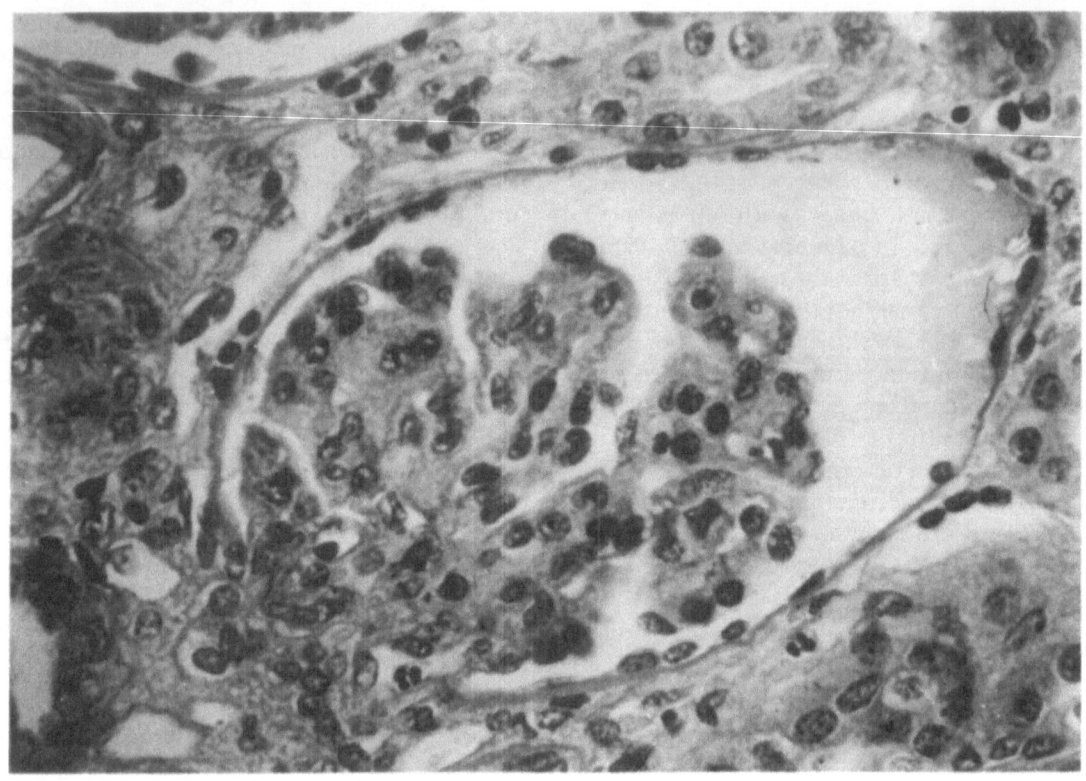

FIGURE 14–3. Ischemic glomerulus. (×250)

sclerosis. In some cases, it could be due to a rapid aggravation of hypertension, which was latent and disregarded. However, in other patients, both adults and children, blood pressure was definitely normal before the onset of malignant hypertension, but renal lesions (giving rise to symptoms) were already present. Renal biopsy shows well-organized endarterial proliferation, which suggests that the arterial wall was damaged prior to onset of malignant hypertension and that these injuries may even be responsible for the hypertension [4]. Similarly, in HUS, which complicates pregnancy, hormonal contraceptive treatment, or scleroderma, renal arterial lesions have been shown to precede the other manifestations of the syndrome. It is therefore possible that an exclusively renal vascular disease could be responsible for some cases of primitive malignant hypertension accompanied by HUS.

2.3.2 *Histopathology* Arteriolar lesions are predominant [5]. In some areas, fibrinoid necrosis covers all the layers of the arteriolar wall.

In others, this wall is not destroyed: the endothelium is hypertrophic, the concentric proliferation of its cells creating onion-like proliferative endarteritis. The remaining lumen is much-reduced or even obliterated. The media contain numerous muscular cells, wedged between the multiple lamellae of elastic fibers. The lumen can be obstructed by cruoric thrombi. The lesions of all the arterioles are always strikingly similar. The flocculi of most glomeruli contain no blood and are retracted to the vascular pole, leaving a vast Bowman's space (figure 14–3). The decrease in the capillary lumen is due to festooned folding of the glomerular basement membrane alone, with neither matting feutrage, argentaffine fibrils, endothelial swelling, nor eosinophilic deposits. Clear deposits, when present, are rare, irregular, and small. Some glomerular loops are ectatic, swollen, and full of red blood cells. The mesangium is retracted, containing few cells. Bowman's capsule is generally thickened.

Later, glomeruli are invaded by an irregular, homogenous sclerosis, but silver staining still reveals thick, festooned, residual basement membranes. These two different aspects are named glomerular simplification and glomerular obsolescence. The glomerular ischemia, which is responsible for these lesions, is closely related to the degree of arteriolar injury [130, 131].

2.3.3 Physiopathology Hypertension is at least partially responsible for the arteriolar lesions of HUS, including fibrinoid necrosis. This is implied by the correlation between the intensity of these lesions and the blood pressure levels [132–134] and by the fact that both essential hypertension and hypertension secondary to Cushing's syndrome, phaeochromocytoma or renal artery stenosis, cause identical damage [135]. Hypertension experimentally induced by angiotensin infusion also produces these lesions. Moreover, early antihypertensive therapy can bring about their reversal: this confirms histologically what has been observed in clinical practice. Hypertension is the pathogenic factor not angiotensin, whose production is always increased in these patients. Indeed, the same typical lesions occur in hypertensive rats whether the plasma renin activity is high or low. It is easy to understand the establishment of a vicious circle of hypertension, producing renal arteriolar lesions, which in turn cause glomerular ischemia stimulating renin and angiotensin II release with increased hypertension. One can therefore conclude that antihypertensive therapy plays more than a purely symptomatic part in the treatment of this syndrome [136–142].

Despite this common pre-eminence of hypertension in the sequence of pathological events, cases where arteriolar lesions antedate hypertension should not be overlooked. Their mechanism is not understood. It is only known that they can follow synthetic estrogen therapy and viral or microbial infections.

2.3.4 Treatment Treatment consists solely of controlling the hypertension, the only known factor that intervenes on the renal vascular lesions, exacerbating them in all cases, probably their only cause when hypertension existed beforehand. As related above, partial recovery of sufficient renal function for autonomous survival is rare. The aim is to maintain a reasonable quality of life with dialysis and, if possible, with transplantation. The modalities of the treatment are described above.

2.4 THE HEMOLYTIC UREMIC SYNDROME AND SCLERODERMA

HUS is a frequent cause of death in scleroderma. In a survey of 358 cases, HUS occurred in 17 patients; in two other surveys, HUS was responsible for half of all deaths [143–147]. Our own experience of four patients confirms these statistics. During the course of scleroderma, vague premonitory manifestations appear; uterine hemorrhages are particularly frequent in this phase. Several weeks later, the onset of HUS is explosive, completed by abrupt anuria. Hypertension is moderate in our experience, the systolic level is less than 180 mm Hg, the diastolic level less than 110 mm Hg, and blood pressure is easily controlled by treatment. This certainly does not fit the classical description of malignant hypertension. An intense retinopathy also contrasts with the modesty of the hypertension. All our patients died within a few months, without recovery of diuresis. Attention has recently been drawn to cases of returned renal function, particularly in patients treated by inhibitors of the angiotensin-converting enzyme. Renal transplantation using a cadaver kidney is possible as recurrence of HUS after transplantation is not systematic. Among ten patients, one still survives after five years with a transplanted kidney [147].

2.4.1 Histopathology Renal arterial lesions are prevalent, with accessory arteriolar injury, as in all cases of scleroderma, with or without hypertension, even in the absence of the clinical and biochemical features of renal failure. The lesions consist of a "mucoid" thickening of the endothelium and cellular proliferation (figure 14–4). A few zones of fibrinoid necrosis can be authenticated. The glomeruli are ischemic and contain scarce clear deposits [21, 148]. Immunofluorescent microscopy shows fibrin deposits in the arteries and arterioles.

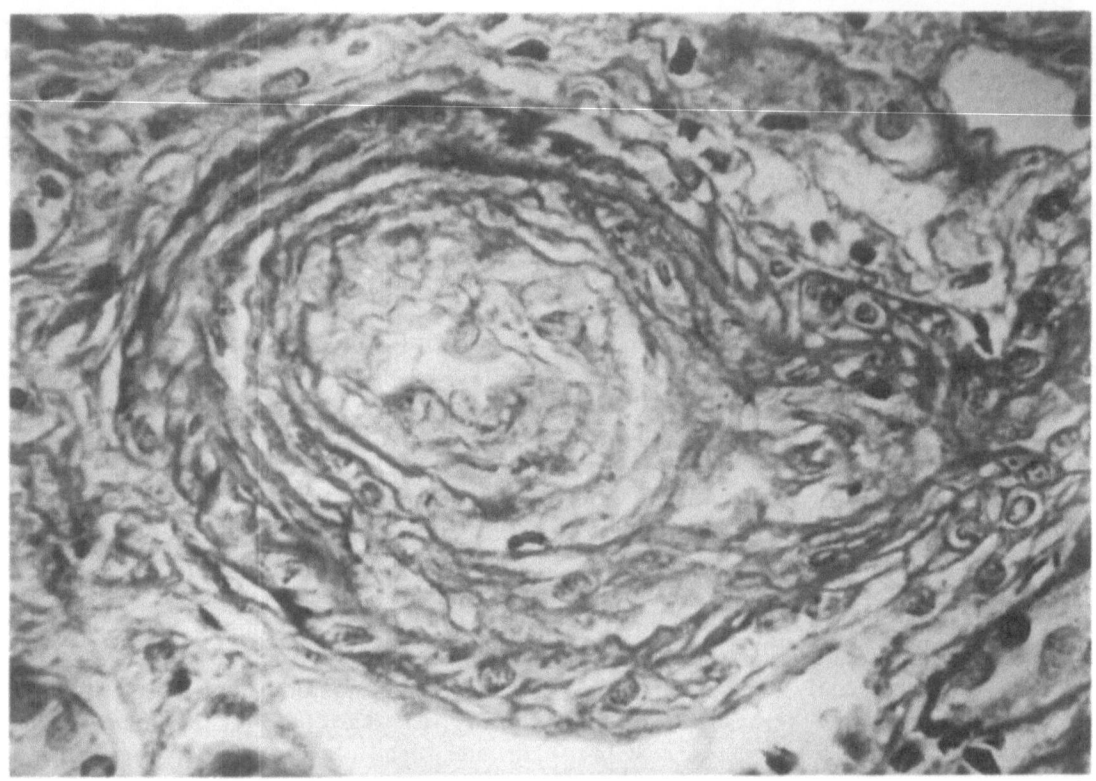

FIGURE 14-4. Renal arterial lesions in scleroderma. (× 400)

It is clear from this clinical and anatomical description that the HUS of scleroderma and secondary malignant hypertension have little in common. On the other hand, there is some similarity with the initial phase of primitive malignant nephroangiosclerosis in cases when hypertension makes a belated appearance: in both syndromes, hypertension follows the renal lesions. The hypothesis of renal arterial spasm is tempting, however vague this term may be, aggravation would then be due to the adjunction of intravascular coagulation [149, 150].

3 Acute Renal Failure in Angiitis

In contrast with the previous renovascular diseases, renal failure in angiitis closely resembles that of glomerulonephritis.

3.1 COMMON FEATURES OF ACUTE RENAL FAILURE IN ANGIITIS

Renal and extrarenal symptomatology is extremely rich.

3.1.1 Renal Manifestations of Angiitis Complicated by Acute Renal Failure In the phase prior to onset of acute uremia, most of the renal signs are those of a progressive glomerulonephritis: proteinuria is frequently is excess of 2 g per day. Hematuria, often gross, is present in 75% of all cases. A clinical and biochemical nephrotic syndrome often accompanies renal failure. Hypertension is usually moderate and rarely bears the characteristic traits of malignant hypertension. Accordingly, retinopathy is rarer than in other forms of acute renal failure of vascular origin. Lastly, in most cases, renal failure can be more precisely termed "rapidly progressive" than "acute," as it occurs at least 30 days after the first clinical sign of uremia [151–155].

3.1.2 The Extrarenal Signs of Angiitis During Acute Renal Failure They are numerous, bearing witness to the vascular lesions in multiple organs. Fever, weight loss, arthralgia, and amyotrophy are present in over 60% of all patients. Peripheral neuropathy, skin lesions, upper respiratory tract disorders and coronary signs are less common. The hematological profile usually combines eosinophilia and various immunological anomalies, for example, positive Rose Waaler and Latex agglutination tests, cryoglobulinemia, circulating immune complexes detected by radio-labeled Clq or Raji cells technique [155–157].

The association of peripheral neuropathy, abdominal pain, and intra- or extrarenal aneurysms on aortography is strongly in favor of polyarteritis nodosa, whereas an upper respiratory tract disorder generally implies Wegener's granulomatosis. These two variants are best distinguished.

The ultimate diagnosis of angiitis is made on the grounds of renal or extrarenal histology. Histological and clinical descriptions and treatment of these diseases are dealt with in the chapter concerning diffuse extracapillary glomerulonephritis (chapter 13).

4 Acute Renal Failure in Essential Cryoglobulinemia

Renal involvement is one of the complications of mixed cryoglobulinemias. In most cases, as Meltzer and Franklin [158, 159] demonstrated in 1967, the renal manifestation is chronic glomerulonephritis. Sometimes ARF can occur secondarily. Occasionally, it is the initial sign of renal disease.

4.1 THE ONSET
ARF is heralded by a short premonitory phase with fever and other extrarenal features. Proteinuria and microscopic or gross hematuria are present from then onward. A nephrotic syndrome is frequent and hypertension usual but not malignant. Within a few days, an acute renal failure, which is habitually anuric, is established [160].

4.2 EXTRARENAL MANIFESTATIONS
The extrarenal manifestations reflect the widespread inflammatory vascular lesions: papular purpura, necrotic ulceration and sundry other skin lesions, seizures, Raynaud's phenomenon,

abdominal pain, hepatosplenomegaly, and enlarged lymph nodes are the main features. Mixed cryoglobulinemia usually consists of IgG and IgM, sometimes IgG and IgA or two IgGs belonging to different groups. When the IgM is monoclonal, cryoglobulinemia is classified type II; when the IgM is polyclonal, it is classified type III. Latex and Rose Waaler agglutination tests are positive with the supernatant and the cryoglobulin. Serum complement components are depressed and circulating fragments of C3 abundant [158, 159, 161–164].

4.3 RENAL HISTOLOGY
Renal histology characteristically shows predominantly glomerular lesions, with an association of endocapillary proliferation, discrete extracapillary proliferation, and endomembranous deposits, which are often voluminous, forming genuine occlusive thrombi. The proliferative cells are mainly mononucleated; it is not known whether they are of mesangial, endothelial, or hematological origin. The deposits contain IgG and IgM or IgA, or IgGs of different types, like the circulating cryoglobulin. Clq and C3 can be detected. However, there are no fibrin deposits, and the term *fibrinoid*, given to the deposits because of their staining characteristics, is misleading [160, 165–168]. Necrotizing angeitis is often disclosed on serial sections.

4.4 EVOLUTION
Evolution is largely dependent on the underlying disease and the trigger that launched the acute episode of cryoglobulinemia, often an infection in our experience. In addition, the course is governed by the complications of extrarenal manifestations, intercurrent infections, and therapeutic incidents, especially when immunosuppressive agents are prescribed systemically. If the patient escapes these multiple dangers, the renal lesions regress simultaneously with the extrarenal features and cryoglobulinemia. The increase in urinary volume is accompanied by profuse proteinuria, which can entail appearance or reappearance of a transitory nephrotic syndrome, which vanishes within a few weeks when urinary albumin leakage decreases. Hypertension ceases within one to three weeks. Renal recovery can be total, with neither functional nor anatomical se-

310

quelae, as we have confirmed by means of iterative biopsies. Sometimes, discrete proteinuria persists, with or without stable renal failure. We have witnessed several cases of recurrent ARF associated with reappearance of cryoglobulinemia and resurgence of the extrarenal manifestations. The cause of these episodes is unclear, but they seem related to a relapse of the underlying disorder, or some intercurrent factor, for example an infection. One of our patients survived five episodes of acute oligo-anuric renal failure, each one reversible, from which recovery was proven anatomically, before dying from a reticulosarcoma [160, 167, 168].

5 Acute Renal Failure Due to Acute Vascular Occlusion

These cases of ARF are exceptionally rare. They occur only on bilateral occlusion or are unilateral with one functional kidney.

5.1 ARTERIAL OCCLUSION
Three types of oriental occlusion can be distinguished.

5.1.1 Cruoric Obstacle in the Large Renal Vessels
This can be due either to embolism or to acute thrombosis on an atheromatous plaque in the renal artery or the aorta at the origin of the former [169–172]. Onset is explosive, marked by violent abdominal and lumbar pain with multiple radiations, sometimes migrating downwards as in nephritic colic. The occasional presence of gross hematuria is a decisive element when the intensity of the gastrointestinal manifestations evokes an acute abdominal emergency. Irreversible total or partial renal infarction is to be feared. Therefore, the obstacle must be removed as soon as possible. The decision to intervene depends on the results of arteriography. This investigation is indicated whenever there are clinical arguments suggesting sudden arterial occlusion, especially if they are completed by etiopathogenic factors such as atherosclerosis, aortic ectasia, emboligenic cardiac conditions or infective endocarditis. Arteriography demonstrates the arterial obstacle, establishing both the cause of ARF and the surgical attitude to be adopted. Even a belated op

eration may now restore renal function in cases despaired of a few years ago.

5.1.2 Dissection of the Aorta
ARF is one manifestation of this disease. In addition to acute abdominal and lumbar pain, the arterial pulses of the lower limbs are abolished. Arteriography is again necessary to establish the diagnosis. Renal failure has obviously little impact on the evolution, which is most often fatal, whatever surgical procedure is adopted.

5.1.3 Occlusion of the Branches of the Renal Artery by Cholesterol Emboli [173–175]
This type of acute vascular renal failure is often ignored. Initially, a slight fever accompanies an inflammatory syndrome. Within a few days, ARF and hypertension appear, together with the manifestations of multiple visceral and cutaneous sites of arterial occlusion. The territories involved depend on the origin of the cholesterol emboli, for example, an ulcerated atheromatous plaques of the aortic arch. On fundoscopy, cholesterol emboli are often mistaken for features of hypertensive retinopathy, and an erroneous diagnosis of malignant hypertension can be suggested. The systematic search for cutaneous lesions, especially of the lower limbs, is helpful. Biopsy of these lesions demonstrates the presence of typical cholesterol crystals; identical crystals are found in the renal vessels on autopsy or exceptionally on renal biopsy.

5.2 ACUTE RENAL FAILURE DUE TO RENAL VEIN OCCLUSION
Isolated renal vein thrombosis does not engender ARF, as human collateral venous circulation is well developed. For this reason, the left renal vein can be used for anastomosis to the splenic vein. If the development of the collateral circulation is hindered, renal vein thrombosis can cause ARF. This is the case when the retroperitoneal tissue is infiltrated due to local extension of a pelvic or abdominal cancer, inflammatory liposclerosis, a retroperitoneal hematoma, or hemorrhagic pancreatitis [176–178]. In these complex situations, there is often a combination of renal vein thrombosis, extrinsic ureteral blockage, and, to a varying de

gree, thrombosis of the inferior vena cava. Diffuse thrombosis of the renal venous system due to extracellular dehydration entailing ARF is observed only in children. However, renal vein thrombosis can cause anuria when it complicates an advanced chronic nephropathy due to a pyelonephritis or amyloidosis [179]. We have observed no case of ARF due to venous thrombosis during membranous glomerulopathy. Diagnostic aids are late arteriography films and inferior vena caval and sometimes selective renal venography. Surgical treatment is ineffective. Heparin therapy has not been proved effective. We have observed one case that evolved favorably when treated with a combination of heparin and streptokinase, but the patient had benign liposclerosis and might well have recovered without therapy [180–182].

References

1. Richet G, Sraer JD, Kourilsky O, Kanfer A, Mignon F, Whitworth J, Morel-Maroger L. La ponction biopsie rénale dans les insuffisances rénales aigues. Ann Med Intern 129: 445–447, 1978.
2. Wilson DM, Turner DR, Cameron JS, Ogg CS, Brawn CB, Chanteler C. Value of renal biopsy in acute intrinsic renal failure. Brit Med J. 2: 459–461, 1976.
3. Bonomini V, Daldrati L, Stefoni S, Vangelista A. Acute renal failure: 10 years experience. In Acute renal failure, Eliahou HE (ed). London: John Libbey, 1982, pp. 149–151.
4. Richet G. The Kidney and malignant hypertension. In Hemostasis, Prostaglandins and Renal Disease, Remuzzi G, Mecca G, de Gaetano G (eds). New York: Raven Press, 1980, pp. 333–335.
5. Sraer JD, Morel-Maroger L, Beaufils P, Ardaillou N, Helenon C, Richet G. Les insuffisances rénales d'origine vasculaire. Etude de 25 cas. J Urol Nephrol 4: 317–329, 1972.
6. Brain MC, Dacie JV, O'Hourihane DO 'B. Microangipathic hemolytic anemia. The possible role of vascular lesions in pathogenesis. Brit J Haematol 8: 858–874, 1962.
7. Pritchard JA, Weisman R, Ratnoff OD, Vosburgh GJ. Intravascular hemolysis, thrombocytopenia and other hematologic abnormalities associated with severe toxemia of pregnancy. N Engl J Med 250: 89–92, 1954.
8. Bithell TC, Wintrobe MM. Disorders of platelets. In Principles of Internal Medicine, Wintrobe MM, Thorn GW, Adams R, Braunwald E, Isselbacher J, Petersdorf RG (eds). New-York: McGraw-Hill, 1978.
9. Vadri J, Fileds GA. Microangiopathic hemolytic anemia in severe pre-eclampsia. Amer J Obstet Clin 119: 617–622, 1974.
10. Brain MC, O'Hourihane DO 'B. Microangiopathic hemolytic anemia: The occurrence of hemolysis in experimentally produced vascular disease. Brit J Haematol 13: 135–142, 1967.
11. Gasser C, Gautier E, Steck A, Siebenmall RE, Dechslin R. Hämolytisch-urämisches Syndrome: bilaterale Nierenrindennekrosen bei akuten erworbenen hämolytischen anämien. Schweiz Med Wochensehr 85: 905–909, 1955.
12. Habib R, Mathieu H, Royer P. Le syndrome hémolytique et urémique de l'enfant. Néphron 4: 139–172, 196.
13. Waddell AJH, Matz LR. Hemolytic uremic syndrome: Report of two cases in adults. Med J Aust 2: 893–897, 1966.
14. Dunea G, Muehrcke RC, Nakamoto S., Schwartz FD. Thrombotic thrombocytopenic purpura with acute renal failure. Amer J Med 41: 1000–1006, 1966.
15. Méry JP, Grunfeld JP. Insuffisance rénale aigue avec microangiopathie thrombotique chez l'adulte. Path Biol 15: 1079–1083, 1967.
16. Richet G. Insuffisances rénales aigues d'origine vasculaire. Rev Med Liege 29: 1–4, 1974.
17. Helenon C, Nochy D, Sraer JD, Michel C, Brutus J, Richet G. Les artères en "collier de perles" au cours des néphropathies vasculaires avec insuffisance rénale aigue. J Radiol Electrol 56: 219–225, 1975.
18. Morel-Maroger L, Kanfer A, Solez K, Sraer JD, Richet G. Prognostic importance of vascular lesions in acute renal failure with microangiopathic hemolytic anemia (hemolytic-uremic syndrome). Clinicopathologic study in 20 adults. Kidney Int 17: 548–558, 1979.
19. Goldstein MH, Churg J, Strauss L, Gribetz D. Hemolytic-uremic syndrome. Néphron 23: 263–272, 1979.
20. Sraer JD, Morel-Maroger L, Beaufils P, Richet G. Vascular nephropathis and acute renal failure. In Glomerulonephritis, Kincaid-Smith P, Mathiew TH, Becker EL (eds). New York: John Wiley, 1973, (vol. 2), pp. 1035–1046.
21. Heptinstall RH. Microangiopathic hemolytic anemia, hemolytic-uremic syndrome, thrombotic thrombocytopenic purpura and Scleroderma. In Pathology of the Kidney. Boston: Little, Brown, 1974, pp. 675–711.
22. Alfrey AC. The renal response to vascular injury. In The kidney, Brenner BM, Rector FC Jr (eds). Philadelphia: WB Saunders, 1981 (2nd ed), pp. 1668–1718.
23. Habib R, Courtecuisse V, Leclerc F, Mathieu H, Royer P. Etude anatomopathologique de 35 observations de syndromes hémolytiques et urémiques chez l'enfant. Arch Franc Ped 26: 391–416, 1969.
24. Bohle A, Helmchen U, Meyer D, Bock KD, Burning L, Edel HH, Heimsoth V, Scheler F. Uber die

primäre and sekundäre maligne Nephrosklerose. Klin Woschenschr 51: 841–857, 1973.

25. Bohle A, Grund KE, Helmchen U, Meyer D. Primary malignant nephrosclerosis. Clin Sci Mol Med 51: 235–259, 1976.

26. Bohle A, Helmchen U, Grund KE, Gartner HV, Meyer D, Bock KD, Bull AM, Bunger P, Diekmann L, Frotscher U, Hayduck K, Kosters W, Strauch M, Scheler F, Christ U. Malignant nephrosclerosis in patients with hemolytic-uremic syndrome (primary malignant hypertension). Curr Top Pathol 65: 81–113, 1977.

27. Thoenes W, John HD. Endotheliotropic (hemolytic) nephroangiopathy and its various manifestation forms (thrombotic microangiopathic, primary malignant nephrosclerosis, hemolytic-uremic syndrome). Klin Wochenschr 58: 173–184, 1980.

28. Symmers W St C. Thrombotic microangiopathic hemolytic anemia (thrombotic microangiopathy). Br Med J 2: 897–903, 1952.

29. Monroe WM, Strauss AF. Intravascular hemolysis: A morphologic study of schizocytes in thrombotic purpura and other diseases. South Med J 46: 837–844, 1953.

30. Gavras H, Brown WCB, Brown JL, Lever AF, Linton AL, McAdam RF, McNichol GP, Robertson JIS, Wardrop C. Microangiopathic hemolytic anemia and the development of the malignant phase of hypertension. Circ Res 28 and 29 (Suppl II): 127–141, 1971.

31. Piel CF, Phibbs RH. The hemolytic-uremic syndrome. Pediatr Clin North Am 13: 295–314, 1966.

32. Shumway CN Jr. Miller G. An unusual syndrome of hemolytic anemia, thrombocytopenic purpura and renal disease. Blood 12: 1045–1052, 1957.

33. Bull BS, Rubenberg ML, Dacie JV, Brain MC. Microangiopathic hemolytic anemia: Mechanisms of red-cell fragmentation: In vitro studies. Brit J Haematol 14: 643–652, 1968.

34. Brain MC. The hemolytic-uremic syndrome. Semin Hematol 6: 162–180, 1969.

35. Bull BS, Kuhn IN. The production of schizocytes by fibrin strands (a scanning electron microscope study). Blood 35: 104–111, 1970.

36. Monnens L, Schretlen E. Intravascular coagulation in infant with hemolytic-uremic syndrome. Acta Paediat Scand 56: 436–441, 1967.

37. Avalos JS, Vitacco M, Molinas F, Penalver J, Gianantonio L. Coagulation studies in the hemolytic-uremic syndrome. J Pediat 76: 538, 1970.

38. Good RA, Thomas L. Studies on the generalized Shwartzman Reaction. II. The production of bilateral cortical necrosis of the kidneys by a single injection of bacterial toxin in rabbits previously treated with Thorotrast or Trypan blue. J Exp Med 96: 625–641, 1952.

39. McKay DG, Jitlin D, Craig JM. Immunochemical demonstration of fibrin in the generalized Shwartzman reaction. Arch Pathol 67: 270–273, 1959.

40. Pappas G, Ross MM, Thomas F. Studies on the Shwartzman reaction. VIII. The appearance by electron microscopy of intravascular fibrinoid in the glomerular capillaries during the reaction. J Exp Med 107: 333–340, 1958.

41. McKay DG, Shapiro SS. Alteration in the blood coagulation system induced by bacterial endotoxin. I. In vivo (generalized Shwartzman reaction). J Exp Med 107: 353–367, 1958.

42. Conte J, Delsol J, Mignon-Conte M, Ton That H, Suc JM. Acute renal failure and intravascular coagulation. In Hamburger J, Crosnier J, Maxwell MH (eds), Adv Nephrol, Vol 3, Year Book Medical, Chicago, 1973, pp. 197–240.

43. Rudenberg ML, Regolli E, Bull BS, Dacie JV, Brain MC. Microangiopathic hemolytic anemia: The experimental production of hemolysis and red-cell fragmentation by defibrination in vivo. Brit J Haematol 14: 627–642, 1978.

44. Vitsky BH, Suzuki Y, Strauss M, Churg J. The hemolytic-uremic syndrome: A study of renal pathologic alterations. Amer J Path 57: 627–647, 1969.

45. Collier HDJ, Denning-Kendall PA, Mc Donald-Gipson WJ, Saeed SA. Plasma proteins that inhibit prostaglandin synthesis. In Hemostasis, Prostaglandins, and Renal Disease, Remuzzi G, Mecca G, de Gaetano G. (eds), New York: Raven Press, 1980, pp. 257–267.

46. Gordon JL, Person JD. Endothelial and plasma factors modulating platelet aggregation. In Hemostasis, Prostaglandins and Renal Metabolism. Remuzzi G, Mecca G, de Gaetano G (eds). New York: Raven Press, 1980, pp. 269–271.

47. Remuzzi G, Marchesi D, Livio M, Schieppati A, Mecca G, Donati MB, de Gaetano G. Prostaglandins, plasma factors and hemostasis in uremia. In Hemostasis, Prostaglandins and Renal Disease, Remuzzi G, Mecca G, de Gaetano G (eds). New York: Raven Press, 1980, pp. 275–281.

48. Donati MB, Misiani R, Marchesi D, Livio M, Mecca G, Remuzzi G, de Gaetano G. Hemolytic-uremic syndrome: Prostaglandins and plasma factors. In Hemostasis, Prostaglandins and Renal Disease, Remuzzi G, Mecca G, de Gaetano G (eds). New York: Raven Press, 1980, pp. 283–290.

49. Remuzzi G, Mecca G, Livio M, de Gaetano G, Donati MB, Pearson JD, Gordon JL. Prostacyclin generation by cultured endothelial cells in hemolytic-uremic syndrome. Lancet 1: 656–657, 1980.

50. Remuzzi G, Misiani R, Marchesi D, Livio M, Mecca G, de Gaetano G, Donati MB. Hemolytic-uremic syndrome: Deficiency of plasma factors regulating prostacyclin activity. Lancet 2: 871–872, 1978.

51. Kincaid-Smith P, Hobbs JB, Friedman A, Mathews DC. Structural and ultrastructural alterations in mesenteric and renal arterioles following incision of vasoactive agents. In Hypertension '72, Genest J,

Koiw E (ed). Berlin: Springer-Verlag, 1972, pp. 97–108.

52. Gaynor E, Bouvier C, Spaet TH. Vascular lesions: possible basis of the generalized Shwartzman reaction. Science 170: 986–988, 1970.

53. Bergstein JM, Michael AF. Cortical fibrinolytic activity in normal and diseased kidneys. J Lab Clin Med 79: 701–709, 1972.

54. Sraer JD, Boelaert J, Mimoune O, Morel-Maroger L, Hornych H. Quantitative assessment of the fibrinolysis on isolated glomeruli. Kidney Int 4: 350–352, 1973.

55. Sraer JD, Delarue F, de Seigneux R, Morel-Maroger L, Kanfer A. Glomerular fibrinolytic activity after thrombin perfusion in the rat. Lab Invest 32: 515–517, 1975.

56. Ardaillou N, Sraer JD, Beaufils P. Fibrinogen kinetics in renal failure of various causes. Biomedicine Express 21: 49–56, 1974.

57. Cameron JS, Vick R. Plasma-C₃ in hemolytic-uremic syndrome and thrombotic thrombocytopenic purpura. Lancet 2: 975, 1973.

58. Kaplan BS, Thomson PD, Macnab GM. Serum-complement levels in the hemolytic-uremic syndrome. Lancet 2: 1505–1506, 1973.

59. Stuhlinger W, Kourilsky O, Kanfer A, Sraer JD. Hemolytic-uremic syndrome: Evidence of intravascular C₃ activation. Lancet 2: 788–789, 1974.

60. Stuhlinger WD, Verroust P, Morel-Maroger L. Detection of circulating immune complexes in patients with various renal diseases. Immunology 30: 43–47, 1976.

61. Kim Y, Miller R, Michael AF. Breakdown products of C₃ and Factor B in hemolytic-uremic syndrome. J Lab Clin Med 89: 845–850, 1977.

62. Wagoner RD, Holley KE, Johnson WJ. Accelerated nephrosclerosis and postpartum acute renal failure in normotensive patients. Ann Intern Med 69: 237–248, 1968.

63. Robson JG, Martin AM, Ruckley VA, Mac Donald MK. Irreversible post-partum renal failure. Quart J Med 137: 423–435, 1968.

64. Gilchrist GS, Lieberman E, Ekert H, Fine RN, Grushkin C. Heparin therapy in the hemolytic-uremic syndrome. Lancet 1: 1123–1126, 1969.

65. Schoolwerth CA, Sandler RS, Kalahr S, Kissan JM. Nephrosclerosis postpartum and in women taking oral contraceptives. Arch Intern Med 136: 178–185, 1976.

66. Luke RG, Talbert W, Siegel RR, Holland N. Heparin treatment for postpartum renal failure with microangiopathic hemolytic anemia. Lancet 2: 750–752, 1970.

67. Donadio JV, Holley KE. Postpartum acute renal failure: Recovery after heparin therapy. Amer J Obstet Gynecol 118: 510–516, 1974.

68. Churg J, Koffler D, Paronetto F, Rorat E, Barnett RN. Hemolytic-uremic syndrome as a cause of postpartum renal failure. Amer J Obstet Gynecol 108: 253–261, 1970.

69. Timor-Tritsch I, Better OS, Tatarsky I, Chaimowitz C, Peretz A, Abramovici H. Successful treatment of postpartum renal failure with heparin. Brit Med J 4: 221–222, 1970.

70. Ponticelli C, Imbasciati E, Tarantino A, Grazan G, Redaelli B. Postpartum renal failure with microangiopathic hemolytic anemia. Néphron 9: 27–41, 1972.

71. Ponticelli C, Imbasciati E, Rivolta E, Rossi E, Manucci PN. Long-term follow-up of postpartum hemolytic-uremic syndrome treated with heparin and antiplatelet agents. In Hemostasis, Prostaglandins and Renal Disease, Remuzzi G, Mecca G, de Gaetano G (eds). New York: Raven Press, 1980, pp. 443–451.

72. Prosmans W, Muaka BK, Van Damme B, Eeckles R. The use of heparin in childhood hemolytic-uremic syndrome. In Hemostasis, Prostaglandins and Renal Disease, Remuzzi G, Mecca G, de Gaetano G (eds). New York: Raven Press, 1980, pp. 407–411.

73. Rossi EC, Green G, del Greco F. The use of inhibitors of platelet functions in thrombotic microangiopathy. In Hemostasis, Prostaglandins and Renal Disease, Remuzzi G, Mecca G, de Gaetano G (eds). New York: Raven Press, 1980, pp. 413–422.

74. Burke HA, Hartmann RC. Thrombotic thrombocytopenic purpura: Two patients with remission associated with the use of large amounts of steroids. Arch Intern Med 103: 105–109, 1959.

75. Jorgensen KA, Moller-Petersen J, Ekelund S, Smith-Pedersen R. Prostacyclin and hemolytic thrombocytopenic microangiopathy. Lancet 2: 530–531, 1981.

76. Burkowski RM, Hewlett JS, Harris JW, Hoffman GC, Battle JD, Silverblatt E, Yang I. Exchange transfusions in the treatment of thrombotic thrombocytopenic purpura. Semm Hematol 13: 219–232, 1976.

77. Myers TJ, Wakem MB, Ball ED, Tremont SJ. Thrombotic thrombocytopenic purpura: Combined treatment with plasmapheresis and antiplatelet agents. Ann Inter Med 92: 149–155, 1980.

78. Bukowski RM, King JW, Hewlett JS. Plasmapheresis in the treatment of thrombotic thrombocytopenic purpura. Blood 50: 413–417, 1977.

79. Misiani R, Trevisan F, Marthesi D, Bertani T, Remuzzi G, Mecca G. Plasmapheresis and plasma infusion in the treatment of hemolytic-uremic syndrome. In Hemostasis, Prostaglandins and Renal Disease, Remuzzi G, Mecca G, de Gaetano G (eds). New York: Raven Press, 1980, pp. 423–431.

80. Arias-Rodriguez M, Sraer JD, Kourilsky O, Smith MD, Verroust P, Meyrier A, Kuntziger HE, Kanfer A, Nessim V, Neuilly G, Morel-Maroger L, Richet G. Renal transplantation and immunological abnormalities in thrombotic microangiopathy of adults. Transplantation 23: 360–365, 1977.

81. Baker NM, Mills AE, Rachman I, Thomas JEP.

Hemolytic-uremic syndrome in typhoid fever. Brit Med J 2: 84–87, 1974.

82. Clarkson AR, Lawrence JR, Meadow R, Seymour AE. The hemolytic-uremic syndrome in adults. Quart J Med 39: 227–244, 1970.

83. Clarkson AR, Sage HE, Lawrence JR. Consumption coagulopathy and acute renal failure due to gram-negative septicemia after abortion. Complete recovery with heparin therapy. Ann Intern Med 70: 1191–1199, 1969.

84. Rapaport SI, Tatter O, Coeur-Barrow N, Hjort PF. Pseudomonas septicemia with intravascular clotting leading to the generalized Shwartzman reaction. N Engl J Med 271: 80–84, 1964.

85. Seger R, Joller P, Baerlocher K, Kennig A, Dulake C, Leumann E, Spierig M, Hitzig WH. Hemolytic-uremic syndrome associated with neuraminidase producing microorganism: Treatment by exchange transfusion. Hael Paediat Acta 35: 359–367, 1980.

86. Koster F, Levin J, Walker L, Taung KSK, Gilman RH, Rahaman MM, Majid MA, Islam SI, Williams RS. Hemolytic-uremic syndrome after Shigellosis. Relation to endotoxemia and circulating immune complexes. N Engl J Med 298: 927–933, 1978.

87. Rahamam MM, Greenough WB. Shigellose and hemolytic-uremic syndrome. Lancet 1: 1051–1052, 1978.

88. Austin TW, Ray CG. Coxsackie virus group B infections and the hemolytic-uremic syndrome. J Infect Dis 127, 698–701, 1973.

89. Davison AM, Thomson D, Robson JS. Intravascular coagulation complicating influenza A 2 infection. Brit Med J 1: 654–655, 1973.

90. Berjstein J, Michael AF, Kjellstrand C, Simmons R, Najarian J. Hemolytic-uremic syndrome in adults sisters. Transplantation 17: 487–490, 1974.

90b. Glasgow LA, Balduzzi P. Isolation of coxsackie virus group A type 4 from a patient with hemolytic-uremic syndrome. N Engl J Med 273: 754–756, 1965.

91. McKay DC, Jewett JF, Reid DE. Endotoxin shock and the generalized Shwartzman reaction in pregnancy. Amer J Obstet Gynecol 78: 546–549, 1959.

92. Benson L, Cuppage FP, Grantham J. Disseminated intravascular coagulation. Postpartum hemolytic-uremic syndrome with recovery of renal functions. J Kans Med Soc 72: 738–741, 1971.

93. Hibbard DM, Jeffcoate TNA. Abruptio placentae. Obstet Gynecol 27: 155–167, 1966.

94. Kleinknecht D, Grunfeld J, Gomez PC, Moreau J, Garcia-Torres T. Diagnostic procedures and long-term prognosis in bilateral renal cortical necrosis. Kidney Int 4: 390–400, 1973.

95. Scheer RL, Jones DB. Malignant nephrosclerosis in women postpartum. J Amer Med Ass 201: 106–110, 1967.

96. Kincaid-Smith P. The similarity of lesions and underlying mechanism in pre-eclamptic toxemia and postpartum renal failure. Studies in the acute stages and during follow-up. In Glomerulonephritis, Kin-

caid-Smith P, Mathew TH, Becker EL (eds). New York: Wiley, 1973, pp. 1013-1025.

97. Vandewalle A, Kanfer A, Kourilsky O. Oliguric thrombotic microangiopathy during the fifth month of pregnancy. Brit Med J 1: 479–480, 1975.

98. Schoolwerth AC, Sandler RS, Klahr S, McConnell JB. Nephrosclerosis postpartum and in women taking oral contraceptives. Arch Intern Med 136: 178–185, 1976.

99. Tobon H. Malignant hypertension, uremia and hemolytic anemia in a patient on oral contraceptives. Obst Gynecol 40: 681–685, 1972.

100. Brown TG, Clarkson AP, Robson JS, Cameron JS, Thomson D, Ogg CS. Hemolytic-uremic syndrome in women taking oral contraceptives. Lancet 1: 1479–1481, 1973.

101. Hauglustaine D, Van Damme B, Vanrenterghen Y, Michielsen T. Recurrent hemolytic uremic syndrome during oral contraception. Clin Nephrol 15: 148–153, 1981.

102. Kanfer A. Risque vasculo-rénal des contraceptifs oraux. Rev Prat 27: 23–25, 1977.

103. Reiner M, Cox J, Bernheim C, Vischer TL. A propos de deux cas de lupus érythémateux disséminé avec syndrome de Moschcowitz terminal. Schwez Med Wschr 98: 1691–1692, 1968.

104. Thomson D, Gardner DL. Thrombotic microangiopathy in rheumatoid arthritis. Scot Med J 14: 190–193, 1969.

105. Kourilsky O, Gubler MC, Morel-Maroger L, Adam-Rordorf C, Sraer JD, Kanfer A, Verroust P, Richet G. A new form of familial glomerulonephritis. Néphron 30: 97–105, 1982.

106. Rumpf KW, Rieger J, Lankisch DG, Von Heyden H, Nagel GA, Scheller F. Letter: Mitomycin-induced hemolysis and renal failure. Lancet 2: 1037–1038, 1980.

107. Amorosi EL, Ultmann JE. Thrombotic thrombocytopenic purpura: Report of 16 cases and review of the litterature. Medicine (Baltimore) 45: 139–159, 1966.

108. Ridolfi RL, Bell WR. Thrombotic thrombocytopenic purpura. Report of 25 cases and review of the litterature. Medicine (Baltimore) 60: 413–428, 1981.

109. Walls J, Schorr WJ, Kerr DNS. Prolonged oliguria with survival in acute bilateral cortical necrosis. Brit Med J 4: 220–222, 1968.

110. Volhard F, Fahr T. Die Brightsche Nierenkrankheit. Berlin: Springer Verlag, 1914.

111. Kincaid-Smith P, McMichael J, Murphy EA. The clinical course and pathology of hypertension with papilledema (malignant hypertension). Quart J Med 27: 117–153, 1958.

112. Sevitt IH, Evans DJ, Wrong OM. Acute oliguric renal failure due to accelerated (malignant) hypertension. Quart J Med 40: 127–144, 1971.

113. Johansson B, Standgaard S, Lassen NA. On the pathogenesis of hypertensive encephalopathy. The hypertensive "break through" of auto-regulation of

cerebral blood flow with forced vasodilatation, flow increase and blood-brain barrier damaged. Circ Res 34 (Suppl. 1): 167–174, 1974.

114. Strandgaard S, Olesen J, Skinoj E, Lassen NA. Auto-regulation of brain circulation in severe arterial hypertension. Brit Med J 1: 507–510, 1973.

115. Skinhoj E, Strandgaard S. Pathogenesis of hypertensive encephalopathy. Lancet 1: 461–462, 1973.

116. Finnerty FA. Hypertensive encephalopathy. Amer J Med 52: 672–678, 1972.

117. Byrom FB. The pathogenesis of hypertensive encephalopathy and its relation to the malignant phase of hypertension. Lancet 2: 201–211, 1954.

118. Buhler FR, Laragh JH, Vaughan ED, Brunner HR, Gavras H, Baer L. The anti-hypertensive action of propranolol. Specific antirenin responses in high and normal renin forms of essential, renal, renovascular and malignant hypertension. In Hypertension Manual, Laragh JR (ed). New York: Dun-Donnelley, 1973.

119. Beaufils P, Sraer JD. Problèmes actuels du diagnostic et du traitement des néphropathies vasculaires avec insuffisance rénale aigue. Vie Med 13: 1543–1547, 1972.

120. Mamdani BH, Lim VS, Mahurkak SD, Katz AJ, Dunea G.: Recovery from prolonged renal failure in patients with accelerated hypertension. N Engl J Med 291: 1343–1344, 1974.

121. Mroczek WJ, Davidov M, Gavrilavich L, Finnerty FA. The value of agressive therapy in the hypertensive patients with azotemia. Circulation 40: 893–904, 1969.

122. Pickering G. Reversibility of malignant hypertension. Lancet 1: 413–418, 1971.

123. Meyrier A, Laaban JP, Kanfer A. Protracted anuria due to active vasoconstriction in malignant hypertension. Brit. Med. Jour under press 1984.

124. Lam M, Ricanati ES, Kahn MA, Kushner I. Reversal of severe renal failure in systemic sclerosis. Ann Intern Med 89: 642–643, 1978.

125. Perera GA. Hypertensive vascular disease, description and natural history. J Chronic Dis 1: 33–47, 1955.

126. Derow HA, Altschule MD. The nature of malignant hypertension. Ann Int Med 14: 1768–1780, 1941.

127. Milliez P, Tcherdakoff P, Samarcq P, Rey LP. The natural course of malignant hypertension. In Essential Hypertension: An International Symposium, Bock KD, Cottier PT (Eds). Berlin: Springer, 1960.

128. Platt R, Davson J. A clinical and pathological study of renal disease. Part II. Diseases other than nephritis. Quart J Med 19: 33–55, 1950.

129. Schurmann P, MacMahon HE. Die maligne Nephrosklerose zugleich ein Beitrag zur Frage der Bedeutung der Blutgewebsschranke. Virchows Arch 291: 48–218, 1933.

130. McGregor L. Histological changes in the renal glomerulus in essential (primary) hypertension. A

study of fifty-one cases. Amer J Path 6: 347–366, 1930.

131. McManus JFA, Lupton CM. Ischemic obsolescence of renal glomeruli. Lab Invest 9: 413–434, 1960.

132. Mandal AK, Frolich ED, Nordquist J. An ultrastructural analysis of renal arterioles in benign and malignant essential hypertension. Ann Clin Lab Sci 7: 158–168, 1977.

133. Heptinstall RH. Renal biopsies in hypertension. Brit Heart J 16: 133–141, 1953.

134. Allison PR, Bleenhan N, Brown W, Pickering CW, Robb-Smith AHT, Russel RP. The production and resolution of hypertensive vascular lesions in the rabbit. Clin Sci 33: 39–51, 1967.

135. Heptinstall RH. Malignant hypertension. A study of fifty-one cases. J Pathol Bacteriol 65: 423–439, 1953.

136. Floyer MA. The effect of nephrectomy and adrenalectomy upon the blood pressure in hypertensive and normotensive rats. Clin Sci 10: 405–421, 1951.

137. McCormack L.J, Beland JE, Schnecklotrh RE, Corcoran AC. Effect of antihypertensive treatment on the evolution of the renal lesions in malignant nephrosclerosis. Amer J Path 34: 1011–1021, 1958.

138. Linton AL, Gavras H, Gleadle RI, Hutchison HP, Lawson DH, Lever AF, Macadam RF, McNicol GP, Robertson JIS. Microangiopathic hemolytic anemia and the pathogenesis of malignant hypertension. Lancet 1: 1277–1282, 1969.

139. Catt KZ, Kimmel PZ, Cain MD, Cran E, Best JB, Clghlan JB. Angiotension II blood levels in human hypertension. Lancet 1: 459–463, 1971.

140. Kahn JR, Skeggs LT, Shumway NP, Wisenbaugh PE. The assay of hypertensin from the arterial blood of normotensive and hypertensive human beings. J Exp Med 95: 523–529, 1952.

141. Asscher AW, Anson SG. A vascular permeability factor of renal origin. Nature (London) 198: 1097–1099, 1963.

142. Thiel G, Huguenin M, Torhorst J, Peters L, Peters G, Brunner F. "Low renin" and "high renin" hypertension in the rat. I. Correlation between blood pressure, plasma renin activities and severity of vascular damage. Kidney Int 3: 273–276, 1973.

143. Medsger TA, Rodnan GP, Benedek TG, Robinson H. Survival with systemic sclerosis (scleroderma) a life-table analysis of clinical and demographic factors in 309 patients. Ann Inter Med 75: 369–385, 1971.

144. Cannon PJ, Hassar M, Case DB, Casarella WJ, Sommers SC, Le Roy EC. The relationship of hypertension and renal failure in scleroderma (progressive systemic sclerosis) to structural and functionnal abnormalities of the renal cortical circulation. Medicine (Baltimore) 53: 1–46, 1974.

145. Heptinstall RH. Scleroderma (progressive systemic sclerosis) Pathology of the Kidney. Boston-Little, Brown, 1974, pp. 687–706.

146. Sayler WR, Sayler DC, Heptinstall RH. Sclero-

derma and microangiopathic hemolytic anemia. Ann Intern Med 78: 895–897, 1973.

147. Richardson JA. Hemodialysis and kidney transplantation for renal failure from scleroderma. Arthr and Rheum 16: 265–271, 1973.

148. D'Angelo WA, Fries JF, Nasi AT, Shulman LE. Pathologic observations in systemic sclerosis (scleroderma). A study of fifty-eight autopsy cases and fifty-eight matched controls. Amer J Med 46: 428–440, 1969.

149. LeRoy EC, Downey JA, Cannon PJ. Skin cappilary blood flow in scleroderma. J Clin Invest 50: 930–939, 1971.

150. Norton WL, Hurd ER, Lewis DC, Ziff M. Evidence of microvascular injury in scleroderma and systemic lupus erythematosus: Quantitative study of the microvascular bed. J Lab Clin Med 71: 919–933, 1968.

151. Davson J, Ball J, Platt R. The kidney in periarteritis nodosa. Quart J Med 17: 175–202, 1948.

152. Richet G, Habib R. Les localisations rñales de la PAN. J Urol Nephrol 65: 177–182, 1959.

153. Kanfer A, Sraer JD, Feintuch MJ, Morel-Maroger L, Beaufils P, Richet G. Insuffisance rénale aigue au cours de la périartérite noueuse. Nouv Presse méd 5: 1883–1888, 1976.

154. Droz D, Noel LH, Leibowitch M, Barbanel C. Glomérulonéphrite et angéites nécrosantes. In Actualités Néphrologiques de l'hôpital Necker, Hamburger J, Crosnier J, Maxwell MH (Eds). Paris: Flammarion, 1978, pp. 199–217.

155. Fauci AS, Haynes BF, Katz P. The spectrum of vasculitis: Clinical, pathologic, immunologic and therapeutic considerations. Ann Intern Med 89: 660–676, 1978.

156. Howel SB, Epstein WV. Circulating immune complexes in Wegener's granulomatosis. Amer J Med 60: 259–268, 1976.

157. Conn DL, Mc Duffie FC, Holley KE, Schroeter AL. Immunologic mechanisms in systemic vasculitis. Mayo Clin Proc 51: 511–518, 1976.

158. Meltzer M, Franklin EC. Cryoglobulinemia. A study of twenty-nine patients. I. IgG and IgM cryoglobulins and factors affecting cryoprecipitability. Amer J Med 40: 828–836, 1966.

159. Meltzer M, Franklin EC, Elias K. Cryoglobulinemia. A clinical and laboratory study. II Cryoglobulins with rheumatoid factor activity. Amer J Med 40: 837–856, 1966.

160. Verroust P, Mery JP, Morel-Maroger L, Clauvel JP, Richet G. Les lésions glomérulaires des gammapathies monoclonales et des cryoglobulinémies idiopathiques IgG-IgM. In Actualitiés Néphrologiques de l'hpital Necker, Hamburger J, Crosnier J, Maxwell MH (Eds). Paris: Flammarion, 1971, pp. 167–202.

161. Brouet JC, Clauvel JP, Danon F, Klein M, Seligmann M. Biologic and clinical significance of cryoglobulins. Am J Med 57: 775–778, 1974.

162. Case report of the Massachussets General Hospital. N Engl Med 292: 1285–1290, 1975.

163. Williams RC. A second look at rheumatoid factor and other "autoantibodies." Am J Med 67: 179–181, 1979.

164. Zimmerman SW, Dreher WH, Burkholder PM, Goldfarb S, Weinstein AB. Nephropathy and mixed cryoglobulinemia: Evidence for an immune complex pathogenesis. Néphron 16: 103–115, 1976.

165. Cordonnier D, Martin H, Groslambert P, Micoin C, Chenais F, Stoebner P. Mixed IgG-IgM cryoglobulinemia with glomerulonephritis. Am J Med 59: 867–872, 1975.

166. Faraggiara T, Parolini C, Previato G. Light and electron microscopic findings in five cases of cryoglobulinemic glomerulonephritis. Virchows Arch A Path Annat Histol 384: 29–44, 1979.

167. Morel-Maroger L, Mery JP. Renal lesions in mixed IgG-IgM essential cryoglobulinemia in proc. 5th Int. Congr Nephrol Mexico, 1972, Basal: Karger 1974, vol. 1, pp. 173–178.

168. Morel-Maroger L, Verroust P. Glomerular lesions in dysproteinemias. Kidney Int 5: 249–252, 1974.

169. Joekes AM, Owen K, Sherwood T. Acute renal failure due to lateral renal artery emboli. Case report. Brit Med J 1: 286–287, 1964.

170. Gill TJ, Dammin GJ. Paradoxal embolism with renal failure caused by occlusion of the renal arteries. Am J Med 25: 780–787, 1958.

171. Duncan DA, Dexter RN. Anuria secondary to bilateral renal artery embolism. N Engl J Med 266: 971–973, 1962.

172. Kaiser TF, Ross RR. Total infarction of the kidney from bilateral arterial emboli. J Urol 66: 500–511, 1951.

173. Heptinstall RH. Infarction, cortical necrosis and papillary necrosis including the kidney of analgesic abuse. In Pathology of the Kidney (2nd ed), Heptinstall RH (ed). Boston: Little, Brown, 1974, pp. 221–272.

174. Gore I, McCombs, Lindquist RL. Observations from the fate of cholesterol emboli. J Atheroscler Res 4: 527–535, 1969.

175. Kassirer JP. Atheroembolic renal disease. N Engl J Med 280: 812–818, 1969.

176. McCarthy LJ, Titus JL, Daugherty GW. Bilateral renal vein thrombosis and the nephrotic syndrome in adults. Ann Intern Med 58: 837–857, 1963.

177. Richet G, Meyrier A. Liposclérose rétropéritonéale/Thrombose des Veines Rénales. Richet G, Meyrier A. Paris: Masson, 1979.

178. Zech P, Blanc-Brunat N, Pinet A, Colon S, Bernheim JL, Berthoux F, Traeger J. Les thromboses veineuses rénales de l'adulte. Schweiz Med Wschr 105: 398–406, 1975.

179. Rosenmann E, Pollack VE, Pirani CL. Renal vein thrombosis in the adult: A clinical and pathological

study based on renal biopsies. Medicine (Baltimore) 47: 269–335, 1968.

180. Pollack VE, Pirani CL, Seskind C, Griffel B. Bilateral renal vein thrombosis. Clinical and electron microscopic studies of a case with complet recovery after anticoagulant therapy. Ann Int Med 65: 1056–1071, 1966.

181. Trew PA, Biava CG, Jacobs RP, Hopper J. Renal vein thrombosis in membranous glomerulopathy: Incidence and association. Medicine (Baltimore) 57: 69–82, 1978.

182. Llach F, Arieff AI, Massry SG. Renal vein thrombosis and nephrotic syndrome. A prospective study of 36 adult patients. Ann Int Med 83: 8–14, 1975.

15. ACUTE RENAL FAILURE ASSOCIATED WITH LEPTOSPIROSIS

Visith Sitprija

1 Introduction

Leptospirosis is one of the common infectious diseases in the tropics caused by leptospires. Leptospira interrogans is the only species divided into two complexes: the interrogans complex and the biflexa complex. The interrogans complex, with its 18 serogroups and 130 serotypes, is pathogenic, while the biflexa complex is saprophytic.

Rodents, especially rats, are the most important reservoir. Transmission is by direct contact with blood, tissue, or urine of infected animals or by exposure to the environment contaminated with leptospires. People working in an environment infested with rats or rodents or with infected material or water are therefore prone to infection. Leptospires enter a host through abrasions in the skin or through the mucosa, including conjunctiva, vagina, and nasopharynx. Penetration through the intact skin is unlikely, although prolonged exposure of the skin to contaminated water may provide an opportunity for invasion [1].

Leptospirosis is in fact worldwide although it is predominantly tropical. The disease is characterized by a broad spectrum of clinical manifestations, which include fever, chills, headache, conjunctivitis, and muscular pains. The kidney is invariably involved, and renal failure is seen in severe infection. In certain geographical areas, leptospiral renal failure accounts for almost 40% of acute renal failure due to tropical diseases [2]. Weil's syndrome denotes leptospirosis with renal failure and

jaundice. It is not serotype specific, but represents severe infection.

2 Renal Pathological Changes

Leptospirosis involves every structure of the kidney. Glomerular and vascular changes, however, are mild and are not of clinical importance. Tubulo-interstitial changes account for the impairment of renal function. In man, renal lesions completely resolve when the disease is brought under control.

2.1 DEMONSTRATION OF LEPTOSPIRES

In biopsy studies, it is often difficult to identify leptospires in the renal tissue since the pathological study is usually performed late in the course of the disease. The organisms may be demonstrable in the renal tubules by Levaditi's stain. In hamsters, leptospires are seen in the glomeruli and interstitium a few hours following inoculation. After nine hours, they are only detectable in the interstitium and proximal tubules. The organisms are found in the antigen form five days after inoculation. The antigen is detected in increasing amounts in proximal and distal tubular cells over a period of two to three weeks.

2.2 GLOMERULAR LESIONS

Glomerular changes in leptospirosis are in general not remarkable. There is usually mild proliferation of the mesangial cells with widening of the mesangial matrix, similar to that observed in the other infectious diseases [3]. In the biopsied kidney, scattered polymorphonuclear cell infiltration may be present when the study is made early in the course of the disease. In animal experiments, polymorphonuclear cells are demonstrable in the glomeruli in the early stage of the disease, but disappear very quickly [4].

By immunofluorescence, deposition of C3 is seen in the mesangial areas and in the capillary loop [4]. Usually, immunoglobulins are not detectable, but in occasional cases IgM deposition may be observed in the mesangial areas.

By electron microscopy, there is focal foot process fusion and focal thickening of the basement membrane due to widening of the lamina rara interna. The cytoplasm of visceral epithelial cells shows prominent Golgi complexes and dilated endoplasmic reticulum. Pseudovilli, representing the long slender projections of the visceral epithelial cells into the urinary space, are observed [3].

2.3 VASCULAR LESIONS

It has been suggested that bacterial toxins increase the fragility of the capillary wall, and hemorrhage is one of the important manifestations of leptospirosis. Although leptospires affect the blood vessels, vascular changes are usually not noticeable by light microscopy. By immunofluorescence, C3 deposition without immunoglobulins is demonstrable in the glomerular afferent arterioles [4]. The significance of the finding is not understood. It is possible that it represents trapping of C3 at the site of injury in the blood vessels. The same finding has been shown in a number of infectious diseases [5].

By electron microscopy nonspecific swelling and vacuolation of the endothelial cells is demonstrable. The endoplasmic reticulum is dilated and the mitochondria are enlarged. Necrotic lesions, characterized by segmental necrosis of the endothelium and the presence of holes that allows the escape of erythrocytes, are also seen in the peritubular capillaries. Platelet aggregation is noted in the corticomedullary capillaries [6]. It is suggested that vascular lesions induced by leptospires begin with increased vascular permeability before endothelial necrosis.

2.4 TUBULAR LESIONS

Degeneration and necrosis occur in both proximal and distal convoluted tubules. Cloudy swelling is the early lesion. The disease primarily involves proximal tubules. Distal tubules are affected as the disease progresses. Disruption of the basement membrane may be noted. Histochemically, impairment of tubular enzyme activity such as alkaline phosphatase, glutamic, isocitric, lactic, malic, and glucose-6-phosphate dehydrogenases may precede the pathological changes [7]. These changes may show focal distribution. An increased number of mitoses may be seen in the tubular epithelial cells. Bile casts and heme casts may be present in the tubular lamen.

Electron microscopy reveals an increased number of cytosomes and an active system of apical vesicles and vacuoles [3]. There are focal dilatations of the intercellular space.

2.5 INTERSTITIAL LESIONS

Although interstitial changes may occur as a secondary phenomenon to acute tubular necrosis, the changes in leptospirosis are more striking and deserve being a distinct pathological entity. Interstitial edema and cellular infiltration are observed, even in the patient without renal failure and tubular necrosis. Infiltration may be diffuse or may occur around the glomeruli and venules [3]. The infiltrate consists mainly of mononuclear cells and a few eosinophils. Neutrophils may be present during the early stage of the disease. Interstitial hemorrhage may occur. Although tubular necrosis and interstitial changes are observed in the patient with renal failure, interstitial changes chronologically precede tubular necrosis. In the hamster, it has been shown that leptospires penetrate the peritubular capillaries to the interstitium and then to renal tubules [4]. Leptospirosis is therefore one of the models of interstitial nephritis due to bacterial infection.

3 Pathogenesis

The clinical features in leptospirosis have been attributed to toxins elaborated by or released from the lysed leptospires [8]. Previous investigations have indicated that renal damage is the result of hemodynamic alteration. The focal distribution of the lesions suggests a relationship with impairment of renal blood flow. Mitochondrial injury and histochemical lesions are also suggestive of hypoxic injury [7]. However, the presence of leptospires in the tissue is prerequisite for the development of renal lesions, the finding indicating direct nephrotoxicity [4]. Three mechanisms are considered in the pathogenesis of renal disease in leptospirosis.

3.1 NONSPECIFIC EFFECTS OF INFECTION

A number of nonspecific factors related to infection can lead to hypoperfusion of the kidney and renal ischemia. These nonspecific factors are responsible for renal failure of ischemic type in various infections.

3.1.1 Hypovolemia In infectious diseases, hypovolemia may occur. Determination of blood volume in leptospirosis in the patients not previously receiving intravenous fluid reveals a decrease in blood volume [4]. The same is true for the other infectious diseases. Hypovolemia is brought about by several mechanisms, including increased insensible fluid loss due to fever, increased sweating, decreased fluid and salt intake, and increased vascular permeability [9]. Increased vascular permeability occurs in a variety of inflammatory processes and is attributed to the presence of chemical mediators released during the inflammatory reaction. Kinins, prostaglandins, serotonin, and histamine are among the known substances produced during inflammation. The other less known substances include fibrinopeptides and fibrin degradation products (FDP), which can also increase vascular permeability [10]. Increased plasma kinin activity and histamine have been shown in infectious diseases [11–13]. The cytotoxin, which is present in the blood early in the course of leptospirosis, is known to have an injurious effect on the vascular endothelium, leading therefore to increased vascular permeability [14, 15].

3.1.2 Blood Hyperviscosity The rise in plasma fibrinogen is a normal response to acute infection. In leptospirosis, the plasma fibrinogen is markedly increased, thus accounting for the increase in blood viscosity and the rise in the erythrocyte sedimentation rate [4]. The plasma fibrinogen may be as high as 1,000 mg/dl. Hypovolemia and hemoconcentration also contribute to blood hyperviscosity. Since the laminar blood flow is inversely related to the blood viscosity, the flow in the microcirculation, including the kidney, is therefore compromised. Without the compensatory mechanism, the renal blood flow would be reduced.

3.1.3 Catecholamine Release In a number of infections, especially in septicemia, catecholamines are released, a response to hypovolemia and kinin stimulation [16]. Although the rise in catecholamines in the blood has not been described in leptospirosis, it is highly possible theoretically because of the common pathophysiologic pathway. Besides the reduction in renal blood flow, catecholamines can also increase vascular permeability [17].

3.1.4 Intravascular Coagulation Because of hyperfibrinogenemia, hemoconcentration, and vascular damage, intravascular coagulation may occur in leptospirosis. The increased serum FDP have been demonstrated, especially when the infection is severe. Platelets may be reduced. In most cases intravascular coagulation is local and of low grade [4]. Disseminated intravascular coagulation (DIC) occurs rarely. The patient may present the picture of hemolytic uremic syndrome (HUS). Whether PGI_2 deficiency plays any role in the pathogenesis of DIC in leptospirosis has not been established. While severe intravascular coagulation can adversely affect the renal blood flow, low-grade intravascular coagulation has no effect.

3.1.5 Intravascular Hemolysis Although leptospires have hemolysin, severe intravascular hemolysis seldom occurs. Mild intravascular hemolysis may be present during the acute phase of infection [4]. However, severe intravascular hemolysis may be observed in the patient with G-6-PD deficiency. DIC may further contribute to hemolysis. Severe intravascular hemolysis may decrease the renal blood flow. In the usual case of leptospirosis, this is uncommon since hemolysis is very mild.

3.1.6 Jaundice Jaundice is not necessarily present in leptospirosis, although its presence indicates severe infection. In a study of renal function in jaundice, it has been found that mild jaundice has no effect on renal function; but when jaundice is severe, renal function may be impaired and, although renal failure may be nonoliguric, severe oliguria may be observed [18]. Hyperbilirubinemia is known to interfere with the renal function, but the/mechanism is not understood. Unconjugated bilirubin [19], conjugated bilirubin [20], and bile acids [21] have been implicated. Natriuresis has been described when there is hyperbilirubinemia [18]. It has been postulated that a high concentration of unconjugated bilirubin in the renal medulla might interfere with sodium chloride transport through the ascending limb in Henle's loop [19]. Jaundice has been shown to increase sensitivity to catecholamines [22] and increase plasma renin activity [23], leading to vasoconstriction. Increased urine uric acid excretion in jaundice might also contribute to nephropathy when the urine is concentrated [24]. Exchange blood transfusion has been shown to improve renal function in hyperbilirubinemic renal failure [25]. On the clinical ground, it is felt that hyperbilirubinemia of over 428 μmol/l (25 mg/dl) contributes to the impairment of renal function.

All these factors are nonspecific and are shared by several infectious diseases. They can lead to renal ischemia and renal failure. Hyperpyrexia [26] and carditis [1] may enhance tubular damage in this clinical setting. In this respect, any severe infection is capable of causing renal failure. In mild cases, renal failure may be prerenal. Prerenal failure has been noted in leptospirosis [27].

3.2 IMMUNOLOGIC MECHANISMS

Immune-mediated nephropathy has been shown in canine leptospirosis [28] However, the evidence is lacking in man [4]. Immune complexes are not detectable in the renal lesions. Only C3 deposition is seen in the afferent arterioles and occasionally in the glomeruli [4]. Occasional demonstration of faint IgM deposition in the mesangium is perhaps nonspecific. Experiments in hamsters also failed to show immune complex deposition [4]. The role of cell-mediated immune response in the pathogenesis of interstitial nephritis is debatable.

The fact that interstitial changes are characterized by mononuclear cell infiltration favors cell-mediated mechanism. However, in animal experiments these changes occur within three hours following leptospire inoculation. The onset is too short for the delayed type of hypersensitivity. The discrepancy in findings between humans and hamsters, on the one hand, and dogs, on the other hand, could reflect the difference in immune response and the clinical course of the disease in different hosts. In dogs, leptospirosis usually runs a chronic course and may lead to chronic renal failure [29]. Autoimmune response to the epithelial antigens released by degenerated tubules might lead to chronic lesions. However, antikidney antibodies are not detectable in the chronic stage of the disease [30]. In man, chronic renal lesion has not been shown in repeat renal biopsies. It seems unlikely that immunologic mechanisms play any important role in the pathogenesis of the renal lesions in man.

3.3 DIRECT NEPHROTOXICITY

Despite the fact that the nonspecific effects of infection can lead to acute tubular necrosis with renal failure, they cannot explain the mild glomerular changes and interstitial nephritis. Since the clinical features of leptospirosis resemble those of endotoxemia, it is tempting to assume that renal lesions are attributed to endotoxemia. However, endotoxin is present only in some serotype [31]. Intravenous and intraperitoneal injections of suspension of killed leptospires into guinea pigs failed to produce renal lesions. Pathologic changes are caused only by viable organisms [1], and the presence of leptospires in the tissue is needed for the development of lesions.

In hamster experiments, leptospires were demonstrable in the glomeruli along with glomerular changes within a few hours after intraperitoneal inoculation. Interstitial changes also occur at the same time, but became more marked during the later stage. Tubular degeneration began later at the sixth hour. Since glomerular changes, interstitial nephritis, and tubular necrosis occur with the presence of leptospires or leptospire antigens in the lesions, it is interpreted that renal lesions are caused by leptospire invasion. The severity of lesions correlates well with the number of organisms. Interstitial changes always preceded tubular changes, and both continued on even though glomerular changes had ceased [4]. It is thus evident that leptospires gain access to the kidney by the blood stream, causing initially glomerular injury that is mild and transient. The organisms then reach the peritubular capillaries and penetrate into the interstitium and tubules producing interstitial nephritis and tubular necrosis. Proximal tubules are first involved. Distal tubules are later affected. The view is contrary to the previous findings that tubular necrosis was initially produced with secondary interstitial changes and that distal tubular degeneration is the main lesion [32]. In man, interstitial nephritis is noted even in the absence of tubular necrosis [3], the finding that supports the animal experiments. Glomerular changes, interstitial lesions, and tubular necrosis are thus pathological reactions to leptospire invasion. However, it remains unclear as to whether these changes are due to leptospire migration per se or to factors inherent to bacterial virulence, such as bacterial enzymes, metabolites, or exotoxins. Both are likely involved. Cytotoxin has been implicated in causing vascular endothelial injury [14, 15]. Although vascular changes are not shown in light microscopy, C3 deposition in the glomeruli and arterioles without immunoglobulins would suggest complement activation through the alternative pathway and trapping of C3 by the injured vessels.

Clinical and experimental evidence suggests that renal failure in leptospirosis is attributed to nonspecific effects of infection and direct nephrotoxicity of leptospires. It represents both ischemic and nephrotoxic models of acute renal failure. This could explain the broad spectrum of renal changes and the conflicts among the pathological reports, which depend on the predominance of factors involved and the time of study.

4 Clinical Manifestations

Renal involvement is observed in all forms of leptospirosis regardless of the severity and the infecting serotype. Impairment of renal function is common. Alterations of renal function

may be profound and out of proportion to the histologic changes. It has been documented that even in relatively mild cases in which the glomerular filtration rate is normal, para-aminohippurate clearance may be low, indicating proximal tubular dysfunction [1]. Abnormal urine findings are noted in 70 to 80% of cases during the septicemic period. Proteinuria is most frequent and is often mild. Hyaline and granular casts with cellular elements are often noted. Bilirubinuria and hemoglobinuria may be observed. Leptospires may be detectable by dark field microscopy. Azotemia may appear as early as three to four days after the onset of the disease. ARF is noted in 67% of cases [33]. Any serotype of leptospires can cause ARF. Jaundice may or may not be present. Although it is often described that ARF occurs in the immunologic phase of the disease, it can in fact occur either in the septicemic phase or immunologic phase. ARF is usually hypercatabolic in type, with rapid rise in blood urea nitrogen, giving the BUN-and-serum-creatinine ratio of more than 10:1. Hyperkalemia, hyperphosphatemia, and hyperuricemia may be present. Severe jaundice is often associated with severe renal function impairment. Nonoliguric ARF is not uncommon. Occasionally, the patient may be severely oliguric or even anuric. Mild intravascular hemolysis and low-grade intravascular coagulation are not infrequent. The serum complement may be decreased during the acute phase along with the rise in plasma fibrinogen and erythrocyte sedimentation rate. The rise of antibody titer may be delayed in severe uremia.

4.1 ANICTERIC RENAL FAILURE

Anicteric renal failure represents a mild form of ARF and may be prerenal due to volume depletion [27]. Blood volume has been found to be diminished prior to fluid administration. There is usually a mild elevation of serum creatinine. The urinary indices are helpful in the diagnosis [34]. The renal failure index (see chapter 7) is below 1 and fractional sodium excretion is less than 1%. Oliguria is often mild and transient and readily resolves following fluid administration.

Acute tubular necrosis also occurs in anicteric leptospirosis. The urinary indices agree with those of acute tubular necrosis due to other causes. Renal failure is usually of mild degree and may resolve without dialysis.

4.2 ICTERIC RENAL FAILURE OR WEIL'S SYNDROME

Weil's syndrome denotes a severe form of leptospirosis with ARF and jaundice or hepatic dysfunction. It may be associated with hemorrhage, vascular collapse, and alteration of consciousness. The syndrome was originally described in icterohemorrhagia infection. It is now not specific, and any serotype in its severe form of infection can cause Weil's syndrome. Jaundice is usually cholestatic in type with high serum alkaline phosphatase and a modest rise in transaminases. In the presence of G-6-PD deficiency, jaundice can be severe due to hemolysis. Renal failure is usually severe. Although it is often nonoliguric, severe oliguria and even anuria may be observed occasionally [35]. Hyperuricemia may be more than 0.70 mmol/l (12 mg/dl). The urine uric acid excretion may be increased, and, interestingly, the urine uric acid and urine creatinine ratio may exceed 1. In the past, Weil's syndrome carried a high mortality rate. However, with the present knowledge on pathophysiology of the disease, the use of dialysis, and exchange blood transfusion, the mortality rate is greatly decreased to almost negligible. The decrease in degree of jaundice is often associated with improvement of renal function.

4.3 HEMOLYTIC UREMIC SYNDROME (HUS)

Rarely is the HUS (see chapter 16) observed. This is characterized by thrombocytopenia, reticulocytosis, bizarre red blood cells, the presence of FDP in the circulation, and ARF. The pathogenesis of the syndrome is not well understood although it is believed to be triggered by intravascular coagulation. Several factors, including immune mechanisms, toxemia, vascular injury, alteration of erythrocyte membrane, and the presence of underlying renal disease, have been implicated in the pathogenesis of the syndrome [36]. The recent hypothesis suggests PGI_2 deficiency [36]. The syndrome has been observed in various infections [37–39]. On the theoretical basis, the observation

of the HUS in leptospirosis is not surprising since there is vascular injury caused by leptospires or toxins. In leptospirosis, the syndrome is less severe, and spontaneous recovery occurs following the conventional treatment. Cortical necrosis has not been observed.

5 Treatment

Renal failure in leptospirosis varies in severity. In the mild form of prerenal failure, good urine flow is restored following fluid administration. The general principle of management of ARF in leptospirosis does not differ from that due to the other causes. However, certain points should be brought to attention. Since renal failure is hypercatabolic, dialysis, when indicated, should be performed frequently. In oliguric renal failure, a high dose of furosemide may be helpful in converting to the nonoliguric phase, which eases in the clinical management. The clinical course of renal failure is, however, unaltered when compared with the control group [40].

In cases with hyperbilirubinemic renal failure (total bilirubin over 428 μmol/l, 25 mg/dl), exchange blood transfusion has been of value in improving the renal function and decreasing the degree of jaundice [25, 35].

On the theoretical ground, heparinization, plasmapheresis, fresh plasma infusion, and PGI_2 infusion could be useful in the management of the HUS. However, the syndrome has a rare incidence, and, in the author's experience with a limited number of cases, only conservative treatment suffices.

Of great importance is the specific treatment of infection. Penicillin, streptomycin, and tetracycline are among the antibiotics known to kill leptospires. Penicillin is preferable since the others are nephrotoxic. Treatment should be instituted during the febrile period or within four to seven days after the onset of the disease when there is septicemia. Parenteral aqueous penicillin G at a dosage of 1,000,000 units at six-hour intervals for a period of one week is recommended in adults. Erythromycin can be used in the patient with penicillin hypersensitivity.

Since ARF is an important cause of death in leptospirosis, dialysis is therefore life saving.

The mortality rate in leptospirosis is greatly reduced to almost negligible by dialysis and our present knowledge in the pathophysiology of the disease.

References

1. Feigin RD, Anderson DC. Human leptospirosis. CRC Crit Rev Clin Lab Sci 5: 413–467, 1975.
2. Sitprija V, Benyajati C. Tropical disease and acute renal failure. Ann Acad Med (Suppl) 4: 112–114, 1975.
3. Sitprija V, Evans H. The kidney in human leptospirosis. Am J Med. 49: 780–788, 1970.
4. Sitprija V, Pipatanagul V, Mertowidjojo K, Boonpucknavig V, Boonpuckhavig S. Pathogenesis of renal disease in leptospirosis. Kidney Int 17: 827–836, 1980
5. Sitprija V. The kidney in acute tropical disease (abstract). Eighth International Congress of Nephrology, Athens, 1981, p. 273.
6. De Brito T, Böhm GM, Yasuda PH. Vascular damage in acute experimental leptospirosis of the guinea pig. J Path 128: 177–182, 1979.
7. Arean VM, Henry JB. Studies on the pathogenesis of leptospirosis. IV. The behavior of transaminases and oxidative enzymes in experimental leptospirosis. A histochemical and biochemical assay. Am J Trop Med Hyg 13: 430–442, 1964.
8. Arean VM, Sarasin G, Green JH. The pathogenesis of leptospirosis: Toxin production by Leptospira icterohemorrhagia. Am J Vet Res 25: 836–843, 1964.
9. Sitprija V. Mechanisms of renal involvement in tropical disease. Proceeding of the 3rd Colloquim in Nephrology, Tokyo, 1979. p. 104.
10. Graeme RB, Majno G. Acute imflammation. A review. Am J Path 86: 185–276, 1977.
11. Srichaikul T, Archararit N, Siriaswakul T, Viriyapanich T. Histamine changes in Plasmodium falciparum infection. Tran Roy Soc Trop Med Hyg 70: 36–38, 1976.
12. Tella A, Maegraith BG. Studies on bradykinin and bradykininogen in malaria. Ann Trop Med Parasitol 60: 304–317, 1966.
13. Stuchly Z, Fal W. The level of kinins in the blood plasma in the course of experimental trichinosis in white rat. Wiad Parazyt 15: 698–699, 1969.
14. Knight LL, Miller NG, White RJ. Cytotoxic factor in the blood and plasma of animals during leptospirosis. Infect Immun 8: 401–405, 1973.
15. Miller NG, Allen JE, Wilson RB. The pathogenesis of hemorrhage in the lung of the hamster during acute leptospirosis. Med Microbiol Immunol 160: 269–278, 1974.
16. Feldberg W, Lewis GP. Action of peptides on adrenal medulla: Release of adrenalin by bradykinin and angiotensin. J Physiol (London) 171: 98–108, 1964.
17. Rosell S. Neuronal control of microvessels. Ann Rev Physiol 42: 359–371, 1980.
18. Sitprija V. Renal failure in obstructive jaundice: A pathophysiologic consideration. J Med Assoc Thai 61 (Suppl 3): 46–49, 1978.
19. Odell GB, Natzschka JC, Storey GNB: Bilirubin nephropathy in the Gunn strain of rat. Am J Physiol 212: 931–938, 1967.
20. Baum BM, Sterling GA, Dawson JL. Further study into obstructive jaundice and ischemic renal damage. Br Med J 2: 229–231, 1969.
21. Aoyagi T, Lowenstein LM. The effect of bile acids and renal ischemia on renal function. J Lab Clin Med 71: 686–692, 1968.
22. Bloom D, McCalden TA, Rosendorff C. Effect of jaundiced plasma on vascular sensitivity to noradrenalin. Kidney Int 8: 149–157, 1975.
23. Melman A, Weinberger MH. Alterations of renin-angiotensin system in bile duct ligated dogs varied sodium diet. Clin Res 24: 407, 1976.
24. Schlosstein L, Kippen I, Bluestone R, Whitehouse MW, Klinenberg JR. Association between hypouricemia and jaundice. Ann Rheum Dis 33: 308–312, 1974.
25. Pochanugool C, Sitprija V. Hyperbilirubinemic renal failure in tropical disease; treatment with exchange transfusion. J Med Assoc Thai 61 (Suppl): 75–77, 1978.
26. Elkon D, Fechner RE, Homzie M, Baker DG, Constable WC. Response of mouse kidney to hyperthermia: Pathology and temperature-dependence of injury. Arch Path Lab Med 104: 153–158, 1980.
27. Sitprija V. Renal involvement in human leptospirosis. Br Med J 2: 656–658, 1968.
28. Morrison WI, Wright NG. Canine leptospirosis: An Immunopathological study of interstitial nephritis due to Leptospira canicola. J Pathol 120: 83–89, 1976.
29. Taylor PL, Hanson LE, Simon J. Serologic, pathologic and immunologic features of experimentally induced leptospiral nephritis in dogs. Am J Vet Res 31: 1033–1049, 1970.
30. Krohn K, Mero M, Oksanen A, Sandholm M. Immunological observations in cainine interstitial nephritis. Am J Pathol 65: 157–172, 1971.
31. Finco DR, Low DG. Endotoxin properties of Leptospira canicola. Am J Vet Res 128: 1863–1872, 1967.
32. Arean VN. The pathologic anatomy and pathogenesis of fatal human leptospirosis (Weil's disease). Am J Pathol 40: 393–423, 1962.
33. Charoonruangrit S, Boonpucknavig S. Leptospirosis at Chulalongkorn Hospital: A report of 54 cases. J Med Assoc Thai 47: 653–659, 1964.
34. Miller TR, Anderson RJ, Linas SL, Henrich WL, Berns AS, Gabow PA, Schrier RW. Urinary diagnostic indices in acute renal failure. Ann Intern Med 89: 47–50, 1978.
35. Sitprija V, Chusilp SK. Renal failure and hyperbilirubinemia in leptospirosis. Treatment with exchange transfusion. Med J Aust 1: 171–172, 1973.

36. Morel-Maroger L. Adult hemolytic-uremic syndrome. Kidney Int 18: 125–134, 1980.
37. Baker NM, Mills AE, Rachman I, Thomas JEP. Hemolytic-uremic syndrome in typhoid fever. Br Med J 2: 84–87, 1974.
38. Ragphupathy P, Date A, Shastry JCM, Sudarsanam A, Jadhav M. Hemolytic-uremic syndrome complicating shigella dysentery in South Indian Children. Br Med J 2: 1518–1521, 1978.
39. Fialam M, Bauer H, Khaleeli M, Giorgio A. Dog bite, bacteroides infection, coagulopathy, renal microangiopathy. Ann Intern Med 87: 248–249, 1977.
40. Borirakchanyavat V, Vongsthongsri M, Sitprija V. Furosemide and acute renal failure. Postgrad Med J 54: 30–32, 1978.

16. HEMOLYTIC UREMIC SYNDROME

Carlos A. Gianantonio

1 Introduction

The hemolytic uremic syndrome (HUS) is a disease entity of unknown cause, characterized by the acute compromise of renal function, red blood cell fragmentation, and injury to the central nervous system. In the average patient, clinical presentation includes acute renal failure (ARF), hemolytic anemia, gastrointestinal bleeding, and compromise of the central nervous system. The association of red cell fragmentation, thrombocytopenia, and evidences of intravascular coagulation is the hallmark of the syndrome.

Although HUS does occur in children and adults (see chapter 14), it predominates in infants, constituting the chief cause of ARF in this age group. The present perspective of HUS must include its late consequences, such as neurologic sequelae, arterial hypertension, and chronic renal failure.

2 History

The first report about the association of hemolytic anemia and bilateral renal cortical necrosis in infants was published by Gasser in 1955 [1]. The second important contribution was that of Brain et al. [2]. They developed the concept of microangiopathic hemolytic anemia and contributed to the understanding of the erythrocyte abnormalities of HUS. Simultaneously, a fast-growing number of publications defined HUS as a clear-cut entity. The clinical and pathologic aspects of the syndrome were described, together with the results of the adequate treatment of these infants [3, 4].

V.E. Andreucci (ed.), ACUTE RENAL FAILURE.
All rights reserved. Copyright © 1984.
Martinus Nijhoff Publishing, Boston/The Hague/
Dordrecht/Lancaster

In more recent years, the participation of intravascular coagulation in pathogenesis of HUS has been established. The importance of early peritoneal dialysis on the immediate prognosis has been recognized, and the late consequences of HUS are now known [5–7]. There has not been much progress in the elucidation of the etiology of the syndrome.

3 Epidemiology

The number of reported cases of HUS has increased steadily in many countries. It is clear, however, that the disease predominates in Argentina [8], where the problem is alarming, South Africa [9], the Netherlands [10], the United States [11], and Australia [12].

During the 1965–1976 period, 1,456 infants with HUS were admitted to pediatric nephrology units in Argentina. They amounted to 65% of the total number of pediatric patients in ARF treated in those centers, and to 92% in the group under than two years of age [8]. An unknown number of patients may have died or recovered, without a correct diagnosis. The increasing incidence of HUS around the world is more likely due to a growing awareness by pediatricians, rather than to a real increment in the attack rate.

In many series, as in ours, the patients are admitted in small "epidemics," although we treat patients rather uniformly throughout the year. There is no special ecologic situation for the families of these infants although, curiously, they belong almost exclusively to the higher socio-economic levels. There are reports on the simultaneous occurrence of HUS in siblings, especially if they are infants or toddlers [13, 14].

HUS is basically a disease of late infancy.

Our patients had a mean age of 12.4 months, with a range of 2 months to 8 years [5]. The incidence is similar in both sexes, and there is no racial predilection. Adults with HUS are a more heterogeneous group. The syndrome is present in women with complications during pregnancy or the puerperium. A similar clinical and pathologic picture has been associated with gram-negative sepsis and the use of oral contraceptives, although many examples of HUS in adults are idiopathic and difficult to discriminate from thrombotic thrombocytopenic purpura [15–19].

4 Etiology

The etiology of HUS is still unknown. The geographical predilection, the occurrence in epidemics (even intrafamilial), and the prodromal symptoms suggest an infectious etiology. Although the search for a specific agent has been generally unrewarding, a number of organisms—such as Coxsackie, Eco, Arena, Influenza, Respiratory syncytial viruses, Shigella, Salmonella, Bacteroides, and Rickettsia—have been implicated in different areas of the world [20–25]. Our previous viral findings have not been confirmed, Evidence of preceding streptococcal infection (either by history or serology) is missing, and the occasional relationship of HUS to vaccinations with live attenuated viruses seems a chance occurrence.

5 Pathogenesis

Although much progress in the elucidation of the pathogenesis of HUS has been made during recent years, the basic mechanism—which must explain not only the renal component of the syndrome but also the widespread vascular compromise, the anemia, and the abnormalities of coagulation—is unknown. An immunological mechanism has been proposed but is not well defined. The histological pattern of the acute lesions in the kidney and other organs do not resemble the immune-mediated patterns of injury. The immunofluorescence studies, done by most authors, reveal only fibrin and platelet material, although C3 and IgM have been demonstrated by others in the glomerular cap-

illaries and small renal vessels [26, 27]. In our experience, the serum levels of C3, C4, and CH50 are normal during the acute phase although they were decreased in other studies [28].

The disturbance of coagulation, combined with microangiopathic hemolytic anemia and thrombosis of small arteries and capillaries, strongly suggests that disseminated or local intravascular coagulation plays a key role in HUS. The coagulation derangements that have been documented vary but depend on the coagulation activity at the time of the study and the nature of the compensating mechanisms that have been brought into play. In the great majority of the patients, we have studied, an initial and single episode of intravascular coagulation was present, and it occurred before admission to hospital. In a few cases, repeated bouts of intravascular coagulation were demonstrated during the acute phase [29].

The microvascular lesions suggest a primary alteration in the vascular endothelia, due to the action of a vasculotropic organism or other agent or mediator, followed by activation of the coagulation mechanism. During recent years, much research has been devoted to vascular endothelium physiology and platelet-vessel interaction. Normally, endothelial cells synthesize prostacyclin, a potent vasodilator and inhibitor of platelet aggregation, whereas platelets produce thromboxane, a vasocontrictor and platelet aggregating agent. Physiologically, there is a balance between the two systems, maintaining normal platelet-endothelium interaction. There is evidence that in HUS and related conditions, the endothelial damage and disruption cause a defect in the synthesis of prostacyclin that leads to adherence of the platelets to the subintima, local platelet clumping, and release of thromboxane, with secondary vasoconstriction and activation of the coagulation pathways [30, 31]. Intravascular deposition of fibrin is the key phenomenon that conditions the ischemic lesions in the kidney and other organs. Bleeding is observed as a consequence of diffuse intravascular coagulation; it is prominent in HUS, especially as a consequence of extensive necrosis of the colonic mucosa.

The altered intima of the small vessels and

the partially occluding thrombi subject the erythrocytes to mechanical stress, followed by rupture, alteration of their morphology, and a marked reduction of their life span. Once circulation stops completely on the infarcted tissues and/or fibrin is lysed, hemolysis stops. On other grounds, fibrinolysis is probably altered in HUS. A circulating factor that inhibits glomerular fibrinolytic activity has been demonstrated in a group of patients, and an inhibitor of platelet aggregation may be absent, not only in the HUS but also in thrombotic thrombocytopenic purpura [32, 33]. Finally, it should be mentioned that endothelial damage (very likely the initial event of HUS) causes local activation of the coagulation mechanism per se and may also locally activate the complement system.

The pathogenesis of the late renal lesions is obscure. The massive renal scarring present in patients who do not recover renal function after the initial phase is the sequel of the multiple infarcts characteristic of the more severe forms of HUS. However, the pathogenesis of the chronic active glomerulopathy that ends in chronic renal failure years after is unclear. Serum complement levels are normal, and immunofluorescent studies did not show a consistent pattern; some gave normal results and others demonstrated mesangial and/or capillary deposits of C3 and immunoglobulins [34]. It is possible that acute fibrin deposition in the glomerular capillaries may be followed, as it is in experimental animals, by proliferative and sclerotic glomerular changes.

6 Clinical Picture

6.1 PRODROMAL PHASE

During this period, the patient is not very ill. The general picture corresponds to a nonspecific infectious disease, with fever, malaise, irritability, vomiting, and moderate diarrhea. Fever runs from 37°5C to 38°5C and is accompanied by pharyngitis and choryza in one-third of patients. However, vomiting is the central problem in this phase: it is profuse, with gastric contents, tinged occasionally with fresh or digested blood. Diarrhea is also a constant finding although it is not severe or prolonged. The

stools are liquid, with abundant mucus and clumps of blood. There is abdominal pain, sometimes intense and intermittent.

The symptoms of the prodromal phase persist for one to seven days and are followed with or without a short interval (one to five days) by the manifestations of the acute stage.

6.2 ACUTE PHASE

The severity of the illness is only discovered during the first few hours of the acute phase. It is abruptly initiated by intense pallor, oliguria, and, in some patients, convulsions. If immediate remedial measures are not implemented, the infant may die without a correct diagnosis.

6.2.1 Hemolytic Anemia The acute anemia is one of the hallmarks of HUS. It is intense from onset, with admission hemoglobin of 1.2 to 7.5 mmol/l ($\bar{x}$ = 4.1 mmol/l) (2 to 12 g/dl; $\bar{x}$ = 6.6 g/dl). Pallor is intense, but there is no jaundice. The anemia per se, or complicated by electrolyte disturbances and hypervolemia, may lead to congestive cardiac failure.

Repeated hemolytic crises are often seen during the first two weeks of the syndrome. However, the intensity of hemolysis does not correlate with the degree of renal and central nervous system involvement. Moreover, in some infants, anemia is the only relevant clinical problem.

6.2.2 Acute Renal Failure (ARF) Although in some infants (the actual proportion is unknown, but may be considerable) the renal injury is minimal—with a transient decrease in urinary volume, abnormal urinary sediment, proteinuria, and slight depression of the glomerular filtration rate—ARF is present in more than 90% of patients referred for admission in our unit. Renal failure is severe, with an average oliguric period of 14 days. In a few infants, oliguria lasts only two or three days while in others it may persist until death (nine weeks in one patient). In one-third of cases (those with grave renal lesions), the oliguric period has a mean duration of 25 days. Anuria of more than four days duration is present in half the patients (mean 10 days, range 4 to 47 days).

The usual metabolic and hemodynamic complications of ARF are frequently observed in these small patients, especially when the diagnosis is delayed. Most of the fatalities are related to these complications, which can be minimized by early diagnosis and comprehensive management. Arterial hypertension is found in one-third of patients. In some, it is related to sodium and fluid overload; in the remainder, hypertension may be severe, with hypertensive encephalopathy, left ventricular failure, and signs of hypertensive vascular damage to the kidneys and other organs.

The diuretic phase is not abrupt, with a stepwise increase in diuresis that requires several days before dialysis may be interrupted.

6.2.3 *Hemorrhagic Diathesis*

Gastrointestinal blood loss is present in every case. Melena of clinical relevance is found in 60% of patients and blood-tinged vomitus in 20%. The association of pallor, abdominal colic, vomiting, and rectal bleeding may suggest intestinal intussusception. It should be kept in mind that this is a rather exceptional complication of the ileal and colonic intramural hemorrhages of HUS. No other obvious sites of bleeding are observed, with the exception of occasional intracranial and retinal haemorrhages. Petechiae are rare, but small dermal hematomas are found in one-third of the patients.

6.2.4 *Neurological Involvement*

All the infants with HUS, with the exception of the mildest cases, manifest signs of central nervous system involvement. In half the patients, the signs are not alarming, consisting of somnolence, irritability, jerkiness, tremor, and ataxia. In other patients, the problems are much more severe and include generalized convulsions, either single or recurrent, prolonged alteration in the level of consciousness, and focal neurological signs. Deep coma that persists days or weeks is also observed and may end in respiratory failure and death. Signs of decerebrate rigidity, muscular hypotonia or hypertonia, transient hemiparesis, nystagmus, pupillary abnormalities, and retinal hemorrhages are found in many of the gravely ill infants.

6.2.5 *Myocardial Failure*

A few patients have signs of myocardial failure, with electrocardiographic evidence of ischemia. There is no clinical evidence of vascular compromise in other organs.

6.3 CHRONIC RENAL DISEASE

Recovery of renal function is attained rapidly after the diuretic phase in most of the patients. However, a normal glomerular filtration rate, and the disappearance of proteinuria and hematuria, usually take more than six months to be complete and stable. A moderate to marked restriction in the capacity to handle the dietary sodium persists for several weeks and may precipitate hypervolemic cardiac failure if a low-sodium diet is not prescribed after the oliguric phase. Asymptomatic hyperkalemia is not uncommon during the first weeks and may require the daily administration of ion-exchange resins in some exceptional cases.

A small group of patients (1 to 5%), with an oligo-anuric period longer than three weeks, never recover adequate renal function and end up in chronic renal failure and death six months to three years after the initial phase. Another distressing group of children have persistent urinary abnormalities, intermittent or permanent arterial hypertension, and slowly deteriorating renal function, leading to terminal uremia five to thirteen years after onset. The overall incidence of chronic renal disease varies from 5 to 40%, depending on the initial severity of the syndrome and the duration of the follow-up period [35].

In our more recent experience, progression to end-stage renal failure during school years and adolescence was observed in about 15% of patients. Severe arterial hypertension poses a critical problem in these children and requires careful management.

7 *Neurological Sequelae*

The great majority of patients recover completely from the neurological manifestations of HUS, in days or weeks. However, signs of permanent neurological impairment are encountered in some patients. The spectrum is wide, ranging from behavioral problems and learning difficulties to severe mental retardation and quadriparesis or hemiparesis. Convulsive episodes, either akinetic, myoclonic, focal, or grand mal, are present in some children, either as an isolated problem or in combination with motor, intellectual, or sensory handicaps. In these cases, electroencephalograms are abnormal, and computerized axial tomography shows single or multiple areas of cerebral atrophy.

8 Laboratory Findings

8.1 ANEMIA

Five to 50% of the erythrocyte population is morphologically abnormal. Those red cells are fragmented, distorted, triangular, helmet-like, burred, or transformed into very small erythrocytes or ghost cells. The number of damaged red cells increases during the hemolytic crisis, but they persist in decreasing proportion for an average of 70 days.

The reticulocyte number is increased (mean 7.8%; range 2.6 to 20%). Serum bilirubin levels are moderately elevated (mean 32 μmol/l, 1.88 mg/dl; range 18 to 60 μmol/l, 1.06 to 3.5 mg/dl) initially and during the recurrent hemolytic crisis. High plasma hemoglobin and depressed haptoglobin levels are indicative of the intravascular nature of hemolysis.

The life span of transfused erythrocytes is markedly shortened during the first two weeks of HUS [36, 37]. Leucocytosis (mean leucocyte count $17 \times 10^9/1$; range $4.6 \times 10^9/1$ to $62 \times 10^9/1$) with an increase in the percentage of neutrophils is found during the same period. Marked erythroblastic and moderate myeloid hyperplasia, together with abundant but immature megakaryocytes, are found in the bone marrow. The Coombs test is negative, and erythrocyte glucose-6-phosphate dehydrogenase and pyruvate kinase and the hemoglobin structure are normal.

8.2 PLATELETS AND COAGULATION FACTORS

Thrombocytopenia is present initially in about 90% of cases, with a mean platelet count of $75 \times 10^9/1$ and a range of $16 \times 10^9/1$ to $175 \times 10^9/1$ [29]. In the remainder, platelet counts are either normal or high, suggesting a

rebound phenomenon after an undetected initial fall. Thrombocytopenia persists for 7 to 15 days and is followed by a stepwise increase in the platelet count, very often to the level of thrombocytosis.

In patients with extremely severe symptoms, the recovery from thrombocytopenia is irregular, transient, or absent until death. Recently, a shortened platelet survival has been documented [38, 39]. Quick's prothrombin time is prolonged in half the cases and is related to decreases in factors II, VII, VIII, IX, and X. In most patients, partial thromboplastin time-kaolin is shorter than normal during the first three weeks. These infants have simultaneously elevated levels of factor VIII, and to a lesser extent of factors IX and XI. Plasma fibrinogen concentrations are elevated in half the patients and normal or low in the remainder. Serum fibrin degradation products (FDP) may be demonstrated in one-third the cases.

When the cases are studied very early—during the first hours of the acute phase—thrombocytopenia, low fibrinogen, depressed levels of factor VIII, IX, and XI, and serum FDP are consistently found. Secondary falls in fibrinogen and factors VIII, IX, and XI are observed in the few patients with relapsing thrombocytopenia and clinical deterioration during the acute phase of HUS. There is an initial and single episode of intravascular coagulation in most infants; since most are studied hours or days after onset, rebound of the coagulation mechanism is the usual finding.

8.3 RENAL ABNORMALITIES

Although renal compromise may be minimal in a group of patients with predominant anemia, metabolic acidosis, hyperkalemia, and high levels of blood urea (mean: 54.28 mmol/l; 326 mg/dl; range: 7.66 to 115.88 mmol/l; 46 to 696 mg/dl) are present from onset in all infants admitted to pediatric renal units. Increment in the blood urea concentration is very rapid (7.66 mmol/l/day, 46 mg/dl/day, in our series) during the first week of oliguria in nondialyzed patients.

Hematuria, either gross or microscopic, is found in every case, together with hyaline, granular and epithelial casts, and proteinuria (2

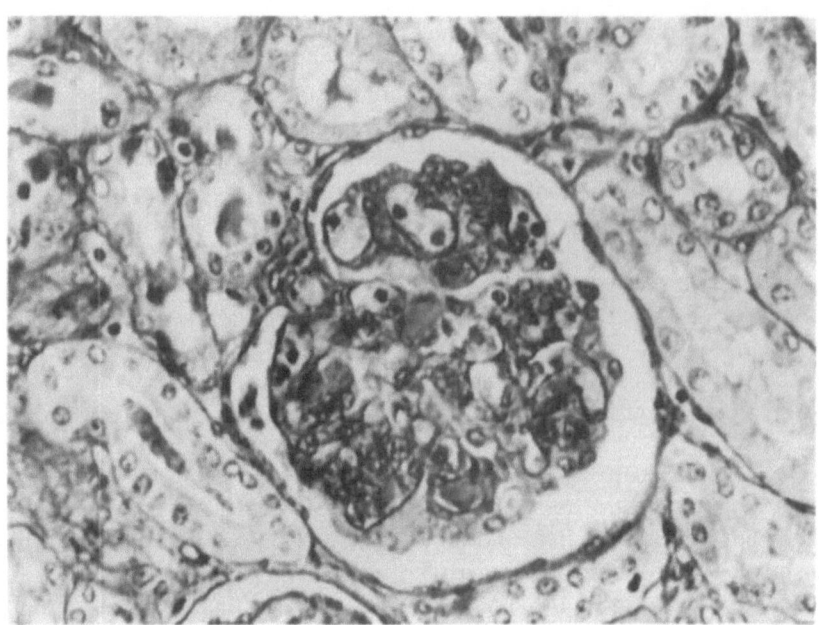

FIGURE 16–1. HUS (Acute): Six days from onset. Glomerulus with several fibrin thrombi. Swelling of endothelial cells and mesangium. Subendothelial clear spaces. (PAS Courtesy Dr. G.E. Gallo, pathologist-Children's Hospital and Italian Hospital, Bs. Aires, Argentina.)

to 12 gr/l). Hemoglobinuria is present in the patients with severe hemolysis.

Serum complement factors (C1q, C4, C3) were consistently normal in our patients although they were low in the infants studied by other groups. The possibility of activation of complement by the alternative pathway has also been described [28, 40].

In the patients with a good late prognosis, the urinary sediment becomes normal in six months and proteinuria subsides in less than one year. Glomerular filtration rates reach normal values about the same time.

The group of patients with massive parenchymal necrosis and renal scarring show critically low glomerular filtration rates immediately after the diuretic phase and run a downhill course over the following months.

The third group of patients with persistent urinary abnormalities and arterial hypertension have proteinuria and slowly declining glomerular filtration rates.

9 Pathological Features

9.1 ACUTE PHASE

9.1.1 The Kidney Pathological findings differ according to timing of specimens [41, 42].

When the autopsy is performed in the first two weeks after onset, the most severe lesion is bilateral renal cortical necrosis, either complete or focal. Frequently, the renal cortex shows multiple pinpoint hemorrhages, together with extensive vascular congestion and edema. In more than half the cases, there are foci of hemorrhagic necrosis in the outer medulla, where they appear as triangles, with the base in the corticomedullar region and the apex toward the papilla.

Microscopically, the lesions affect the glomeruli, convoluted tubules, arteries, collecting tubules, and the interstitium. The basement membrane of the glomerular capillaries is normal, but a clear space is present between the membrane and the endothelium. The endothelial cells are swollen, narrowing the capillary lumen. Capillary thrombi are constant, affecting more than 80% of the glomeruli in severe cases (figure 16–1). Initially, they are lax and consist of fibrin and platelets; later on, they become more dense and intensely eosinophilic, PAS-positive, and bright red with Masson's

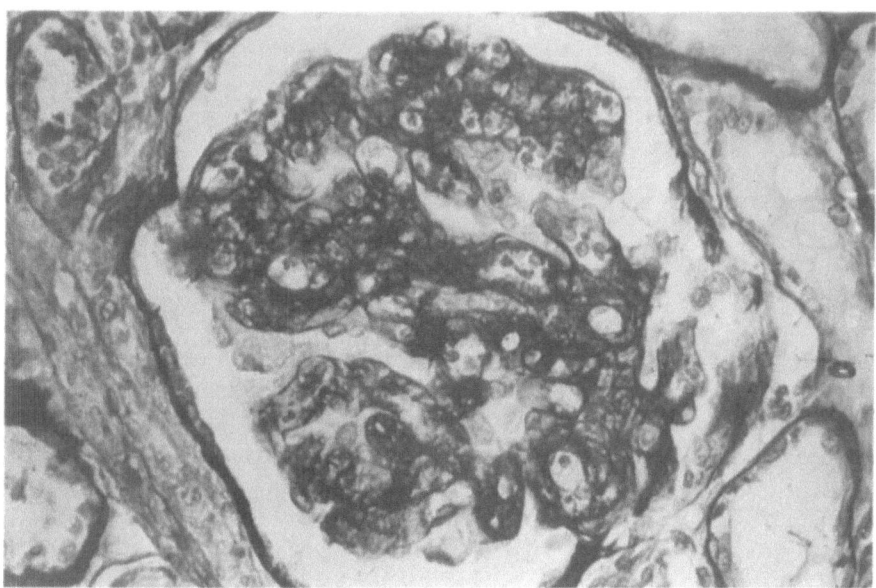

FIGURE 16–2. HUS (Acute): 14 days from onset. Glomerulus with increase in the mesangial matrix and "reduplications" ("double contours") in the peripheral capillary walls. (PAS. Silver methenamine. Courtesy Dr. G.E. Gallo).

stain. The initial mesangial abnormalities are mild, consisting of swelling and scattered clear deposits. During the second week, an increase in the mesangial matrix is observed, together with slight hypercellularity. Visceral epithelial cells are swollen, with hyaline droplets, but some are necrotic and detached from the basement membrane. Epithelial crescents are uncommon.

Many afferent arterioles have luminal thrombi, with subendothelial fibrin deposits and endothelial swelling. In one-third of the cases, the interlobular arteries are thrombosed or show patches of fibrinoid necrosis, with ischemic necrosis of the renal tissue. The confluence of such infarcts is the cause of bilateral renal cortical necrosis. The convoluted tubules show hyaline droplets. It is common to observe small foci of necrotic tubules and many granular casts in the collecting ducts.

When renal cortical necrosis is present, there is initially nuclear pyknosis, followed by disappearance of the nuclear structures and persistence of "ghost" cellular structures. A chronic inflammatory reaction with eventual fibrosis and calcification develops at the periphery of the infarcted areas. The irregular distribution of ischemic areas poses a severe limitation on the prognostic value of the percutaneous kidney biopsies obtained during the acute phase of HUS.

When the kidneys are examined after the second week, there are no thrombi in the glomerular capillaries, with the uncommon exception of cases with secondary bouts of intravascular coagulation. There is a marked increased in the mesangial matrix, with mesangial interposition inside the capillary walls, which gives images of "reduplication" or "double contour" (figure 16–2). The clear subendothelial space becomes more prominent while glomerular scarring and foci of tubular atrophy begin to appear. On the other hand, the mild cases of HUS may show normal kidneys when biopsed weeks after onset.

Immunofluorescence studies performed in our laboratory and elsewhere have shown fibrin/fibrinogen deposits in the glomeruli (capillary walls, mesangium, and capillary thrombi) and in the arterial walls. Deposits of IgM and C3 may be observed. They are always focal and light, without a consistent pattern.

The electron microscopy studies confirm the findings of optical microscopy. The glomerular basement membrane shows a normal structure,

334

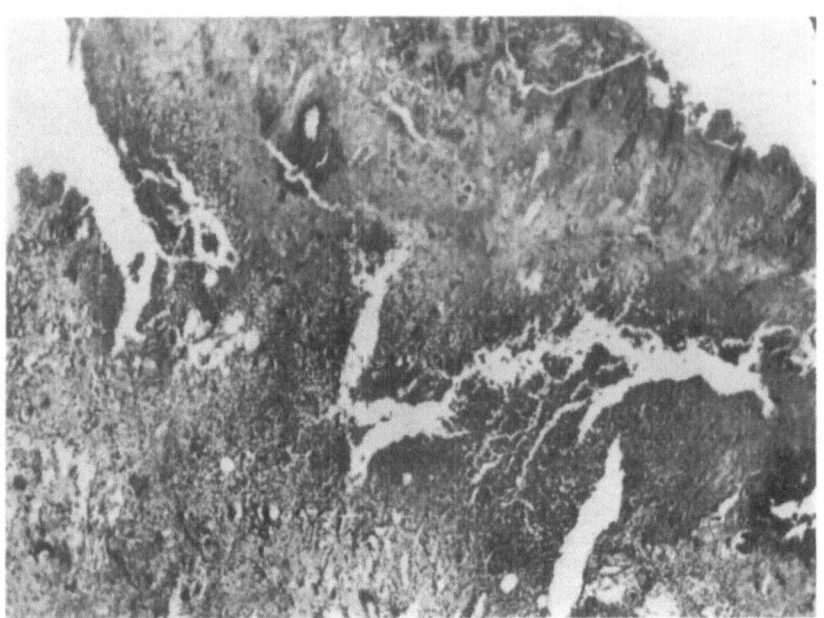

FIGURE 16–3. HUS (Acute): Seven days from onset. Colon, with hemorrhage and necrosis of the mucosa and submucosa; fibrin thrombi in the small vessels. (Autopsy; Phosphotungstic acid-hematoxilin. Courtesy Dr. G.E. Gallo).

with no electron-dense deposits. The clear space between the basement membrane and the endothelium is filled with cotton-like deposits, lipid droplets, platelets, red cell fragments, fibrin strands, and extensions of the mesangial cytoplasm and mesangial matrix. The epithelial cells present scattered fusion of the foot processes.

9.1.2 The Gastrointestinal Tract In one-third of the autopsies, thrombotic occlusion of small arteries and capillaries in the colonic wall is accompanied by areas of hemorrhagic necrosis of variable extension (figure 16–3). These lesions predominate in the ascending colon and are also occasionally present in the stomach, esophagus, and the small bowel. Several patients developed intestinal intussusception and a few, extensive colonic necrosis with perforation.

9.1.3 The Heart One-fourth of the autopsied patients show fibrin thrombi in the myocardial arterioles and capillaries, associated with small foci of ischemic necrosis. These lesions may be extensive enough to be the cause of death of some infants. Similar abnormalities are found in the pancreas, adrenals, lungs, and exceptionally in other organs [43, 44].

9.1.4 The Brain Two-thirds of the autopsied patients show punctate cerebral hemorrhages or small but multiple foci of necrosis. Fibrin thrombosis of small vessels predominates in the choroid plexuses. An occasional patient may show extradural or subdural hematoma.

In summary, nearly all the patients who died during the first week of HUS presented extrarenal vascular lesions. They disminished rapidly thereafter unless (and exceptionally) the initial course was followed by repeated bouts of intravascular coagulation. Pathologically, HUS is not merely a renal disease but a widespread and generalized injury to the microvascular structures of the body.

9.2 LATE PHASE
Kidney biopsies are normal for an average of two years after the acute stage in patients who have stable and normal renal function, blood pressure, and urinary sediment.

Infants with prolonged acute renal failure who never recover normal renal function and

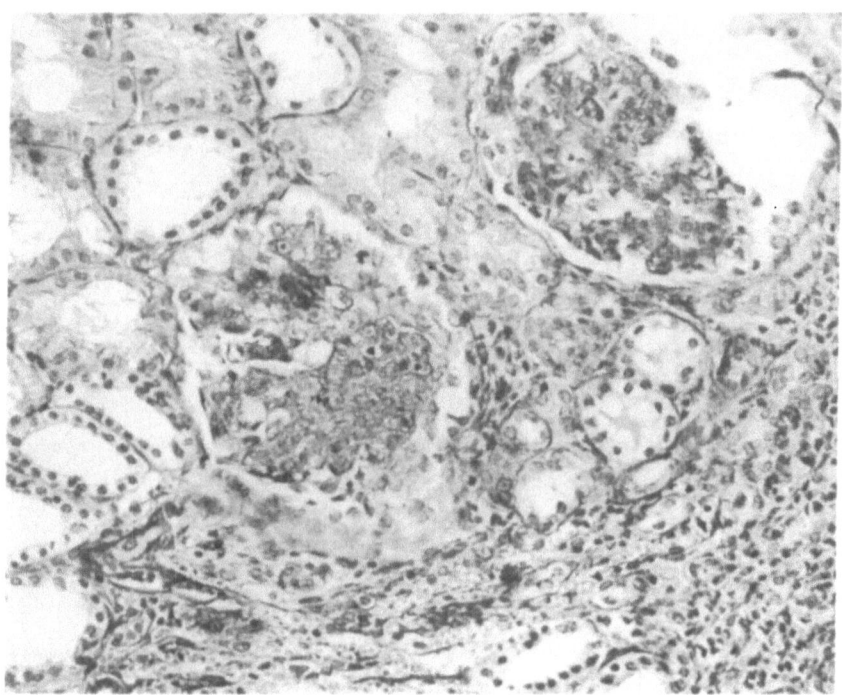

FIGURE 16–4. HUS (Late): Three years after onset. Diffuse proliferative mesangial glomerulonephritis. (PAS. Courtesy Dr. G.E. Gallo).

have persistent proteinuria, hematuria, and arterial hypertension develop end-stage kidneys. In many of them, multiple infarcts and calcium deposition permit a correlation with the histologic findings of the initial stage.

In the patients with evidence of chronic and progressive glomerulopathy, the most frequent histological findings are diffuse mesangial proliferation (figure 16–4) and/or focal and segmental glomerular sclerosis (figure 16–5). Repeated biopsies of these cases show progression to end-stage kidneys.

10 Diagnosis

Diagnosis of HUS during infancy and childhood depends on the pediatrician's awareness of this entity. In the average case, the syndrome is so dramatic and clear-cut that the diagnosis is easily made. Although the diagnosis may be suspected when a well baby, 6 to 14 months old, becomes ill with blood-streaked diarrhea

and persistent vomiting, the confirmation comes when, suddenly, an intense pallor or a generalized convulsion initiates the acute phase of the syndrome. An increase in body weight, related to unrecognized oliguria, is often observed. At this time, proteinuria and abnormal urinary sediment, a markedly elevated BUN, and a typical blood smear confirm the diagnosis.

The differential diagnosis includes acute tubular necrosis, either toxic or ischemic, renal vein thrombosis, acute glomarulonephritis, Schonlein-Henoch nephritis, lupus nephritis, and thrombotic thrombocytopenic purpura.

Difficult diagnostic problems are presented by patients in whom one symptom predominates, such as extreme anemia, grave neurological disturbance, or profuse rectal bleeding. Anemia may be erroneously ascribed to blood loss or to other causes of hemolysis, such as erythrocyte enzymatic defects, abnormal hemoglobins, congenital microspherocytosis, immunohemolytic anemias, poisoning, bacterial sepsis, or malignancy. Erythrocyte fragmentation may also be present in thrombotic thrombocytopenic purpura, cavernous hemangioma,

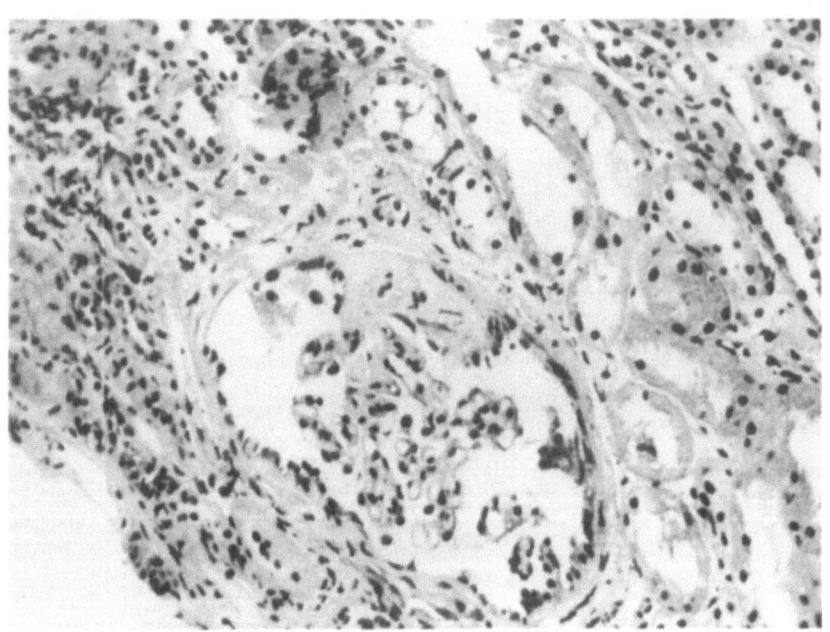

FIGURE 16–5. HUS (Late): Five years from onset. Glomerulus with focal and segmental sclerosis and hyalinosis. (Masson's Trichrome. Courtesy Dr. G.E. Gallo).

metastatic tumor, gram-negative sepsis, congenital heart disease, and surgical repair of heart defects. Neurological symptoms may be taken as evidence of viral or bacterial infection of the central nervous system, acute metabolic brain dysfunction, poisoning, or trauma.

11   Treatment

Treatment of HUS, although very effective, is symptomatic. Of prime importance is the early introduction of peritoneal dialysis in the management of acute renal failure. In our initial experience (1957), conservative treatment and late dialysis brought a mortality of 50%. Our present mortality of 3.5% is related to a correct indication of peritoneal dialysis and to a much greater experience in the management of the many problems intrinsic to the syndrome and its complications. Hyperkalemia, hypervolemia, and metabolic acidosis can be effectively treated or prevented by peritoneal dialysis and careful conservative measures.

It is essential to prevent hospital-acquired infections and to promote a loving atmosphere in the management of these infants during the difficult weeks of the acute phase. Parents are routinely included in the process of care of their children. Anemia often requires repeated transfusions of packed red blood cells. Neurological manifestations of the syndrome, such as status epilepticus, deep coma, and respiratory depression, require the usual treatment for these states, together with peritoneal dialysis.

There is ample literature on anticoagulation with heparin, with poor or no results in the majority of recent studies [45–47]. In a controlled study, in which supportive measures were compared with similar management plus heparin, no advantage of anticoagulant therapy was observed [45]. Most of the reports are difficult to evaluate because of the different standards of care (especially peritoneal dialysis) and the inclusion of patients with unequal severity of the disease. In the vast majority of the patients with a single initial episode of intravascular coagulation, the administration of heparin was of necessity begun too late to be effective. The value of heparin treatment in the prevention of late renal complications of HUS is unknown.

Removal of deposited fibrin is theoretically a

TABLE 16–1. Clinical grading of severity

Condition	Mild	Moderate	Severe
Oliguria (days)	<7	7–14	>14
Anuria (days)	—	<7	>7
CNS symptoms	0 to +	0 to + + +	+ + to + + +
Arterial hypertension	0 to +	0 to + +	+ to + + +
G.I. bleeding	0 to +	0 to + +	+ + to + + +
Anemia	+ to + + +	0 to + + +	0 to + + +
Mortality (%)	1	2	25
Chronic renal disease* (%)	2	15	60

*Estimated rates.

more rational approach than anticoagulation. Although there are several reports on fibrinolytic treatment of the syndrome employing streptokinase, the effectiveness, as well as the limitations and dangers of such therapy, are not well established [48]. In one study, however, there was the suggestion that streptokinase therapy had a beneficial effect on the subsequent incidence of proteinuria and hypertension [10].

Aspirin and dipyrridamole have been employed in small groups of patients. The results of the studies were not conclusive, even when these drugs were associated with fibrinolysis. It has been suggested that prolonged anticoagulation and antiplatelet drugs may be beneficial in adults [49].

There are recent reports on the good results of plasmapheresis and exchange transfusions in patients with thrombotic thrombocytopenic purpura [50]. Remuzzi et al. [51] treated two adult patients with HUS with plasma exchange and dialysis; there was improvement in platelet count and recovery of antiplatelet aggregating activity, although no apparent effect on renal function could be demonstrated.

In summary, there is no doubt that the early and aggressive management of ARF by dialysis is the basis of the present treatment of HUS. Whether other types of therapy may result in an improved long-term prognosis has not yet been demonstrated.

There are no reports on the medical treatment of the chronic glomerular disease although several children have been transplanted with good initial results.

12 Prognosis

Although there are no easy ways to establish an accurate prognosis during the first one or two days of HUS, there is no doubt that anuria and severe central nervous system symptoms imply a more guarded prognosis. On the other hand, the preeminence of anemia and lack of oliguria are usually associated with rapid and complete recovery. In any case, the retrospective grading of severity is of great help to anticipate the long-term prognosis (table 16–1). Mortality approaches zero in infants with mild disease while it rises to 25% in those with more than 25 days of oliguria. Anuria of more than four days' duration is also a sign of bad prognosis since it often coincides with rather extensive cortical necrosis. Some of these patients, with prolonged coma and convulsions, have little chance of survival. Apparently, the syndrome is more severe in toddlers and school-aged children than in infants and has a significant mortality in the adult.

Factors of prime importance are the quality of care and the experience of the professional team in the management of ARF in infancy.

Chronic renal insufficiency can be expected immediately to follow the initial phase in 1 to 5% of patients. They all belong to the severe group and present massive renal scarring. Late renal failure, with terminal uremia during childhood or early adolescence developed in about 15% of the patients. Within this group, the severity of HUS varied from mild to severe.

The present challenge is the prevention of these late sequelae, either through new approaches in the management of the acute phase, or in the treatment of the chronic glomerular disease.

References

1. Gasser, C von, Gautier E, Steck A, Sieberman RE, Oeschlin R. Hämolytisch-uramische syndrome. Bilaterale nierenrindennekrossen bei akuten erworbenen hämolytischen anamien. Schweiz Med Wochenschr 85: 905–909, 1955.
2. Brain MC, Dacie JV, Hourinane D O'B. Microangiopathic hemolitic anemia: The possible role of vascular lesions in pathogenesis. Brit J Haematol 8: 358–371, 1962.
3. Gianantonio CA, Vitacco M, Mendilaharzu F, Rutty AH, Mendilaharzu J. The hemolytic-uremic syndrome. J Pediatr 64: 478–491, 1964.
4. Lieberman E, Heuser E, Donnell GN, Landing BH, Hammond GD. Hemolytic-uremic syndrome. N Engl J Med 275: 227–236, 1966.
5. Gianantonio CA, Vitacco M, Mendilaharzu F, Gallo GE, Sojo ET. The hemolytic-uremic syndrome. Nephron 11: 174–192, 1973.
6. Piel C. Hemolytic-uremic syndrome. Pediat Clin North Am 13: 295–314, 1966.
7. Habib R, Mathieu H, Royer P. Le syndrome hémolitique et urémique de l'enfant. Nephron 4: 139–172, 1967.
8. Gianantonio CA. Epidemiology and prevention of kidney disease (South America). Abstracts, 1977 Meeting International Pediatric Nephrology Association, Helsinski Finland.
9. Kaplan BS, Thompson PD, de Chadarevian JP. The hemolytic-uremic syndrome. Pediat Clin North Am 23: 761–775, 1976.
10. Monnens L, Van Collenburg J, De Jong M. Treatment of the Hemolytic-uremic syndrome. Helv Pediat Acta 33: 321–328, 1978.
11. Lieberman E. Hemolytic-uremic syndrome. J Pediat 80: 1–11, 1972.
12. Robertson SEJ. Hemolytic anemia associated with acute glomerulonephritis in infancy. Med J Aust 2: 686–693, 1957.
13. Kaplan BS, Chesney RW, Drummond KN. Hemolytic uremic syndrome in families. N Engl J Med 292: 1090–1093, 1975.
14. Tune BM, Groshong T, Plumer IB. The hemolytic-uremic syndrome in siblings: A prospective survey. J Pediat 85: 682–683, 1974.
15. Alfrey AC. The renal response to vascular injury. In The kidney, Brenner BM, Rector FC Jr (eds). Philadelphia: WB Saunders, 1976, pp. 1145–1192.
16. Clarkson AR, Lawrence JR, Meadows R, Seyour AE. The hemolytic-uremic syndrome in adults. Quart J Med 39: 227–244, 1970.
17. Finkelstein FD, Kashgarian M, Hayslett JP. Clinical spectrum of postpartum renal failure. Am J Med 57: 649–654, 1974.
18. Brown CG, Clarkson AP, Robson JS, Cameron JS, Thompson D, Ogg CS. Hemolitic-uremic syndrome in women taking oral contraceptives. Lancet 1: 1479–1489, 1973.
19. Ponticelli C, Maestri O, Imbasciati E, Brancaccio D, Rossi E. Late recovery of renal function in a woman with the hemolytic-uremic syndrome. Clin Nephrol 8: 367–373, 1977.
20. Austin TW, Ray CG. Coxsackie virus group B infection and the hemolytic-uremic syndrome. J Infect Dis 127: 698–701, 1973.
21. Ray CG, Tucker VL, Harris DJ. Enteroviruses associated with the hemolytic uremic syndrome. Pediatrics 46: 378–388, 1970.
22. Chan JCM, Eleff MG, Campbell RA. The hemolytic uremic syndrome in nonrelated adopted siblings. J Pediat 75: 1050–1053, 1969.
23. Koster F, Levin J, Walker L, Taung KSK, Gilman RH, Rahaman MM, Majid MA, Islam SI, Williams RS. Hemolytic-uremic syndrome after Shigellosis. Relation to endotoxemia and circulating immune complexes. N Engl J Med 298: 927–933, 1978.
24. Fiala M, Bauer H. Dog bite, bacteroides infection, coagulopathy, renal microangiopathy. Ann In Med 87: 248–249, 1977.
25. Mettler N, Gianantonio CA. Aislamiento del agente causal del sindrome urémico-hemolítico. Medicina 23: 139–144, 1963.
26. Miller K, Dresner IG, Michael AF. Localization of platelet antigens in human kidney disease. Kidney Int 18: 472–479, 1980.
27. Gervais M, Richardson JB, Chiu J. Inmunoflourescent and histologic findings in the hemolytic-uremic syndrome. Pediatrics 47: 352–359, 1971.
28. Kim Y, Miller K, Michael AF. Breakdown products of C_3 and factor B in hemolytic-uremic syndrome. J Lab Clin Med 89: 845–850, 1977.
29. Avalos JS, Vitacco M, Molinas F, Penalver J, Gianantonio I. Goagulation studies in the hemolytic-uremic syndrome. J Pediatr 75: 538–548, 1970.
30. Remuzzi G, Misiani R, Marchesi D, Livio M, Mecca G, deGaetano G, Donti MB. Hemolytic-uremic syndrome: Deficiency of plasma factor(s) regulating prostacyclin activity. Lancet 2: 871–872, 1978.
31. Moncada S, Vane JR. Archidonic acid metabolities and the interaction between platelets and blood vessel walls. N Engl J Med 300: 1142–1147, 1979.
32. Berstein JM. Circulating inhibitor of glomerular fibrinolytic activity in human renal disease. 12th Ann meeting ASN, November 1979.
33. Lyan ECY, Harkness DR. The presence of a platelet aggregating factor in the plasma of patients with TTP and its inhibition by normal plasma. Blood 53: 333–338, 1979.
34. Cossio PM, Laguens RP, Pantin DJ. Persisting glomerulonephritis following the hemolytic uremic syndrome. Immunologic and morphologic studies. Clin Exper Immunol 29: 361–368, 1977.
35. Gianantonio CA, Vitacco M, Mendilaharzu F, Gallo GE. The hemolytic uremic syndrome—Renal status

of 76 patients at long-term follow up. J Pediat 72: 757–765, 1968.

36. Katz J, Krawitz S, Sacks P, Levin SE. Platelet, erythrocyte and fibrinogen kinetics in the hemolytic uremic syndrome of infancy. J Pediat 83: 739–745, 1973.

37. Metz J. Observations on the mechanisms of the hematologic changes in the hemolytic remic syndrome of infancy. Brit J Haematol (Suppl) 23: 53–59, 1972.

38. George CRP, Slighter SJ, Quadracci LJ, Striker GE, Harker LA. A kinetic evaluation of hemostasis in renal disease. N Engl J Med 291: 1111–1115, 1974.

39. Montgomery RR, Hathaway WE. The Hemolytic Uremic Syndrome in Kidney Disease; Hematological and Vascular Problems. New York: Wiley Medical, 1977, pp. 89–105.

40. Stuhlinger W, Kourilsky O, Kanfer A, Sraer JD. Hemolytic uremic syndrome: Evidence for intravascular C_3 activation. Lancet 11: 788–790, 1974.

41. Churg J, Spargo BH, Mostophi FK, Abell MR. The hemolytic uremic syndrome. In Kidney Disease: Present Status. Baltimore: Williams & Wilkins, 1979, pp. 142–157.

42. Levy M, Gagnadoux MF, Habib R. Pathology of the hemolytic-uremic syndrome in children. In Hemostasis, Prostaglandins and Renal Disease, Remuzzi G, Mecca G, de Gaetano G (eds). New York: Raven Press, 1980, pp. 383–397.

43. Gallo GE, Mendilaharzu F, Delgado N, Sojo ET. Extrarenal lesions in the hemolytic uremic syndrome. Abstract 18th meeting Lat Am Soc Ped Res, Sao Paulo, Brazil, 1980.

44. Upadhyaya K, Barwick K, Fishaut M. The importance of nonrenal involvement in hemolytic uremic syndrome. Pediatrics 65: 115–120, 1980.

45. Vitacco M, Sanchez Avalos J, Gianantonio CA. Heparin therapy in the hemolytic uremic syndrome. J Pediat 83: 271–275, 1973.

46. Kaplan BS, Katz J, Krawitz S, Lurie A. An analysis of the results of therapy of 67 cases of the hemolytic-uremic syndrome. J Pediat 78: 420–425, 1971.

47. Proesman W, Eeckels R. Has heparin changed the prognosis of the hemolytic uremic syndrome? Clin Nephrol 2: 169–173, 1974.

48. Stuart J, Winterborn MH, White RHR, Flinn RM. Thrombolytic therapy in hemolytic uremic syndrome. Brit Med J 3: 217–221, 1974.

49. Ponticelli C, Rivolta E, Imbasciati E, Rossi E, Mannucci PM. Hemolytic uremic syndrome in adults. Arch Int Med 140: 353–357, 1980.

50. Byrnes JJ, Lyan ECY. Recent therapeutic advances in thrombotic thrombocytopenic purpura. Sem Thromb Hemost 5: 199–215, 1979.

51. Remuzzi G, Misiani R, Marchesi D, Livio M, Mecca G, de Gaetano G, Donati MB. Treatment of the hemolytic uremic syndrome with plasma. Clin Nephrol 12: 279–284, 1979.

17. ACUTE RENAL FAILURE IN PREGNANCY

Dieter Kleinknecht,

Gérard Bochereau,

Paul Chauveau

During the past 20 years, a changing pattern has been observed in acute renal failure (ARF) complicating pregnancy. During the decade 1960–1970, most cases were due to septic abortion, and a great majority of patients had a potentially recoverable lesion. During the following decade, the incidence of septic abortion progressively declined in industrialized countries, due to more liberal abortion laws and the availability of contraceptives. In parallel, there was also a reduction in pre- and postpartum accidents occurring in late pregnancy, due to earlier detection and better management of obstetric complications [1]. Consequently, the total percentage of obstetrical patients with ARF fell from 40% in 1965 to 4% in 1980 [1–4] (table 17–1). According to Lindheimer and Katz [5], ARF occurs in one of every 2,000 to 5,000 pregnancies; but several years ago, the Department of Obstetrics at the Foch Hospital in Suresnes, France, recorded no cases of ARF among 12,000 delivered women, 2,041 of whom followed high-risk pregnancies [1]. As stated by Chapman and Legrain [1], obstetrics is probably the field in which the most striking progress has been made in ARF.

Paradoxically, the mortality of ARF due to pregnancy is now higher although remaining lower than that observed in nonobstetric cases of ARF (table 17–1). This may reflect an increased severity of the diseases affecting these young women [6].

ARF during pregnancy occurs generally either in the first trimester as a complication of septic abortion or later at 30 to 40 weeks as a complication of abruptio placentae or uterine hemorrhage, carrying a high risk of renal cortical necrosis [7]. In addition, ARF may occur after delivery and is often termed then "idiopathic postpartum ARF" [8–10]. These cases fit into the more serious prognostic categories, including thrombotic microangiopathy and cortical necrosis.

The main causes and renal pathology of ARF in pregnancy are listed in table 17–2 and will be successively considered. Recent and comprehensive reviews can be consulted for further details [5, 11, 12].

1 Sodium and Water Loss

Hyperemesis gravidarum and late vomiting of pregnancy may induce ARF due to hypovolemia and hypotension [13, 14]. Acute tubular nephropathy may develop when urinary tract infection is present or when early correction of water and electrolyte losses is not achieved.

2 Infection

2.1 SEPTIC ABORTION
Ten years ago, septic abortion was the main cause of obstetric cases of ARF and of septi-

TABLE 17–1. The changing incidence of acute renal failure (ARF) in pregnancy during the past 15 years in France

	Kleinknecht and Ganeval, 1973 [2]	Chapman, 1978 [3]	Kleinknecht, 1982 [4]
Period	1966–1972	1974–1977	1977–1980
Total patients with ARF	760	2102[b]	263
Obstetrical patients with ARF	184 (24,2%)	95 (4,6%)	8 (3%)
Septic abortion	141 (18,5%)	51 (2,4%)	4 (1,5%)
Pre- and postpartum[a]	43 (5,7%)	44 (2,2%)	4 (1,5%)
Mortality			
Total patients	274 (36,1%)	1251 (59,5%)	147 (55,9%)
Obstetrical patients	20 (10,9%)	22 (23,1%)	2 (25,0%)

[a]Septic abortion excluded.
[b]Oliguric patients only.

cemia during pregnancy, but such cases now tend to disappear in Western countries. We observed only four cases of ARF related to septic abortion during the past four years [4]. Kincaid-Smith and Fairley [15] did not see a single case in their department in the 10-year period 1970–1979. In other countries, however, many cases of ARF due to septic abortion have continued to present during the past decade [16, 17], mainly in communities with poor economic conditions.

Presenting features are often severe infection and hemolysis with hemoglobinemia, uterine bleeding, shock, and intravascular coagulation. The bacteria responsible (usually clostridium welchii) may be found in blood and uterine discharge cultures. Emergency treatment includes antibiotics, intensive control of shock, and di-

TABLE 17–2. Causes and renal pathology of acute renal failure (ARF) in pregnancy

Causes of ARF	Possible renal pathology
Sodium and water loss	(Prerenal failure)
Infection	
Septic abortion	Tubular necrosis, cortical necrosis
Acute pyelonephritis	Acute interstitial nephritis
Diseases not specifically related to pregnancy	
Acute glomerulonephritis	Proliferative glomerulonephritis
Drug nephrotoxicity	Tubular necrosis
Mismatched blood transfusion	Tubular necrosis
Bacterial endocarditis	Focal or diffuse glomerulonephritis
Obstructive uropathy	
Toxemia of pregnancy	
Eclampsia	Glomerular endotheliosis, Tubular necrosis, Cortical necrosis
Abruptio placentae	
Intrauterine fetal death	Cortical necrosis
Amniotic fluid embolism	Tubular necrosis
Uterine hemorrhage	
Postpartum ARF	Malignant nephrosclerosis
(Hemolytic-uremic syndrome)	Thrombotic microangiopathy
	Cortical necrosis
Acute fatty liver	Focal tubular necrosis
	Glomerular fibrin deposits

alysis when required. Conservative measures with a minimum surgical intervention are now recommended [18]. Hysterectomy is occasionally indicated when uterine perforation is present.

The oliguric phase may last from a few days to several weeks. Nonoliguric forms of ARF are less frequent. In most patients, the underlying renal pathology is tubular necrosis. A great majority of patients surviving the acute phase will recover fully, and most will have normal renal histology on long-term follow-up biopsy [1, 19]. In the experience of one of us [7], renal cortical necrosis was not more frequent in these patients (1.5%) than in those with ARF of nonobstetric origin. These results differed from those of Chugh et al. [17], who found up to 18.6% of cortical necrosis after abortion. This proportion of cortical necrosis and the high mortality observed seemed due to late referral, high incidence of infection, and prolonged hypotension.

2.2 ACUTE PYELONEPHRITIS

Acute pyelonephritis occurs in 1 to 2% of all gravidas and is probably the most common infectious complication of pregnancy [5, 11]. Unilateral or bilateral pyelonephritis of ascending origin is favored in pregnant women by ureteral dilatation and by a considerable increase of the ureteral deadspace. Transient but marked decrements in GFR are commonly observed [20]. Severe uremia due to bilateral renal parenchymal involvement is rare [12]; in these cases, pathological examination shows edematous kidneys with some polymorph infiltration and sometimes cortical abscesses; tubules may be filled with polymorphs, and glomeruli may show inflammatory changes even with cellular proliferation [21]. Prompt antibiotic treatment is required since renal scarring is one of the possible sequelae. In other patients, pregnancy may reveal an asymptomatic congenital hydronephrotic kidney that has become infected.

It has been stated that pyelonephritis may lead to maternal death or to fetal growth retardation and prematurity. Fortunately, under adequate surveillance and treatment, the great majority of women will deliver living babies and will have a further benign course [21].

Asymptomatic infections may be largely prevented by treatment of bacteriuric pregnant women. Bladder catheterization during labor should also be avoided whenever possible [20].

3 Diseases Not Specifically Related to Pregnancy

3.1 ACUTE GLOMERULONEPHRITIS

Acute glomerulonephritis is a very rare complication of pregnancy. Its calculated incidence is approximately one in 40,000 pregnancies [22]. When it occurs, recovery of renal function is complete and the gestation is usually successful, provided blood pressure and fluid balance are controlled [11, 20]. No evidence of renal disease is seen in the babies. If superimposed eclampsia is present, delivery of the fetus may be indicated when blood pressure remains high and renal function declines [11]. Acute glomerulonephritis may be differentiated from preeclampsia by the presence of microscopic hematuria with red blood cell casts and low serum complement. A renal biopsy would be useful but is exceptionally indicated in this setting.

A previous history of acute glomerulonephritis is not a contraindication for pregnancy [11, 20]. However, patients with such a history should be followed closely during pregnancy, even in cases where no evidence of activity of the disease is registered.

3.2 OTHER DISEASES

ARF may be occasionally related to coincidental factors, such as drug nephrotoxicity, blood transfusion, and bacterial endocarditis. A good maternal prognosis is usual in these cases.

4 Obstructive Uropathy

Although women with solitary kidneys tolerate pregnancy well [20], anuria due to pressure from the gravid uterus has been reported in a few cases [23]. Bilateral hydronephrosis has also been documented [24]. Treatment modalities for ARF have included nephrostomy, ureteral catheterization, amniocentesis, hemodialysis, and bed rest in the appropriate lateral decubitus position, leading to decompression of the affected ureter [23].

5 Toxemia of Pregnancy and Related Obstetric Complications

The frequency distribution of ARF during pregnancy shows a peak during the thirtieth through the fortieth week of gestation [20], mainly due to preeclampsia and local complications such as abruptio placentae and uterine hemorrhage.

5.1 PREECLAMPSIA AND ECLAMPSIA

The development of ARF in late pregnancy is associated with hypertension or preeclampsia in one-third to two-thirds of women, preferentially in older gravidas who are often multiparas [12]. The underlying renal pathology ranges from swelling of the glomerular endothelial cells (glomerular endotheliosis) in benign cases, to acute tubular necrosis and eventually to cortical necrosis in more severe cases. The latter condition will be further discussed. The respective role of renal hemodynamic changes, tubular obstruction, intravascular hemolysis, and intravascular coagulation in inducing ARF is still debated [12].

5.2 OBSTETRIC COMPLICATIONS

In the study by Sheehan and Lynch [25], as well as in that of Grünfeld et al. [12], 50% of the gravidas with ARF complicating abruptio placentae had cortical necrosis. Other conditions inducing ARF (and often cortical necrosis) are prolonged intrauterine fetal death, amniotic fluid embolism, and uterine hemorrhage. Low plasma volume and renal blood flow, high pressor responsiveness to catecholamines and angiotensin II, and an increase in clotting factors have been recorded in preeclamptic women [26–28]. These abnormalities possibly facilitate the development of ARF by enhancing the sensitivity of these women to blood loss.

6 Postpartum Renal Failure (Postpartum Hemolytic Uremic Syndrome)

Since 1966, numerous cases of idiopathic postpartum ARF (also termed postpartum hemo-

lytic uremic syndrome, HUS) have been recorded in the literature [8–10, 29–34]. After a normal or nearly uneventful pregnancy, the syndrome begins several days to 10 weeks postpartum, sometimes preceded by a flu-like illness. In exceptional instances, it occurred during pregnancy or appeared several months postpartum. It may recur after subsequent pregnancies [12]. The characteristic features of the illness are a sudden and severe anuria with a microangiopathic hemolytic anemia and thrombocytopenia. The blood pressure may be normal, but in most cases hypertension develops later in the course. In some cases, without the help of renal biopsy, it may be difficult to differentiate idiopathic postpartum ARF from severe preeclampsia with microangiopathic anemia and ARF [31]. Other features may include fever, without sepsis, seizures, and heart failure.

According to a recent review [32], end-stage renal failure developed in 73% of reported cases, the outcome being more severe when the features appeared after a symptom-free period than in patients who developed the syndrome immediately after pregnancy. Long-term studies have shown that prognosis may be variable, some patients recovering appreciable renal function even after prolonged anuria; but severe hypertension and progressive renal failure may appear later in recovering patients [35].

The use of renal biopsy is an important guide for prognosis and therapeutic measures. In some cases, the medium-sized arteries are more severely involved, the vascular lesions being characteristic of malignant nephrosclerosis; glomeruli are often ischemic. In this form, termed *postpartum nephrosclerosis* [10, 34], it may no longer be possible to differentiate these lesions from primary nephrosclerosis with malignant hypertension [32]. In other cases, the lesions are suggestive of thrombotic microangiopathy, involving glomerular capillaries and arterioles; in typical instances, the glomeruli show double-contoured capillary loops due to endothelial swelling and translucent subendothelial deposits; on electron microscopy, these deposits appear granular-like with fibrin or fibrillar material. Fibrin thrombi are also found in glomerular capillaries and in arterioles [12, 32, 33, 36]. Sludging of red blood cells in capillary lumen and polymorphonuclear in-filtration, epithelial crescents, ischemic glomeruli, or even scattered areas of cortical necrosis are less common findings. In late cases, glomerular ischemia and sclerosis are prominent, as in malignant nephrosclerosis, although changes suggestive of thrombotic microangiopathy may still be present [12]. Further details may be found in chapter 14.

Many authors see a good correlation between the pathological findings and the clinical outcome. Recovery is to be expected in patients with minor renal abnormalities. The degree of renal insufficiency is related to the number of glomeruli involved. Severe hypertension and poor renal prognosis is often associated with important arterial intimal thickening, especially of the medium-sized arterioles [12, 32, 33, 36].

The pathophysiology of the syndrome is unclear but probably involves primary endothelial damage, with subsequent local renal intravascular coagulation. Such a phenomenon is supported by the high coagulable state occurring in pregnancy and by platelet consumption, glomerular fibrin deposits, and activation of the fibrinolytic system (suggested by elevated fibrin degradation products), sometimes found in cases of thrombotic microangiopathy. The significance of slight hypocomplementemia. probably due to local C3 activation via the alternate pathway found by some authors, has been questioned [32]. Remuzzi et al. [37] and others [38, 39] proposed that thrombotic microangiopathy may be due to a deficiency of a plasma factor(s) stimulating vascular prostacyclin (PGI_2) activity since no PGI_2 activity was recorded during the acute phase of the disease and since the deficiency of the plasma factors(s) may persist one year after clinical remission from HUS [40]. This plasma defect might be genetically determined [40]. It is to be noted that PGI_2 production by the fetal and maternal vessels is depressed in preeclampsia and even in late normal pregnancy, and this may be a facilitating factor. A decrease in plasma antithrombin III has been found in another case of postpartum HUS [41]. Further studies are needed in this field.

A high predominance of women is observed in adults with HUS. Of the 37 cases reported in the literature between 1966 and 1973, only 3 were men, 13 women were within 10 weeks of delivery, and 9 women were taking oral contraceptives [30]. Women developing late postpartum ARF are sometimes taking contraceptives, and it is puzzling whether in these cases the HUS is postpill or really postpartum [12, 33]. Renal changes of postpill HUS also include malignant nephrosclerosis and thrombotic microangiopathy [10]. It is not known whether postpill and postpartum HUS share the same pathogenetic mechanism(s). Severe renal failure was recorded in women taking the pill with previous uneventful pregnancies [12]. HUS can be triggered by oral estrogen intake in predisposed individuals since recurrence of the syndrome was observed eight years later after resumption of the estro-progestogen contraception [42]. The estrogen component likely acts as a trigger for HUS since Ylikorkala recently presented evidence for a reduced prostacyclin production in normal women after prolonged use of estro-progestogens, but not after use of pure progestogens [43].

Some authors have advocated a beneficial effect from the use of heparin and/or antiplatelet agents in postpartum HUS. According to a recent review, only 24% of untreated patients survived while the percentage of survival reached 60% in heparin-treated patients [32]. However, a thorough evaluation of this treatment appears difficult in the absence of controlled series. In short series, the value of heparin and/or antiplatelet agents is either emphasized [15, 35, 44] or questioned [12], considering also the risk of bleeding when heparin is prescribed a few days after renal biopsy. In the absence of unquestionable results, it seems advisable to consider first conservative management, including dialysis (hemodialysis rather than peritoneal dialysis) and antihypertensive drugs when necessary [12, 32, 36]. Thrombolytic therapy is disappointing, even by endarterial infusion [45]. Interesting results have been observed after intravenous antithrombin III infusion [41], prostacyclin infusion [40], plasma exchange, or plasma infusion in some patients [37]. Successful renal transplantation was performed in a few cases of postpartum ARF without recurrence of the disease [12].

7 Acute Fatty Liver of Pregnancy

Acute fatty liver (or acute yellow atrophy of the liver) is a rare complication of pregnancy, occurring in the prepartum or in the postpartum period. It is marked by rapid appearance of jaundice, with only minimal elevation of SGOT and SGPT, and a high incidence of ARF [12, 46, 47]. Toxemic and multisystemic symptoms are frequent. Prognosis is fatal in most instances for both the fetus and the mother, with death resulting from acute hepatic failure. Immediate evacuation of the uterus is the recommended treatment when possible.

On pathologic examination, the liver is infiltrated by fatty vacuoles without necrosis or infiltrates. Renal histological changes resemble those reported in toxemic patients or in HUS. Clinical and pathologic evidence of intravascular coagulation is obvious in some patients.

8 Renal Cortical Necrosis (RCN)

The incidence of renal cortical necrosis (RCN) is high in ARF, occurring in late pregnancy and ranging from 27 to 38% of women [12, 17, 48]. As was already emphasized, this incidence, exceeding then 50%, is particularly high in cases with abruptio placentae and retention of dead fetus. In addition, abruptio placentae accounts for more than half the cases of RCN in the literature [49]. It is likely that the real incidence of RCN may be underestimated if only autopsy material is available since the frequency of patchy cortical necrosis with partial or almost complete recovery has been well documented during the last decade (7).

Comparison of patients with RCN and those with ARF occurring in late pregnancy, and recovering fully, shows that in women with RCN (a) toxemic symptoms are less common; (b) ARF appears earlier in gestation (mean of 29 weeks), mainly in cases with retention of a dead fetus; and (c) prolonged oliguria is significantly more frequent. Age or parity are not discriminant features [7]. The diagnosis of RCN relies on renal biopsy and/or selective arteriographic data. The two methods may give accurate information on the extent of necrosis. Total cortical necrosis is characterized by a large percentage of destroyed glomeruli and the lack of a cortical nephrogram (figure 17–1). In patchy cortical necrosis, many glomeruli are spared, and the percentage of spared glomeruli correlates well with the degree of functional recovery; in addition, on selective arteriography, the cortical nephrogram appears heterogeneous and sometimes striated [7]. Cortical calcifications may be inconstantly seen on x-ray films and appear only after a few weeks.

The high frequency of RCN in obstetrical complications during late pregnancy has been linked to coagulation disorders. It is well known that normal pregnant women have high levels of plasma fibrinogen, factors II, VII, VIII, IX and X, and a reduced fibrinolytic ac-

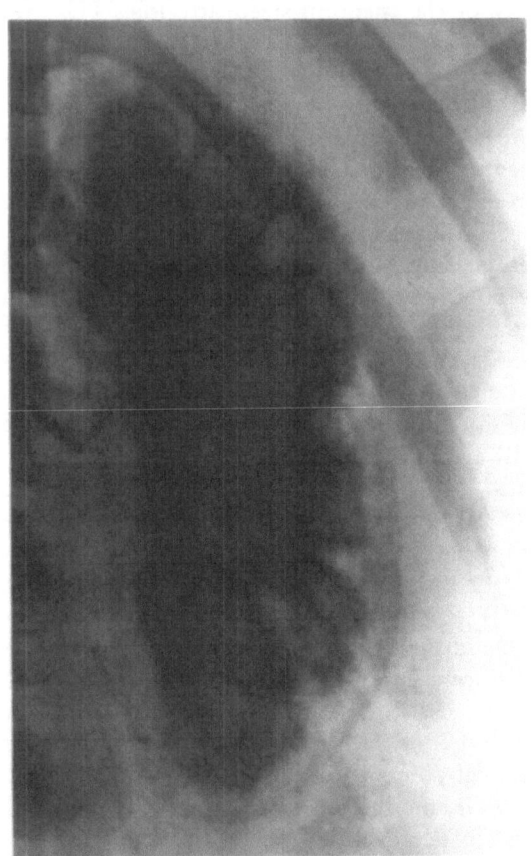

FIGURE 17–1. Patient with total cortical necrosis. Selective renal arteriography. Cortical nephrogram is absent. The outer edge of the cortex is outlined and separated from the inner layer by a clear, nonvascularized area. (Reprinted from *Kidney International* 4: 396, 1973, with permission.)

tivity [26, 28], thus facilitating the development of intravascular coagulation. When severe preeclampsia occurs, there is a decrease in the number of circulating platelets, an increase in the level of serum fibrin degradation products, and an enhanced thrombin activity. All these disturbances disappear several days after delivery [27]. Severe preeclampsia is accompanied by glomerular deposits of granular fibrin and platelets, which tend to occlude intrarenal vessels, particularly when antifibrinolytic drugs are inadvertently prescribed. Local or generalized intravascular coagulation may thus be induced by the release of thromboplastin from a placental or amniotic site and facilitate the development of ARF, depending on the importance of the triggering event, the duration and the severity of the clotting disturbances, the degree of endothelial cell injury that favors the formation of platelet thrombi and fibrin deposition, the rate of organ blood flow, and the rate of clearing of the various clotting breakdown products [12]. Little is known about the significance of other substances simultaneously released, such as serotonin, histamine, kallikrein, and the complement system. These points were extensively developed in chapter 6.

In patients dying during the acute phase of RCN, extensive renal and extrarenal thrombi are a common finding at postmortem examination. They may, however, be found in patients with obstetrical ARF without cortical necrosis, and their significance has been questioned [7]. There is little doubt that their presence within the kidneys indicates a poor prognosis.

Although it has been stated that RCN represents the human counterpart of the generalized Schwartzman reaction, there are no convincing data demonstrating the primary role of intravascular coagulation in obstetric ARF. In a recent study, Conger et al. [50] examined postpartum ARF in Munich-Wistar rats using intravenous endotoxin. Decline in renal function occurred prior to intrarenal fibrin deposition and was associated with marked increases in afferent and lesser increases in efferent arteriolar resistances; glomerular filtration rate and glomerular capillary pressure also fell, suggesting that cogulation within the kidney per se was not the initial event in postpartum rats

with ARF, and that the role of changes in glomerular dynamics was probably more important. Another study emphasized the primary role of endotoxin on the renal vascular endothelium in inducing experimental cortical necrosis and the subsequent formation of thrombi [51].

Renal cortical necrosis does not have a uniformly poor outcome. When renal biopsy and selective arteriograms indicate a "patchy" variety, some recovery may be expected [7]. Even after a prolonged oliguric episode, renal function may slowly improve over a one-year period due to the compensatory hypertrophy of the remaining nephrons. A stable period of moderate renal insufficiency then follows. Subsequent uneventful pregnancies have even been reported [12]. Years later, however, renal function deteriorates again in more than half the recovering patients, requiring chronic hemodialysis and renal transplantation [7]. Some authors have pointed out the high risk of acute rejection in patients with previous RCN [52], but successful transplantation has been reported [7].

9 Nonspecific Treatment of ARF in Pregnancy

The first aim of treatment should be prevention of toxemia, hypovolemia and hemorrhage in pregnant women. Valuable attempts in preventing oliguria in eclamptic women, are the use of intravenous or intramuscular injection of magnesium sulphate, intravenous hydralazine and clonidine without heparin, and vaginal delivery as soon as the woman has regained consciousness. [53]. Plasma volume expansion and sustained natriuresis by saline drinking significantly protect pregnant rats against ARF [54]. In hypovolemic women, plasma expanders (human albumin, low-molecular weight dextran, or other colloid solutions) or whole blood may be indicated [55–57]. In one case of postpartum hemorrhage, hysterectomy was averted by a controlled reduction of arterial blood pressure with sodium nitroprusside [58].

Pregnant women with ARF should be treated conservatively whenever possible, and reversible causes of ARF should be detected and treated when present. In some instances, dialysis has to be performed. Hemodialysis may be preferred to peritoneal dialysis, provided fluid balance and anticoagulation is monitored [12]. The belief that an enlarged uterus is a contraindication to peritoneal dialysis is not shared by Lindheimer and Katz [20]. In their opinion, this procedure is not technically difficult early in pregnancy, but later in gestation it is preferable that the catheter be inserted surgically under direct vision. The peritoneal route may be preferable in cases with circulatory instability or a bleeding diathesis. In any case, delivery should be obtained as soon as possible, but the prognosis is often poor for the fetus [5].

References

1. Chapman A, Legrain M. Acute tubular necrosis and interstitial nephritis. In Nephrology, Hamburger J, Crosnier J, Grünfeld (eds). New York: John Wiley, 1979, pp. 383–410.
2. Kleinknecht D, Ganeval D. Preventive hemodialysis in acute renal failure. Its effect on mortality and morbidity. In Proceedings Conference on Acute Renal Failure, Friedman E, Eliahou HE (eds). Washington, DHEW, 1973, pp. 165–184.
3. Chapman A. Etiologie et pronostic actuel de l'insuffisance rénale aiguë en France. Résultats d'une enquête. In L'insuffisance Rénale Aiguë. Paris: Expansion Scient, 1978, pp. 37–54.
4. Kleinknecht D. Les insuffisances rénales aiguës. In Principes de Réanimation Médicale. Paris: Flammarion Médicine-Sciences, 1982, 3rd ed, pp. 155–194.
5. Lindheimer MD, Katz AI. Kidney Function and Disease in Pregnancy. Philadelphia: Lea and Febiger, 1977.
6. Cameron JS, Brown CB. The investigation and management of acute uremia. In Nephrology, Hamburger J, Crosnier J, Grünfeld JP (eds). New York: John Wiley, 1979, pp. 255–280.
7. Kleinknecht D, Grünfeld JP, Cia-Gomez P, Moreau JF, Garcia-Torres R. Diagnostic procedures and long-term prognosis in bilateral renal cortical necrosis. Kidney Int 4: 390–400, 1973.
8. Robson JS, Martin AM, Ruckley VA, Mac Donald MK. Irreversible post-partum renal failure. Quart J Med 37: 423–435, 1968.
9. Wagoner RD, Holley KE, Johnson WJ. Accelerated nephrosclerosis and postpartum acute renal failure in normotensive patients. Ann Intern Med 69: 237–249, 1968.
10. Schoolwerth AC, Sandler RS, Klahr S, Kissane JM. Nephrosclerosis postpartum and in women taking oral contraceptives. Arch Intern Med 136: 178–185, 1976.
11. Ferris TF. The kidney in pregnancy. In Strauss and Welt's Diseases of the Kidney, Earley LE, Gottschalk CW (eds). Boston: Little, Brown, (3rd ed), 1979, pp. 1321–1356.
12. Grünfeld JP, Ganeval D, Bournérias F. Acute renal failure in pregnancy. Kidney Int. 18: 179–191, 1980.
13. Soyannowo MAO, Armstrong MJ, McGeown MG. Survival of a fetus in a patient with acute renal failure. Lancet 2: 1009–1011, 1966.
14. Cole EH, Bear RA, Steinberg W. Acute renal failure at 24 weeks of pregnancy: A case report. Can Med Ass J 122: 1161–1162, 1980.
15. Kincaid-Smith, PS, Fairley KF. The changing spectrum of acute renal failure in pregnancy and the postpartum period. Contr Nephrol 25: 159–165, 1981.
16. Seedat YK, North-Coombes D, Sewdarsen M. Acute renal failure in Indian and black patients. S Afr Med J 49: 1907–1910, 1975.
17. Chugh KS, Singhal PC, Sharma BK, Pal Y, Mathew MT, Dhall K, Datta BN. Acute renal failure of obstetric origin, Obstet Gynecol 48: 642–646, 1976.
18. Hawkins DF, Sevitt LH, Fairbrother PF, Tothill AU. Management of septic chemical abortion with renal failure. N Engl J Med 292: 722–725, 1975.
19. Emmanouel D, Katz AI. Acute renal failure in obstetric septic shock. Current views on pathogenesis and management. Amer J Obstet Gynecol 117: 145–159, 1973.
20. Lindheimer MD, Katz AI. The kidney in pregnancy. In Nephrology, Hamburger J, Crosnier J, Grünfeld JP (eds). New York: John Wiley 1979, pp. 1141–1166.
21. Kincaid-Smith P. Pyelonephritis, chronic interstitial nephritis, and obstructive uropathy. In Nephrology, Hamburger J, Crosnier J, Grünfeld JP (eds). New York: John Wiley, 1979, pp. 553–582.
22. Nadler N, Salinas-Madrigal L, Charles AG, Pollak VE. Acute glomerulonephritis during late pregnancy. Obstet Gynecol 34: 227–237, 1969.
23. Homans DC, Blake GD, Harrington JT, Cetrulo CL. Acute renal failure caused by ureteral obstruction by a gravid uterus. J Amer Med Ass 246: 1230–1231, 1981.
24. Marwood RP. Anuria in pregnancy. Brit Med J 2: 931, 1978.
25. Sheehan HL, Lynch JB. Pathology of toxemia of pregnancy. Baltimore: Williams and Wilkins, 1973.
26. Kleinknecht D, Kanfer A, Josso F. Intravascular coagulation and heparin therapy in acute renal failure. A reappraisal. Eur J Clin Biol Res 17: 695–700, 1972.
27. Bonnar J, Redman CWG, Denson KW. The role of coagulation and fibrinolysis in preeclampsia. In Hypertension in Pregnancy, Lindheimer MD, Katz AI, Zuspan FP (eds). New York: John Wiley, 1976, pp. 85–93.
28. Mc Kay DG. Chronic intravascular coagulation in normal pregnancy and preeclampsia. Contr Nephrol 25: 108–119, 1981.
29. Clarkson AR, Meadows R, Lawrence JR. Postpartum

renal failure? The generalized Schwartzman reaction. Three further cases and a review. Aust Ann Med 18: 209–216, 1969.

30. Finkelstein FO, Kashgarian M, Hayslett JP. Clinical spectrum of post-partum renal failure. Amer J Med 57: 649–654, 1974.

31. Kanfer A, Morel-Maroger L, Vandewalle A, Godin M, Sraer JD, Kourilsky O, Richet G. Diagnosis of hemolysis and uremia in late pregnancy and puerperium. Acute tubular nephritis or thrombotic microangiopathy. Kidney Int 13: 436, 1978.

32. Segonds A, Louradour JM, Suc JM, Orfila C. Postpartum hemolytic uremic syndrome: A study of three cases with a review of the literature. Clin Nephrol 12: 229–242, 1979.

33. Morel-Maroger L, Kanfer A, Solez K, Sraer JD, Richet G. Prognostic importance of vascular lesions in acute renal failure with microangiopathic hemolytic anemia (hemolytic-uremic syndrome): Clinicopathologic study in 20 adults. Kidney Int 15: 548–558, 1979.

34. Larcan A, Lambert H, Laprevote-Heully MC, Hesse JY, Gerbaux A, Grignon M. Néphroangiosclérose accélérée du post-partum. J Urol Néphrol (Paris) 85: 831–840, 1979.

35. Ponticelli C, Rivolta E, Imbasciati E, Rossi E, Mannucci PM. Hemolytic uremic syndrome in adults. Arch Intern Med 140: 353–357, 1980.

36. Goldstein MH, Churg J, Strauss L, Gribetz D: Hemolytic-uremic syndrome. Nephron 23: 263–272, 1979.

37. Remuzzi G, Misiani R, Marchesi D, Livio M, Mecca G, De Gaetano G, Donati MB. Hemolytic-uremic syndrome: Deficiency of plasma factor(s) regulating prostacyclin activity? Lancet 2: 871–872, 1978.

38. Donati MB, Misiani R, Marchesi D, Livio M, Mecca G, Remuzzi G, De Gaetano G. Hemolytic-uremic syndrome, prostaglandins, and plasma factors. In Hemostasis, Prostaglandins and Renal disease, Remuzzi G, Mecca G, De Gaetano G (eds). New York: Raven Press, 1980, pp. 283–290.

39. Wiles PG, Solomon LR, Lawler W, Mallick NP, Johnson M. Inherited plasma factor deficiency in hemolytic-uremic syndrome. Lancet 1: 1105–1106, 1981.

40. De Gaetano G, Livio M, Donati MB, Remuzzi G. Platelet and vascular prostaglandins in uremia, thrombotic microangiopathy, and preeclampsia. Phil Trans R Soc Lond B 294: 339–342, 1981.

41. Brandt P, Jespersen J, Gregersen G. Post-partum hemolytic-uremic syndrome treated with antithrombin-III. Nephron 27: 15–18, 1981.

42. Hauglustaine D, Van Damme B, Vanrenterghem Y, Michielsen P. Recurrent hemolytic uremic syndrome during oral contraception. Clin Nephrol 15: 148–153, 1981.

43. Ylikorkala O, Puolakka J, Viinikka L. Estrogen containing oral contraceptives decrease prostacyclin production. Lancet 1: 42, 1981.

44. Thorsen CA, Rossi EC, Green D, Carone FA. The treatment of the hemolytic uremic syndrome with inhibitors of platelet function. Amer J Med 66: 711–716, 1979.

45. Jones RWA, Morris MC, Maisey MN, Saxton HM, Chantler C. Endarterial urokinase in childhood hemolytic uremic syndrome. Kidney Int 20: 723–727, 1981.

46. Holzbach RT. Jaundice in pregnancy—1976. Amer J Med 61: 367–376, 1976.

47. Blétry O, Roche-Sicot J, Rueff B, Degott C. Stéatose hépatique aiguë gravidique. Nouv Presse Méd 8: 1835–1838, 1979.

48. Smith K, Browne JC, Shackman R, Wrong OM. Renal failure of obstetric origin: An analysis of 70 patients. Lancet 2: 351–354, 1965.

49. Schreiner GE: Bilateral cortical necrosis. In Nephrology, Hamburger J, Crosnier J, Grünfeld JP (eds). New York: John Wiley, 1979, pp. 411–430.

50. Conger JD, Falk SA, Guggenheim SJ. Glomerular dynamics and morphologic changes in the generalized Shwartzman reaction in postpartum rats. J Clin Invest 67: 1334–1346, 1981.

51. Raij L, Keane WF, Michael AF: Unilateral Shwartzman reaction: Cortical necrosis in one kidney following in vivo perfusion with endotoxin. Kidney Int 12: 91–95, 1977.

52. Gelfand MC, Friedman EA, Knepshield JH, Karpatkin S. Detection of antiplatelet antibody activity in patients with renal cortical necrosis. Kidney Int 6: 426–430, 1974.

53. Pritchard JA, Pritchard SA. Standardized treatment of 154 cases of eclampsia. Amer J Obstet Gynecol 123: 543–552, 1975.

54. Bidani A, Churchill PC, Mc Donald FD, Fleischmann L. Glycerol-induced myohemoglobinuric acute renal failure in pregnant rat. Nephron 26. 35–40, 1980.

55. Cloeren SE, Lippert TH, Hinselmann M. Hypovolemia in toxemia of pregnancy: Plasma expander therapy with surveillance of central venous pressure. Arch Gynäk 215: 123–132, 1973.

56. Goodlin RC, Cotton DB, Haesslein HC. Severe edema-proteinuria-hypertension gestosis. Amer J Obstet Gynecol 132: 595–598, 1978.

57. Sehgal NN, Hitt JR. Plasma volume expansion in the treatment of preeclampsia. Amer J Obstet Gynecol 138: 165–168, 1980.

58. Jackson SH, Liebermann MC, Smith DE. Sodium nitroprusside-induced hypotension as a supplemental therapeutic modality in post-partum hemorrhage. Obstet Gynecol 58: 649–651, 1981.

18. ACUTE RENAL FAILURE IN INFANCY AND CHILDHOOD

George B Haycock

The general characteristics of acute renal failure (ARF) in childhood have much in common with those encountered in the adult patient. Many of the causes of ARF in the adult, such as glomerulonephritis, post-ischemic and toxic nephropathy, and burns, may also affect children, although the relative importance of different diseases and injuries as causes of the syndrome may differ greatly according to age. Furthermore, the differences in physiology, metabolism, and nutritional requirements, which are dependent on the age and size of the patient, exert a crucial influence on management; and it is certainly not appropriate simply to "scale-down" the treatment that would be appropriate for an adult in proportion to the age or size of the child. This is especially true with regard to newborn infants, in whom ARF is a relatively common event, particularly in those of low birth weight or who suffer complications of labor and delivery. Proper understanding and successful management of ARF in very young patients therefore requires an appreciation of the physiology of the developing individual and its implications with respect to fluid and electrolyte balance and nutrition. These subjects are comprehensively covered in standard textbooks of general pediatrics [1–3] as well as in more specialized works of reference [4, 5].

1 Fluid Balance in Childhood

In the absence of abnormal losses, the nutritional water requirement is directly proportional to energy expenditure. Under specified conditions of activity, metabolic rate is closely correlated with body surface area (SA); it is therefore convenient to relate water requirement either to estimated energy consumption or more directly to the calculated SA. The system of units conventionally used for meaning energy and volume has resulted, by coincidence, in the convenient relationship that the expenditure of one kilocalorie requires the consumption on one ml exogenous water. Since basal metabolic activity requires the expenditure of approximately 1,000 kilocalories per m^2 SA, it follows that the basal water requirement is approximately one liter m^2. Normal activity or, alternatively, the conditions usually encountered in a hospital ward increase energy consumption by about 50%; therefore a good first estimate of normal daily water requirement is 1,500 ml/m^2. SA may be estimated from the formula:

$$SA \ (m^2) = \text{weight (kg)}^{0.5378} \times \text{height (cm)}^{0.3964} \times 0.024265,$$

or from the published nomograms on it [6]. Of this total intake, approximately 400 ml/m^2 is accounted for by insensible losses, in the non-pyrexial patient not subject to extreme ambient temperatures. This figure may therefore be taken as the basal water requirement of the anuric patient, and in patients with impaired renal function who are not absolutely anuric, a first estimate of daily water requirement may be made on the basis of 400 ml/m^2/day added to the measured losses.

An alternative formulation for total water intake, avoiding the necessity for surface area calculations, is as follows: for each of the first 10

352

kg body weight, 100 ml/kg/day; for the second 10 kg, 50 ml/kg/day; and for each additional kg (over 20 kg), 20 ml/kg/day. Insensible loss may be taken at 25% of the resulting total. This formula is not applicable to small infants, in whom it leads to an underestimation of needs. Babies in the weight range of 5 to 10 kg need 120 ml/kg/day, while those of 2.5 to 5 kg require 150 ml/kg/day. Low birth weight (less than 2.5 kg) infants may need even more, sometimes in excess of 200 ml/kg/day; however, it is entirely inappropriate to consider managing such infants anywhere other than in a competent intensive care baby unit, where such considerations are part of daily routine. It should be noted that however the water requirement is arrived at, it increased by about 12% for every 1°C *body* temperature above 37°C, and by 30 ml/kg for every 1°C *ambient* temperature above 30°C, the temperature at which thermal sweating normally begins under resting conditions.

It will be immediately obvious from the above considerations that the smaller the individual, the larger the ratio SA to weight; consequently, water turnover, expressed in relation to body weight, is very much higher in small individuals than in larger ones. Thus, whereas an adult man normally requires a quantity of water equivalent to 2 to 3% of his weight each day, the corresponding figure for a healthy baby in the first six months of life is 15%. It follows that serious derangements of hydration and extracellular fluid chemistry are liable to occur much more rapidly in infants and in small children with renal failure than in adults, and these parameters must be monitored extremely closely if homeostasis is to be preserved.

The normal requirement for sodium and potassium is 1 to 3 mmol/kg/day, with chloride making up most of the attendant anion. However, since most of this is replacement of urinary output, in the oliguric patient intake should be based on measured urinary, gastrointestinal, and other losses and on measured plasma concentrations.

Energy needs are directly proportional to surface area and therefore to normal water requirement. The importance of meeting the nu-

tritional demands of the child in ARF cannot be exaggerated and will be discussed below.

2 Causes of Acute Renal Failure in Infancy and Childhood

The first suspicion that ARF may be present is usually occasioned by the appearance of oliguria in association with a raised blood urea concentration. It is both useful and customary to divide such patients into three preliminary categories, sometimes known as prerenal, postrenal and intrinsic renal failure.

2.1 PRERENAL FAILURE

Prerenal failure is more appropriately considered as physiological oliguria, being the situation in which the capacity of the kidney to function is preserved, but this capacity is not realized due to a (reversible) reduction in perfusion; oliguria results from maximal renal conservation of salt and water in response to dehydration. Restoration of adequate circulating volume is promptly followed by return of urine flow, the widespread metabolic derangements characteristic of intrinsic renal failure being generally absent. The cause is a contraction of effective arterial volume, as may be found in association with dehydration, blood loss, hypotension due to trauma or severe infection, and other similar disorders. Differentiation of physiological oliguria from true renal failure is discussed below.

2.2 POSTRENAL FAILURE

Postrenal failure refers to oliguria due to obstruction of the urinary tract. Acquired obstruction is distinctly unusual in children, but congenital obstruction, usually due to posterior urethral valves in male newborn infants [7], may present as ARF and is a most important condition to be considered in a differential diagnosis of oliguria in the newborn. Whatever the cause of the obstruction, its relief is followed by diuresis and the return of normal renal function, provided that secondary renal damage has not yet occurred. If the obstruction is incomplete, it may unfortunately be missed; in which case progressive renal damage is likely to ensue, and the child will probably present years later with chronic, irreversible renal insufficiency.

2.3 INTRINSIC OR TRUE RENAL FAILURE

Intrinsic renal failure refers to the consequences of intrinsic disease of, or injury to, the kidney itself. In contrast to the situation in physiological oliguria, rehydration is not followed by diuresis; recovery of renal function will occur only after resolution or healing of the underlying cause. The term ARF as used subsequently in this chapter refers specifically to this class of disease. Numerous specific diseases and injurious events may give rise to ARF, the more important of these being listed in table 18–1. The term *acute tubular necrosis* (ATN) has been employed in the knowledge that some experts prefer other terms such as *vasomotor nephropathy* [8]. The various hypotheses regarding the pathophysiology of this condition are discussed at length in chapter 1; but although of great theoretical interest, this is of little clinical importance, and the term ATN remains the most widely used label in clinical practice. It will be noted from table 18–1 that the causes of ATN are similar to those responsible for physiological oliguria, and there is no doubt that the latter may progress to true ATN if the underlying cause is not corrected sufficiently and quickly. The diagnostic categories listed in table 18–1 are not always as clearly separated as this kind of listing suggests. For example, ATN and renal vein thrombosis almost certainly represent part of the same spectrum of response to renal injury, at any rate in the newborn; similarly, glomerulonephritis and interstitial nephritis commonly coexist in a patient with poststreptococcal disease.

Glomerulonephritis and interstitial nephritis are conspicuously rare in the new born period and early infancy, ARF in this age group being in the great majority of cases due to ATN secondary to asphyxia, sepsis, or a combination of the two [9–11]. Unilateral or bilateral renal vein thrombosis is occasionally seen in very sick newborns; tender enlargement of one or both kidneys and evidence of consumption of clotting factors (e.g., thrombocytopenia) may provide a clue to this very serious complication. As mentioned above, congenital obstructive lesions, with or without associated sepsis, must always be considered as a possibility [12], and congenital dysplasia or hypoplasia of the kidneys, although not strictly a cause of ARF, may present in an indistinguishable manner in the neonatal period [13].

In contrast, after the first year of life the major causes of intrinsic renal failure are glomerulonephritis, the hemolytic uremic syndrome, and ATN, the last usually following major surgery [14–16]. In units where cardiothoracic surgery is performed, bypass and other major intrathoracic procedures are one of the most important causes of ARF [17], the incidence in one series being as high as 8% of all heart operations, of which the majority died [18]; this high mortality almost certainly reflects the seriousness of the underlying disease or disturbance, rather than being the consequence of the renal failure itself.

TABLE 18–1. Causes of acute renal failure

Primary glomerular disease (glomerulonephritis)
    Acute postinfectious glomerulonephritis
    The nephritis of Henoch-Schönlein purpura
    Systemic lupus erythematosus
    Others
Interstitial nephritis
    Drug-induced (methicillin, diuretics)
    Postviral
    Idiopathic
Acute tubular necrosis—renal damage due to:
    Anoxia/ischemia/hypovolemia/hypotension
    Septicemia (especially Gram-negative organisms)
    Nephrotoxins, e.g., mercury, myoglobin
    Combination of above (burns, crush injuries, surgery)
Vascular disorders
    Hemolytic-uremic syndrome
    Renal vein thrombosis
    Disseminated intravascular coagulation
Crystalluria
    Uric acid (following antitumor therapy)
    Sulphonamides
    Oxalic acid (ingestion of polyethylene glycol or methanol)
Miscellaneous (rare) causes

3 Pathophysiology

The pathophysiology of ARF is complex and incompletely understood. Various aspects of it are discussed elsewhere in this book (chapters

1, 4, 5, 6, and 10); in addition, a number of excellent reviews have been published recently [8, 19–21]. The suggestion that tubuloglomerular feedback may play a central role in mediating the oliguria of ARF [19] may go some way toward explaining the peculiar vulnerability of the newborn kidney [11] to ARF in response to a variety of insults.

Glomerular filtration rate is low at birth, rising rapidly in the early postnatal period in both premature and term human infants [22–25]. Morphological studies in several species [26–29] have consistently shown a centrifugal pattern of renal development, with the juxtamedullary glomeruli being the first formed and the more superficial layers of the cortex added later. Measurements of intrarenal distribution of blood flow [30–32], glomerular capillary volume [33], and nephron filtration rate [34, 35] show clearly that functional development follows the same pattern; in addition, the study of Spitzer and Brandis [35] yielded the intriguing finding that not only was glomerulotubular balance for salt and water demonstrable at the single nephron level, but nephron filtration rate was strongly correlated with proximal tubular length. Taken together with the fact that the healthy newborn has a highly developed capacity to conserve sodium [23], this strongly suggests that the low GFR in the newborn period is the consequence of suppression of superficial nephron filtration by tubuloglomerular feedback, in order that the filtered load may not exceed the reabsorptive capacity of the immature proximal tubules. According to this synthesis, tubular functional reserve is so small that even a relatively slight further impairment might lead to complete renal shutdown; by comparison with the adult organ, the neonatal kidney is half way to ARF even before any injury has occurred.

After the newborn period, there is no reason to believe that the pathophysiology of ARF in childhood differs significantly from that in adults.

4 Clinical Features

To a considerable extent, clinical features will depend on the cause. Where renal failure is due to primary renal disease (e.g., glomerulonephritis, hemolytic uremic syndrome), the oliguria and uremia previously referred to are usually associated with edema and hypertension secondary to salt and water retention. The urine contains blood, protein, and casts. Fluid retention may be severe enough to cause pulmonary edema or convulsions, which may be the presenting feature. Specific details of history and physical findings may indicate a particular cause (previous respiratory infection or gastrointestinal disturbance, rashes, etc.); descriptions of the individual diseases will be found in standard textbooks of pediatric nephrology [36, 37].

In ATN, the patient's condition will reflect the causative disorder. Typically, the patient will be dehydrated, ill, and possibly shocked; the contributing causes will in most cases be apparent from the history. Acidotic respiration, tetany, and other consequences of the complex metabolic disturbance that is likely to be present may be seen. Sometimes, particularly when ATN has occurred unrecognized in a hospital setting, overenthusiastic rehydration therapy will have led to fluid overload, but with adequate medical and nursing supervision, the condition should be suspected before this has occurred. Sepsis will frequently be present and must be carefully sought in all cases.

The natural history of ATN is distinctive and may be divided into four main phases:

a. Inciting cause or insult (see above).
b. Oliguric (occasionally anuric) phase.
c. Polyuric (diuretic) phase.
d. Recovery.

In a minority of cases, for reasons not well understood, the oliguric phase is omitted and urine output is high from the outset (polyuric or high output ATN, see chapter 10). This variant may be more common than generally realized, particularly if milder episodes of ATN are considered, perhaps accounting for as many as 25% of the total. The cause is failure of tubular reabsorption of filtrate out of proportion to the fall in glomerular filtration rate; in such cases, the urine, though abundant in quantity, is abnormal in quality (see below). According to one view, this can be interpreted as a failure of suppression of filtration by tubuloglomerular feedback [19].

5 Diagnosis

The usual starting point in the investigation of ARF is a patient who, either in the context of pre-existing illness or without prior warning, becomes oliguric (occasionally polyuric) and is found to have disordered extracellular fluid chemistry, including a high blood urea concentration. The diagnostic process may then be divided into two phases:

a. Establishing whether the uremia is of prerenal, renal, or obstructive origin (see above).
b. Identifying the underlying cause.

The first step is of extreme urgency since it dictates the immediate management of the patient. Unless the cause of the condition is clear at the outset, obstruction must be excluded without delay. It is useful to perform, as soon as possible after admission, (a) abdominal ultrasound examination, (b) plain abdominal x-ray and micturating cystourethrogram, and (c) dynamic ^{99m}Tc DTPA renal scan. Taken together, these provide the following information: the size and general shape of the kidneys: the presence of absence of dilatation of pelvicalyceal systems, ureters, and bladder; the presence or absence of radioopaque calculi; whether or not the urethra is obstructed; and some indication of the perfusion and functional state of the kidneys. In particular, by these means obstruction may be excluded with confidence.

The distinctive functional characteristics of acute intrinsic renal failure are reduced GRF and impaired tubular reabsorption of sodium. In contrast, although GFR is reduced to a variable degree due to reduction of renal perfusion, sodium reabsorption is avid in prerenal failure. These facts allow a clear distinction to be made between the two on biochemical grounds. Formal demonstration of low GFR by clearance or other techniques, although useful, does not provide a result quickly enough to be helpful in the management of the acute situa-

tion, and a number of simpler (and much quicker) tests are available.

The plasma urea concentration is of almost no value in this context; simple dehydration alone will produce levels similar to those seen in renal failure due to enhanced tubular reabsorption of urea under conditions of low urine flow rate. The plasma creatinine concentration, on the other hand, is a reliable guide to GFR [38, 39] and if grossly elevated, suggests the presence of intrinsic renal insufficiency although values substantially higher than the upper limit of normal for age [40] may be encountered in severely hypovolemic patients with prerenal failure. Frequently, the patient will be investigated very early in the course of the disease, before the creatinine has had time to rise to diagnostic levels; thus, while a very high creatinine confirms the presence of renal failure, a lower one does not exclude it. Examination of the urine is then helpful. The urine in ATN has the following characteristics: high sodium and low nitrogen (urea and creatinine concentration and approximate isosmolality with plasma (250–400 mOsmol/kg water; specific gravity about 1010). The oliguric patient with prerenal failure produces urine with exactly opposite composition: high urea, creatinine and osmolality, and low sodium concentration.

Various permutations of these urinary and plasma values have been explored in an attempt to add precision to the biochemical diagnosis of ARF. Of these, the calculated fractional sodium excretion (FE_{Na}) [41] has been clearly shown to be the most effective, that is, the proportion of filtered sodium that is excreted in the urine. This is obtained by dividing sodium clearance by creatinine clearance and reduces to the simple formula:

$$FE_{Na} (\%) = \frac{U_{Na} \times P_{Cr}}{P_{Na} \times U_{Cr}} \times 100,$$

where FE_{Na} is fractional sodium excretion and the other terms represent the urine and plasma concentrations of sodium and creatinine, respectively. Note that timed urinary collections are not required; a "spot" blood and urine sent immediately that the presence of ATN is suspected is sufficient. The value of this calculation has been documented in adults, children, and the newborn [42, 43]. The so-called renal failure index (RFI), obtained by dividing the urinary sodium concentration by the urine–plasma creatinine ratio [44], reduces in effect to a calculation of FE_{Na} assuming a plasma sodium concentration of 100 mmol/l. Since the actual plasma sodium will invariably be known when such calculations are made, there seems little reason to prefer RFI to FE_{Na} since the former has no real physiological meaning. It is important to recognize that both FE_{Na} and RFI are only helpful in the oliguric, volume-depleted patient in whom the diagnosis lies between physiologic oliguria and acute renal failure. The volume-expanded, polyuric patient may well have high values of both these "diagnostic indices" in the presence of good renal function; however, in such patients, the plasma creatinine concentration will be normal, so confusion is unlikely to arise in practice. The tests that may be used in the differentiation of ATN from physiological oliguria are listed in table 18–2.

The child who when first seen has no recent history of a disease or event likely to predispose to ATN, and who is well hydrated or over-

loaded at presentation, presents a somewhat different diagnostic problem. Assuming obstruction has been excluded and ultrasound examination shows the kidneys to be of normal size, the likely diagnoses are: (a) some form of glomerulonephritis, (b) acute interstitial nephritis, (c) hemolytic uremic syndrome, or (d) a drug-induced or toxic form of ATN. If there is no clinical or serological clue to help discriminate among these, urgent renal biopsy is indicated since early specific therapy of some of these possibilities may influence the eventual outcome. If the kidneys are not seen well on intravenous urography (as is probable in this setting), the procedure should be performed either under ultrasound control or as a formal open biopsy; in either case it is essential that an experienced operator obtain the tissue and that clotting defects be corrected first.

In addition to tests designed to establish the presence and cause of ARF, the patient should be assessed to evaluate the effects of ARF on the patients general condition and, in particular, on the composition of the extracellular fluid. This topic is discussed further in the next section.

6 *Metabolic Consequences of Acute Renal Failure*

Since the primary function of the kidney is regulation of the volume and composition of the extracellular fluid (homeostasis), interruption of renal function leads to predictable disturbances in body chemistry. Homeostasis is achieved by adjustment of the rate of urinary output of the substances that make up the extracellular fluid in response to changes in the rate of input, the two routes of entry into the system being diet and metabolism. The changes typically resulting from ARF are listed in table 18–3.

The alterations in salt and water balance are variable and depend largely on the patient's intake during the interval between onset of ARF and its clinical recognition. By the time the diagnosis is made, continuing intake in the face of diminished output has often led to overload of salt and water, usually with water predominating. Thus, the patient is frequently edematous, hypertensive, and hyponatremic.

TABLE 18–2. Biochemical differentiation of prerenal and renal failure

	Prerenal failure	Renal failure
Plasma urea	raised	raised
Plasma creatinine	usually raised*	raised
Urine urea	high	low
Urine creatinine	high	low
Urine osmolality	high (>500)	low (200–400)
Urine specific gravity	high (>1025)	low (1008–1012)
U:P urea	high (>10)	low
U:P creatinine	high (>40)	low
U:P osmolality	high (>2)	low (1)
FE_{Na}	low (<1%)	high (>3%)
RFI	low (<1%)	high (>4%)

Note: U:P = urine-plasma ratio; FE_{Na} = fractional sodium excretion; RFI = renal failure index.
*Although plasma creatinine may be relatively normal in mildly dehydrated patients, the reversible fall in GFR seen in more severely volume-depleted subjects may cause it to rise considerably, and this measurement alone cannot be relied on to distinguish between the two conditions.

TABLE 18–3. Typical changes in plasma composition in acute renal failure

Increased
creatinine
urea
uric acid
potassium
hydrogen ion (acid)
phosphate
osmolality
Decreased
bicarbonate (metabolic acidosis)
calcium
Variable
sodium
chloride

Since patients with ARF are usually ill as a result of the precipitating cause of the failure, they are likely to be catabolic; this condition leads to increased production of urea and other nitrogenous products, hydrogen ion, potassium, and phosphate, exaggerating the increase in plasma concentration of these substances. In consequence, the conservative management of ARF is largely aimed at reducing the effective input of these substances into the system, while management by dialysis is directed toward removing them by artificial means.

7 Conservative Management

Conservative management consists of adjusting the input of various dietary components in response to the damaged kidneys' limited capacity to excrete and regulate them. In addition, specific treatment may need to be given for the underlying disease, and attention must be directed to the general care and maintenance of the child, especially to nutrition.

Circulating blood volume, if depleted, must be restored as a matter of urgency. This is best done with blood or plasma in the first instance, and the circulation should be monitored by means of measurement of central venous pressure and the central-peripheral temperature gap [45]. If peripheral perfusion is poor in the face of high venous pressure, the judicious use of vasodilator drugs is often helpful. It is not unusual for the correction of volume depletion to be followed by the prompt restoration of urine flow [11, 14], thus establishing the diagnosis of physiological oliguria in anticipation of the results of the diagnostic tests, which may not yet be available. If circulatory insufficiency is allowed to persist, the effects may be very damaging; not only may further damage be sustained by the kidneys but acidosis and hyperkalemia may become uncontrollable due to release of hydrogen ion and potassium from hypoxic tissues. The alternative problem of circulatory overload can, if mild, be reversed by reducing input below normal requirements, but if more than mild is an indication for dialysis without delay. Occasionally, a patient may be admitted with severe congestion and pulmonary edema, in which case positive pressure ventilation may be life saving and should be instituted immediately. This maneuver will buy time for dialysis or for ultrafiltration to be effective in reversing the overload. If this problem should be encountered in a setting where neither ventilation nor dialysis is immediately available, then the old-fashioned measure of venesection may tide the patient over until arrangements can be made for definitive treatment to be instituted.

When the circulation is secure, external balance for water is achieved by restricting input in insensible loss (see above) plus a volume equivalent to measured urinary and other output. In the oliguric or anuric patient whose general condition is stable, fluid intake may be calculated on a daily basis according to the previous day's output, but the polyuric patient must be reassessed at much more frequent intervals; it may be necessary to adjust the rate of infusion hourly or half-hourly in order to "chase" an obligate diuresis. This is not a task that can safely be delegated to a nurse; close medical supervision is mandatory. The patient who is well enough to drink presents a particular problem in approximately inverse proportion to age, in that it is often extremely difficult or impossible to prevent a thirsty child from drinking. In a busy ward, the only person who can be relied on to exercise the necessary continuous control may well be the mother, who should be actively recruited into the treatment team whenever possible.

Sodium input is adjusted in accordance with the estimated degree of overload or deficiency at presentation and measured output. Although patients with ARF are frequently hyponatremic when first seen, this condition more commonly reflects water overload than sodium depletion. Therefore, a careful clinical estimate of volume status should be made as part of the initial assessment, and subsequent management will depend on this. Such factors as the presence or absence of edema, arterial blood pressure, central venous pressure, and peripheral skin temperature in a thermoneutral environment (a reliable indicator of tissue perfusion) should enable the clinician to form an accurate judgment in this respect. If extracellular fluid volume is increased, the more usual finding, the appropriate response to hyponatremia is water restriction; ongoing insensible losses will tend gradually to restore plasma sodium concentration to normal. As discussed elsewhere, if volume overload is severe, the early institution of dialysis will correct both hypervolemia and the sodium concentration. The occasional patient who is both volume depleted and hyponatremic should be managed initially by volume repletion and the judicious administration of sodium. The sodium deficit is best calculated on the assumption that the sodium space represents one-third of body weight (30 to 35%) in infants less than one year of age and 20 to 25% in older children. The redistribution of body water that occurs in hyponatremic states may lead to an underestimate of total body sodium deficit; but it is safer to correct in this manner and then to repeat the assessment than to risk a sodium overload in a patient who, by the nature of his condition, is unable to excrete excess salt. The consequence of accidentally induced hypernatremia may well be uncontrollable thirst, which will induce a child to drink his way into dangerous volume overload and pulmonary edema if he is allowed to do so.

Alkali (usually sodium bicarbonate) is given in amounts sufficient to correct acidosis, the dose being calculated on the basis of estimated extracellular fluid volume as for sodium. Frequently, the amount of alkali required exceeds that which can be given without endangering the patient's sodium status, in which case dialysis should be instituted.

Potassium is severely restricted unless (unusually) the plasma concentration is low. If dangerously high levels are present (6mmol/l or more), emergency measures must be taken to prevent cardiac arrhythmias; these measures are listed in table 18–4. A cardiac monitor (showing waveform as well as rate) should be employed until the emergency is contained. The first three steps should be taken in the order listed while dialysis is simultaneously instituted. It should be noted that, of the options given, only the ion-exchange resin and dialysis actually achieve the net removal of potassium from the body. It therefore follows that hyperkalemia in the context of ARF is always an indication for dialysis, even if conservative measures as successful in temporarily normalizing the plasma potassium concentration. For the same reason, there is probably no advantage in attempting to control potassium levels with glucose and insulin infusions; the underlying need for dialysis remains, and anything that delays it should be regarded as a form of potentially hazardous displacement activity.

Phosphate absorption from the gut is reduced by giving aluminum hydroxide gel by mouth, which forms insoluble aluminum phosphate in the lumen. This is worth doing in the hyperphosphatemic patient who is not eating since a significant amount of phosphate is present in gastrointestinal secretions, particularly saliva. The low-protein diet the patient will be receiving (see below) will already be low in phosphate, and little further can be achieved in this respect by dietary manipulation.

Calcium may need to be given to correct severe hypocalcemia, which should not be allowed to persist, particularly in the presence of hyperkalemia. A combination of hypocalcemia and marked hyperphosphatemia will not be

TABLE 18–4. Treatment of acute hyperkaloemia

1. IV sodium bicarbonate (1 mmol/kg)
2. IV calcium gluconate (0.1–0.2 ml 10% solution/kg)
3. Oral and/or rectal calcium resonium (1 g/kg)
4. Dialysis

corrected by the administration of calcium alone and is another indication for dialysis.

Detailed attention to nutritional requirements forms an essential part of the management of any sick child, and the child with renal failure is no exception. The exact policy to be adopted will vary somewhat according to the cause and duration of the renal failure; energy requirements must be met as fully as possible in all cases, while protein and vitamin and trace element intake becomes progressively more important as time passes. If renal failure persists for more than a few days, modern practice requires that dialysis will routinely be instituted, so the need to provide full nutrition in the context of conservative management is rarely encountered.

A child who is well enough should be fed orally if at all possible. If the child cannot (or will not) eat, intragastric or jejunal tube feeding should be attempted, with intravenous feeding reserved for failure of enteral alimentation. The usual limiting factor in the oliguric patient is volume. It is not easy to pack sufficient energy into a volume not much more than 400 ml/m^2 daily, but a good approach to this ideal can be made by using modern highly concentrated energy supplements. Table 18–5 shows the composition of a "renal feed" based on glucose polymer [46] as a carbohydrate source and arachis oil emulsion [47] as fat. Mixed in these proportions it provides 1,385 calories in a total water volume of 465 ml (65 ml water being contained in 130 ml Prosparol). The mixture may be flavored with chocolate or milk-shake flavoring for oral consumption or may be given unflavored down a tube. The aqueous phase of the feed is hyperosmolar with respect to plasma, and it is therefore wise to start with a quarter- or half-strength prepa-

ration, working up to the full concentration over three or four days. Small amounts of protein can be added as required, using either milk-based protein, for example, "Clinifeed" [48] or amino acid preparations; the latter are very expensive and offer no theoretical or actual advantage over protein unless digestive function is impaired. The specific named products suggested here can, of course, be replaced by similar alternatives according to local availability.

The object of intensive nutritional therapy in ARF is threefold: (a) to support the child's general condition and prevent cachexia, (b) to minimize catabolism and thus limit the increase of urea, potassium, hydrogen ion, and phosphate concentrations in the extracellular fluid, and (c) theoretically, to accelerate healing of the renal lesion. There is no experimental evidence in support of the last objective, but the importance of the first two is well established.

Once the cause of the renal failure is known, there may be an indication for specific treatment of the underlying disease, such as steroids [49] or "cocktail" therapy [50] for glomerulonephritis (chapter 13), plasma infusions for the hemolytic uremic syndrome [51] (chapter 16), or antibiotics for septicemia associated with ATN. If antibiotics or other drugs are to be used, special attention must be directed to the metabolism or excretion of the drug in question. If excretion is wholly or partly via the kidney, appropriate modifications must be made to dosage, and blood levels, where relevant, should be obtained. A very valuable review of the effects of renal failure on drug metabolism and dosage has been published [52].

The use of powerful loop diuretics, particularly frusemide, has been advocated as a means of accelerating the resolution of ATN. However, there is no convincing evidence of any benefit in man, and very little in animals, resulting from the administration of frusemide (or mannitol) after the onset of ARF. A variable protective effect has been demonstrated when the drug is given before renal failure is induced but probably no more so than can be achieved by simple saline diuresis. Frusemide is known to potentiate the toxic effects of an-

TABLE 18–5. Composition of "renal feed"

Caloreen (46)	200 g
Prosparol (47)	130 ml
Water	400 ml

Note: This provides 1,385 calories in a total water content of 465 ml (see text). Protein may be added as, e.g., Clinifeed [48] which contains 4 g protein in 100 ml.

imo glycosides and other nephrotoxic drugs and therefore has no place in the routine management of ARF in childhood. This question is considered at length in chapters 3 and 21.

8 Treatment by Dialysis

The general principles governing the use of dialysis techniques in ARF are discussed in chapters 23 and 24. The same methods used in adult patients can be applied to children, but various adaptations must be made with respect to the smaller size and different metabolism of the child if good results are to be obtained.

Indications for dialysis are summarzied in table 18–6. Frequently, multiple indications will be present, and the need for dialysis obvious from the outset. On other occasions, the choice between conservative management and dialysis may be difficult, but certain generalizations may be made as a result of experience. First, the ill child who is catabolic and in renal failure should be dialyzed early since the probability of succeeding with conservative management alone in such patients is remote; further, if dialysis is delayed until the last possible moment, the risks are greatly increased. Second, very small infants and children are less readily controlled conservatively than large individuals and should be dialyzed for less indications than might be required in the latter, that is, the threshold for dialysis is relatively low. Third, once the decision has been made that dialysis will be required for a particular patient, it should be commenced immediately—delay can only increase risk. Fourth, if you are in doubt that dialysis is indicated, it probably is. Pro-

TABLE 18–6. Indications for acute dialysis

---

1. Hyperkalemia
2. Severe acidosis
3. Salt and/or water overload (manifest as hypertension; generalized or pulmonary edema)
4. Hyperphosphatemia/hypocalcemia
5. Failure of early improvement on conservative management
6. The very sick patient with impairment of other systems

Note: The presence of two or more of these indications at the time of presentation suggests that dialysis should probably be instituted immediately, without prior attempts at conservative management.

vided that the staff concerned are properly trained in the techniques, both peritoneal and extracorporeal dialysis are relatively low-risk procedures. Patients are much more often lost through failure to begin dialysis in time than through dialyzing someone who might have survived without it.

The choice of methods lies between peritoneal dialysis (PD) and hemodialysis (HD). Both are highly effective as a means of managing ARF, and local practice will to some extent determine which is selected in a particular case. In general, the smaller the child the more difficult it is to establish access to the circulation; thus PD is almost universally used as the treatment of choice in babies. Very small patients aside, HD is advantageous (a) in very prolonged ARF since much less time is spent on dialysis and a much greater degree of mobility and activity is possible; (b) in hypercatabolic patients, in whom even continuous PD may not be efficient enough to keep pace with the rate of accumulation of urea and other metabolic products; and (c) arguably, in the hemolytic uremic syndrome since the same shunt used for dialysis can be used for the administration of the large volumes of plasma that have recently been advocated as active treatment for the disease [51].

The basic technique of PD in infants and children is much the same as for adults (see chapter 24). Special cannulae are available for pediatric use, being essentially miniature versions of the adult ones. If they are not available, the perforated end of an adult cannula can be shortened with a pair of scissors, the ideal length being the maximum that can be accommodated inside the peritoneal cavity. The cut end should be flamed with a match to remove sharp edges, and the cannula should be mounted on its trochar in the usual way but with the short length that has been cut off behind it; thus, the total length of tubing on the introducer remains the same. The conventional subumbilical placement of the cannula is not always satisfactory in infants and small children, allowing insufficient length of intra-abdominal tubing for efficient dialysis. The preferred site is in either flank and above and anterior to the anterior superior iliac spine, lateral to the inferior epigastric artery at the level of the umbilicus. Great care must be taken to avoid injury to the liver, the spleen, and the great vessels when using these high insertion sites; the most skilled operator available should place the cannula, and beginners should learn the technique firsthand from an expert. Catheter insertion is made easier and probably safer if a volume of fluid equivalent to about half the intended cycle volume is infused into the peritoneal cavity through an intravenous needle beforehand. This separates the viscera and creates a space into which the dialysis cannula can be placed.

The cycle volume must, of course, be reduced in proportion to the size of the patient. Effective dialysis usully requires 20 to 50 ml/kg/cycle, or approximately one litre m^2 body surface area. The most efficient volume is the maximum that can comfortably be tolerated without abdominal pain, respiratory embarrassment, or interference with venous return from the lower half of the body. Rapid exchanges, up to three to four per hour, increase the efficiency of dialysis but are more uncomfortable for the patient; one to two per hour is usually adequate when the patient's condition is stable. A mechanical dialyzer is an immense help in relieving nursing staff of much of the burden of supervision of the procedure, and a number of satisfactory models are available. That manufactured by the LKB Corporation [53] has been found to be safe and reliable and can be adapted to instill volumes as small as 125 ml per cyle.

The duration and frequency of dialysis must be determined on a day-to-day basis according to the patient's condition. If renal failure is prolonged, a routine of about 12 hours of treatment in every 24 is usually satisfactory, the procedure being performed overnight for convenience if adequate nursing supervision is available. This schedule may not be sufficient for ill patients, and continuous dialysis for days or weeks may be required. If treatment is likely to be needed for a prolonged period, a soft Tenckhoff catheter, surgically placed, is better tolerated than the more rigid "acute" type; alternatively, a change to HD may be considered.

Larger children may be hemodialyzed via shunts placed as in the adult patient or by the Shaldon technique using intermittent femoral venous catherization [54]. The smaller the child, however, the greater the problem of circulatory access, and it is this that limits the use of the technique in infancy. If hemodialysis is essential, it is nearly always possible to gain access by a variety of techniques. A shunt may be inserted using the femoral vessels; this has the obvious disadvantage of the eventual sacrifice of the femoral artery, but experience shows that the collateral circulation to the leg is sufficient in infants and young children to prevent acute ischemic damage. Possible long-term effects on the limb, however, have not as yet been documented. A preferable alternative is to cannulate the internal or external jugular vein using a short umbilical catheter, and then to dialyze using the single-needle technique [55, 56]; effective dialysis can be maintained for quite long periods using this method.

The choice of equipment for the extracorporeal circulation can be difficult in smaller children and is constrained by two considerations. First, not more than 8 to 10% of the calculated blood volume should be outside the body at one time. Assuming a blood volume of 85 ml/kg, the smallest commercially available equipment is unsatisfactory for infants smaller than 8 kg since the priming volume of the circuit is about 70 ml. This can be reduced by improvizing a set of tubing lines on an ad hoc basis, but this is difficult and time consuming. Work currently in progress in several centers should result in the general availability of a smaller set in the near future, which will greatly simplify the problem of HD in infants.

Second, because metabolic rate is more closely related to body surface area than weight, the smaller the patient the greater the excretory and homeostatic load on the kidney per unit weight; this is clearly reflected in the development of the normal kidney, GFR being closely related to surface area. The logical solution to this problem in the child with renal failure is to use a proportionately larger dialyzer (considered per unit body weight) the smaller the patient. In practice, this approach is limited by the size of the extracorporeal cir-

362

cuit, as discussed above [57]. The only alternative is to increase the time spent on dialysis, and experience shows that infants and small children require either longer periods on the machine or, preferably, shorter interdialytic intervals than larger subjects. Daily dialysis is therefore the optimal regime in such patients and should be employed electively if resources (i.e., the availability of skilled staff) permit. A further reason for daily dialysis is the need to remove fluid in order to make room for the provision of adequate nutrition, which, as discussed above, may be critically important in supporting the patient's general condition. Usually a daily dialysis of three to four hours is sufficient but it is not possible to lay down such hard and fast rules as is the case for chronic dialysis; adequacy of treatment must be assessed on an individual basis according to the degree of control of extracellular fluid volume and chemistry.

Providing proper account is taken of the differences in metabolism and physiology between individuals at different stages of development, application of the above principles should allow children in ARF to be managed with results at least as good as can be obtained in adult practice, perhaps better in view of the child's superior ability to heal damaged tissues and the lower incidence of unrelated disease in other systems. It must be recognized, however, that the appropriate place for sick children to be treated is a pediatric unit equipped with all the specialized expertise relevant to the child's condition. In the particular case of ARF, this means a pediatric intensive care unit with more than occasional experience of management of renal failure, in particular dialysis of pediatric patients. The optimal treatment is therefore to transfer the child to such a center as soon as acute renal failure is diagnosed, unless circumstances make this impossible.

References

1. Rudolph AM (ed). Pediatrics. New York: Appleton-Century-Crofts (16th ed), 1977.
2. Forfar JO, Arneil GC (eds). Textbook of Pediatrics. Edinburgh: Churchill Livingstone (2nd ed), 1978.
3. Vaughan VC, McKay RJ Jr, Behrmann RE (eds). Nelson Textbook of Pediatrics. Philadelphia: Saunders (11th ed), 1979.
4. Winter RW (ed). The Body Fluids in Pediatrics. Boston: Little, Brown, 1973.
5. McLaren DS and Burman D (eds). Textbook of Pediatric Nutrition. Edinburgh: Churchill Livingstone (2nd ed), 1982.
6. Haycock GB, Schwartz GJ, Wisotsky DH. Geometric method for measuring body surface area: A height-weight formula validated in infants, children and adults. J Pediatr [93]: 62–66, 1978.
7. Moore ES, Galvez MB. Delayed micturition in the newborn period. J Pediatr [80]: 867–873, 1972.
8. Oken DE. Pathogenetic Mechanisms of Acute Renal Failure (Vasomotor Nephropathy). In Pediatric Kidney Disease, Edelmann CM Jr (ed). Boston: Little, Brown, 1978, pp. 189–205.
9. Bernstein J, Meyer R. Congenital abnormalities of urinary system. II. Renal cortical and medullary necrosis. J Pediatr [59]: 657–668, 1961.
10. Anand SK, Northway JD, Grussi FG. Acute renal failure in newborn infants. J Pediatr [92]: 985–988, 1978.
11. Norman ME, Asadi FK. A prospective study of acute renal failure in the newborn. Pediatrics [63]: 475–479, 1979.
12. Sheldon CA, Gonzalez R, Mauer SM, Fraley EE. Obstructive uropathy, renal failure and sepsis in the neonate—A surgical emergency. Urology [16]: 457–463, 1980.
13. Reimold EW, Don TD, Worthen HG. Renal failure during the first year of life. Pediatrics 59 (Suppl 6 part 2) [987]: 994, 1977.
14. Counahan R, Cameron JS, Ogg CS, Spurgeon P, Williams DG, Winder E, Chantler C. Presentation, management, complications and outcome of acute renal failure in childhood: Five years experience. Brit med J 1: 599–602, 1977.
15. Hodson EM, Kjellstrand CM, Mauer SM. Acute renal failure in infants and children: Outcome of 53 patients requiring hemodialysis treatment. J Pediatr [93]: 756–761, 1978.
16. Ellis D, Gartner JC, Galvis AG. Acute renal failure in infants and children: Diagnosis, complications and treatment. Crit Care Med [9]: 607–617, 1981.
17. John EG, Levitsky S, Hastreiter AR. Management of acute renal failure complicating cardiac surgery in infants and children. Crit Care Med 8: 562–569, 1980.
18. Chesney RW, Kaplan BS, Freedom RS. Acute renal failure: An important complication of cardiac surgery in infants. J Pediatr 87: 381–388, 1975.
19. Thurau K and Boylan JW. Acute renal success: The unexpected logic of oliguria in acute renal failure. Am J Med 61: 308–315, 1976.
20. Stein JH, Lifschitz MD and Barnes LD. Current concepts on the pathophysiology of acute renal failure. Am J Physiol 234: F171–F181, 1978.
21. Schrier RW. Acute renal failure. Kidney Int 15: 205–216, 1979.
22. Sertel H, Scopes J. Rates of creatinine clearance in babies less than one week of age. Arch Dis Child 48: 717–720, 1973.

23. Siegel SR, Oh W. Renal function as a marker of human fetal maturation. Acta Pediatr Scand 65: 481–485, 1976.

24. Aperia A, Broberger O, Elinder G, Herin P, Zetterstrom R. Postnatal development of renal function in pre-term and full-term infants. Acta Pediatr Scand 70: 183–187, 1981.

25. Leake RD, Trygstad CW. Glomerular filtration rate during the period of adaptation to extrauterine life. Pediat. Res 11: 959–962, 1977.

26. Arataki M. On the postnatal growth of the kidney, with special reference to the number and size of the glomeruli (albino rat). Am J Anat 36: 399–436, 1926.

27. Potter EL, Thiersen ST. Glomerular development in the kidney as an index for fetal maturity. J Pediatr 22: 695–706, 1943.

28. Ljundquist A. Fetal and postnatal development of intrarenal pattern in man. Acta Paediat 52: 443–464, 1963.

29. Fetterman GH, Shuplock NA, Philipp FJ, Gregg HS. The growth and maturation of human glomeruli and proximal convolutions from term to adulthood. Studies by microdissection. Pediatrics 35: 601–619, 1965.

30. Jose PA, Logan AG, Slotkoff LM, Lilienfield LS, Calcagno PL, Eisner GM. Intrarenal blood flow distribution in canine puppies. Pediat Res 5: 335–344, 1971.

31. Olbing H, Blaufox MD, Aschinberg LC, Silkalns GI, Bernstein J, Spitzer A, Edelmann CM Jr. Postnatal changes in renal glomerular blood flow distribution in puppies. J Clin Invest 52: 2885–2895, 1973.

32. Aschinberg LC, Goldsmith DI, Olbing H, Spitzer A, Edelmann CM Jr, Blaufox MD. Neonatal changes in renal blood flow distribution in puppies. Am J Physiol 228: 1453–1461, 1975.

33. John E, Goldsmith DI, Spitzer A. Quantitative changes in the canine glomerular vasculature during development: Physiologic implications. Kidney Int 20: 223–229, 1981.

34. Horster M, Valtin H. Postnatal development of renal function: Micropuncture and clearance studies in the dog. J Clin Invest 50: 779–795, 1971.

35. Spitzer A, Brandis M. Functional and morphological maturation of the superficial nephrons. Relationship to total kidney function. J Clin Invest 221: 1431–1435, 1971.

36. Rubin MI, Barratt TM. Pediatric Nephrology. Baltimore: Williams & Wilkins, 1975.

37. Edelmann CM Jr (ed). Pediatric Kidney Disease. Boston: Little, Brown, 1978.

38. Schwartz GJ, Haycock GB, Edelmann CM Jr, Spitzer A. A simple estimate of glomerular filtration rate in children derived from body length and plasma creatinine. Pediatrics 58: 259–263, 1976.

39. Counahan R, Chantler C, Ghazali S, Kirkwood B, Rose F, Barratt TM. Estimation of glomerular filtration rate from plasma creatinine concentration in children. Arch Dis Child 51: 875–878, 1976.

40. Schwartz GJ, Haycock GB, Spitzer A. Plasma creatinine and urea concentration in children: Normal values for age and sex. J Pediatr 88: 828–830, 1976.

41. Espinel CH. The FENa test. JAMA 236: 579–581, 1976.

42. Miller TR, Anderson RJ, Linas SL, Henrich WL, Berns AS, Gabow PA, Schrier RW. Urinary diagnostic indices in acute renal failure: A prospective study. Am Int Med 89: 47–50, 1978.

43. Mathew OP, Jones AS, James E, Bland H, Groshong E. Neonatal renal failure: Usefulness of diagnostic indices. Pediatrics 65: 57–60, 1980.

44. Handa SP, Marrin PAF. Diagnostic indices in acute renal failure. Can Med Assoc J 96: 78–82, 1967.

45. Aynsley-Green A, Pickering D. Use of central and peripheral temperature measurement in care of the critically ill child. Arch Dis Child 49: 477–481, 1974.

46. Roussel Laboratories Ltd., Roussel House, North End Road, Wembley, London, England.

47. Duncan, Flockhard & Co. Ltd., London E2 6LA, England.

48. Laboratories Sopharga, Puteaux, France.

49. Cole BR, Brocklebank JT, Kienstra RA, Kissane JM, Robson AM. "Pulse" methylprednisolone therapy in the treatment of severe glomerulonephritis. J Pediatr 88: 307–314, 1976.

50. Brown CB, Wilson D, Turner D, Cameron JS, Ogg CS, Chantler C, Gill D. Combined immunosuppression and anticoagulation in rapidly progressive glomerulonephrtis. Lancet 2: 1166–1172, 1974.

51. Remuzzi G, Misiani R, Marchesi D, Livio M, Mecca G, de Gaetano G, Donati MB. Treatment of the hemolytic uremic syndrome with plasma. Clin Nephrol 12: 279–284, 1979.

52. Bennett WM, Singer I, Coggins CJ. A guide to drug therapy in renal failure. JAMA 230: 1544–1553, 1974.

53. LKB Instruments Ltd, 232 Addington Road, Selsdon, South Croydon, Surrey CR2 8YD, England.

54. Shaldon S, Silva H, Pomeroy J, Rae AI, Rosen SM. Percutaneous femoral venous catheterization and reusable dialyzers in the treatment of acute renal failure. Trans Am Soc Artif Internal Organs 10: 133–135, 1964.

55. Mauer SM, Lynch RE. Hemodialysis techniques for infants and children. Pediatr Clin North Am 23: 843–856, 1976.

56. Bock GH, Campos A, Thompson T, Mauer SM, Kjellstrand CM. Hemodialysis in the premature infant. Am J Dis Child 135: 178–180, 1981.

57. Donckerwolcke RA, Chantler C, Broyer M, Brunner FP, Brynger H, Jacobs C, Kramer P, Selwood NG, Wing AJ. Combined report on regular dialysis and transplantation of children in Europe, 1979. In Robinson BHB, Hawkins JB (eds), Proceedings of the European Dialysis and Transplant Association, Volume 17. Bath, Pitman Medical, 1980. pp. 100–104.

19. ACUTE OBSTRUCTIVE RENAL FAILURE (POSTRENAL FAILURE)

Antonio Dal Canton,

Vittorio E. Andreucci

1. Etiology

Obstruction has been recognized since antiquity as a common cause of urinary disorder [1]. It is, indeed, one of the most frequent causes of chronic renal failure [2].

Yet, obstruction is a relatively uncommon cause of acute renal failure (ARF) since, for this to take place, urine flow must be suddenly and simultaneously interrupted from the whole functioning renal mass. Possible causes of so-called "postrenal" ARF are listed in table 19–1.

Postrenal ARF may occur quite easily in patients with a single functioning kidney, when almost every kind of urinary obstacle, whatever the location along the urinary tract, may determine total obstruction. In patients with a solitary kidney, renal stones, which are the most common cause of obstructive uropathy in the general population [3, 4], are the most common cause of postrenal ARF. A notable exception is the patient with a kidney transplant; even though cases of obstruction due to calculous formation have been reported [5, 6], postrenal ARF is usually secondary to surgical complications [7, 8].

In patients with two functioning kidneys, obstructive anuria may occur when urine flow is stopped distal to the sites where the urinary tract becomes unique. In many instances, this anuria is of short duration and is better defined as acute urinary retention rather than postrenal ARF. Sometimes, however, a true renal failure

with azotemia may ensue (figure 19–1). This may occur when a stone is wedged into the urethra, but usually renal calculi that arrive at the bladder are easily expelled, unless there is an urethral stricture. Rarely is the urethra obstructed by primary urethral tumors or by neoplasms originating from pelvic organs, vagina, vulva, or penis [9]. In the adult male, how-

TABLE 19–1. Causes of "postrenal" acute renal failure

I Distal urinary tract (urethra and bladder)
urethral stone
primary urethral tumor
neoplasm from pelvic organs, vagina, vulva, penis
prostatic enlargement
ovarian cyst, pessary, pelvic, or vulvar hematoma secondary to obstetrical trauma
(in infants and children:) urethral atresia, valves, hypertrophy of the colliculus, ectopic ureterocele, hydrometrocolpos, pelvic neuroblastoma
rectal distension due to constipation
bullous and interstitial cystitis
neurogenic bladder
II Proximal urinary tract (ureter and pelvis)
stones
invasion by contiguous malignant tumors (prostate, bladder, cervix, pancreas)
ureteric metastases from malignant distant tumors (lung, breast, stomach)
compression by iliac or para-aortic lymph nodes
retroperitoneal fibrosis
diffuse malignant infiltration of retroperitoneum
gynecological causes: uterine prolapse, pregnancy, gynecological operations
aortic aneurysm
aortic or iliac bypass surgery
primary ureteric tumors
intraurinary bleeding
fungus balls
traumatic hematoma of abdominal wall

ever, prostatic enlargement is the prevalent cause of obstruction of the lower urinary tract. In females, common causes of urethral obstruction are a gravid retroverted uterus, a fibroid, an ovarian cyst, a pessary, or obstetrical traumas causing pelvic or vulvar hematomas [10]. These masses may obstruct urine flow either by exerting an extrinsic pressure on the bladder neck or the urethra or by overstretching these structures.

In infants and children, intrinsic urologic diseases accounting for distal urinary obstruction are urethral atresia, posterior or anterior urethral valves, hypertrophy of the colliculus, and a prolapsing ectopic ureterocele [11–13]. Nonurologic conditions include trauma, hydrometrocolpos, uterine and prostatic sarcomata, pelvic neuroblastoma, and fecal impaction [14–17].

Rectal distension due to constipation may also result in acute obstruction in the adult, especially in the elderly and in psychiatric patients, either by directly compressing the urethra or by angulating the urethrovescical junction [18, 19].

Distal obstruction has also been reported as an uncommon manifestation of bullous cystitis, when this acute inflammation causes marked bullous edema involving the trigone and the ureteral ostia [20]. A similar mechanism may account for rapidly progressive obstruction of the vescicalureteral junctions in the course of chronic cystitis, such as interstitial cystitis [21]. Finally, acute urinary retention may be the first symptom of neurologic diseases, such as demyelinating disorders, herniated nucleus pulposus, and Landry-Guillain-Barrè syndrome [22, 23]; psychogenic urinary retention may also exceptionally result in renal failure [24].

The acute and simultaneous obstruction of both kidneys proximally to the bladder is an improbable event. Frequently, however, postrenal ARF may appear as if it were secondary to simultaneous obstruction of both ureters; actually, a disorder may have already interrupted urine flow from one kidney without clinical symptoms; the subsequent occlusion of the contralateral ureter will result in anuria. Usually, this occurs when the ureters are either compressed or invaded by malignant tumors of

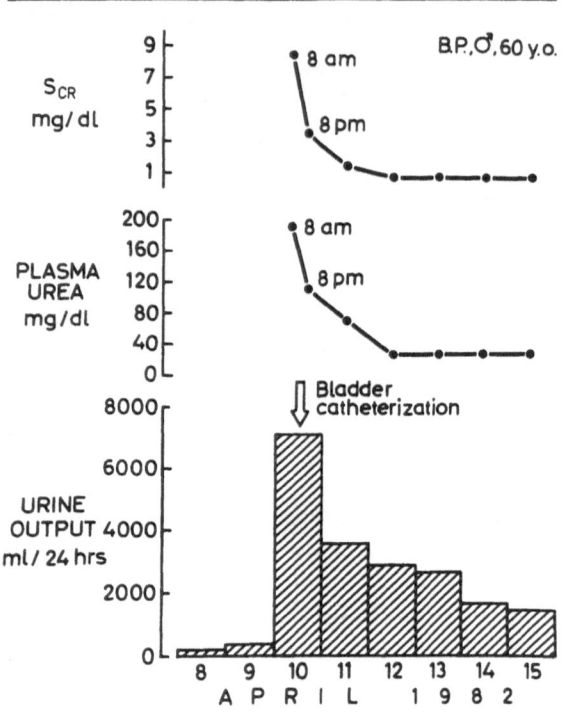

FIGURE 19–1. Postrenal ARF due to prostatic enlargement. B.P., a 60-year-old man was operated for inguinal hernia on 1 April 1982. Preoperatory serum creatinine (S_{Cr}) was 88.40 μmol/l (1.0 mg.dl). Postsurgical course was normal until April 8 when the patient became oligoanuric. Total urine output was less than 300 mls/24 hours. On April 10, at 8 a.m., S_{Cr} was 751 μmol/l (8.5 mg/dl) and plasma urea (P_{urea}) 32.47 mmol/l (195 mg/dl). The insertion of a catheter into the bladder allowed the collection of 1.5 liters of urine in the next 12 hours that reached about 7 liters at the end of the 24 hours. At 8 p.m. of the same day, S_{Cr} had already fallen to 327 μmol/l (3.7 mg/dl), and P_{urea} to 19.48 mmol/l (117 mg/dl). Both S_{Cr} and P_{urea} were completely normalized on April 12, while a moderate polyuria persisted until April 14.

prostate, cervix, bladder, or, more rarely, pancreas [25, 26].

Complete anuria may result also from hematogenous or lymphatic ureteric metastases from distant tumors (lung, breast, cervix, and, more frequently, stomach and prostate) [27–29]. These metastases appear on the mucosal surface of the ureters as nodules protruding into the lumen.

Another mechanism of postrenal ARF is by encasement or compression of the ureters by iliac or para-aortic lymph nodes, either invaded by metastases (e.g., seminoma) [30] or affected by primary tumors [31–33].

In a few cases, the postrenal ARF has been shown to be due to diffuse infiltration of the retroperitoneal space, with malignant cells causing a functional but not mechanical obstruction of the ureters [34]. In such circumstances, a retrograde catheter could be introduced freely to the kidney to allow urine drainage, but urine could not pass spontaneously down into the bladder when the catheter was removed. Presumably, this occurred because the ureteral peristalsis, which moves the urine from the pelvis to the bladder, was abolished due to malignant infiltration and rigidity of ureteral wall and surrounding tissues. An analogous mechanism may explain the anuria that sometimes occurs in patients affected by retroperitoneal fibrosis [35–38]. This disorder may be either idiopathic or associated with such heterogeneous conditions as drug abuse [38]; aortic and iliac artery aneurism [39–41]; Chron's disease [42]; retroperitoneal infections [42–44]; extravasation of urine, blood, or aqueous contrast in retroperitoneum [45, 46]; retroperitoneal arteritis [47]; radiation therapy [48]; and local application of Avitene, a microfibrillar collagen used in surgical hemostasis [49]. In all these disorders, the fibrosis is secondary to chronic inflammation of retroperitoneal tissues.

Uterine prolapse is a well-known gynecological cause of bilateral ureteral obstruction [50–52] that may occasionally cause anuria [10, 53]. Due to uterine prolapse, the obstruction has been attributed to compression of the lower ureters either by the uterus between the bladder and the marginis of the hiatus genitalis (the levator muscles) or by the uterine artery (which lies in the broad ligament anterior to the ureter) [52]. The most probable mechanism, however, is that the uterus carries with it the base of the bladder so that the ureters are compressed against the inferior pubic rami [51].

Another gynecological cause of bilateral ureteral obstruction is pregnancy: the gravid uterus may compress both ureters to such an extent as to cause anuria [54, 55].

Post renal ARF may also occur as a complication of gynecological operations [56–58]; the ureters are usually injured at the site of ligation of the uterine arteries; their occlusion may result from partial transfixation and kinking, angulation caused by suture of neighboring tissues, or crushing due to gripping by artery forceps. Sometimes the ureters may be erroneously ligated.

Bilateral ureteric obstruction may follow aortic or iliac bypass surgery [59]. In such a case, the renal failure may occur some weeks or even months after the operation, the obstruction being caused either by organization of a hematoma secondary to bleeding from the vascular anastomosis or by ureteral strictures ensuing as late complications of ureteric devascularization [60].

Exceptionally, postrenal ARF is the first symptom of bilateral primary ureteric tumors [61, 62]. Other rare causes of anuria are intraurinary bleeding secondary to papillary necrosis [63], in the course of anticoagulant treatment [64], and "fungus balls" consisting of chunky clumps of Candida hyphae in patients with deficient immunity [65–67]. Anedoctal cases of anuria due to traumatic hematoma of the abdominal wall compressing the ureters have been reported [68].

A debated question is whether the acute, mechanical obstruction of a single kidney may evoke a reflex anuria due to marked ureteral spasm or ischemia of the contralateral kidney. In the few cases in which this condition was apparently documented [69, 70], severe colicky pain was thought to be essential to raise the reflex. It cannot be excluded, however, that another undetected disorder was also affecting the apparently sound kidney, such as a small radiolucent calculus or a pyeloureteral junction syndrome, that was acutely decompensated by the sudden increase in water load, secondary to contralateral functional shutdown [71].

The contrast between the exceptional occurrence of anuria and the frequency of renal colic in clinical practice argues against the existence of a "true" reflex anuria. Animal studies, however, have shown that acute ligation of a ureter may cause moderate contralateral ischemia [72]. In man, with colicky pain due to unilateral ureteral occlusion, a similar reflex ischemia may be associated with vomiting, fever, and feeding difficulty. A transient oliguria may thus result from the combination of acute loss of function of the obstructed kidney with reduced function of contralateral kidney due to reflex ischemia and dehydration.

2 Pathophysiology

Acute, mechanical interruption of urine flow is rapidly followed by profound modifications both in urodynamics and in renal hemodynamics. Persistent urinary obstruction ultimately leads to structural alterations of the urinary tract and to renal damage.

2.1 EFFECTS OF OBSTRUCTION ON URODYNAMICS

Transport of urine within the normal urinary tract is accomplished by both active and passive forces. The active forces result from peristalsis within the calyces, renal pelvis, and ureter, while the passive force is the hydrodynamic pressure gradient between Bowman's capsule and the bladder. Peristaltic contractions cause the various tracts of the urinary conduit to shorten and to oppose their walls. Shortening plays only a minimal role in urine transport. More important is the opposition of the walls that is brought about by a force termed *wall tension*. The mechanism by which this force determines urine transport has been experimentally studied in detail in the ureter [73]. In the ureter, segmental increases in wall tension form the urine into boluses. Intraluminal pressure within each constricting segment, and therefore behind each bolus, is markedly increased. This rise in pressure propels the bolus toward the bladder as contractions pass distally. When the ureter is acutely occluded, urine accumulates behind the obstruction, rapidly increasing intraluminal pressure. This may rise to about 80 mm Hg within 60 minutes in man [74] and may even cause, in rare cases, spontaneous pelvic rupture and urine extravasation [75–78].

The response of both pelvis and ureter to this rise in intraluminal pressure is similar initially and consists of an increase in wall tension to resist dilatation, while peristaltic contractions become more forceful and are generated at an increasing rate [79, 80]. With further

accumulation of urine and an ever increasing intraluminal pressure, the responses of ureter and pelvis become different. In the pelvis, in fact, an adaptation to stretch occurs ("stress relaxation"), for which the pelvis dilates, while wall tension and the frequency of contractions decrease, returning toward the original values [80]. In the ureter, greater and greater amounts of the tensile force of the wall are applied to oppose dilatation. Therefore, less force is available for peristaltic contractions, which become weaker and weaker, until all the muscular force of the ureter is spent to maintain the structural integrity and no more contractions are generated [73]. When occlusion continues for days, however, the ureter, as well as the pelvis, is overdistended by the retained urine. Stretching overwhelms the elastic capacity of the walls, and structural changes take place, such as loss of continuity of muscle cells and collagen deposition [73, 81]. Finally, the elastic and tensile properties of the walls are modified, and large volumes of urine are contained within the dilated system at low intraluminal pressure [82].

For this reason, the intrapelvic and endoureteric pressures are commonly found normal in chronically hydronephrotic kidneys [74]; undoubtedly, renal ischemia (see below) and increased fluid egress through pyelovenous, and pyelolymphatic backflow [83] greatly contribute to this normal pressure. With normalization of intraluminal pressure, the chronically obstructed ureter regains its ability to generate peristaltic contractions, but these contractions are less forceful than normal due to scar formation and collagen replacement of smooth muscle units. These structural changes account for impairment of active transporting function of the ureter, even after the obstruction has been relieved [73].

Vesical dynamics in acute urinary retention have been studied in dogs in which the bladder has been acutely distended by both endogenous urine secretion and instillation of fluid. Over a period of 12 to 18 hours, intravesical pressure rose to a peak and then slowly fell, tracing a bell-shaped curve that fitted the requirements of an elastic system. The descending part of the curve indicated that overstretching had occurred and that the bladder had lost its normal elastic properties [84]. Similarly, in man with acute vesical retention, small bladders, which contain less than 1 liter of urine, respond to withdrawal of 100 ml of urine with a much greater fall in intraluminal pressure than larger bladders. Conversely, small bladders respond more vigorously to refilling, with a mean increase in pressure of 25 cm H_2O, than bladders originally containing larger volumes, in which no increase in pressure occurs [85]. These observations indicate that overdistended bladders lose their normal elasticity. Overdistension, instead, does not influence the response to bethanecol chloride, indicating that normal muscular properties are retained.

2.2 EFFECTS OF OBSTRUCTION ON RENAL HEMODYNAMICS

Experimental studies in rats and dogs have shown that within a short time after acute obstruction of one or both ureters, renal blood flow (RBF) is markedly increased [86–89]. Micropuncture studies have shown that the rise in RBF is secondary to a dilatation of the afferent arteriole, which also accounts for a significant rise in glomerular capillary hydrostatic pressure (P_G). The increase in P_G blunts the reduction in effective filtration pressure ensuing from the enhanced intratubular pressure (ITP) and, in association with the increased glomerular plasma flow, maintains the single nephron GFR at values that are only moderately reduced with respect to normal [86]. This hemodynamic adaptation explains why urine continues to be formed and to accumulate in the collecting system despite very high values of ITP (up to 45 mm Hg in the rat) observed as early as two hours after ureteral ligation [90]. Indirect evidence suggests that vasodilatation in the acutely obstructed kidney is mediated by increased PGE_2 synthesis since the phenomenon is inhibited by indomethacin administration [91] (see chapter 1).

As complete ureteral obstruction persists, RBF begins to decrease [89, 90, 92], probably due to increased renal synthesis of Thromboxane A_2, a potent vasoconstrictor prostaglandin [93–95] (see chapter 1). The fall in RBF is striking in rats with 24-hour unilateral ureteral

obstruction (UUO) and intact contralateral kidney [96]. In this animal model, micropuncture studies have shown that glomerular blood flow is reduced to 40% of normal, due to a marked increase in afferent arteriolar resistance [96]. The fall in glomerular blood flow is less marked in rats with 24-hour bilateral ureteral obstruction (BUO) [97], either because anuria is followed by extracellular fluid volume (ECV) expansion or because of retention of unidentified vasodilating substances that are normally excreted in urine. In this animal model (which resembles more strictly postrenal ARF in man), P_G is normal while ITP is elevated; a reduction in effective filtration pressure, therefore, accounts for the fall in GFR [97].

Unfortunately, experimental data on renal hemodynamics in BUO longer than 24 hours are not available. Therefore, to evaluate the hemodynamic effects of more prolonged obstruction, we can refer only to the unilateral model, bearing in mind that this is not a completely satisfactory experimental counterpart of postrenal ARF. Studies in UUO, however, have shown a progressive decrease in RBF over a period of a few weeks. In rats, RBF is reduced to 10% of control after 14 days of obstruction and falls further to 5% after 35 days [98]. Similar results have been obtained in dogs [99].

In the acutely obstructed kidney, during the initial phase of vasodilatation, an intrarenal redistribution of blood flow has been shown, with a relative decrease in outer cortical and an increase in inner cortical blood flow [100, 101]. A similar redistribution has been observed in other states of renal vasodilatation [102, 103]. Both in dogs [104] and in rats [105], however, redistribution of blood flow to inner cortex persists even after 24 hours of obstruction, when RBF is reduced. In rats, inner medullary plasma flow has been found to be strikingly decreased both in UUO and in BUO (to 22% and 12% of normal, respectively) at 18 hours [106].

The hemodynamic changes that occur following urinary obstruction are associated with an increase in renin secretion [107, 108]. Both in UUO [109] and in BUO [110], this occurs immediately, while RBF is higher than normal. At this stage, the increased renin production has been attributed either to reduced NaCl delivery to the macula densa [111] or to increased PGE release [112]. As obstruction persists, however, the renal ischemia may play a role in maintaining high renin secretion. This may become responsible for arterial hypertension in patients with stabilized urinary obstruction [113–116].

2.3 EFFECTS OF OBSTRUCTION ON RENAL MORPHOLOGY AND METABOLISM

2.3.1 Morphologic Changes Early morphologic changes in the obstructed kidney have been thoroughly studied in rabbits [117]. Twenty-four hours after obstruction, the kidney appears swollen and deeply congested, especially in the outer strip of the medulla. The majority of proximal convoluted tubules exhibit obliteration of the lumina and fine vacuolation of the epithelial cells. Some cells have a diminution in basilar interdigitation. This phenomenon is much more marked in the ascending thick segment of Henle's loop, whereas the descending thick segment and the thin limb are normal. Distal convoluted tubules and collecting ducts are dilated and lined by a flattened epithelium. At the tip of the papilla, necrosis of cells lining the collecting ducts may be seen. The cortical interstitial space is enlarged and contains extravasated red blood cells and enlarged fibroblasts with both morphologic and autoradio-micrographic (enhanced incorporation of tritiated thymidine) signs of increased proliferation [118]).

On the fourth day of obstruction, all the changes described are more prominent. In addition, there is obvious necrosis of epithelial cells of the thin limb of Henle's loop near the papilla; in the medulla, intercellular spaces are enlarged and often occupied by mononuclear cells, and capillaries are markedly congested and occasionally closed by microtrombi.

With further prolongation of obstruction, the most prominent changes occur in the renal interstitium. By the seventh day of obstruction, in fact, the interstitial space is diffusely increased and contains numerous fibroblasts that synthesize and lay down increased amounts of collagen. These fibroblasts contain numerous actin-like filaments and, by the sixteenth day, clearly react with fluorescin-labeled antismooth muscle antibodies [119]. As a result of these structural modifications, stripes of renal cortex may contract when stimulated in vitro by vasoactive substances [120]. Should a similar contraction be operating in vivo in obstructed kidneys, it might lead to changes in local microcirculation and potentiate the cortical ischemia secondary to afferent arteriole constriction. Ischemia is probably the cause of progressive interstitial fibrosis and tubular damage that result in final disruption of the normal microarchitecture of the kidney.

An important question is how long after total obstruction the kidney is still able to recover its original integrity. The morphologic changes observed in the rabbit suggest that irreversible renal damage occurs from the second week of obstruction. On the other hand, a permanent reduction in renal function has been observed in rats after two weeks of obstruction [98]. In dogs, GFR returns to 70% of normal after two weeks of obstruction, but only to 30% of normal after four weeks [99]. No conclusive information is available in man, due to incomplete description of the reported cases concerning duration of obstruction and return to normal function. However, a two-week total obstruction may reasonably be considered the time limit beyond which the kidney is unlikely to return to full function [121] although longer periods may be followed by partial recovery [58, 122].

2.3.2 Metabolic Changes In rats, ureteral obstruction causes a host of derangements in renal cell metabolism. Renal medullary Na-K-ATPase activity is reduced after 24 hours of obstruction [123]. The levels of ATP, ADP, and AMP in renal tissue fall to 67% of control within six hours of obstruction and remain low thereafter. In renal tubules, glucose production from α-ketoglutarate is significantly reduced after 24 hours of obstruction, indicating impaired gluconeogenesis. The rates of glucose production from glycerol, malate, and pyruvate are also suppressed [124].

In dogs, the renal ability to accumulate α-

ketoglutarate after α-ketoglutarate and/or β-hydroxybutyrate infusion is decreased by two weeks of obstruction. Six weeks of obstruction are associated with the inability to produce or accumulate α-ketoglutarate, lactate, citrate, or malate after infusion of α-ketoglutarate and/or β-hydroxybutyrate [125]. These metabolic changes indicate that aerobic metabolism is inhibited, with the virtual elimination of many aerobic reactions in the six-week obstructed kidney.

In rabbits, histochemical studies have shown an increase in acid phosphatase reaction and a reduction in alkaline phosphatase, adenosine triphosphatase, glucose 6-phosphatase, succinic dehydrogenase, leucine aminopeptidase, and DPNH and TPNH dehydrogenase activities in proximal tubules after four days of obstruction. The ascending thick segment reveals consistent reduction in ATP-ase, succinic dehydrogenase, and α-glycerophosphate dehydrogenase activities [117].

One may speculate that these metabolic derangements interfere with energy-dependent renal tubular functions, mainly the active reabsorption processes. This is suggested in rabbits [117] and in rats [126] by a correlation between reduced alkaline phosphatase reaction in proximal tubules and decreased glucose reabsorption. In dogs, the rate of renal sodium reabsorption correlates with renal α-ketoglutarate utilization [127]. In rats, the reduced renal PAH uptake observed after 48 hours of obstruction may be reasonably accounted for by reduced cytosolic ATP or by Na-K-ATP-ase inhibition [124].

2.4 PATHOPHYSIOLOGY OF THE POSTOBSTRUCTED KIDNEY

The relief of acute obstruction is not followed by immediate return to normality of renal function. The postobstructed kidney, in fact, presents functional derangements, as altered handling of salt and water, impaired concentrating ability, and defective urine acidification. In the clinical setting of postrenal ARF, the most impressive postobstructive manifestation is a polyuria that is occasionally of alarming volume. A more than academic question is whether these changes in renal function, espe-

cially the polyuria, are secondary to intrinsic renal defects or are merely accounted for by modifications of the internal environment caused by anuria. Unfortunately, in man it has been difficult to obtain information about the mechanisms involved in postobstructive changes in renal function. Therefore, most of our present knowledge is derived from animal studies.

2.4.1 Animal Studies The function of the postobstructive kidney has been extensively investigated in rats.

2.4.1.1 THE POSTOBSTRUCTIVE KIDNEYS FOLLOWING BILATERAL URETERAL OBSTRUCTION (BUO) It has been demonstrated that massive diuresis and natriuresis occur after relief of 24-hour BUO, but not after relief of 24-hour UUO [128], unless the contralateral kidney has been previously removed [129]. There is no doubt, therefore, that a period of anuria is essential to the occurrence of postobstructive polyuria.

Balance studies have shown that polyuria continues for a few days. Water balance, in fact, is negative until four days after release of the obstruction, while sodium and potassium balances are negative for three and five days, respectively [130]. Creatinine clearance is reduced to one-sixth of normal and remains low for the next four days. Urine osmolality is abnormally low throughout the recovery period (five days) [130].

Micropuncture studies have shown that following either BUO or UUO, the relieved kidney is markedly ischemic due to afferent arteriolar vasoconstriction [96, 97]. The consequent fall in glomerular plasma flow and in effective filtration pressure will cause the reduction in single nephron GFR [90]. These results clearly indicate that the polyuria occuring in BUO is entirely accounted for by defective tubular reabsorption. Micropuncture studies have given evidence that this defect is not limited to a single tubular site, but occurs in proximal and distal tubules and in the ascending limb of Henle's loop [130, 131]. In these tubular segments, both absolute and fractional reabsorption of salt and water are significantly reduced. Due to the marked fall in filtration rate, however, the absolute amount of salt and water delivered through the distal tubule is normal or only moderately increased. Therefore, the marked postobstructive polyuria following BUO must be accounted for by altered handling of sodium and water beyond the end of the distal tubule, i.e., in the collecting duct. Alternatively, the polyuria might result from alterations in fluid reabsorption in deep nephrons; but the finding that almost half of deep nephrons are not filtering after relief of BUO [132] argues against this hypothesis. Evidence for a critical role of the medullary collecting duct has been given by Sonnenberg and Wilson [133], who have shown, by direct microcatheterization techniques, a net addition of sodium and water to this nephron segment during the postobstructive polyuria that follows BUO. Consistent with these findings are the results of micropuncture studies, which have shown a greater fraction of filtered sodium in final urine than at the end of the distal tubule [130].

2.4.1.2 THE POSTOBSTRUCTIVE KIDNEY FOLLOWING UNILATERAL URETERAL OBSTRUCTION (UUO). As mentioned above, the relieved kidney after UUO is markedly ischemic, with consequent fall in GFR. In contrast with the findings following BUO, fractional tubular reabsorption along superficial proximal and distal tubules is markedly enhanced [131]. Also in UUO, fractional excretion of sodium and water in final urine is increased even in the absence of polyuria [129, 131]. These findings indicate that in this condition also, the reduction in sodium and water reabsorption occurs beyond the distal tubule, i.e., in the collecting duct. In keeping with this hypothesis, Sonnenberg and Wilson [133] found net addition of sodium to the collecting duct also after relief of UUO. The phenomenon did not occur when natriuresis and diuresis similar to that observed in postobstructive conditions were induced by continuous intravenous reinfusion of urine [133].

On the basis of these experimental studies we may conclude that anuria is an essential prerequisite to the development of postobstructive polyuria, since it does not occur after relief of UUO. The effects of anuria consist of an inhibition of tubular reabsorption both in proximal and distal tubules, so that fluid delivery to the

most distal part of the nephron is not reduced, despite a marked fall in filtration rate. Postobstructive diuresis, however, is largely accounted for by impaired reabsorptive capacity in the collecting duct; the latter defect appears to be a direct consequence of obstruction, independent of complete cessation of renal excretory function since it occurs after both BUO and UUO. Even though this explanation appears satisfactory, some reservations should be maintained, in view of micropuncture studies in weanling rats (with accessible collecting ducts), which suggest that collecting duct function is not markedly altered following release of obstruction [134]. Whether or not this discrepancy reflects an age-related difference, however, requires further investigation.

The mechanism responsible for the functional defects occurring in the collecting duct after relief of ureteral ligation has not been clarified. Several factors could interact to produce the observed changes in sodium and water reabsorption:

a. *Increased permeability of the epithelial wall,* similar to that observed after ureteral obstruction in more proximal parts of the nephron [130]. Increased permeability could reduce net reabsorption by increasing back-diffusion.

b. *Loss of normal medullary osmotic gradient.* A loss of medullary hypertonicity has been demonstrated after a brief period of obstruction [135, 136] and may account for the impaired concentrating ability of postobstructive kidneys, which is not modified by infusion of vasopressin [128]. Medullary solute concentration gradient may be dissipated either by abnormal permeability to sodium and/or water in the loop of Henle and collecting duct or by a washout effect due to increased postobstructive inner medullary plasma flow [137] and blood flow redistribution to deep cortex [105].

c. *Loss of normal hormonal effects,* such as unresponsiveness to aldosterone [128], which is known to modulate sodium reabsorption in medullary collecting ducts [138, 139].

Some uncertainty also exists about the mechanisms by which anuria exerts its critical role in postobstructive diuresis. ECV expansion is a possible mechanism, not only because of its well-known inhibitory effect on proximal tubular reabsorption, but also because it has been shown that ECV expansion exaggerates the reabsorptive defect of the collecting duct in the hydronephrotic kidney [140]. Postobstructive diuresis, however, takes place even if a contraction of ECV is present [130]. Another mechanism is the retention of diuretic and natriuretic factors that are normally excreted in urine. Experimental evidence indicates that urea is one of these factors [129]. The osmotic urea diuresis, however, is transient and self-limited, being rapidly antagonized by ECV depletion [129]. Therefore, other more potent factors are probably retained in blood or enter systemic circulation from urine during total urinary obstruction. Evidence that this is the case derives from experiments showing that i.v. reinfusion of urine in normal rats produced renal vasodilatation and massive increase in urine volume and sodium excretion [141]. The role of circulating substances in postobstructive diuresis was confirmed in experiments involving cross-circulation of blood between rats [142].

Experiments in dogs [143] and in rats [144] have shown a postobstructive defect in urinary acidification. In dogs with UUO, this defect consisted of excretion of urine from the obstructed kidney with a higher pH than from the contralateral kidney. No titratable acid was excreted from the obstructed kidney, even after administration of a sodium sulphate load. These abnormalities were associated with, but not dependent on, reduced phosphate excretion. The acidification defect, in fact, persisted following normalization of urinary phosphate levels with sodium phosphate infusion. Fractional bicarbonate reabsorption during bicarbonate load was more elevated in the obstructed kidney, suggesting that the urinary acidification defect was localized exclusively in the distal part of the nephron. The distal defect appeared secondary to a generalized disorder of distal transport, in that K^+ secretion and steroid-responsive Na^+ reabsorption were impaired in the postobstructive kidney [143]. Similar results were obtained in micropuncture experiments in rats [144]. These studies, in fact, failed to demonstrate decreased proximal bicarbonate reabsorption in surface nephrons

and suggested that the acidifying defect was due either to decreased H^+ secretion in distal tubule or to marked alteration in bicarbonate reabsorption in juxtamedullary nephrons.

2.4.2 Clinical Studies Few studies are available on renal function following relief of postrenal ARF. Seven reports, describing a total of ten patients with clearly inappropriate salt loss following release of acute prostatic obstruction have been recently reviewed [145]. All these patients were azotemic at the moment when the obstruction was relieved. In the recovery period, peak urine flow averaged 30 ml/min, and average maximal fractional sodium excretion was 21%. All patients recovered completely normal renal function in a few days, suggesting that postobstructive polyuria was accounted for by extrarenal factors, such as increased urea load and ECV expansion. Peterson et al. [146] reported five patients with postrenal ARF due to prostatic enlargement of short duration. A three-to-five-day postobstructive diuresis occurred in all patients: soon after relief of obstruction, GRF ranged from 23 to 157 ml/min, renal plasma flow from 137 to 633 ml/min, and fractional Na^+ excretion from 4 to 21%. A peak daily diuresis of 35.6 liters occurred in an azotemic patient in whom negative fluid balance and ECV depletion were witnessed by a fall in both body weight and central venous pressure. An osmotic urea load, therefore, may have been the main factor responsible for polyuria in this patient. Peak daily diuresis, however, was extraordinarily elevated (18.8 liters) in one nonazotemic patient; according to the authors, this was a typical example of polyuria independent of osmotic diuresis due to urea load, inappropriate fluid administration, or lack of ADH.

The possibility that postobstructive polyuria is due to the retention of unknown substances that are normally excreted in urine is suggested by studies showing that a natriuretic factor is identifiable in the serum of uremic patients [147, 148].

Whether postobstructive diuresis is also due to tubular dysfunction caused by obstruction per se has been studied in patients with unilateral obstruction and normal overall renal function. In most of these studies, the pathological setting of the obstructed kidney was quite different from that occurring in ARF, the obstruction being only partial and of long duration. With these limits, the present evidence is against a critical role of intrinsic tubular defects in postobstructive polyuria. In the unilaterally obstructed kidney, in fact, postobstructive fractional water and salt excretion is normal [149] or only moderately increased [122]. In the absence of complicating urinary infection, we have also found a normal ability to generate both positive (C_{H_2O}) and negative ($T^C_{H_2O}$) free-water per unit GFR; a lower maximal urine osmolality was the only functional defect observed [150].

3 Diagnosis

The recognition of obstruction as the pathogenic mechanism of ARF should be considered a diagnostic emergency. A prompt diagnosis of this mechanism and localization of urinary obstruction will give the chance for a rapid recovery of renal function; the removal of the obstruction, in fact, will avoid the risk of prolonged anuria and the occurrence of irreversible renal damage. While approaching a patient with ARF, therefore, the clinician should always face the question: has this patient a postrenal ARF?

3.1 ANAMNESTIC CLUES

With this question in mind, a careful past and recent history must be collected.

3.1.1 Past History The existence of a solitary functioning kidney should be investigated. Unfortunately, this condition is often totally unknown to the patient, not only when a kidney is congenitally absent but also when the function of a kidney is obscured by acquired diseases, such as large pelvic stone, tuberculosis, or neoplasm. These disorders, however, are only rarely completely silent: more frequently, instead, past history will disclose episodes of colicky pain, passage of stones, macroscopic hematuria, dysuria, or a persistent backache. Symptoms related to stones are of special interest not only because calculi are the single most frequent cause of unilateral loss of a kidney,

but also because this same disorder may recur in the other side and suddenly obstruct the contralateral organ.

Infravescical obstruction may be heralded by a progressive decrease in the force of the urinary stream, intermittency, postvoid dribbling, urgency with frequent urination, and urinary incontinence ("overflow" incontinence). Sensory deficits, muscular weakness, or incoordination may be the first symptoms of a neurologic demyelinating disorder, such as multiple sclerosis, accounting for acute urinary retention. Vaginal or rectal hemorrhage may indicate pelvic tumors invading the bladder or the ureters.

Retroperitoneal fibrosis should be suspected in patients with a long history of methysergide consumption, a drug used in treatment of postgastrectomy dumping syndrome and of migraine. Other agents mentioned in the literature as possible cause of retroperitoneal fibrosis are atenolol [151], hydralazine, lysergic acid diethylamide, dexamphetamine, methyldopa and colchicine [152], analgesics [38], and avitene [49]. Retroperitoneal fibrosis may be associated with a pain along the costal margin, between the posterior axillary and midclavicular lines, nonradiating, lasting for several minutes, and then subsiding, unrelated to meals, micturition, or activity [152].

A persistent or intermittent pain in the middle or lower belly, often radiating to the lower back, is a frequent presenting symptom of an aortic abdominal aneurysm.

Finally, all retroperitoneal operations should be carefully registered, holding in mind that obstructive anuria may sometimes occur as a late complication of retroperitoneal surgery [60].

3.1.2 Recent History The sudden onset of complete anuria is considered the hallmark of postrenal ARF [153]. In our experience, however, obstruction cannot be excluded as the pathogenic mechanism of ARF simply because total anuria is lacking. Some urine, in fact, may be excreted from a chronically ill and severely damaged kidney, when the contralateral kidney that bears the burden of almost total renal function becomes acutely occluded. More pathognomonic for postrenal ARF is the intermittency of oliguria, that is, the excretion of large volumes of urine interposed between oliguric intervals.

Anuria due to ureteric obstruction is often preceded by or associated with excruciating colicky pain in the loins, radiating to the lower abdominal quadrants, the testes, or the labia. A periumbilical localization of colicky pain may occur in children. Gross hematuria, fever, nausea, and vomiting may accompany this colicky pain.

3.2 PHYSICAL SIGNS AND LABORATORY FINDINGS

When the obstruction has stabilized, usually no more colicky pain is present. The patient may feel well, except for a dull backache, due to stretching of the pelvis and the renal capsule, and/or a lateral abdominal or soprapubic discomfort due to distension of the ureter or the bladder, respectively. This backache may be increased by pressing one finger into the costovertebral angle, between the spine and the twelfth rib. Similarly, the abdominal tenderness may be enhanced by manual palpation. Sometimes, abdominal examination is difficult, due to generalized abdominal distension that may simulate paralytic ileus. Bimanual palpation of the upper quadrants of the abdomen should be performed, with one hand pushing into the abdomen and the other one lifting from the back. With this maneuver, a hydronephrotic kidney may be disclosed as a tender mass moving with inspiration. The abdominal profile should be carefully inspected, searching for a distention of the lower third that may result from pelvic tumors and for a pulsatile mass, indicating aortic aneurysm.

The overdistended urinary bladder may be detected by palpation as a soprapubic mass with a global shape; amazingly, this mass may extend up to the level of the umbelicus. The distended bladder can be detected also by auscultatory percussion: with the patient supine, place the stethoscope above the symphisis pubis, in the midline, at a constant point. Then, percuss the abdominal wall with the pulp of a finger, starting from above the umbelicus and proceeding toward the stethoscope

along the midline. The upper border of the bladder is indicated by a sharp, loud change in the percussion note [154]. The distended bladder, however, is not always detectable on abdominal examination; in the male patient, it may be suggested by priapism.

Careful rectal and, in the female, pelvic examination should never be neglected. The former may disclose a rectal cancer, as a plateau-like, nodular, annular, or cauliflower mass. It also allows the appreciation of prostatic enlargement due either to benign hyperplasia or to carcinoma. Benign prostatic hyperplasia, however, is difficult to diagnose when it is limited to the median lobe. In this case, in fact, the bulk of the lobe may protrude anteriorly and produce urethral obstruction, without being palpable. Vaginal inspection may reveal neoplasm either primary or extending from the uterus, rectum, or bladder. Bimanual pelvic examination may reveal uterine and ovarian tumors.

Postrenal ARF can not be differentiated from other types of ARF by means of laboratory investigations. This negative statement must be held in mind, especially when the patient is not totally anuric and a sample of urine is collected for examination. In some cases, the small amount of urine may derive from a chronically ill kidney contralateral to the acutely occluded one; in this urine, sodium concentration will be relatively high and osmolality will equal that of plasma, suggesting intrinsic ("renal") ARF (ATN). In other cases, the small amount of urine may derive from the acutely obstructed kidney(s) shortly before the occlusion becomes complete, as when ARF is the final event of a progressive invasion by retroperitoneal tumors; in this urine, sodium concentration may be very low, and osmolality elevated, mimicking sodium depletion and functional ("prerenal") ARF [155, 156].

Of interest is the experimental observation of Hiatt et al. [157], who found in dogs with BUO a markedly decreased ability to transfer potassium from extracellular to intracellular fluid. This phenomenon was neither dependent on anuria per se since it did not take place in nephrectomized dogs, nor on the renin-angiotensin system. Whether these experimen-

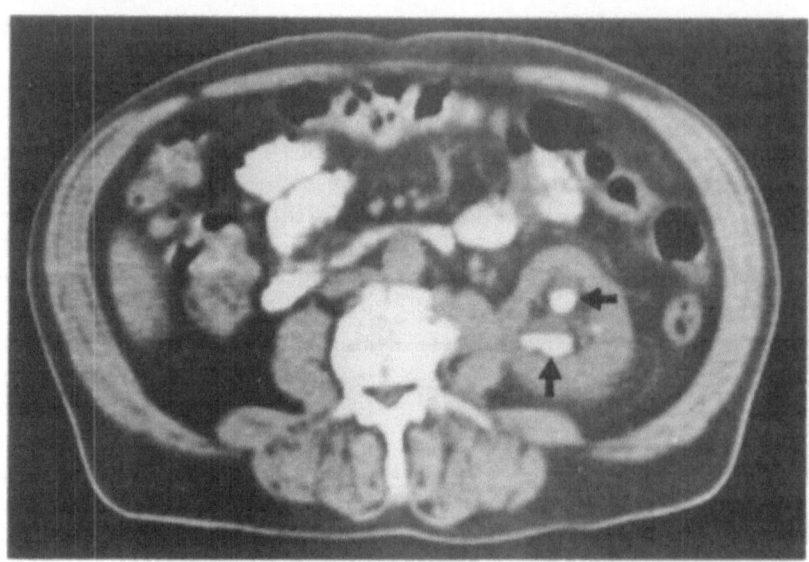

tal findings have any clinical correspondence, in the sense that patients with postrenal ARF are more easily prone to hyperkalemia than other anuric patients, deserves investigation.

3.3 RADIOLOGIC FINDINGS

3.3.1 Plain Film of the Abdomen The plain film of the abdomen, possibly with tomography, is a simple and safe investigation that may show obvious causes of obstruction, such as radiopaque stones. Hydronephrosis can occasionally be suggested from the findings of an enlarged kidney and a soft tissue "mass" effect produced by enlarged renal pelvis [158]. Paravertebral linear calcifications may raise the suspect of aortic abdominal aneurysm.

3.3.2 Echography Renal sonography should be carried out whenever possible since it is absolutely safe and highly effective in ruling out obstruction. Obstruction causes a well-visible splaying of normally compact central echo complex, with sonolucent "fluid-filled" areas representing the dilated calyces and renal pelvis [159]. In addition, stones as small as 1.5 × 1.5 cm may be identified [160]. The ultrasonic properties of renal calculi are a strong reflection at the surface of the stone, with significant absorption of sound and distal acoustic shadowing.

FIGURE 19–2. E.G., a 69-year-old hypertensive man had for several years a serum creatinine (S_{Cr}) around 124–133 μmol/l (1.4–1.5 mg/dl). No intravenous pyelography was performed at any time. Suddenly, a marked rise in S_{Cr} occurred to reach, in a few weeks 1,149 μmol/l (13 mg/dl), with progressive decrease in urine output to 100 ml/24 hours. Plain film tomograms did not show renal stones. CT demonstrated the absence of the right kidney, while a renal stone (arrows) was identified in the left renal pyelocalyceal system that was clearly dilated, as observed in this figure. A retrograde pyelography confirmed a nonradioopaque obstructing stone (uric acid stone) in the pelvis; ureteral catheterization could overcome the obstacle and allow resumption of urine output. The catheter was left in place for two weeks; meanwhile, a treatment with allopurinol per os and sodium bicarbonate i.v. was performed. S_{Cr} gradually decreased. Before withdrawing the ureteral catheter, the injection of contrast material revealed the complete dissolution of the uric acid stone; meanwhile, S_{Cr} had returned to baseline values (124–133 μmol/l, 1.4–1.5 mg/dl).

3.3.3 Computed Tomography Computed tomography (CT) is of limited hazard to the patient because the dilated renal collecting system may be visualized clearly without using contrast media (figure 19–2). Due to its high cost, however, this investigation is not usually performed as the first radiologic step for ruling out the existence of obstruction. The main indication for performing CT is the suspicion that postrenal ARF is caused by an aortic aneurysm, retroperitoneal fibrosis, or retroperitoneal malignancies. In such instances, in fact, CT has proven valid not only to disclose obstruction, but also to define the underlying disorder [161, 162].

3.3.4 Renography

The radioisotopic renogram is used sometimes with the aim of visualizing urinary obstruction. However, we believe that in contrast with its proven utility in chronic obstruction [163], this investigation is of no value in the diagnosis of postrenal ARF. In anuric patients, in fact, the renogram frequently shows an "obstructed" pattern that is a marked delay in excretory phase, even if the ARF is due to nonobstructive mechanism [164].

3.3.5 Intravenous Pyelography

Intravenous pyelography (IVP) is invaluable in the recognition of obstructive ARF (see also chapter 9). In this condition, clear urograms and pyelograms are usually obtained (figure 19–3). Pyelograms are often surprisingly good, particularly in delayed films (24–36 hours), when not only the existence but also the level of the obstruction may be identified. A diagnostic pyelogram is so common in postrenal ARF that its absence suggests a nonobstructive pathogenesis [165]. On occasion, IVP may also indicate the cause of obstruction, as when this is accounted for by endoureteral or pelvic obstruction or by retroperitoneal fibrosis; in the latter condition, in fact, the ureters are characteristically tortuous and are deviated toward the midline in the lower third.

3.3.6 Antegrade Percutaneous Pyelography

Antegrade percutaneous pyelography can be performed by placing a 22-gauge needle directly into the pelvis under ultrasonic guidance. Contrast medium is injected to opacify the collecting structures and ureter to the point of obstruction. The limit of this investigation is that it can be safely carried out only when a large pelvis is easily visible with echography. Antegrade pyelography is very useful to determine the site and, on occasion, the etiology of obstruction.

3.3.7 Retrograde Pyelography

In the last decade, the need for this investigation has diminished markedly thanks to the other imaging modalities, which are preferable because retrograde pyelography is painful, bears a great risk of infection, and may cause traumatism and even perforations of the urinary tract. In some instances, however, retrograde pyelography remains invaluable both to diagnose obstruction and to delineate the exact site of urinary obstacle. In addition, cystoscopy, which is preliminary to retrograde pyelography, can directly visualize vescical causes of obstruction as neoplasms or rare occlusive types of cystitis.

4 Treatment

In this section, we shall deal only with the therapeutic problems that are peculiar to postrenal ARF. A distinctive feature of this disorder, in contrast with other types of ARF, is the possibility of greatly influencing its course and duration by interrupting the pathogenic mechanism, that is, by relieving the obstruction.

4.1 INFRAVESCICAL OBSTRUCTION

Since acute urinary retention may be asymptomatic and the enlarged bladder is not always easily recognized, an attempt to verify whether the bladder is empty should be done in all patients with sudden anuria of unknown origin. Bladder catheterization should be first attempted with a Foley's catheter of adequate size. Due to their flexibility, however, Foley's catheters cannot be passed through tight urethral strictures. When this occurs, Couvelaire's rigid catheters may be successfully used, maneuvering gently to avoid trauma or even perforation. Should even this attempt be unsuccessful, small ureteral catheters or Phillip's followers may succeed in establishing urinary drainage. Finally, when the obstruction cannot be bypassed through the urethra, a stab cystomy has to be performed.

When an overdistended bladder is drained too rapidly, hemorrhage "e vacuum" may occur. To avoid sudden decompression, therefore, the bladder should be emptied slowly, for example, by draining 50 ml of urine at a time and then clamping the catheter for 20 to 30 minutes.

Infection is a frequent complication of catheterization; it occurs more frequently the longer indwelling catheters are left in the blad-

378

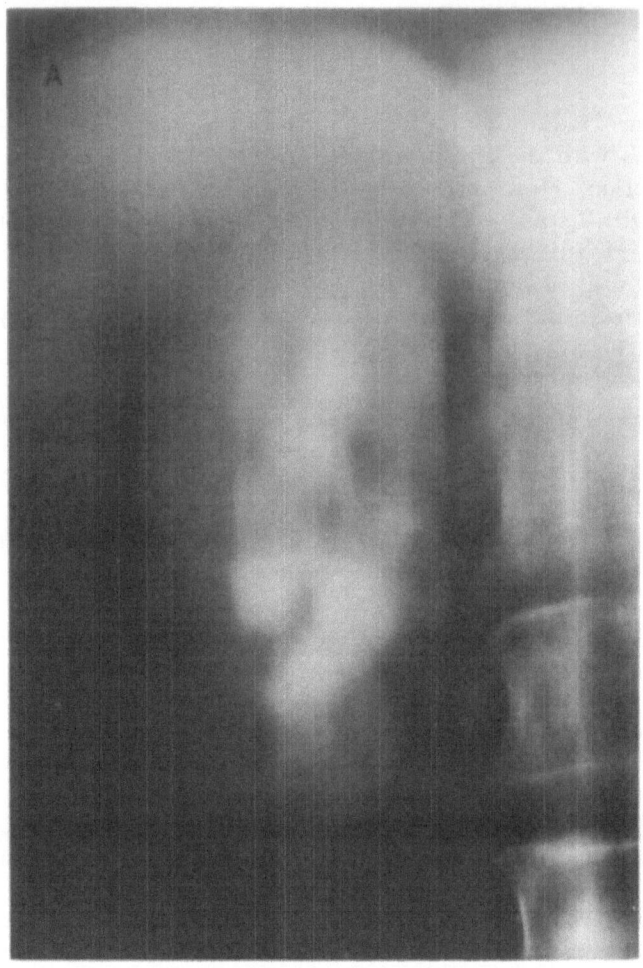

FIGURE 19–3. Postdialysis intravenous pyelograms with nephrotomography in a patient with postrenal ARF. Immediate adequate visualizatoin of the pyelocaliectasis was obtained in both kidneys. **A.** The right kidney. **B.** The left kidney.

der. Preventive efforts should be particularly focused on aseptic care of the bladder catheter—that is, aseptic insertion, observation of handwashing by personnel before any manipulation of the catheter site or apparatus, and maintenance of a closed sterile system [166]. Perineal and pericatheter cleansing is recommended while meatal care regimens have proved of scant utility [167]. The collecting bag should be emptied regularly, and the catheters should be replaced only when they malfunction or become contaminated [168]. In addition, the likelihood of cross-infection is decreased by separating infected and uninfected patients [169]. Other procedures, such as daily bacteriologic monitoring and maintenance of a high-volume urine flow, may be useful. Bladder irrigation with antibacterial solutions is of

little value in reducing the occurrence of infection and appears to select for more resistant microorganisms [170].

The final objective of treatment of patients with infravescical obstruction is the establishment of bladder emptying without an indwelling catheter. This can be obtained with transurethral resection of the prostate, in case of hypertrophy or operable tumor. Vaginal hysterectomy or simply a pessary is indicated for procidentia. Usual treatment of neurogenic bladder ranges from sympatholytic agents [171], such as phenoxybenzamine, to transure-

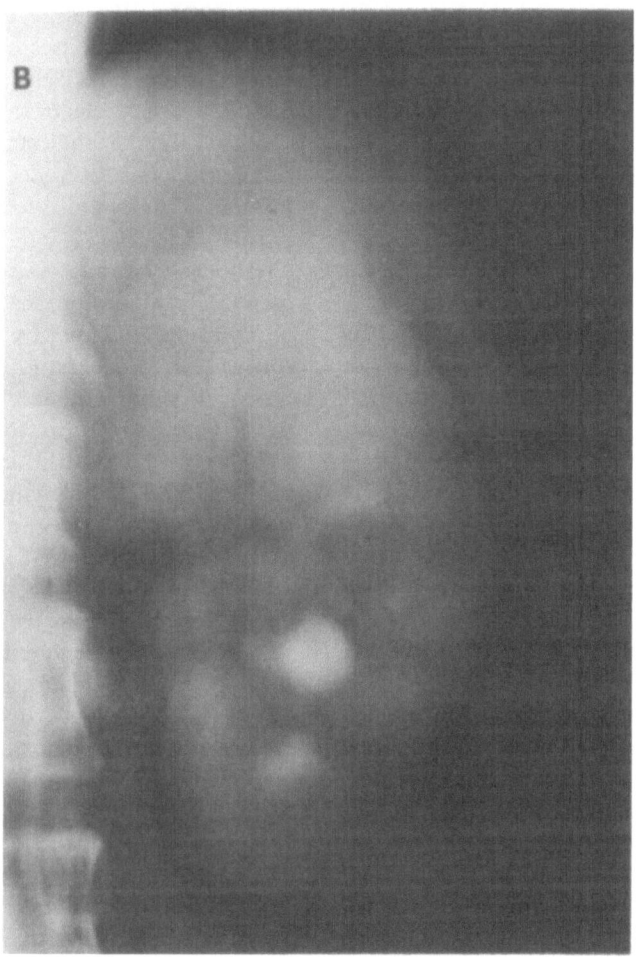

thral bladder neck resection [172, 173]. In children, urethral valves may be treated with sharp excision, cold disruption, or electrofulguration.

4.2 SUPRAVESCICAL OBSTRUCTION

Treatment of supravescical obstruction has the immediate objective of relieving the patient from uremic symptoms and the final objective of ensuring a durable urinary drainage. Both objectives can be attained simultaneously when (a) the cause of obstruction is rapidly diagnosed, (b) the basic disorder is curable surgically, and (c) the patient is in good condition, with mild uremia and low operative risk. This may be the case, for example, in a patient with radiopaque stone. More often, however, a two-step strategy has to be followed; this occurs when (a) the cause of obstruction is not established, or (b) the patient is at high operative risk, or (c) a medical treatment is indicated, beneficial effects of which will occur slowly. In these cases, in order to prevent life-threatening complications of uremia, emergency relief of the obstruction should be attempted and precede the final treatment. This may be performed either by means of ureteral catheterization or by percutaneous pyelostomy under echographic control. Usually, we prefer the latter procedure since it is less traumatic and carries less risk of infection. Should both percutaneous pyelostomy and ureteric catheterization fail, a surgical pyelostomy may be carried out. This, however, is a true surgical intervention (needing general anesthesia), the validity of which as a transitory drainage procedure is questionable. Today, in fact, dialysis facilities are widely available to ensure the survival of the patient and the achievement of that good clinical condition that will allow the definitive treatment to be performed on the basis of the cause and the site of obstruction [174].

In most cases of supravescical obstruction, treatment consists of surgical intervention, selection and actuation of which is a matter for the skilled urologist. Usually, ureterolysis is performed when obstruction is accounted for by extrinsic, noninvasive disorders encasing or compressing the ureter, such as retroperitoneal fibrosis, aortic aneurism, or enlarged para-aortic lymph nodes. While carrying out ureterolysis, special attention is needed to completely free the ureter(s), thus preventing recurrences [175]. An uretero-neocystostomy may be indicated to repair traumatic ureteric occlusion or to obviate obstruction of intramural part of the ureters due, for example, to prostatic cancer [176] or to cystitis glandularis [177]. When obstruction is caused by advanced, invasive retroperitoneal tumors, a palliative surgical procedure is selected among nephrostomy, ureterostomy, or the implantation of pyelo- or ureteralvescical prostheses. Nephrostomy is the treatment indicated for patients with a life expectancy longer than a few months. Internal prosthetic diversions, being of short duration but much more comfortable, are to be chosen for patients with poor prognosis [178].

In some instances, the obstructive disorder may be treated without surgery. Thus, uric acid calculi may be dissolved by administration of allopurinol and alkalinization of urine; sometimes catheter irrigation of the renal pelvis with sodium bicarbonate solution is necessary [179]. Calculi in the lower urinary tract may be eliminated by means of physical methods, such as ultrasound-lithotrypsy or administration of electrohydraulic waves. These methods require direct contact between the energy source and the stone. Recently, a promising technique has been developed to disintegrate stones by externally administered shock waves [180]. The patient is placed in a heated bathing tube, having an ellipsoidal section, at the bottom of which lays an energy source consisting of a high-voltage condensor spark discharge. The discharge electrodes are placed in one of the two focuses of the ellipsoid, and the renal stone is precisely positioned in the focus opposite to the electrodes by an x-ray scanning system. Thus, the shock waves originating from one focus are reflected from the surrounding wall and collected in the other focus against the stone.

Another condition when nonsurgical treatment of obstruction may be indicated is when obstruction is caused by advanced or inoperable tumors. Radiotherapy (4,000 to 6,000 rads during a period of four to six weeks) may relieve obstruction due to prostatic carcinoma [181, 182]. This tumor may also be sensitive to endocrine treatment (diethylstilbestrol, 3 mg/day, or cyproterone acetate, 200 mg/day) [181], especially when estrogens are associated with orchiectomy [183, 184]. Some patients with hormone-sensitive tumor respond very well to this therapy, and relief of obstruction may become evident in two or three days [183]. External radiotherapy is also an effective treatment of bladder carcinomas [185], while chemotherapy may dramatically resolve a condition of complete renal shutdown secondary to lymphomata [33, 186]. Finally, steroids (prednisone 60 to 80 mg/day for two to four weeks) have been shown to prevent recurrence and even to reverse obstruction due to perianeurismal or idiopathic retroperitoneal fibrosis [187, 188].

References

1. Lud Dureto, Segusiano (Interprete et Narratore): Hippocratis Magni Coacae, Lutetiae Parisiorum, Io Meiat, 1621.
2. Peacock M, Robertson WG, Heyburn PJ, Rutheford A. Urinary tract stone disease. Proc EDTA 16: 556–565, 1979.
3. Boyce WH, Garvey FK, Strawviter HE. Incidence of urinary calculi among patients in general hospitals. JAMA 161: 1437–1442, 1956.
4. Tschöpe W, Ritz E, Haslbeck M, Mehnert H, Wesch H. Prevalence and incidence of renal stone disease in a German population sample. Klin Wochenschr 59: 411–412, 1981.
5. Robson AJ, Calne RY. Complications of urinary drainage following renal transplantation. Brit J Urol 43: 586–590, 1971.
6. Malek GH, Uehling DT, Daouk AA, Kisken WA.

Urological complications of renal transplantation. J Urol 109: 173–176, 1973.

7. Kiser WS, Hewitt CB, Moutie JE. The surgical complications of renal transplantation. Surg Clin North Am 51: 1133–1140, 1971.

8. Rattazzi LC, Simmonds RL, Miller J, Casali R, Najarian JS. Acute ureteric obstruction of kidney transplant. Urology 4: 384–388, 1974.

9. Rao MS, Bapna BC, Bhat VN, Vaidyanathan S. Multiple urethral metastases from prostatic carcinoma causing urinary retention. Urology 10: 566–567, 1977.

10. Doran J, Roberts M. Acute urinary retention in the female. Brit J Urol 47: 793–796, 1976.

11. Firlit RS, Firlit CF, King LR. Obstructing anterior urethral valves in children. J Urol 119: 819–821, 1978.

12. Shapiro SR, Stratton ML, Adelman RD. Anuria in infants and children. J Urol 120: 227–228, 1978.

13. McGuire EJ, Weiss RM. Secondary bladder neck obstruction in patients with urethral valves. Urology 5: 756–758, 1975.

14. Touloukian RJ, Weiss RM. The obstructed bladder syndrome in the neonate. Surg Gynecol Obst 143: 965–969, 1976.

15. Harshman MW, Cromie WJ, Wein AJ, Duckett JW. Urethral stricture disease in children. J Urol 126: 650–654, 1981.

16. Willich E, Halsband H. Subvesicale Harnabflussstörungen im kindesalter und ihre Folgen für die harnableitenden Wege. Der Urologe 8: 279–288, 1969.

17. Gallo D, Presman D. Urinary retention due to fecal impaction in children. Pediatrics 45: 292–294, 1970.

18. Nelson RP, Brugh R. Bilateral ureteral obstruction secondary to massive fecal impaction. Urology 16: 403–406, 1980.

19. Rovich L. Constipation: A cause of urinary tract obstruction and infection. Urology 7: 236–237, 1976.

20. Shackelford GD, Manley CB. Acute ureteral obstruction secondary to bullous cystitis of the trigone. Radiology 132: 351–354, 1979.

21. Weisman MH, McDonald EC, Wilson CB. Studies of the pathogenesis of interstitial cystitis, obstructive uropathy, and intestinal malabsorption in a patient with systemic lupus erythematosus. Am J Med 70: 875–880, 1981.

22. Gangai M. Acute urinary obstruction secondary to neurologic diseases. J Urol 95: 805–808, 1966.

23. Kogan BA, Solomon MH, Diokno AC. Urinary retention secondary to Landry-Guillain-Barré syndrome. J Urol 126: 643–644, 1981.

24. Margolis GJ. A review of literature of psycogenic urinary retention. J Urol 94: 257–258, 1965.

25. Wanuck S, Schwimmer R, Orkin L. Carcinoma of the pancreas causing ureteral obstruction. J Urol 110: 395–396, 1973.

26. Vandendris M. Complete bilareral ureteral obstruc-

tion secondary to pancreatic carcinoma. Eur Urol 2: 43–44, 1976.

27. Tock EPC, Wee AST. Bilateral ureteric metastases causing complete anuria. Brit J Urol 40: 421–424, 1968.

28. Geller Se, Lin CS. Ureteral obstruction from metastatic breast carcinoma. Arch Pathol 99: 476–478, 1975.

29. Presman D, Ehrlich L. Metastatic tumors of the ureter. J Urol 59, 312–325, 1948.

30. O'Flynn JD. Seminoma with ureteric obstruction. Irish J Med Sci 379: 333–334, 1957.

31. Koziol I. Reticulum Cell Sarcoma. Unusual cause of ureteral obstruction. Urology 4: 456–458, 1974.

32. Loening S, Carson CC, Faxon DP, Morin LJ. Ureteral obstruction from Hodgkin's disease. J Urol 111: 345–349, 1974.

33. Abeloff MD, Lenhard RE. Clinical management of ureteral obstruction secondary to malignant lymphoma. J Hopkins Med J 134: 34–42, 1974.

34. Kay RG. Metastatic malignant, functional, postrenal anuria. Brit J Urol 34: 194–199, 1962.

35. Chantrie M, Vandendris M, Schulman CC. Management of ureteric obstruction in the solitary kidney by a segmental suspended ureteric prosthesis. Eur Urol 2: 286–288, 1976.

36. Pearlman CK, Mackey JF. Anuria resulting from abdominal aneurysm. J Urol 83: 184–187, 1960.

37. Marzo Franco JE, Alarcon Zurita A, Sala O'Shea E, Beltran la Torre J, Piza Bunola C, Dalmau Diana M, Morey Molina A, Ozonas Moragues M. Fracaso renal agudo de origen retroperitoneal. Rev Clin Espan 154: 37–42, 1979.

38. Lewis CT, Molland EA, Marshall VR, Tresidder GC, Blandy JP. Analgesic abuse, ureteric obstruction and retroperitoneal fibrosis. Brit Med J 2: 76–78, 1975.

39. Schumacker HB, Garret R. Obstructive uropathy from abdominal aortic aneurysm. Surg Ginecol Obst 100: 758–761, 1955.

40. Abercrombie GF, Hendry WF. Ureteric obstruction due to peri-aneurysmal fibrosis. Brit J Urol 43: 170–173, 1971.

41. Safran R, Sklenica R, Kay H. Iliac artery aneurysm: A common cause of ureteral obstruction. J Urol 113: 605–609, 1975.

42. Isaacson P, Jenning M. Bilateral ureteric obstruction in a patient with ileocecal Crohn's disease complicated by actinomycosis. Brit J Urol 49: 410, 1977.

43. Bentley PG, Higgs DR. Peritoneal tuberculosis with ureteric obstruction, mimicking retroperitoneal fibrosis. Brit J Urol 48: 170, 1976.

44. Willscher MK, Mozden PJ, Olsson CA. Retroperitoneal fibrosis with ureteral obstruction secondary to Actinomyces Israeli. Urology 12: 569–571, 1978.

45. Landes RR, Hooker JW. Sclerosing lipogranuloma and periureteral fibrosis following extravasation of urographic contrast media. J Urol 68: 403–408, 1952.

46. Ohlsen L. Retroperitoneal fibrosis due to leakage of urine. A contribution to the etiology of idiopatic retroperitoneal fibrosis. Acta Societatis Medicorum Upsaliensis 70: 231–240, 1966.

47. Partridge REN, Colvin RB. Necrotizing glomerulitis and arteritis, pulmonary nodules and ureteral obstruction. N Engl J Med 297: 1164–1172, 1977.

48. Debled G, Nercier G. La sclerose rétropéritonéale pelvienne d'origine radique associée à un fibrome utérin. Acta Urol Belg 46: 23–31, 1978.

49. Chung AF, Menou J, Dillon TF. Acute postoperative retroperitoneal fibrosis and ureteral obstruction secondary to the use of Avitene. Am J Obstet Gynecol 132: 908–909, 1978.

50. Elkin M, Goldman SM, Meng CH. Ureteral obstruction in patients with uterine prolapse. Radiology 110: 289–294, 1974.

51. Riddle PR, Shawdon HH, Clay B. Procidentia and ureteric obstruction. Brit J Urol 47: 387–390, 1975.

52. Stabler J. Uterine prolapse and urinary tract obstruction. Brit J Radiol 50: 493–498, 1977.

53. Gregoir W, Schulman CC, Chantrie M. Les obstructions urétérales dans les prolapsus utérine. J Urol Nephrol 82 (suppl 2): 414–420, 1976.

54. O'Shaughnessy R, Weprin SA, Zuspan FP. Obstructive renal failure by an overdistended pregnant uterus. Obstet Gynecol 55: 247–249, 1980.

55. Goldberg KA, Kwart AM. Intermittent urinary retention in first trimester of pregnancy. Urol 17: 270–271, 1981.

56. Wesolowki S. Bilateral ureteral injuries in gynecology. Brit J Urol 41: 666–675, 1969.

57. Lloyd-Davies. A case of bilateral ureteric obstruction following obstetrical trauma. Brit J Urol 41: 689–691, 1969.

58. Raney AM. Ureteral trauma: Effects of ureteral ligation with and without deligation. Experimental studies and case reports. J Urol 119: 326–329, 1978.

59. Rajfer J, Smith GW. Bilateral ureteral obstruction after repair of aortic aneurysm. J Urol 122: 255–256, 1979.

60. Rastogy SP, Reid JS. Bilateral ureteral obstruction following aortic bypass surgery. Clin Nephrol 14: 250–255, 1980.

61. Raymond G, Toubol J, Pastorini P, Mattei M. A propos d'un cas de tumeur bilatérale de l'uretère révélée par une anurie. J Urol Nephrol 84: 618–621, 1978.

62. Barroso CH Jr, Florence TJ, Scott C Jr. Bilateral papillary carcinomas of the ureters: Presentation of a case and 2-year follow-up report. J Urol 96: 451–454, 1966.

63. Simpson A, Ashby EC. Anuria due to ureteric obstruction by blood clot. Brit J Urol 38: 177–181, 1966.

64. Sitprija V, Nakamoto S, Kolff WJ. Hemodialysis in obstructive disease as a preliminary to urologic diagnosis. J Urol 89: 149–155, 1963.

65. Levin DL, Zimmerman AL, Ferder LF, Shapiro WB, Wax SH, Porush JG. Acute renal failure secondary to ureteral fungus ball obstruction in a patient with reversible deficient cell-mediated immunity. Clin Nephrol 5: 202–210, 1975.

66. Schindera F, Pringsheim W. Postrenales Nierenversagen infolge beidseitiger Ureter-Obstruktion durch Candida-albicans Pyelonephritis bei einem Säugling. Mschr Kinderheilk 125: 797–799, 1977.

67. Biggers R, Edwards J. Anuria secondary to bilateral ureteropelvic fungus balls. Urology 15: 161–163, 1980.

68. Masson JC, Bollack C, Renaud R, Gandar R. Uropathie obstructive par hématome de la gaine de droits de l'abdomen. J Urol Nephrol 81: 246–249, 1975.

69. Hull JD, Kumar S, Pletka PG. Reflex anuria from unilateral ureteral obstruction. J Urol 123: 265–266, 1980.

70. Shearlock KT, Howards SS. Post-obstructive anuria: A documented entity. J Urol 115: 212–213, 1976.

71. Mausion C, Petit J, Remond A, Lambrey G, Fournier A, Quichaud J. Décompensation d'un syndrome de jonction pyélo-urétérale, mécanisme de l'anurie "réflexe" a une obstruction pyélo-urétérale lithiasique controlatérale? Sem Hop Paris 53: 1711–1713, 1977.

72. Francisco LL, Hoversten LG, Di Bona GF. Renal nerves in the compensatory adaptation to the ureteral occlusion. Am J Physiol 238: F229–F234, 1980.

73. Rose JG, Gillenwater JY. Effects of obstruction on ureteral function. Urology 12: 139–145, 1978.

74. Michaelson G. Percutaneous puncture of renal pelvis, intrapelvic pressure and concentrating capacity of the kidney in hydronephrosis. Acta Med Scand (suppl) 559: 1–26, 1974.

75. Aubert J. Anurie calculeuse et rupture spontanée du bassinet. Intérêt de l'urographie intraveineuse chez l'anurique. Acta Urol Belg 41: 396–403, 1973.

76. Rovinescu I, Belanger PM, Fleurent B, Desbiens R. Considération sur la stase urétérale prolongée et ses conséquences. J Urol Nephrol 1–2: 67–74, 1974.

77. Rittemberg GM, Schabel SI, Nelson RP. Bilateral spontaneous urinary extravasation in ureteral obstruction. Radiology 127: 648, 1978.

78. Rao MS, Bapna BC, Subudhi CL, Rajendran LJ, Shrikhande VV, Rao KMK, Vaidyanathan S. Spontaneous rupture of renal pelvis during postobstructive diuresis. Eur Urol 5: 214–215, 1979.

79. Rose JG, Gillenwater JY. Pathophysiology of ureteral obstruction. Am J Physiol 225: 830–837, 1973.

80. Djurhuus JC. Dynamics of upper urinary tract. III. The activity of renal pelvis during pressure variations. Invest Urol 14: 475–477, 1977.

81. Gosling JA, Dixon JS. Functional obstruction of the ureter and renal pelvis. A histological and electron microscopic study. Brit J Urol 50: 145–152, 1978.

82. Koff SA. The diagnosis of obstruction in experi-

mental hydroureteronephrosis. Mechanism for progressive urinary tract dilatation. Invest Urol 19: 85–88, 1981.

83. Bhagavan BS, Wenk RE, Dutta D. Pathways of urinary backflow in obstructed uropathy. Hum Path 10: 669–683, 1979.

84. Lawson JD, Schneeberg AL, Tombinson WB. Observations on dynamics of acute urinary retention in the dog. J Urol 66: 678–685, 1951.

85. Osins TG, Hinman F Jr. Dynamics of acute urinary retention: A manometric, radiographic and clinical study. J Urol 90: 702–712, 1963.

86. Dal Canton A, Stanziale R, Corradi A, Andreucci VE, Migone L. Effects of acute ureteral obstruction on glomerular hemodynamics in rat kidney. Kidney Int 12: 403–411, 1977.

87. Moody TE, Vaughan ED, Gillenwater JY. Relationship between renal blood flow and ureteral pressure during 18 hours of total unilateral ureteral occlusion. Invest Urol 13: 246–251, 1975.

88. Gaudio KM, Siegel NJ, Hayslett JP, Kashgarian M. Renal perfusion and intratubular pressure during ureteral occlusion in the rat. Renal Fluid Electrol Physiol 7: 205–209, 1980.

89. Moody TW, Vaughan ED, Gillenwater JY. Comparison of the renal hemodynamics response to unilateral and bilateral ureteral occlusion. Invest Urol 14: 455–459, 1977.

90. Dal Canton A, Andreucci VE. Glomerular hemodinamics in ureteral obstruction. In Renal Pathophysiology, Leaf A, Giebish G, Bolis L, Gorini S (eds). New York: Raven Press, 1980, pp. 189–201.

91. Blackshear JL, Wathen RL. Effects of indomethacin on renal blood flow and renin secretory responses to ureteral occlusion in the dog. Mineral Electrolyte Metab 1: 271–278, 1978.

92. Saphasan S, Saraggananda B. Renal blood flow after bilateral ureteral ligation in the rat. Pflügers Arch 381: 165–169, 1979.

93. Morrison AR, Nishikawa K, Needleman P. Thromboxane A$_2$ biosynthesis in the ureteral obstructed isolated perfused kidney of the rabbit. J Pharmacol Exp Ther 205: 1–8, 1978.

94. Yarger WE, Schoken DO, Harris RH. Obstructive nephropathy in the rat. Possible roles for the renin-angiotensin system, prostaglandins, and thromboxanes in postobstructive renal function. J Clin Invest 65: 400–413, 1980.

95. Morrison AR, Benabe JE. Prostaglandins and vascular tone in experimental obstructive nephropathy. Kidney Int 19: 786–790, 1981.

96. Dal Canton A, Corradi A, Stanziale R, Maruccio GF, Migone L. Effects of 24-hour unilateral ureteral obstruction on glomerular hemodynamics in rat kidney. Kidney Int 15: 457–462, 1979.

97. Dal Canton A, Corradi A, Stanziale R, Maruccio GF, Migone L. Glomerular hemodynamics before and after release of 24-hour bilateral ureteral obstruction. Kidney Int 17: 491–496, 1980.

98. Huguenin ME, Thiel GT, Brunner FP, Thorhorst J, Flückiger EW, Wirz H. Regeneration du rein

après levée d'une occlusion de l'uretère chez le rat. Kidney Int 5: 221–232, 1974.

99. Vaugham ED, Gillenwater JY. Recovery following complete chronic unilateral ureteral occlusion: Functional, radiographic and pathologic alterations. J Urol 106: 27–35, 1971.

100. Miyazaki M, Mc Nay J. Redistribution of renal cortical blood flow during ureteral occlusion and renal venous constriction. Proc Soc Exp Biol Med 138: 454–461, 1971.

101. Abe Y, Kishimoto T, Yamamoto K, Ueda J. Intrarenal distribution of blood flow during ureteral and venous pressure elevation. Am J Physiol 224: 746–751, 1973.

102. Stein JH, Ferris TF, Huprich JE, Smith TC, Osgood RW. Effect of renal vasodilatation on the distribution of cortical blood flow in the kidney of the dog. J Clin Invest 50: 1429–1438, 1971.

103. Mc Nay JL, Abe Y. Pressure-dependent heterogeneity of renal cortical blood flow in dogs. Circ Res 27: 571–588, 1970.

104. Huland H, Leichtweiss HP, Augustin HJ. Changes in renal hemodynamics in experimental hydronephrosis. Invest Urol 18: 274–277, 1980.

105. Siegel NJ, Feldman RA, Lytton B, Hayslett JP, Kashgarian M. Renal cortical blood flow distribution in obstructive nephropathy in rats. Circ Res 40: 379–384, 1977.

106. Solez K, Pouchak S, Buono RA, Vernon N, Finer PM, Miller M, Heptinstall RH. Inner medullary plasma flow in the kidney with ureteral obstruction. Am J Physiol 231: 1315–1321, 1976.

107. Aluli E, Davis RS, Cockett ATK. Renin-angiotensin I activity in renal lymph during acute ureteral obstruction. Surg Forum 25: 536–537, 1974.

108. Eide I, Løyning E, Langård Ø, Kiil F. Mechanism of renin release during acute ureteral constriction in dogs. Circ Res 40: 293–299, 1977.

109. Freeman RH, Davis JO, Gotshall RW, Johnson JA, Spielman WS. The signal perceived by the macula densa during changes in renin release. Circ Res 35: 307–315, 1974.

110. Stitzer SO, Martinez-Maldonado M. Mechanism of decrease in plasma renin activity during volume expansion. Am J Physiol 230: 1550–1554, 1976.

111. Nascimento L, Harris AP, Ayala JM, Opawa-Stitzer S, Martinez-Maldonado M. Renin release: Effects of vasodilators and bilateral ureteral obstruction. J Pharmacol Exp Ther 212: 481–486, 1980.

112. Blackshear JL, Wathen RL. Effects of indomethacin on renal blood flow and renin secretory responses to ureteral occlusion in the dog. Mineral Electrolyte Metab 1: 271–278, 1978.

113. Gabriel R, Heslop RW. Reversible hypertension and hyperreninemia after accidental ureteric ligation. Brit Med J 2: 999–1000, 1977.

114. Riehle RA Jr, Vaughan ED Jr. Renin participation in hypertension associated with unilateral hydronephrosis. J Urol 126: 243–246, 1981.

115. Andaloro VA. Mechanism of hypertension produced

by ureteral obstruction. Urology 5: 367–371, 1975.

116. Squittieri AP, Ceccarelli FE, Wurster JC. Hypertension with elevated renal vein renins secondary to ureteropelvic junction obstruction. J Urol 111: 284–287, 1974.

117. Nagle RB, Bulger RE, Cutler RE, Jervis HR, Benditt EP. Unilateral obstructive nephropathy in the rabbit. I. Early morphologic, physiologic and histochemical changes. Lab Invest 28: 456–467, 1973.

118. Nagle RB, Johnson ME, Jervis HR. Proliferation of renal interstitial cells following injury induced by ureteral obstruction. Lab Invest 35: 18–22, 1976.

119. Nagle RB, Kneiser MR, Bulger RE, Benditt EP. Induction of smooth muscle characteristics in renal interstitial fibroblast during obstructive nephropathy. Lab Invest 29: 422–427, 1973.

120. Nagle RB, Ewans LW, Reynolds DG. Contractility of renal cortex following complete ureteral obstruction. Proc Soc Exp Biol Med 148: 611–614, 1975.

121. Erlam RJ. Recovery of renal function after prolonged ureteric obstruction. Brit J Urol 39: 58–62, 1967.

122. Better OS, Arieff AI, Massry SG, Kleeman CR, Maxwell MH. Studies on renal function after relief of complete unilateral ureteral obstruction of three months' duration in man. Am J Med 54: 234–240, 1973.

123. Wilson DR, Knox WH, Hall E, Sen AK. Renal sodium- and potassium-activated adenosine triphosphatase deficiency during post-obstructive diuresis in the rat. Can J Physiol Pharmacol 52: 105–113, 1974.

124. Nito H, Descoeudres C, Kurokawa K, Massry SG. Effect of unilateral ureteral obstruction on renal cell metabolism and function. J Lab Clin Med 91: 60–71, 1978.

125. Panko WB, Beamon CR, Middleton GW, Gillenwater JY. Effects of obstruction on renal metabolism. Renal tissue metabolite concentration after α-ketoglutarate infusion. Invest Urol 15: 331–339, 1978.

126. Novikoff AB. The proximal tubule cell in experimental hydronephrosis. J Biophys Biochem Cytol 6: 136–138, 1959.

127. Stecker JF, Panko WB, Gillenwater JY. Relationship of renal substrate utilization and patterns of renal excretion. Invest Urol 11: 221–224, 1973.

128. Yarger WE, Aynedjan HS, Bank N. A micropuncture study of postobstructive diuresis in the rat. J Clin Invest 51: 625–637, 1972.

129. Harris RH, Yarger WE. The pathogenesis of postobstructive diuresis. The role of circulating natriuretic and diuretic factors, including urea. J Clin Invest 56: 880–887, 1975.

130. Mc Dougal WS, Wright FS. Defect in proximal and distal sodium transport in post-obstructive diuresis. Kidney Int 2: 304–317, 1972.

131. Buerkert J, Alexander E, Purkerson ML, Klahr S. On the site of decreased fluid reabsorption after release of ureteral obstruction in the rat. J Lab Clin Med 87: 397–410, 1976.

132. Harris RH, Yarger WE. Renal function after release of unilateral obstruction in rats. Am J Physiol 227: 806–815, 1974.

133. Sonnenberg H, Wilson DR. The role of medullary collecting ducts in postobstructive diuresis. J Clin Invest 57: 1564–1574, 1976.

134. Buerkert J, Martin D, Head M. Effect of acute ureteral obstruction on terminal collecting duct function in the weanling rat. Am J Physiol 236: F260–F267, 1979.

135. Kessler RH. Acute effects of brief ureteral stasis on urinary and renal papillary chloride concentration. Am J Physiol 199: 1215–1218, 1960.

136. Houda N, Aizawa C, Morikawa A, Yoshitoshi Y. Effect of elevated ureteral pressure on renal medullary osmolal concentration in hydropenic rabbits. Am J Physiol 221: 698–703, 1971.

137. Buerkert J, Martin D, Head M, Prasad J, Klahar S. Deep nephron function after release of acute unilateral ureteral obstruction in young rats. J Clin Invest 62: 1228–1239, 1978.

138. Uhlich E, Baldamus C, Ullrich K. Einfluss von Aldosteron auf den Natriumtransport in den Sammelrohren der Säugetierniere. Pflügers Arch 308: 111–126, 1969.

139. Uhlich E, Habbach R, Ullrich KY. Einfluss von Aldosteron auf den Ausstrom markierten Natriums aus den Sammelrohren der Ratte. Pflügers Arch 320: 261–264, 1970.

140. Wilson DR. The influence of volume expansion on renal function after relief of chronic unilateral ureteral obstruction. Kidney Int 5: 402–410, 1974.

141. Harris RH, Yarger WE. Urine-reinfusion natriuresis: Evidence for potent natriuretic factors in rat urine. Kidney Int 11: 93–105, 1977.

142. Wilson DR, Honrath U. Cross circulation study of natriuretic factors in postobstructive diuresis. J Clin Invest 57: 380–389, 1976.

143. Thirakomen K, Kozlov N, Arruda JAL, Kurtzman NA. Renal hydrogen ion secretion after release of unilateral ureteral obstruction. Am J Physiol 231: 1233–1239, 1976.

144. Walls J, Buerkert JE, Purkerson ML, Klahar S. Nature of acidifying defect after the relief of ureteral obstruction. Kidney Int 7: 304–316, 1975.

145. Wright FS, Howards SS. Obstructive injury. In The Kidney, Brenner BM, Rector FC Jr (eds). Philadelphia: WB Saunders, 1981 (2nd ed) pp. 2026–2027.

146. Peterson LJ, Yarger WE, Shocken DD, Glenn JF. Post-obstructive diuresis: A varied syndrome. J Urol 113: 190–194, 1975.

147. Bourgoignie JJ, Hwang KH, Espinel C, Klahar S, Bricker NS. A natriuretic factor in the serum of patients with chronic uremia. J Clin Invest 51: 1514–1527, 1972.

148. Bricker NS, Bourgoignie JJ, Klahar S. A humoral inhibitor of sodium transport in uremic serum. Arch Intern Med 126: 860–864, 1970.

149. Gillenwater JY, Westervelt FB, Vaughan ED Jr, Howards SS. Renal function after release of chronic unilateral hydronephrosis in man. Kidney Int 7: 179–186, 1975.

150. Dal Canton A, Conte G, Balletta M, Meccariello S, Sabbatini M, D'Armiento M, Mirone V, Fina E, Andreucci VE. La funzione renale in pazienti con idronefrosi cronica unilaterale. Min Nefrol 28: 247–250, 1981.

151. Bullimore DWW. Retroperitoneal fibrosis associated with atenolol. Brit Med J 281: 564, 1980.

152. Kaplan WE, Schoenberg HW, Lyon ES, Strass FH, Gill WB. Flank pain in early renal failure. J Urol 121: 348–351, 1979.

153. Merril JP. Acute renal failure. In Disease of the kidney, Strauss MB, Welt LG (eds). Boston: Little Brown, 1971 (2nd ed), pp. 637–666.

154. Guarino JR. Auscultatory percussion of the bladder to detect urinary retention. N Engl J Med 305: 701, 1981.

155. Suki WN, Guthrie AG, Martinez-Maldonado M, Eknoyan G. Effects of ureteral pressure elevation on renal hemodynamics and urine concentration. Am J Physiol 220: 38–43, 1971.

156. Hoffman LM, Suki W. Obstructive uropathy mimicking volume depletion. JAMA 236: 2096–2097, 1976.

157. Hiatt N, Chapman LW, Davidson MB, Sheinkopf JA, Miller A. Inhibition of transmembrane K transfer in ureter-ligated dogs infused with KCl. Am J Physiol 231: 1660–1664, 1976.

158. Older RA, Van Moore A, Foster WL, Ladwig SH. Urinary tract obstruction. Current methods of evaluation. JAMA 245: 1854–1857, 1981.

159. Ellenbogen PH, Scheible FW, Talner LB, Leopold GR. Sensitivity of Gray Scale Ultrasound in detecting urinary tract obstruction. Am J Roengenol 130: 731–733, 1978.

160. Pollack HM, Arger PH, Goldberg BB, Mulholland SG. Ultrasonic detection of nonopaque renal calculi. Radiology 127: 233–237, 1978.

161. Vint VC, Usselman JA, Warmath MA, Dilley RB. Aortic perianeurismal fibrosis: CT density enhancement and ureteral obstruction. Am J Radiol 134: 577–580, 1980.

162. Pahira JJ, Wein AJ, Barker CF, Banner MP, Arger PH, Mulhern C, Pollack H. Bilateral complete ureteral obstruction secondary to an abdominal aortic aneurysm with perianeurysmal fibrosis: Diagnosis by computed tomography. J Urol 121: 103–106, 1979.

163. Stage KH, Lewis S. Use of radionuclide washout test in evaluation of suspected upper urinary tract obstruction. J Urol 125: 379–382, 1981.

164. Mayo ME, Hilton PJ, Jones NF, Lloyd-Davies RW, Croft DN. ^{131}I Hippuran Renogram in Acute Renal Failure. Brit Med J 3: 516–517, 1971.

165. Fry IK, Cattel WR. Radiology in the diagnosis of renal failure. Brit Med Bull 27: 148–152, 1971.

166. Turck M, Stamm W. Nosocomial infection of the urinary tract. Am J Med 70: 651–654, 1981.

167. Burke JP, Garibaldi RA, Britt MR, Jacobson JA, Conti M, Alling DW. Prevention of catheter-associated urinary tract infections. Efficacy of daily meatal care regimens. Am J Med 70: 655–658, 1981.

168. Garibaldi RA, Burke JP, Dickman ML, Smith CB. Factors predisposing to bacteriuria during indwelling urethral catheterization. N Engl J Med 291: 215–219, 1974.

169. Stamm WE. Guidelines for prevention of catheter-associated urinary tract infections. Ann Intern Med 82: 386–390, 1975.

170. Warren JW, Platt R, Thomas RJ, Rosner B, Kass EN. Antibiotic irrigation and catheter-associated urinary tract infections. N Engl J Med 299: 570–573, 1978.

171. Krane RJ, Olsson CA. Phenoxybenzamine in neurogenic bladder dysfunction. J Urol 110: 650–656, 1973.

172. Mollard P, Romagny G, Monfort G, Maréchal JM, Meunier P, Mélère G. Traitement des obstacles infra-vesicaux des vessies neurologiques. J Urol Nephrol 6: 349–358, 1975.

173. Petri E, Walz PH, Jonas U. Transurethral bladder neck operation in neurogenic bladder. Eur Urol 4: 189–191, 1978.

174. Fox M, Parsons FM. Value of dialysis in obstructive lesions of the upper urinary tract. Brit J Urol 41: 197–204, 1969.

175. Whitaker RH. Urodynamic assessment of ureteral obstruction in retroperitoneal fibrosis. J Urol 113: 26–29, 1975.

176. Leff RG, King DG. Ureteroneocystostomy for bilateral ureteral obstruction in carcinoma of prostate. Urology 11: 633–635, 1978.

177. Rao KG. Cystitis glandularis causing bilateral ureteric obstruction and hydronephrosis. Brit J Urol 47: 398, 1975.

178. Arvis G. Que peut-on attendre des prothèse en urologie? Acta Urol Belg 46: 43–57, 1978.

179. Eason AE, Sharlip ID, Spaulding JT. Dissolution of bilateral uric acid calculi causing anuria. JAMA 240: 670–671, 1978.

180. Brendel W, Chaussy C, Schmiedt E. Extracorporeally induced destruction of kidney stones by shock waves. Lancet 2: 1265–1268, 1980.

181. Michigan S, Catalona WJ. Ureteral obstruction from prostatic carcinoma: Response to endocrine and radiation therapy. J Urol 118: 733–738, 1977.

182. Megalli MR, Gursel EO, Demirag H, Veenema RJ, Guttman R. External radiotherapy in ureteral obstruction secondary to locally invasive prostatic cancer Urology 3: 562–564, 1974.

183. Khan AU, Utz DC. Clinical management of carcinoma of prostate associated with bilateral ureteral obstruction. J Urol 113: 816–819, 1975.

184. Abbou CC, Becquemin JP, Chopin D, Auvert J. Obstruction urétérale au cours du cancer de la prostate. Intérêt du traitement médical. Nouv Presse Med 8: 3025–3027, 1979.

185. Greiner R, Zaunbauer W, Skaleric K, Veraguth P. Lymphknotenmetastasen und Ureterobstruktion als

prognostische Parameter der perkutanen strahlentherapie des Harnblasen-Karzinoms. Strahlentherapie
154: 617–621, 1978.

186. Turner A, Osborn DE. Obstructed uropathy treated
by chemotherapy. Brit J Urol 51: 164, 1979.

187. Huben RP, Schellhammer PF. Steroid therapy for
ureteral obstruction after aortoiliac graft surgery. J
Urol 125: 881–883, 1981.

188. Arger PH, Stolz JL, Miller WT. Retroperitoneal
fibrosis: An analysis of the clinical spectrum and
roentgenographic signs. Am J Roentgenol Radium
Ther Nucl Med 119: 812–821, 1973.

20. ACUTE RENAL FAILURE FOLLOWING RENAL TRANSPLANTATION

Brian H. B. Robinson

1 The Special Problems Associated with Transplantation

Two problems unique to organ transplantation are the preservation of the functional integrity of the organ during transfer from donor to recipient and the prevention of subsequent immunological interaction with the new host. Thus, ischemic damage and immunological graft rejection are major causes of acute renal failure (ARF) following transplantation. To these crucial problems of transplantation must be added technical problems associated with vascular and ureteric anastomosis, the complications of opportunist infections secondary to immunosuppressive therapy and of nephrotoxic drugs, as well as many of the causes of ARF discussed elsewhere in this book.

Table 20–1 summarizes the major causes of ARF after renal transplantation.

The prevention and management of ARF following transplantation vary according to the time after grafting. Loss of renal function may, for convenience, be considered as (a) immediate, with no significant renal graft function from the time of transplantation; (b) early renal failure, with immediate or early onset of graft function but subsequent deterioration within the subsequent four to six weeks; (c) delayed renal failure between four weeks and three months after transplantation; and (d) late ARF developing more than three months after estab-

lishment of apparently adequate graft function. The probable causes and clinical management of graft failure vary with the chronology of the event in relation to initial operation. These aspects of ARF after transplantation are considered under these headings later in the chapter.

2 Pathogenesis and Prevention of Renal Failure After Transplantation

2.1 ISCHEMIC DAMAGE DURING ORGAN HARVESTING

The major cause of damage to the transplanted organ prior to establishing adequate perfusion by the circulation of the recipient is ischemia due to interruption of blood supply during organ harvesting, although infections, nephrotoxins, hyper- or hypotension, anoxia, and acidosis in the donor may cause serious agonal damage. Prolonged ischemia causes progressive cellular damage and autolytic changes in the kidney, which becomes no longer viable and unsuitable for organ grafting. The problem is how to obtain organs that are viable and avoid the hazards of transplanting organs that will not function. Nonviable kidneys have been suggested as the cause of graft failure in as many as 4.6% of recipients in one series [1], but, hopefully, such a high incidence is rare today.

The first histological change is loss of the brush border of the tubules, with subsequent cell swelling, disintegration, and interstitial edema. More severe ischemic damage leads to cortical necrosis. Not infrequently, there may

388

TABLE 20–1. Causes of acute renal failure after transplantation

Immediate	Early	Delayed
Hypovolemia (Blood loss, salt and water depletion, etc.)	Hypovolemia	Late acute tubular necrosis (secondary)
Ischemic and agonal injury	Acute rejection	Acute rejection
Acute tubular necrosis	Vascular occlusion	Arterial thrombosis
Cortical necrosis	Arterial	Arterial stenosis
Vascular occlusion	Venous	Venous thrombosis
Arterial	Allograft rupture or hematoma	Ureteric complications
Venous	Ureteric obstruction or leakage	Stenosis
Hyperacute rejection	Nephrotoxic drugs	Leakage
Ureteric obstruction or leakage	Septicemia or graft infection	Clot or calculus obstruction
	Viral infections	Nephrotoxic drugs
		Bacterial and fungal infections and septicemia
		Cytomegalovirus infection
		Lymphocele
		Recurrent glomerulonephritis
		Hypovolemia—salt-losing nephropathy

be an initial diuresis after restoration of circulation, but as a consequence of the ischemic injury, subsequent cell swelling and disorganization and interstitial edema develop and urine flow temporarily ceases.

Tubular changes may be found even when graft function appears good; more severe changes are associated with more prolonged oliguria, followed by gradual restoration of urine output and by slower restoration of urinary concentrating ability similar to the pattern in acute tubular necrosis from other causes. Very severe damage with cortical necrosis is likely to be irrecoverable; but with lesser degrees of ischemic damage, the majority of grafted kidneys, unless rejected, eventually recover to reach normal or near normal levels of renal function. The more severely damaged kidneys might be expected to develop later changes, such as interstitial fibrosis, and sclerosed glomeruli are frequent; but it is difficult to distinguish late changes that may be the result of acute ischemic damage from chronic minor rejection changes or the results of infection, drug toxicity, or even changes pre-existing in the donor kidney before removal. Some kidneys never recover more than moderate filtration rates after grafting, in the absence of obvious rejection, as a result of damage sustained during graft retrieval, yet such organs may con-

tinue without significant loss of function for many years. In general, it seems that if donor kidneys sustain more than minor damage because ischemia is prolonged or preservation techniques are inadequate, the donor tissues rapidly pass from a recoverable state to one of total nonviability. The emphasis in organ harvesting must therefore be on identifying the best techniques for retrieval and preservation. The major damage to a graft occurs while it is warm. Kidney survival improves exponentially with lowering of temperature, and preservation is better at 0°C than at 5°C [2, 3, 4]. Functional preservation is greatly prolonged, therefore, by graft cooling. The critical factor in organ retrieval is therefore the warm ischemic time [5, 6].

The length of time over which the arterial blood flow to a human kidney can be interrupted without producing severe damage is about one hour in surgical situations, such as aortic grafting, in which the flow may have to be interrupted by vascular clamping.

The major risk of ischemic damage to the kidney graft obviously arises during the period between clamping the artery of the organ to be transplanted and the completion of the vascular anastomosis with the recipient's circulation.

The use of a living donor requires satisfactory donor selection, skilled surgery, and close proximity to the prepared recipient. Both donor and recipient should be in ideal condition. The main difficulty is the need to ensure the safety of the donor even more than the satisfactory removal of the donor organ and its attached blood vessels and ureter.

Adequate preoperative hydration of the donor is important to ensure good early function after completion of the anastomosis in the recipient. With this proviso, immediate graft function is almost invariably the rule in live donor transplantation.

With cadaveric transplantation, apart from the technical need to reanastomose the organ into a foreign circulation, the problems are obviously more complex than with a living donor. By definition, the donor is "dead," and the premortal condition of the renal circulation may have been far from ideal. Circulation may have ceased for a variable length of time before nephrectomy is possible.

Graft injury may thus result from agonal damage even before organ removal [7].

The first requirement to minimize ischemic damage is obviously to harvest the organ for grafting under the best possible conditions. In cadaveric transplantation, the surgical niceties of live donor nephrectomy scarcely apply, although technique must be swift but careful. There are several recognized methods of removing cadaveric kidneys for transplantation [8], and they are not a subject for this review. Suffice it to say that damage to the kidney and attached blood vessels and ureter must be avoided, with due attention to the presence of polar arteries, if necessary by providing aortic patches. At nephrectomy, the viability and suitability of the donor organ must be assessed.

It is not so much the technique of harvesting as the circumstances of organ procurement that influence the extent of ischemc damage at this stage, and it is in attending to these circumstances that the ethical problems of cadaveric transplantation become most controversial.

The need for minimizing the period between circulatory arrest and organ harvesting raises qustions; questions about the diagnosis of death, the stage at which it is justifiable to remove the organs and in what conditions and in which situations, who is to give permission for organ removal, and who is to confirm that the donor is dead. These decisions are both ethical and legal. The legal definition of death varies from country to country, as does the definition of the designated legal owner of the cadaver, and as do the rights concerning the granting of consent to remove organs for transplantation.

There is growing acceptance, not only by the legal as well as the medical profession, but also by the lay public, of the concept of "brain death." With more assured criteria [9, 10] for ascertaining irrecoverable brain damage and legal acceptance of the diagnosis of brain death, it has been increasingly the practice in many countries to harvest kidneys from individuals with severe brain injuries, intracranial hemorrhages, etc., while the heart is still beating and the kidneys are adequately perfused. While kidneys taken after cardiac arrest may prove very satisfactory [11], there is no doubt that the use of kidneys from "heart beating" cadavers has greatly increased the percentage of grafts giving immediate renal function. In our own experience, in the early 1970s, diuresis was usually delayed for 5 to 20 days after grafting. Nowadays, early diuresis is almost the rule as a result of the improved circumstances of organ harvesting. It could be argued that if the potential donor is considered to be dead and the life support systems are to be withdrawn, it is illogical and even perhaps unethical to await final cardiac arrest after a period of anoxia and impaired or absent renal perfusion. Unfortunately, the law in some countries requires that cardiac arrest must take place. Removal of a well-perfused kidney ensures better graft survival, and the early diuresis prevents many of the diagnostic dilemmas of the early posttransplant period (see below), makes management easier, and almost certainly improves the well-being of the patient at this stage.

Another clinical dilemma surrounding cadaveric kidney harvesting concerns the desirability of donor pretreatment [12]. Ensuring adequate hydration and urine flow is clearly good treatment for the donor, but whether the use of mannitol infusions or drug therapy such as phenoxybenzamine is justifiable is an ethical question. Most groups would accept the theory that treatment is acceptable, as long as it can do no harm and particularly does not hazard the survival of a potential donor. Once a diagnosis of brain death is established, the decision to intervene becomes less questionable, but there should be no undue delay in organ procurement both to save distress to relatives and to diminish the risks of infection and other complications in the donor.

Following organ removal, a variable time must inevitably elapse before vascular anastomosis can be completed and circulation restored. If the best use is to be made of a kidney graft by selecting and preparing a recipient and if necessary transporting the kidney to the recipient—not merely across a city, but, as now sometimes happens, across a continent or continents—then some mode of preservation is required.

It is important to distinguish "warm ischemia time" from "cold ischemia time." The former comprises the sum of the time from cessation of renal circulation to the time at which the kidney is cooled and the time spent after removing the kidney from cold preservation to completion of vascular anastomosis in the donor and removal of the arterial clamps. Cold ischemia time is that time spent in cold preservation. Clearly, warm ischemia time must be as short as possible, but many earlier studies were concerned with how long the kidney would remain viable after cessation of effective circulation and removal from the donor.

Studies in dogs suggest that warm ischemia time (a) less than one hour is followed by early recovery, (b) up to two hours, is followed by delayed recovery, and (c) of periods longer than two hours result in permanent loss of function [13]. Similar figures seem to apply in man [6, 14] although warm ischemic times should be less than 30 minutes.

When warm ischemic time has been kept brief, storage of the cooled kidney can still result in a viable graft after 12 hours with simple cooling in ice alone. More effective cooling and preservation is produced by perfusion with ice-cold solutions. Considerable debate has continued as to the best solution for preservation, whether simple Ringer-lactate, or solutions of predominantly "extracellular," or "intracellular" fluid composition are preferable.

During ischemia and cooling, potassium is lost from cells, and sodium tends to enter. Both research studies and clinical experience suggest that fluids of intracellular composition, sometimes made hyperosmolar with a poorly diffusible solute such as mannitol or sucrose, give the best results [15, 16]. The solution most often used is that of Collins [15] (see table 20–2).

Perfusing the kidney has the advantage of rapid cooling and undoubtedly can enhance survival of a viable organ as well as give some idea of the quality of the vasculature of the organ—although conclusions drawn about viability from ease of perfusion can be misleading. The drawbacks are that poor perfusion technique can damage the graft artery or introduce infection.

The use of equipment to maintain continuous perfusion, either normothermic or hypothermic with oxygenated solutions, has been widely practised, especially in the United States. The hope is that prolonged graft preservation by such techniques will allow more careful selection and preparation of recipients. The drawbacks, aside from technical failures, are the difficulty of transporting kidneys complete wth perfusion machine and technician and the risk of damage to the transplant artery. In fact, some reports suggest that continuous machine perfusion confers little benefit and may result in poorer graft survival than simple cold rinsing [17, 18]. Apart from damage to the graft vessels, microembolism by thrombus, platelet aggregates, denatured colloid, and lipid in the perfusion fluid may have deleterious effects. In fact, careful harvesting and cooling with ice-cold "intracellular" solutions prolongs viable graft survival well beyond 24 hours [16] and is quite adequate to permit transport over long distances, HLA matching, cytotoxicity cross-matching, and even DR

TABLE 20–2. Collins' c_3 solution

	mmol/liter		mmol/liter
Sodium	10	Sulphate	30
Potassium	15	Phosphate	50
Magnesium	30	Chloride	15
		Bicarbonate	10
Glucose	139 mmol/liter	pH	7.0

matching. Machine perfusion, particularly with solutions containing colloid, may prolong graft survival, but it is doubtful whether machine perfusion adds any real advantages in the present state of the art. Prolonged storage at low temperatures seems a possibility for the future. This would permit transplantation on a much more elective basis and in theory better organ matching, but the feasibility for human grafting as well as the balance of advantage remain to be established even when the techniques are available.

Perioperative prevention of ischemic damage includes the restoration of adequate perfusion as soon as possible. This implies not only good surgical technique—though not necessarily hasty technique—but a recipient in ideal condition. In fact, both donor and recipient should be adequately hydrated, whether the former is a live or potential cadaveric donor. A previously diuresing kidney would seem to be less readily damaged by ischemia during transfer [12]. Over enthusiastic preoperative dialysis of the recipient may leave him hypovolemic, and the consequent poor graft perfusion may augment ischemic damage as well as increase the chances of graft artery or vein thrombosis (see below).

Finally, although we have been concerned here with minimizing ischemic damage, it has been suggested that a period of tubular necrosis after grafting might in some way protect against early immunological rejection. Theoretically, this might arise either because of the continuing immunosuppressive effect of uremia or because circulatory impairment diminishes the rate of immune recognition of graft antigen and the rate at which antibody and immune effector cells are carried to the graft. Later studies have failed to confirm that a period of oligo-anuria protects against early rejection in comparison with grafts that function immediately, and our Birmingham experience does not suggest that there is a protective effect of early oliguria.

Finally, concerning prevention, one must discuss the role not only of adequate hydration, but also of the use of loop diuretics such as furosemide in reducing or overcoming ischemic damage. It is doubtful whether these agents have any effect on established ischemic damage, but they may have a role in minimizing

the effects of such damage before oliguria is established, as well as being helpful in assessing the degree of functional impairment. It is not uncommon for an initial brisk diuresis to be followed after a few hours—up to 24 hours—by a sharp cutback in urine output. One has the clinical impression that this cutback in urine production may be diminished or prevented by timely administration of furosemide or other potent diuretics, so long as subsequent salt depletion is avoided.

The clinical management of ischemic graft damage will be discussed later in this chapter.

2.2 GRAFT REJECTION

A detailed review of the immunological mechanisms of graft rejection is out of place in this review concerned with acute renal failure. There have been a number of reviews of knowledge concerning the immune response to allografting [19, 20] and the immunogenetics of tissue grafting [21, 22].

In individuals not previously sensitized to histocompatibility antigens, the earliest histological changes usually appear about 48 hours after grafting with infiltration by mononuclear leucocytes along the capillaries and into the interstitium with subsequent proliferation. The majority of the infiltrating lymphoid cells are T cells but include B cells [23, 24]. Capillary walls fragment, and ischemic changes affect the glomeruli. The humoral component of the immune response, the formation of circulating antibody by sensitized cells, is thought to be mainly responsible for the vascular changes of rejection, including fibrinoid necrosis of arterioles, clumping of platelets with occlusion of small vessels, and reduplication and fibrosis of the endothelium of larger vessels seen in chronic rejection. Following early tissue damage from rejection, fibrosis follows later on.

The clinical expression of allograft rejection may appear as follows:

(a) *Hyperacute rejection.* This term is applied to rejection occurring within the first 48 hours of transplantation [25]. It is due to humoral antibody in individuals already immunized against histocompatibility antigens [26] or transplanted across ABO blood group incompatibility [27].

The phenomenon can often be diagnosed before the completion of the transplant operation; a kidney having become pink after revascularization then appears cyanosed and flabby. Hyperacute rejection is usually accompanied by high fever, even rigors, some systemic upset, and occasionally a microangiopathic hemolytic anemia [28, 29].

Microscopy reveals polymorphonuclear infiltration, platelet aggregation, and fibrin in capillaries, leading to thrombosis of arterioles and small arteries (see chapter 6), interstitial edema, and hemorrhage with later cortical necrosis. The condition has been likened to the Schwarzman reaction.

Hyperacute rejection is irreversible.

(b) *Acute rejection.* Characteristically, acute rejection occurs between 7 and 21 days after transplantation although in presensitized individuals it may occur sooner. Later episodes of acute rejection may occur several months or up to a year after grafting, and occasionally later if immunosuppressive drugs are reduced or withdrawn, or sometimes in response to infection. Acute rejection usually presents with fever, swelling of the graft with local tenderness, malaise, and fall in urinary output and rise in serum urea and creatinine. The blood pressure may rise. The majority of cadaver graft recipients have one episode of acute rejection, which is usually reversed by a short course of high-dose steroid therapy, but the condition may recur, either becoming irreversible or necessitating such repeated high doses of steroids or other immunosuppressive agents as to increase the risk of secondary infection.

Histologically, the acutely rejecting kidney shows, in varying degrees, interstitial edema, infiltration by lymphoid cells, and swelling of the endothelial cells of the peritubular capillaries with splitting of the basement membranes. These are the changes of cell-mediated rejection. They are usually accompanied and frequently overshadowed in the immunosuppressed patient by the changes of humoral rejection, which include platelet aggregation in the capillaries and arterioles progressing to fibrinoid necrosis of arterioles.

The chances of reversal by therapy are usually greater when the picture is one of predominant cellular rejection. Probably, many minor episodes of the latter reverse spontaneously [30].

(c) *Chronic rejection.* After the first few months, rejection changes tend to show as gradual deterioration in function rather than episodes. There is slow loss of glomerular filtration rate, and proteinuria is sometimes heavy enough to produce the nephrotic syndrome. Hypertension may become a major clinical problem. The main changes are in the arterioles and arteries of any size, with intimal thickening from continuing deposition of platelets and fibrin [31]. These changes are followed by interstitial fibrosis and tubular atrophy. There is focal thickening of glomerular basement membranes, and epithelial crescents may form. This type of rejection is rarely reversible.

From the above account it is clear that the main problem in differential diagnosis of acute renal failure arises with the first two types of rejection; the approach to diagnosis will be discussed later.

2.3 PREVENTION OF ACUTE RENAL FAILURE FROM REJECTION

Research into prevention of rejection has concentrated on three aspects: the achievement of close histocompatibility, the use of nonspecific suppression of the immune response to the graft, and attempts to achieve donor-specific immunosuppression.

2.3.1 Histocompatibility Matching The importance of avoiding ABO blood group incompatibility has been indirectly mentioned above. The discovery of the major human histocompatibility antigen systems genetically controlled by the HLA system raised the hope that careful matching for the HLA A and B antigens between donor and recipient would enhance survival. Despite promising early studies, more recent large-scale surveys suggest that although there is a correlation between HLA-A, B matching, and graft survival, the effect is not large [32, 33, 34] perhaps of the order of up to 20%. More recently, there has been increasing interest in the influence of matching for HLA-DR on graft survival [34, 35] since these antigens may be the major stimulant for immune response to a graft. To date, the results of the best DR matches are encouraging for the chances of improved graft survival [36, 37].

Other histocompatibility systems, such as the Lewis system, remain to be evaluated or discovered.

For the present, in the field of cadaver grafting, histoincompatibility of some degree has to be accepted, usually with, as yet, no great influence on the chances of graft survival within a reasonable range of incompatibilities. However, sensitization to histocompatibility antigens may result from previous failed transplants, blood transfusion, or pregnancies. Earlier studies suggested that if the patient's antibodies cross-react with donor lymphocytes, hyperacute rejection is likely [26]. Later it was suggested that positive B cell cross-matches might be less significant if the T-cell match is negative. It seems desirable to avoid transplantation in the presence of a positive cross-match, but for some patients with a high titre of antibodies, a more sophisticated study of the nature of the antibodies may be necessary if they are to receive a graft [38].

2.3.2 Nonspecific Immunosuppresion Although various techniques—such as irradiation, lymphocyte depletion by thoracic duct drainage, total lymphoid irradiation, and the administration of antilymphocyte globulin (ALG)—have been used in human transplantation, the latter in particular with some possible long-term advantage [39], the mainstay of imunosuppressive therapy in human renal transplantation has been prednisolone and azathioprine. Both drugs have toxic effects and increase the risk of opportunistic infections. In recent years, there has been a tendency in many centers to start with more moderate doses of steroid [40] with improved patient survival. Acute rejection episodes are treated with large oral doses of prednisolone for two to four days or with bolus injections or methylprednisolone. ALG has also

been used in the therapy of rejection.

Because of the side effects and not infrequent failures of conventional immunosuppression, the search has continued for alternative therapies. One promising new agent is cyclosporin A, isolated from the fungus Trichoderma polysporin. The effect is nonspecific, but cyclosporin A, usually initially combined with prednisolone, has proved effective in a number of patients with cadaveric renal grafts [41]. Unfortunately, the drug has proved to be nephrotoxic [41, 42]. Personal experience suggests the drug has value, but some impairment of overall graft renal function seems to be almost the rule. The true role and value of cyclosporin A remains to be determined, but it seems particularly valuable in diabetics, permitting withdrawal of steroids.

One other finding in recent years has been the effect of blood transfusion. Formerly avoided because of the risks of sensitization, it became clear during the 1970s that prior blood transfusion enhances the overall rate of successful grafting [34, 38], and many centers will not contemplate cadaveric grafting in patients who have not previously received blood transfusion. The ideal protocol is still the subject of research, and the means by which transfusion influences graft survival remains, at the time of writing, the subject of much speculation and study.

2.3.3 Donor-specific Immunosuppression This is the ideal, the aim being to suppress immunity to the graft but leave the recipient's overall immune system intact, particularly to infection and to potentially malignant cells. So far in human cadaveric transplantation, this goal seems far away, but techniques such as enhancement and the induction of anti-idiotypic immunity [43] offer some promise of success. The use of donor-specific blood transfusion in human live donor transplantation may come under the heading of specific immunosuppression.

2.4 SURGICAL AND MECHANICAL PROBLEMS AS A CAUSE OF GRAFT FAILURE

2.4.1 Vascular Complications The vascular anastomosis of the donor organ to the recipient's vessels may be complicated by difficulties and damage during organ procurement, by atheroma in the recipient's iliac vessels and by the presence of multiple vessels, especially small polar vessels. Arterial thrombosis complicates 1 to 2% of grafts [44], and at least some of these incidents are precipitated by intimal tears during surgery, perfusion cannula damage, awkward "lie" of the kidney in situ after grafting, or are secondary to acute rejection. Careful attention to these details must be the major line of prevention.

Later, arterial stenosis may develop but is more likely to cause hypertension and slowly progressive renal failure rather than an acute episode.

Venous occlusion has a slightly lower incidence in most series and in our experience is more often suspected than found. The causes include angulation of the vein after anastomosis, extension of thrombosis in a hypercoagulable subject, pressure from a lymphocele or urinary extravasation or proximity to infection. Acute thrombosis may present with oliguria, proteinuria, hematuria, and graft enlargement. There may be signs of iliac vein occlusion. Apart from technical considerations, prophylactic anticoagulation may, rarely, be indicated in predisposed subjects.

2.4.2 Ureteric Complications The incidence of these complications varies between 2 and 8% of grafts. A major factor in prevention is care of the ureter in organ procurement, to avoid damge to the tenuous blood supply, and great care in making the anastomosis to avoid narrowing or kinking. The two major problems are disruption or the ureteric anastomosis with extravasation of urine and obstruction to the ureter by kinking or stenosis. The latter may be early or late. Obstruction by thrombus is an occasional problem.

Late obstruction may be due to stricture from fibrosis, either ureteral or periureteral secondary to previous urinary extravasation or infection or to a lymphocele. Ureteric calculi are rare but in one of our 800 patients caused ureteric obstruction. It is not altogether unknown for an inexperienced transplant surgeon to anastomose the ureter to the peritoneal cavity instead of the bladder—fortunately a rare cause for anuria!

Ureteric leakage is probably more often due to ischemia than to rejection changes involving the ureter, which seem less common than once supposed.

2.5 MISCELLANEOUS COMPLICATIONS OF TRANSPLANTATION LEADING TO ARF

2.5.1 Fluid Depletion and Related Problems The ischemically damaged organ is susceptible to further damage from insults, such as hypovolemia secondary to salt and water loss or hemorrhage. Recurrence of acute tubular necrosis can occur in a graft that has recovered from the initial ischemia.

Apart from the obvious restitution of blood volume in the event of hemorrhage, salt and water depletion may follow sustained diuresis after grafting if the full extent of fluid requirement is not appreciated. Some transplanted kidneys become significantly salt losing for several weeks after establishment of satisfactory diuresis; salt supplements are therefore necessary. Many patients have avoided salt during their previous years on dialysis and may need considerable encouragement to take salt once a functioning graft is established. On the other hand, many patients continue to retain sodium, particularly while on high doses of steroids.

2.5.2 Infections and Drugs Overwhelming septicemia complicating renal failure may be associated with impaired renal function, sometimes by inducing disseminated intravascular coagulation. Overwhelming renal infection with bacteria or fungi in the immunosuppressed patient may directly depress graft function. Virus infections, particularly cytomegalovirus (CMV), involve the kidney [45, 46]. There has been interest in polyoma virus as a possible factor in renal impairment or even in ureteric obstruction in transplanted patients [47, 48].

Unfortunately, many drugs, including che motherapeutic agents used for infection in transplanted patients, are nephrotoxic and can themselves harm the graft. Examples include the aminoglycoside antibiotics such as genta-mycin, some cephalosporins (notably cephalor-idin), and amphotericin B and the immunosup-pressive agent cyclosporin (see chapter 2). These drugs must be used with caution and only if essential in the transplanted patient. Their nephrotoxic potential is often enhanced, in the diuresing patient, by the use of potent diuretics such as furosemide.

3 Clinical Management of Acute Renal Failure After Transplantation

The problems presented by renal failure after transplantation differ according to time at which the renal failure follows the operation. The timing can be conveniently considered un-der four headings:

a. *Immediate renal failure*, in patients who re-main anuric after transplantation or fail to pass more urine after operation than that produced previously by their own kidneys.
b. *Early postoperative acute renal failure*, where the fall in urine output occurs 24 hours to 21 days after grafting.
c. *Delayed postoperative acute renal failure*, devel-oping between three weeks and three months after grafting.
d. *Late renal failure*, developing more than three months after grafting.

3.1 IMMEDIATE RENAL FAILURE

This is probably the most difficult diagnostic situation following renal transplantation. In this situation, we include those patients who have an immediate diuresis at the time of sur-gery but whose urinary flow falls within 24 hours. The most common cause of immediate posttransplant renal failure is acute tubular ne-crosis due to ischemic damage. The incidence varies from more than 50% of grafts down to less than 10%. The incidence has become much lower with improved techniques of organ procurement and preservation. The diagnosis of this condition is sometimes made difficult in the first few days because the patient's own kidneys continue to secrete urine; it is therefore useful to have established the normal level of residual renal function in the recipient before

grafting. The residual urine volume may even be augmented as a result of an increased post-operative urea load. Some centers use high doses of furosemide or other loop diurectis, hoping to augment urine flow, in an attempt to distinguish if the transplant function is re-covering. What is more important is attention to the adequacy of fluid balance in the postop-erative period. Preoperative dialysis, blood loss, and restriction of fluids before, during, and after surgery can contribute to hypovole-mia and be responsible for postoperative oli-guria and even for the aggravation of ischemic tubular damage. Conversely, fluid overload must also be avoided.

One early concern is to recognize vascular occlusion, which may require immediate sur-gery or hyperacute or accelerated acute rejec-tion, which may pose a risk to the patient. Re-jection at this early stage is usually accom-panied by high fever and malaise. These two symptoms are very suggestive of rejection be-cause severe infection at this time is unusual unless it be due to postoperative chest compli-cations. Arterial occlusion is uncommon but more difficult to recognize.

In the diagnosis of early anuria or oliguria, an isotope scan of the transplant (usually with ^{99m}Tc DTPA) is very helpful. Arterial occlu-sion, irrecoverable ischemic damage with cor-tical necrosis, or hyperacute rejection will ap-pear as a "cold" scan, the region of the allograft remaining poorly perfused and showing no iso-tope uptake compared with the background (figure 20–1). Such a scan is an indication for early surgical exploration. The scan in ATN will show a vascular phase, but little accumu-lation of urine nor delineation of ureter or blad-der. The scan of a functioning transplant is il-lustrated for comparison in figures 20–2 and 20–3.

The evaluation of graft tenderness in the first few postoperative days may be difficult, al-though any change for the worse or evidence of graft swelling is likely to be significant of re-jection, hemorrhage, leakage of urine, or ve-nous occlusion.

Acute tubular necrosis per se is not accom-panied by systemic upset; indeed, the improve-ment in well-being of the patient in compari-

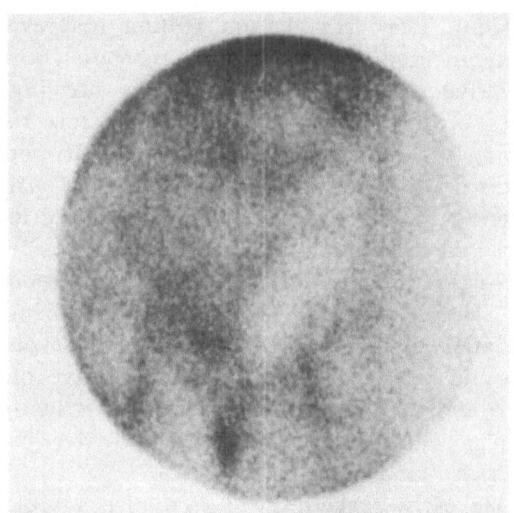

FIGURE 20–1. Use of ^{99m}Tc DTPA scanning after renal transplantation: "cold" scan showing no uptake of radioactivity in the region of an irreversibly rejected graft.

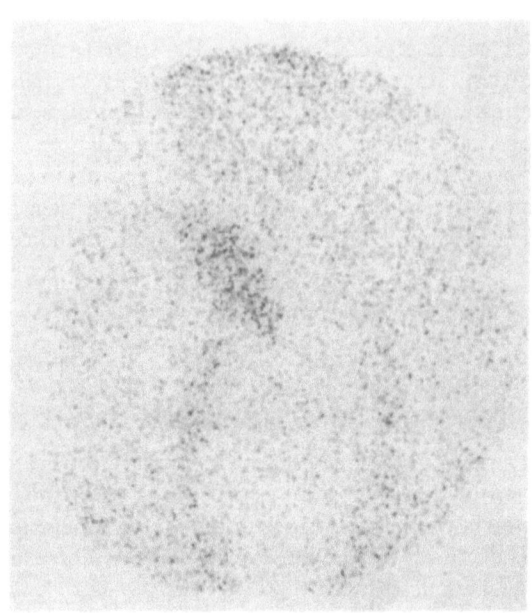

FIGURE 20–2. Use of ^{99m}Tc DTPA scanning after renal transplantation: scan of a functioning transplant showing early uptake of activity by the graft (iliofemoral vessels appear in the background).

son with the preoperative condition is sometimes very striking despite the continuing oliguria. This may in part be psychological or due to the euphoria of steroid therapy, but the restoration of metabolic and endocrine functions of the kidney may play a part.

As long as the patient remains well and the isotope scan confirms a well vascularized graft, there is no immediate indication to intervene in the face of continuing oligo-anuria. This phase, due to ischemic ATN, may last an average of seven to ten days, but longer periods of three to four weeks with subsequent excellent graft function are by no means rare. Our personal record, with eventual recovery of satisfactory renal function, is 12 weeks. The problem, in the face of continuing oliguria, is to recognize the development of acute but potentially reversible rejection. This is one reason why early graft function is so valuable, since the signs of reduction in urine volume and rise in serum creatinine, which may herald rejection in the diuresing patient, are not available in oliguria. The clinically suspicious signs are the appearance of fever, tachycardia, and graft swelling and tenderness in the absence of evidence of infection. Many tests have been devised to detect early rejection (table 20–3), but not all of these are valid in the presence of

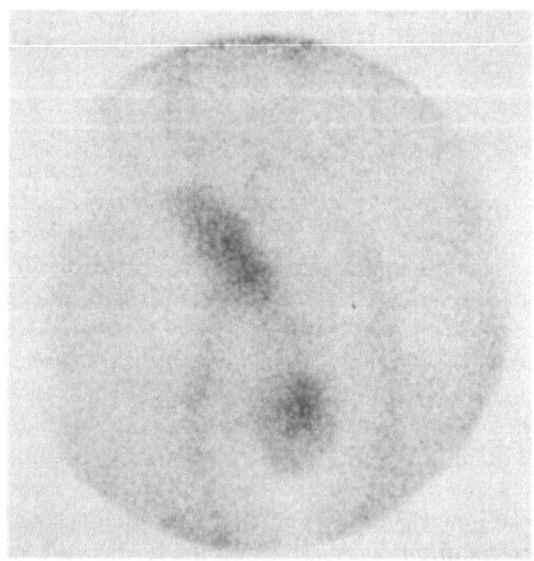

FIGURE 20–3. Use of ^{99m}Tc DTPA scanning after renal transplantation: later scan than that in figure 20–2 showing well-defined graft and outlining bladder, confirming satisfactory drainage of the urine secreted by the graft.

ATN nor do they all give the rapid and reliable answers so often required clinically. Isotope scanning does not give a very positive answer until vascular rejection is well advanced although ultrasound scanning, a commendably safe and easy investigation, may be of value not only in detecting obstruction with distention of the renal pelvis and calyces, but also in recording the increased kidney size, prominent medullary pyramids, and disturbed echogenicity said to be associated with rejection but not seen with ATN [56] (see chapter 9). In the absence of a quick, reliable bedside test, acute rejection initially has to remain a clinical diagnosis.

Renal biopsy is very valuable in confirming and assessing the development of rejection but does carry a small risk of damage to the graft. Transplant centers therefore differ in their enthusiasm for the technique. Fine-needle aspiration [57] is safe but requires expert interpretation. The latter is undoubtedly a very promising line of investigation.

TABLE 20–3. Tests for detecting early rejection

Clinical (see text)
  Falling urine volume and fluid retention; graft
    enlargement
  and tenderness, fever, rising blood pressure
Routine laboratory tests
  Leucocytosis and platelet count, rising blood urea or
    creatinine values
  Proteinuria
  Urine cytology (lymphocytes)
Immunological
  Serum complement or immunoconglutinin levels
  Activated lymphocytes in peripheral blood
  Mixed lymphocyte culture
  Macrophage migration inhibition [49]
  Rosette inhibition [50]
  Leucocyte aggregation
  Fibrin degradation products [51]
Biochemical
  Urine enzymology—Lysozyme, N-acetyl-β-D-
    glucosaminadase [52]
  Beta$_2$-microglobulin monitoring [53]
Radionuclide scanning
  Radionuclide renography
  Radio-labeled fibrinogen uptake [54]
  Uptake of [III]Indium labeled platelets [55]
Ultrasound scanning [56]
Histology
  Renal biopsy
  Fine-needle aspiration [57]

If there is clinical eason to suspect rejection is developing (and 60 to 70% of such acute episodes are accompanied by fever), it is usually safe to give a short sharp course of high dose prednisolone or bolus methylprednisolone. If there is not a brisk response or infection is present, the diagnosis is best confirmed by needle biopsy.

Should there be no clinical hint of rejection but oliguria continues, the clinician enters a phase of dilemma between the need to intervene and assess progress and the desirability of avoiding unnecessary "trauma" to patient and graft. A good guideline is the general well-being of the patient. The appearance of any increase in urine volume is an encouraging sign; some centers reduce the frequency of maintenance dialysis to avoid dehydration and provide a greater osmotic load to encourage diuresis. It is important, however, not to prejudice the patient's well-being and resistance to infection. When useful renal function returns, it usually soon becomes evident and may be more safely tested by administering a loop diuretic.

During the oliguric phase, therefore, careful clinical monitoring and occasional ultrasound scanning may be augmented by isotope scanning when doubt is present. After 10 to 14 days oliguria, a needle biopsy may reveal unsuspected rejection or may provide a clue to the severity of ischemic tubular changes and some guide to the likely rate of recovery.

Obstruction to ureteric drainage may at first be difficult to detect. Graft tenderness and fever may be mistakenly diagnosed as rejection until extravasated urine appears from the wound. Some surgeons leave a fine Tizzard catheter in the ureter at operation, by which retrograde radiological studies may be performed, but the results are not always reliable and obstruction may develop after such a catheter is removed. Ultrasound scanning may reveal a collection of fluid, and isotope scanning may reveal whether urine is being formed and collecting (figure 20–3). Further evidence as to the drainage of the graft may sometimes be obtained by cystography, for transplant ureters not infrequently show vesico-ureteric reflux. The demonstration of free reflux from bladder to renal pelvis excludes the presence of obstruction.

In this early oliguric phase, problems such as infection and drug nephrotoxicity are less likely to arise, although the considerations discussed in the next section should be borne in mind.

3.2 EARLY ACUTE RENAL FAILURE

Although oliguria due to acute tubular necrosis can develop after a brief initial diuresis, the most common cause of renal failure after transplant diuresis is established is acute allograft rejection. The cardinal signs of rejection in the diuresing kidney are reduction in urine volume and decreased excretion of urea, creatinine, and sodium reflected in increasing weight and rise in blood urea and creatinine, fever, tachycardia, malaise, and enlargement and tenderness of the graft. There may be detectable increases in proteinuria and in numbers of lymphocytes in the urine. The blood pressure not infrequently rises. Some or all of these signs suggest the need for antirejection therapy, although the usual careful clinical assessment is required to exclude salt and water depletion, infection, hemorrhage, obstruction, or other incidental complications. Acute rejection may be mimicked by ureteric leakage with extravasation of urine in the region of the graft, acute venous occlusion, or rupture of the allograft [12]. Acute pain, tenderness, and shock usually make the latter diagnosis easy, but oliguria sometimes develops and the symptoms are not always so acute as to make the diagnosis immediately apparent.

In the previously well, diuresing patient, the diagnosis of acute rejection may appear clearcut, confirmed if necessary by biopsy. Greater difficulty lies in recognizing rejection if fever and other signs are absent. Some of the tests listed in table 20–3 were designed to detect very early rejection although how early one needs to start therapy is dubious. Many well-functioning kidneys show some changes of rejection, and minor episodes that reverse without additional steroid therapy are probably common [30]. Nevertheless, oliguria without fever and graft tenderness poses a diagnostic problem. Salt and water depletion should be

excluded, the drug chart scanned for nephrotoxic agents, and evidence for ureteric obstruction or vascular complications sought. Venous occlusion may be accompanied by edema extending into the thigh or clear evidence of iliofemoral thrombosis. Ultrasound scan and isotope scanning may be particulary helpful in differentiating obstruction from rejection.

In the patient who has recovered renal function, excretion urography may be added as a technique sometimes helpful in identifying obstruction or extravasation of urine. This may be helpful, too, if ultrasonic scanning suggests a fluid collection because hemorrhage, abscesses, or lymph collections may cause extrinsic obstruction.

The real challenge in diagnosis and management arises in the patient who develops fever and oliguria in the presence of overt infection. Inappropriate antirejection therapy may jeopardize the life of the patient. In this situation, the investigative tools already discussed must be fully employed. The contribution of infection to recurrent acute tubular necrosis or intravascular coagulation and renal failure must be assessed, and nephrotoxic drugs such as gentamycin or amphotericin B used only where appropriate. Dosage and effect must be carefully monitored. It may be necessary to decide whether it is justifiable to proceed with treatment for rejection if infectious complications are progressing and the graft is failing or whether the risks to the patient outweigh the chances of recovery. Biopsy may be helpful here: extensive vascular changes with fibrinoid necrosis suggest that response is likely to be poor; predominantly cellular changes suggest a potentially reversible situation. Unfortunately, the needle biopsy may occasionally be unrepresentative of the whole.

We have made little mention of surgical exploration in these two sections. Surgical exploration of the graft is necessary if obstruction, ureteric leak, vascular occlusion, total rejection, or capsular splitting are diagnosed or suspected. But it is as well to base these diagnoses on firm evidence. Needless exploration may be complicated by poor wound healing, and infection can further complicate the patient's recovery.

3.3 DELAYED ACUTE RENAL FAILURE

Acute renal failure developing more than three weeks after grafting is rarely due to acute tubular necrosis although the latter may be due to severe hypovolemia, hemolysis, or nephrotoxins. Acute rejection remains a common problem at this stage and may in fact be precipitated by reduction in steroid dosage, or the use of drugs such as anticonvulsants, which interfere with steroid metabolism, or by discontinuation of azathioprine because of leucopenia. The diagnostic features of acute rejection described earlier still apply, but the picture may be complicated by more chronic and often progressive changes, although acute rejection at this stage may still be reversible.

Urinary obstruction may develop several weeks after transplantation as a result of necrosis or stenosis at the site of anastomosis or secondary to extrinsic pressure from a lymphocele. The latter condition is often associated with edema of the ipsilateral leg and may be detected ultrasonically.

Patients at this stage of recovery occasionally have a salt-losing nephropathy, and azotemia may develop secondarily as a result of the hypovolemia. Overuse of potent diuretics may produce a similar result.

To the many causes of deteriorating renal function a few weeks after transplantation must be added the possibility of recurrent (or even de novo) glomerulonephritis, particularly focal segmental glomerulonephritis. Recurrent disease is uncommon at this early phase, however, and is more likely to manifest as proteinuria rather than as renal failure [58, 59].

Deterioration in renal function at this stage demands full investigation, and biopsy may be helpful if obstruction has been excluded. Frequently, any deterioration is multifactorial, with the combined effects of rejection, infection, ischemic or obstructive damage, and potentially nephrotoxic antibiotics. The coincidence of infection and rejection is particularly difficult to handle because of the need to maintain immunosuppression yet control infection. Sometimes, when overwhelming infection remains uncontrolled by antimicrobial agents, it is necessary to make a decision to sacrifice the graft in order to save the patient's life by withdrawing immunosuppressive drugs.

A note is required here about cytomegalovirus (CMV), which may infect as many as 60 to 96% of transplant patients within the first month to one year [48]. Often this is an asymptomatic infection or may be a reactivation of latent virus. CMV infection is one of the most common causes of fever in the period of one to six months after transplantation. Radiologically, these patients show patchy lung changes in the lower lobes, sometimes spreading to focal or more generalized consolidation. Leucopenia and thrombocytopenia are serious complications, and superinfection with other opportunist agents and gastrointestinal bleeding are the major threats to life.

There is increasing evidence that CMV may itself induce renal lesions, either a diffuse glomerulopathy with endothelial cell enlargement and necrosis and accummulation of mononuclear cells [45] or tubulo-interstitial changes [46]. Such renal lesions may mistakenly encourage an increase in immunosuppressive therapy on the basis that the failing renal function reflects rejection, whereas a reduction in immunosuppression might be more beneficial. Renal biopsy, a search for other evidence of CMV infection, and possibly a search for viral induced changes in the T-cell subsets [48] will help to differentiate.

A further complication in the management of renal transplantation arises with the use of cyclosporin A as an immunosuppressive agent. Although this agent can be very effective in renal transplantation and may have certain advantages, it does have the serious drawback over conventional immunosuppresion (steroids, azathioprine, ALG) that it is nephrotoxic [60]. Experience suggests that acute rejection reactions are less florid with cyclosporin A, but deterioration in renal function during treatment with this drug may occur either from direct nephrotoxicity or rejection and is difficult to distinguish on clinical grounds. Further use of some of the tests listed in table 20–3 may be particularly valuable in this clinical dilemma. Reduction in cyclosporin A dosage with temporary increase in prednisolone dosage may be the only simple way of resolving the clinical situation. In the absence of coicident rejection, renal biopsies do not show the cellular infiltrate characteristic of the latter but reveal focal epithelial cell degeneration and interstitial edema, tubular casts, and, in the longer term, interstitial fibrosis and proximal tubular atrophy [61]. Sometimes the changes are slight or absent despite functional deterioration. Renal tubular damage often manifests as systemic acidosis and hyperkalemia.

When serious doubt remains, it is necessary either to reduce dosage or to change to steroids and azathioprine. The latter maneuver is not without the risk of precipitating acute rejection, on the one hand, or excessive immunosuppression, on the other. Probably, such transfers of therapy need to be gradual.

3.4 LATE RENAL FAILURE

Acute renal failure is a much rarer complication three months or more after transplantation, gradual loss of renal function from chronic rejection being much more common, although this may present as "acute on chronic" failure if the patient has escaped supervision or in consequence of a coincidental medical or surgical problem.

Acute rejection episodes may nevertheless develop, sometimes inexplicably but more often because of interference with immunosuppressive medication or failure of patient compliance. Such episodes are not always reversible.

Obstruction due to ureteric stenosis may develop after months or years. Transplant artery stenosis is a late complication that may present as hypertension, but in our experience more often as insidious renal failure. Acute arterial occlusion remains a rare possibility.

Full investigation, including pyelography and if indicated arteriography, is indicated if acute renal failure supervenes at this late stage since surgical correction of ureteric or even arterial stenosis is usually possible.

4 Prospects in Prevention and Management

The prevention of graft failure must be a high priority. The preservation of cadaver organs has reached a satisfactory standard in the best centers, and further advances here must await the development of long-term preservation techniques and of simple tests for graft viability.

Closer identification of the vital factors in histocompatibility matching is needed; currently, attention is being given to the evaluation of DR matching. In the field of specific immunosuppression, elucidation of the mechanism of the blood transfusion effect may give important clues, particularly with the promising results from donor specific transfusions.

We require improved immunosuppressive drugs with less toxicity. Cyclosporin A suggests, at least, that such drugs exist, but the nephrotoxicity of this drug remains a drawback. Increasing skill is being acquired in handling opportunist infections, but agents for safe control of CMV are required.

The apparent graft tolerance shown by long-term recipients suggests that such tolerance might be induced in potential recipients if the mechanism were understood.

In clinical management, the major advance will be a simple bedside test for rejection. Quite possibly, simplification and refinement of some of the tests in table 20–3 will meet this need.

References

1. Jacobs C, Brunner FP, Chantler C, Donckerwolcke RA, Gurland HJ, Hathway RA, Selwood NH, Wing AJ. Combined report on regular dialysis and transplantation in Europe, VII, 1976. Proc Eur Dial Transpl Assoc 14:4–67, 1977.
2. Schloerb PR, Waldorf RD, Welsh JS. The protective effect of kidney hypothermia on total renal ischemia. Surg Gynecol Obstet 109: 561–565, 1959.
3. Harvey RB. Effect of temperature on function of isolated dog kidney. Amer J Physiol 197: 181–186, 1959.
4. Marshall V. Organ preservation. In Tissue Transplantation, Morris PJ (ed). Edinburgh and London; Churchill Livingstone, 1982, pp. 40–59.
5. Hall CL, Sansom JR, Obeid M, Dawson-Edwards P, Robinson BHB, Barnes AD, Blainey JD. Agonal phase, ischemic times, and renal vascular abnormalities and outcome of cadaveric kidney transplants. Brit Med J 3: 667–670, 1975.
6. Marshall VC, Ross H, Scott DF, McInnes S, Thomson N, Atkins RC. Preservation of cadaveric renal allografts—Comparison of flushing and pumping techniques. Proc Eur Dial Transpl Assoc 14: 302–309, 1977.
7. Marshall VC. Organ preservation. In Clinical Organ

Transplantation, Calne RY (ed). Oxford and Edinburgh; Blackwell, 1971, pp. 55–103.

8. Sells RA. The selection of cadaver donors and removal of kidneys for transplantation. In Clinical Organ Transplantation, Calne RY (ed). Oxford and Edinburgh; Blackwell, 1971, pp. 183–198.

9. Report of the Ad Hoc Committee of the Harvard Medical School to examine the definition of brain death. JAMA 205: 337–340, 1968.

10. Diagnosis of brain death: Conference of the Medical Royal Colleges and their faculties in the United Kingdom. Br Med J 2: 1187–1188, 1976.

11. van der Vliet JA, Sloof MJH, Kootstra G, Krom RAF, Rijkmans BG. Non-heartbeating donors, is it worthwhile? Proc Eur Dial Transpl Assoc 17: 445–448, 19

12. Clunie G. Renal transplantation I. Selection and preparation of donors, immunosuppression and surgical complications. In Organ Transplantation, Chatterjee SN (ed). Littleton, Ma, and Bristol: Wright PSG, 1982, pp. 151–219.

13. Friedman SM, Johnson RL, Friedman CL. The pattern of recovery of renal function following renal artery occlusion in the dog. Circ Res 2: 231–235, 1954.

14. Gibson GR, Storey BG, Rogers JH, May J, Sheil APR. Early function in renal allografts from cadaver donors. Aust New Z J Surg 39: 35–37, 1969.

15. Collins GM, Bravo-Shugarman M, Terasaki PI. Kidney preservation for transport. Initial perfusion and 30 hours ice storage. Lancet 2: 1219–1222, 1969.

16. Bany JM, Lieberman S, Wickre C, Lieberman C, Fisher S, Craig D: Human kidney preservation by intracellular electrolyte flush followed by cold storage for over 24 hours. Transplantation 32: 485–487, 1981.

17. Opelz G, Terasaki PI. Advantages of cold storage over machine perfusion for preservation of cadaver kidneys. Transplantation 33: 64–68, 1982.

18. Spees EK, Oakes DD, Hill GS, Light JA, Williams GM, Ernst CB. Why some preserved kidneys do not function: A review of preservation-related endothelial injuries. Transpl Proc 14: 80–85, 1982.

19. Calne RY. The immunological background of organ grafting. In Organ Grafts. Current Topics in Immunology, Turk J (ed). London: Arnold, 1975, pp. 11–21.

20. Steinmuller D. The immune response to a tissue allograft. In Tissue Transplantation, Morris PJ (ed). Edinburgh: Churchill Livingstone, 1982, pp. 14–27.

21. Ketel BL, Stuart FP. Immunology of transplantation. In Organ Transplantation, Chatterjee SN (ed). Littleton, Ma, and Bristol: Wright PSG, 1982, pp. 15–44.

22. White AG. Histocompatibility antigens. In Organ Transplantation, Chatterjee SN (ed). Littleton Ma, and Bristol: Wright PSG, 1982, pp. 45–92.

23. Haskill JS, Häyry P, Radov LA. Systemic and local immunity in allografts and cancer rejection. Con-

temp Top in Immunobiol 8: 107–170, 1978.

24. Graves M, Janossy G. Elicitation of selective T and B lymphocyte response by cell surface binding ligands. Transplant Rev 11: 87–130, 1972.

25. Williams GM, Hume DM, Hudson RP Jr, Morris PJ, Kano K, Milgrom F. Hyperacute renal-homograft rejection in man. N Engl J Med 279: 611–618, 1968.

26. Kissmeyer-Neilson F, Olsen S, Petersen VP, Fjeldborg O. Hyperacute rejection of kidney allografts, associated with pre-existing humoral antibodies against donor cells. Lancet 2: 662–665, 1966.

27. Starzl TE, Marchioro TL, Holmes JH, Hermann G, Brittain RS, Stonington OH, Talmage DW, Waddell WR. Renal homografts in patients with major donor-recipient blood group incompatibilities. Surgery 55: 195–200, 1964.

28. Williams GM. Clinical course following renal transplantation. In Kidney Transplantation: Principles and Practices, Morris PJ (ed). London: Academic Press; New York: Grune and Stratton, 1979, pp. 203–214.

29. Katz J, Lurie A, Kaplan BS, Krawitz S, Metz J. Coagulation findings in the hemolytic-uremic syndrome of infancy. Similarity to hyperacute renal allograft rejection. J Pediatr 78: 426–434, 1971.

30. Kreis H, Noël LH, Lacombe M, Crosnier J. Spontaneously reversible steroid-independent "rejection" episode following cadaver kidney transplantation. Transpl Proc 11: 1220–1221, 1979.

31. Porter KA. Renal transplantation. In Pathology of the Kidney, Heptinstall RH (ed). Boston: Little, Brown, 1974, pp. 977–1041.

32. Patel R, Mickey MR, Terasaki PI. Serotyping for homotransplantation. XVI. Analysis of kidney transplants from unrelated donors. N Engl J Med 279: 501–506, 1968.

33. Opelz, G. Mickey MR, Terasaki PI. HLA and kidney transplants: Re-examination. Transplantation 17: 371–382, 1974.

34. Van Rood JJ, Persijn GG, Lansbergen Q, Cohen B, van Leeuwen A, Bradley BA. How can HLA matching improve kidney graft survival? Proc Eur Dial Transpl Assoc 16: 297–304, 1979.

35. Ting A, Morris PJ. Matching for B-cell antigens of the HLA-DR series in cadaver renal transplantation. Lancet 1: 575–577, 1978.

36. Ting A, Morris PJ. Powerful effect of HLA-DR matching on survival of cadaveric renal allografts. Lancet 1: 282–283, 1980.

37. Svejgaard. DR matching and cadaver kidney transplantation. Transplantation 33:1–2, 1982.

38. Ting A. HLA and organ transplantation. In Tissue Transplantation, Morris PJ (ed). Edinburgh; Churchill Livingstone, 1982, pp. 28–39.

39. Salaman JR. Non-specific immunosuppression. In Tissue Transplantation, Morris PJ (ed). Edinburgh; Churchill Livingstone, 1982, pp. 60–69.

40. Buckels JAC, Mackintosh P, Barnes AD. Controlled trial of low- versus high-dose oral steroid therapy in

100 cadaver renal transplants. Proc Eur Dial Transpl Assoc 18: 394–398, 1981.

41. Morris PJ. Cyclosporin A. Transplantation 32: 349–354, 1981.

42. Hamilton DV, Evans DB, Henderson RG, Thiru S, Calne RY, White DJG, Carmichael DJS. Nephrotoxicity and metabolic acidosis in transplant patients on cyclosporin A. Proc Eur Dial Transpl Assoc 18: 400–407, 1981.

43. Fabre JW. Specific immunosuppression. In Tissue Transplantation, Morris PJ (ed). Edinburgh; Churchill Livingstone, 1982, pp. 80–94.

44. Vidne BA, Leapman SB, Butt KM, Kountz SL. Vascular complications in human renal transplantation. Surgery 79: 77–81, 1976.

45. Richardson WP, Colvin RB, Cheeseman SH, Tolkoff-Rubin NE, Herrin JT, Cosimi AB, Collins AB, Hirsch MS, McCluskey RT, Russell PS, Rubin RH. Glomerulopathy associated with cytomegalovirus viremia in renal allografts. N Engl J Med 305: 57–63, 1981.

46. Cameron J. Rigby RJ, van Deth AG, Petrie JJ JB. Severe tubulo-interstitial disease in a renal allograft due to cytomegalovirus infection. Clin Nephrol 18: 321–325, 1982.

47. Mackenzie EFD, Poulding JM, Harrison PR, Amer B. Human polyoma virus—A significant pathogen in renal transplantation. Proc Eur Dial Transpl Assoc 15: 352–359, 1978.

48. Rubin RH, Tolkoff-Rubin NE. Viral Infection in the Renal Transplant Patient. Proc Eur Dial Transpl Assoc 19: 513–526, 1982.

49. House AK, Boak JL, Hulme B. An in vitro study of renal allograft recipients for cellular delayed type hypersensitivity to GBM and disrupted spleen cells. Clin Exp Immunol 11: 165–172, 1972.

50. Thomas F, Lee HM, Lower RR, Thomas JM. Value of immunologic monitoring studies of human E, EA, and EAC rosetting lymphocyte subpopulations in renal and cardiac transplantation. Transpl Proc 13: 1599–1603, 1981.

51. Hall CL, Pejhan N, Thomson RW, Dawson-Edwards P, Barnes AD, Robinson BHB, Meynell MJ, Blainey JD. Serial estimation of urinary fibrin/fibrinogen degradation products in kidney transplantation. Br Med J 3: 204–207, 1973.

52. Wellwood JM, Ellis BG, Hall JH, Robinson DR, Thompson AE. Early warning of rejection? Br Med J 2: 261–265, 1973.

53. Schweizer RT, Moore R, Bartus SA, Bow L, Hayden J. Beta 2-microglobulin monitoring after renal transplantation. Transpl Proc 13: 1620–1613, 1981.

54. Yeboah ED, Chisholm GD, Short MD, Petrie A. The detection and prediction of acute rejection episodes in human renal transplants using radioactive fibrinogen. Br J Urol 45: 273–280, 1973.

55. Griño JM, Alsina J, Martin J, Roca M, Castelao A, Romero R, Caralpi A. Indium-III labelled autologous platelets as a diagnostic method in kidney allograft rejection. Transpl Proc 14:198–200, 1982.

56. Cruz C, Hricak H, Eyler WR, Levin NW, Uniewski M. Sonographic features of ATN and of acute rejection in renal allografts. Proc Eur Dial Transpl Assoc 17: 413–427, 1980.

57. Häyry P, von Willebrand E. Transplant aspiration cytology in diagnostic evaluation of renal allografts. Transpl Proc 13: 1574–1578, 1981.

58. Cameron JS, Turner DR. Recurrent glomerulonephritis in allografted kidneys. Clin Nephrol 7: 47–54, 1977.

59. Pinto J, Lacerda G, Cameron JS, Turner DR, Bewick M, Ogg CS. Recurrence of focal segmental glomerulosclerosis in renal allografts. Transplantation 32: 83–89, 1981.

60. Calne RY. Cyclosporin. Nephron 26: 57–63, 1980.

61. Hamilton DV, Evans DB, Thiru S. Toxicity of cyclosporin A in organ grafting. In Cyclosporin A, White DJG (ed). Amsterdam; Elsevier Biochemical Press, 1982, pp. 393–411.

21. CONSERVATIVE MANAGEMENT AND GENERAL CARE OF PATIENTS WITH ACUTE RENAL FAILURE

Vittorio E. Andreucci

1 Treatment of Prerenal ARF

Physicians must bear in mind that prerenal ARF, if untreated, may progress to acute tubular necrosis [ATN] [1]. Thus, prerenal ARF must be treated as early as possible.

1.1 HYPOVOLEMIA DUE TO RENAL FLUID LOSS

In addition to the possibility of severe loss of blood in the urine (e.g., gross hematuria in uremic patients with polycystic renal disease), hypovolemia may follow urinary losses of salt and water. This may, for instance, occur in salt-losing nephritis and in diabetic ketoacidosis.

1.1.1 Hypovolemia in Salt-Losing Nephritis
The so-called "salt-losing nephritis" may cause prerenal ARF with hypotension (see chapter 2, section 2). This renal impairment is readily reversed by i.v. infusion of normal saline solution (0.9 g/dl, 154 mmol/1 NaCl) (table 21–1) and maintained by a high oral intake of salt; the improvement in renal function is mirrored by the fall in serum creatinine (see figure 21–1). As much as 25 grams of oral salt daily may be necessary to maintain stable renal function.

1.1.2 Hypovolemia Due to Severe Diabetic Ketoacidosis As described in chapter 2 (section 2), patients with severe diabetic acidosis de-velop marked renal loss of salt and water leading to ECV contraction and prerenal ARF; hyperglycemia also causes osmotic diffusion of water from cells to the extracellular fluid with consequent hyponatremia and intracellular dehydration [2].

Under such circumstances, since urinary losses of water and salt are hypotonic, water and salt replacement should also be hypotonic; if too much salt is given, hypernatremia may result, which prevents cell rehydration and maintains excessive osmotic diuresis even when hyperglycemia has been corrected [2].

Some authors prefer the i.v. infusion of one-half normal saline solution (0.45 g/dl, 77 mmol/l NaCl) [2]. In order to avoid the possible occurrence of hemolysis with hypotonic solutions, it is preferable to alternate normal (isotonic) saline (0.9 g/dl, 154 mmol/l, NaCl) with 5 g/dl (278 mmol/l) dextrose (or fructose) while providing adequate insulin therapy. The infusion rate may vary between 500 and 1,000 ml/hour, depending on severity of dehydration and degree of shock. In patients with severe hypotension or hypovolemic shock, isotonic saline should be given first and in large volume (2 to 3 liters i.v.), since glucose solutions (or hypotonic saline solutions) will not adequately correct ECV contraction because of a rapid shift of water to the intracellular compartment [2].

Whether or not diabetic ketoacidosis should be treated by bicarbonate administration while giving insulin is still a matter of debate. Insulin therapy, which should be given by i.v. in-

TABLE 21–1. Composition of commonly used parenteral solutions

Solutions g/dl	Concentration mmol/l	Concentration of ions mmol/l					Osmolality mOsm/kg H$_2$O
		Na$^+$	K$^+$	Ca^{++}	Cl$^-$	HCO$_3^-$(*)	
DEXTROSE (D-GLUCOSE) OR FRUCTOSE (mol. wt. 180.16)							
5 g/dl	278	—	—	—	—	—	278
10 g/dl	555	—	—	—	—	—	555
20 g/dl	1,110	—	—	—	—	—	1,110
30 g/dl	1,665	—	—	—	—	—	1,665
50 g/dl	2,775	—	—	—	—	—	2,775
MANNITOL (mol. wt. 182.17)							
5 g/dl	275	—	—	—	—	—	275
20 g/dl	1,098	—	—	—	—	—	1,098
25 g/dl	1,372	—	—	—	—	—	1,372
SODIUM CHLORIDE (SALINE) SOLUTIONS (NaCl, mol. wt. 58.45)							
0.45g/dl (half-normal, hypotonic)	77	77	—	—	77	—	154
0.9 g/dl (normal, isotonic)	154	154	—	—	154	—	308
3 g/dl (hypertonic)	513	513	—	—	513	—	1,026
5 g/dl (hypertonic)	855	855	—	—	855	—	1,710
SODIUM BICARBONATE SOLUTIONS (NaHCO$_3$, mol. wt. 84.00)							
1.4g/dl (1/6M) (isotonic)	167	167	—	—	—	167	334
5g/dl (0.6M) (hypertonic)	595	595	—	—	—	595	1,190
7.5g/dl (0.9M) (hypertonic)	893	893	—	—	—	893	1,786
8.4g/dl (1M) (hypertonic)	1,000	1,000	—	—	—	1,000	2,000
SODIUM LACTATE SOLUTION (NaC$_3$H$_5$O$_3$, mol. wt. 112.07)							
1.87g/dl (1/6M) (isotonic)	167	167	—	—	—	167	334
RINGER'S SOLUTION (NaCl,KCl,CaCl$_2$)		147	4	5	156	—	312
RINGER'S LACTATE SOLUTION (NaCl,KCl,CaCl$_2$, NaC$_3$H$_5$O$_3$)		130	4	3	109	28	274
DARROW'S SOLUTION (NaCl,KCl, NaC$_3$H$_5$O$_3$)		121	35	—	103	53	312
THAM (TRIS) (C$_4$H$_{11}$NO$_3$, mol. wt. 121.14)							
3.6g/dl (0.3M)		30	5	—	35	300	370

(*)HCO$_3^-$ or equivalent.

fusion (e.g., 4–8 U/hour) particularly in hypotensive patients (hypoperfused muscles may impede absorption of insulin given intramuscularly), reverses the diabetic ketoacidosis by metabolizing beta-hydroxybutyrate and acetoacetate to bicarbonate [2]. However, when arterial blood pH is less than 7.15 and serum bicarbonate less than 8 mmol/l, 40 to 80 mmol of sodium bicarbonate should be given i.v. [2]; this may be done by i.v. infusion of isotonic sodium bicarbonate (250 to 500 ml of 1.4 g/dl, 1/6 M NaHCO$_3$ solution, with 167 mmol/l). Should the hypovolemic hypotension and shock not be corrected after the first hour of salt and water replacement, blood or plasma should be given immediately.

Diabetic patients with ARF due to volume depletion (secondary to osmotic diuresis) are frequently potassium depleted. During osmotic diuresis, potassium is lost in the urine. Factors favoring this renal loss include (a) lean-tissue breakdown (3 mmol of potassium are liberated for each gram of nitrogen); (b) depletion of tissue glycogen (1 mmol of potassium is liberated for every 3 grams of glycogen); (c) cellular loss of potassium (favored by cellular dehydration and insulin deficiency); and (d) increased aldosterone secretion (secondary to hypovolemia) [2]. Furthermore, anorexia (through reduced intake) and vomiting (10–20 mmol of potassium are lost with each liter of vomitus) will contribute to potassium depletion. In oliguric ARF, however, serum potassium may be in the normal range (despite potassium depletion) because of both severe metabolic acidosis and potassium shift from the cells brought about by extracellular hypertonicity due to hyperglycemia [3].

With an increase in urine output, improvement of renal function and correction of hyperglycemia and metabolic acidosis, serum potassium decreases, requiring potassium replacement. If urinary output is adequate, potassium may be given i.v. at a dosage of 20 to 40 mmol/hour: in oliguric patients, more caution is necessary.

1.2 HYPOVOLEMIA DUE TO EXTRARENAL FLUID LOSS

The amount and nature of fluid replacement in patients with hypovolemia due to extrarenal fluid loss is an individual problem that has to be faced on the basis of the clinical features and fluid and electrolyte balance.

1.2.1 Hemorrhage and Shock When reduction of blood volume or shock predominates, colloidal solutions should be infused intravenously in the form of whole blood, plasma, or dextran (in addition to saline solutions).

Whole blood transfusion is undoubtedly the best way to replace blood loss or correct hypovolemic shock. Massive blood transfusion may cause transient acidosis, possibly followed by alkalosis because of metabolism of the citrate contained in the transfused blood [4].

Plasma may also be used as a volume expander following severe hemorrhage or in shocked patients. Alternatively, in dehydrated patients, human serum albumin can be used. The 25 g/dl albumin solution may be diluted with normal saline or 278 mmol/l (5 g/dl) dextrose to obtain a 5 g/dl albumin solution.

It should be stressed that whole blood may transmit hepatitis virus, cytomegalovirus, and other infectious agents; plasma can also transmit hepatitis; human albumin solution will not transmit hepatitis, but may have side effects (e.g., hyperpyrexia). However, these therapeutic measures are life saving in shock and conditions of severe hypovolemia.

Low-molecular-weight dextran (Dextran 40, Rheomacrodex) is a sucrose polysaccharide with a mean molecular weight of 40,000 which may be used as a plasma volume expander when whole blood, plasma, and human albumin are not available. Dextran 40 is usually available as 10 g/dl solution (either in normal saline or in 278 mmol/l, 5 g/dl, dextrose solution) which is a hyperoncotic solution; in patients with hypovolemic shock, it should be infused i.v. together with isotonic saline solution. Its efficacy is time limited since most of dextran molecules leave the vascular space in a few hours (about 80% is eliminated with urine in 12 hours when renal function is preserved). However, its use in shock appears useful both in decreasing red blood cell sludging and agglutination and in reducing blood viscosity and increasing capillary blood flow; these effects reduce the tendency of shocked patients to coagulation in the capillaries and to tissue ischemia [4].

It should be stressed that Dextran 40 may have important adverse effects, such as urticaria, nausea, fever, and anaphylaxis; cases of death have been reported [4]. Dextran 40 may even cause ARF, probably because it can precipitate in renal tubules [5]. It is therefore suggested that large quantities of Dextran 40 should be avoided, particularly is severely dehydrated and/or old patients.

1.2.2 Vomiting and Nasogastric Suction The ECV depletion with hypokalemic, hypochloremic metabolic alkalosis resulting from prolonged vomiting or nasogastric suction (or spontaneous gastric fistula) requires fluid replacement, mainly in the form of isotonic normal saline (0.9 g/dl, 154 mmol/l, NaCl). Should correction of alkalosis not occur (because of continued nasogastric drainage of large volumes of fluid), i.v. infusion of an acidifying agent (O.1N HCl solution) becomes necessary (see section 3 of this chapter) with careful monitoring of arterial blood pH and serum bicarbonate concentration. Should urine output increase to more than 500 ml/day and serum potassium remain low, potassium chloride (40 to 100 mmol/day) should be added to the infusion solutions with frequent monitoring of serum potassium level. It should be stressed that in postsurgical patients with high gastric secretion (e.g., following surgical intervention in patients with peptic ulcer), continuous nasogastric drainage may maintain high gastric secretion and fluid loss: under such circumstances, it is better to avoid continuous suction and to aspirate gastric juice as infrequently as possible.

1.2.3 Diarrhea and Intestinal Drainage The ECV depletion with hyponatremic, hypokalemic metabolic acidosis resulting from diarrhea or intestinal drainage (or intestinal fluid sequestration because of obstructed bowel) should be immediately treated with i.v. infusion of normal saline; as much as 4 to 6 liters of 0.9 g/dl (154 mmol/l) may be required to restore blood pressure and urine output [6]. Meanwhile, acidosis should be treated with 1/6M NaHCO$_3$ (1.4 g/dl, 167 mmol/l), and hypokalemia with potassium chloride.

1.2.4 Prerenal ARF in Burns When second- and third-degree burns involve 15% or more of the body surface, i.v. fluid replacement becomes necessary to correct the severe fluid loss (see chapter 2, section 2). This may be carried out with Ringer's lactate solution (Na$^+$ 130 mmol/l, K$^+$ 4 mmol/l, Ca^{++} 3 mmol/l, Cl$^-$ 109 mmol/l, lactate 28 mmol/l; 274 mOsm/Kg H$_2$O) or with normal saline (0.9 g/dl, 154 mmol/l, NaCl solution), and 5 g/dl (278 mmol/l) dextrose solution.

Plasma or human serum albumin should also be given. It has been stated that patients with extensive third-degree burns may exhibit as much as 350 to 400 grams of protein loss per day from a combination of direct thermal injury, tissue catabolism, and exudation from the burned wound [7]. Obviously, these losses must be replaced, and plasma or human serum albumin represent the best source of proteins. In emergency, Dextran 40 may also be used.

Marked hemoconcentration occurs because the loss of plasma protein is greater than the decrease in erythrocyte mass resulting from hemolysis and agglutination of RBC damaged during burning. Therefore, blood transfusion should not be given until a fall in hematocrit is observed.

Several formulae, based on the surface area of the burn, have been suggested for calculating fluid requirements of burned patients. A rough estimation of the body surface area involved by burns in adults is the "rule of nines" suggested by Hartford [8]: the body may be divided into 11 areas, each representing 9% of the total body surface; the head and each arm represent three areas of 9%; back, anterior torso, and each leg represent four areas of 18% (i.e., eight areas of 9%). The extent of patchy burns may be roughly estimated by considering that the area of the patient's flat hand is about 1% of the total body surface [8].

The volume of fluid to be given i.v. in the first 24 hours to adult patients with second- or third-degree burns should be (a) Ringer's lactate solution (see table 21–1), 2.9 ml/Kg b.w./% of the burned body surface area; this amount should be infused i.v. as rapidly as possible and is sufficient to maintain an adequate circulatory volume and to cause an urine output between 30 and 50 ml/hour [8]. Planas et al. [9] used only Ringer's lactate solution in an amount of 3 ml/Kg b.w./% of the burned body surface area in the first 24 hours; in the second 24-hour period, they gave single-donor plasma associated with 5 g/dl (278 mmol/l) dextrose at a rate to maintain a minimum urine volume of 0.5 ml/Kg b.w./hour. Once circulatory integrity and urine output have been restored, volumes of intravenous fluid should be decided on the basis of hourly assessment of urine output, blood pressure, pulse rate, respiratory rate, body weight (a bed scale will be useful in these patients), serum creatinine, and hematocrit (or blood hemoglobin). Satisfactory urine output should range between 30 and 50 ml/hour. In planning fluid replacement, the predominant loss of water should be borne in mind (see chapter 2, section 2). Water loss from the burn may be reduced by increasing the room temperature (to body temperature) and by saturating the air with water vapor [7].

If metabolic acidosis occurs, sodium bicarbonate may be given i.v. When adequate urine output is maintained, hypokalemia may occur as a result of potassium loss (usually in the second postburn week); in these cases, potassium should be given i.v. (up to 150 mmol/day) [7].

1.3 PRERENAL ARF AND HYPONATREMIA

Normovolemic hyponatremia and hyponatremia occurring in conditions of mild salt depletion are usually iatrogenic in their origin due to increased water intake and/or i.v. infusion of salt-free solutions (see chapter 7, section 8). Under these conditions, water restriction is mandatory to correct the retention of water in excess of sodium. In prerenal ARF, hyponatremia may reflect severe salt depletion in which hypothalamic-renal factors cause a disproportionate retention of ingested water; the resulting hypotonicity and hyponatremia are frequently worsened by mistakenly replacing sodium-rich fluids with sodium-free solution (see chapter 7). Under such circumstances, both water restriction and i.v. infusion of salt solutions are necessary to normalize ECV.

As described in chapter 7, a reduction in effective circulating blood volume may be seen in edematous states, such as congestive heart failure, cirrhosis with ascites, nephrotic syndrome, severe burns, and posttraumatic conditions. Excessive tubular reabsorption of salt and water (low urine output) associated with retention of ingested water may lead to hypervolemic hyponatremia. When the basic pathophysiology of this condition is congestive heart failure, treatment should be directed to improve myocardial function, the derangement of which is responsible for the impairment of renal perfusion and the resulting prerenal ARF. In hypoproteinemic states, a re-expansion of effective circulating blood volume should be obtained by hyperoncotic colloidal solutions;

these will mobilize extravascular fluid (edema fluid), increase blood pressure and cardiac output, and improve renal perfusion. For this purpose, 25 g/dl human albumin solution should be used; 300 to 400 ml of fluid are rapidly drawn (in about 30 minutes) from the interstitial space into the vascular bed by 100 ml of 25 g/dl albumin [4, 10]. A similar beneficial effect may be obtained with the plasma volume expander Dextran 40; when using a 10g/dl solution, it will pull twice its volume of fluid into the intravascular space [10].

1.4 PRERENAL ARF AND HYPERNATREMIA

As described in chapter 7 (section 8), hypovolemic hypernatremia may occur as a result of losses of hypotonic body fluids (by vomiting, gastric suction, diarrhea, or intestinal drainage, severe sweating, and, as already mentioned, polyuria of diabetic ketoacidosis) that have remained either unreplaced or partially replaced by relatively hypertonic solutions. This condition should be corrected with hypotonic saline solutions, such as one-half normal saline (0.45 g/dl, 77 mmol/l NaCl) or even more dilute solutions.

1.5 THERAPEUTIC ROLE OF DOPAMINE IN SHOCK

Despite massive i.v. infusion of colloidal solutions (whole blood, plasma, human albumin, dextran 40) and saline solutions, patients in shock may remain severely hypotensive and require the use of catecholamines. Under such circumstances, the drug of choice is dopamine.

1.5.1 Dopamine Dopamine is an endogenous catecholamine, the direct biochemical precursor of norepinephrine. It is formed in high concentration in adrenal glands and in sympathetic nerves.

The use of dopamine as a drug has been greatly investigated in recent years because of its peculiar effects. In 1964, in fact, Eble [11] reported that i.v. infusion of dopamine induced a vasoconstriction in some vasular beds (femoral and carotid), but vasodilation in others (mesenteric and renal vessels) where it stimulated specific "dopaminergic" receptors.

All of the three sympathomimetic amines—

norepinephrine, epinephrine, and dopamine—increase myocardial contractility by a beta-adrenergic mechanism; they have, however, different peripheral hemodynamic effects. Norepinephrine has strong generalized alpha-adrenergic effects in all peripheral vessels, including renal vessels, thereby causing a decrease in RBF [11] and fall in glomerular capillary pressure and in GFR [12, 13]. Epinephrine has both alpha and beta effects on the periphery but with predominant vasoconstriction in the renal vessels [13, 14]. Dopamine, even in low doses (1 to 5 μg/Kg b.w./min), causes vasodilation in the renal, mesenteric, coronary, and intracerebral vessels [13–15]; this vasodilating effect is unique for catecholamines and is due to stimulation of specific dopaminergic vascular receptors; it is not antagonized, in fact, by propranolol, atropine, and antihistamines, but is attenuated by haloperidol and phenothiazines [16]. When given in greater doses (5 to 15 μg/Kg b.w./min), dopamine exerts its inotropic effect by stimulating cardiac beta-adrenergic receptors; this cardiac action is antagonized by propranolol and other beta-blocking agents [15]. At large doses (greater than 15 μg/Kg b.w./min), the predominant effect of dopamine in all vascular beds is vasoconstriction due to stimulation of alpha-adrenergic receptors [15, 16].

1.5.2 Use of Dopamine in Shocked Patients In experimental studies in dogs, hemorrhage has been shown to cause a marked decrease in renal cortical blood flow. Intravenous infusion of dopamine induced renal cortical vasodilation with a clear increase in blood flow through the cortex [17]. Micropuncture studies in rats have demonstrated a clear fall in glomerular capillary pressure following hemorrhagic hypotension; under such circumstances, dopamine (but not epinephrine or norepinephrine) normalized both systemic blood pressure and glomerular capillary pressure [13].

These experimental studies can readily explain the beneficial effects on blood pressure and renal perfusion (with maintained or even increased urine output) obtained with dopamine in patients with shock [18].

Today, dopamine is successfully used in pa-tients with cardiogenic, septic, and traumatic shock, particularly when infusion is started soon after the onset of shock. Dopamine has been shown to increase cardiac output, systemic blood pressure, and urine output in shocked patients unresponsive to other sympathomimetic amines, with survival of patients after the shock episode [16].

Continuous i.v. drip infusion of dopamine should frequently be prolonged for several days. Because of the wide variation among shocked patients in cardiac output, peripheral resistance, and responsiveness to the drug, dosage of dopamine should be adjusted to the blood pressure response of the individual patient. Obviously, systemic blood pressure should be frequently monitored, and the lowest infusion rate of dopamine consistent with adequate organ perfusion should be maintained [16].

For a better control of dopamine infusion, the drug should be adequately diluted. Diluting solution for i.v. drip infusion may be either 5g/dl (278 mmol/l) glucose solution, or 0.9 g/dl (154 mmol/l) sodium chloride solution, or 1/6 M sodium lactate (167 mmol/l) solution; sodium bicarbonate or any other alkaline solutions cannot be used since dopamine is inactivated at alkaline pH [16].

1.6 FURTHER MEASURES FOR PREVENTING RENAL DAMAGE

1.6.1 Early Administration of Sodium Bicarbonate As mentioned in chapter 1 (section 4), a low intracellular pH seems to play a crucial role in the pathogenesis of ARF following an ischemic insult [19, 20]. On the other hand, studies on the isolated perfused kidney have demonstrated that when intrarenal pH is increased by selected buffers, renal function may significantly improve [21, 22].

These observations suggest a possible protective effect on the kidney of early i.v. administration of sodium bicarbonate following ischemic insults, such as hypotension, hemorrhage, and severe ECV contraction.

1.6.2 Correction of Hypoxia and Hypercapnia Patients with pulmonary edema and systemic hypoxia may develop renal impairment or exacerbation of pre-existing renal failure. Hypoxia causes peripheral vasodilation with a secondary increase in sympathetic tone and activation of the renin-angiotensin system; on the other hand, hypercapnia stimulates the sympathetic nervous system; the result will be severe renal vasoconstriction and a fall in GFR [23]. Therapy with oxygen and normalization of blood gases will decrease the sympathetic tone and improve cardiac output and renal function [23].

1.6.3 The Danger of Prostaglandin Inhibitors There is evidence that prostaglandins balance the vasoconstrictive effects of angiotensin and renal nerve stimulation during hemorrhagic hypotension in dogs [24]. The use of acetylsalicylic acid as an antipyretic drug should therefore be avoided in hypovolemic hypotensive patients since it may favor the onset of ARF through its inhibition on prostaglandin synthesis [25]. The same precaution is necessary with all nonsteroidal anti-inflammatory drugs.

2 Diuretic Treatment of ARF

The most impressive feature of oliguric ARF is undoubtedly the very low urine output. It is therefore not surprising that physicians have always attempted to increase urine output with diuretics. The first drug used for this purpose was an osmotic diuretic, mannitol (see chapter 3, section 4). The discovery of loop diuretics, such as furosemide (see chapter 3, section 5) and ethacrynic acid, has led to their use both in replacement of and in addition to mannitol.

Some authors have reported a beneficial effect of mannitol and furosemide in reversing ARF. Others have limited their claims for the efficacy of these diuretics to the conversion of the oliguric form of ARF to a milder nonoliguric form. It is commonly believed that nonoliguric ARF has a better prognosis [26–28]. It is, however, possible that the diuretic response of oliguric ARF to mannitol or furosemide occurs only in cases intrinsically less severe with a better prognosis. The dispute has not yet been settled. In my opinion, since the

treatment of ARF is undoubtedly simplified when urine output is high, even if the beneficial effect of mannitol or furosemide is limited to the increase in diuresis, their use should be recommended in all oliguric forms of ARF.

2.1 FUROSEMIDE

2.1.1 Effect of Furosemide in the Early Phase of ARF We have already discussed how to reverse prerenal ARF by correcting impaired renal hemodynamics. On some occasions, however, when all necessary measures to correct renal hypoperfusion have failed to reverse renal impairment, powerful loop diuretics in high doses have been reported to be successful (unfortunately, in uncontrolled studies), at least in increasing urine output. Thus, ethacrynic acid increased urine output in six out of six patients in whom oliguria had lasted less than 22 hours [29]. Similarly, furosemide, when given in doses up to 1,000 mg i.v., increased diuresis in 17 out of 42 patients (40% incidence) whose oliguria had lasted less than 24 hours [30]. When 250 to 1,000 mg of furosemide were given i.v. to 49 patients following surgical operations, a urine output greater than 1,500 ml daily was obtained in 13 patients; in 4 of these responders, dialysis seemed to have been averted by this therapy [31]. But in another retrospective study of 82 cases of postsurgical ARF in which 29 patients had received furosemide intraoperatively, mortality was higher (21 out of 29 patients) in treated patients than in patients not given furosemide (27 out of 53 patients); in this study, however, the administration of furosemide during surgery probably reflected a grave intraoperative event [26].

In order to verify whether short-term administration of furosemide could improve intrarenal hemodynamics and modify the clinical course of ARF, the diuretic was injected directly into one renal artery (280 mg of furosemide infused in 30 minutes) in five patients between two and nine days after the onset of oliguric ARF [32]: under such circumstances, furosemide not only failed to alter RBF or its intrarenal distribution (as evaluated by xenon washout technique) during and up to 40 minutes after the infusion, but did not increase urine output nor decrease serum creatinine during four days after furosemide. Only in the sixth patient with nonoliguric ARF was an increase in diuresis and decrease in serum creatinine observed after the intrarenal administration of furosemide [32]. We have had similar experience; when 200 mg of furosemide were infused into a renal artery of a patient with nonoliguric ARF during renal angiography, a significant but slight increase in inulin clearance, urine volume, and FE_{Na} was observed, but without apparent improvement of renal angiograms [1].

Whether the increase in urine output is associated with improvement in renal function is still a matter of debate. Only 7 of the abovementioned 17 patients who diuresed after furosemide (when the diuretic was given within 24 hours of oliguria) also exhibited an increase in GFR (an incidence of 17% of all treated patients) [30].

Recently, Levinsky et al. [33] have analyzed the data available from the literature in order to evaluate the clinical course of ARF in patients who increased urine output (responders) when diuretics were given in the early phase of ARF: 65 out of 92 responders survived (incidence of 71%) against 34 out of 72 nonresponders (incidence of 47%); the difference was statistically significant by the chi-square test. Whether the diuretic response indicates a real improvement in prognosis [27] or simply identifies an intrinsically less severe ARF has still to be determined [33].

Some reports in the literature (mostly retrospective studies) do not support the efficacy of furosemide even on urine output in oliguric ATN. Thus, Minuth et al. [26] have reported that 51 out of 79 patients (64%) failed to have a diuretic response to furosemide (40 to 500 mg) given i.v. at some point of their clinical course; in the remaining 36%, the diuretic response was not accompanied by a reduced mortality, even though only 46% of patients responding to furosemide needed dialysis therapy against 73% of nonresponders and 60% of patients not treated with furosemide.

Only in the clinical setting of prerenal ARF occurring in cardiogenic shock and left ventricular failure (see chapter 2) is it well established

that furosemide reverses ARF by improving left ventricular function and, consequently, renal perfusion [30, 34]. A diuretic response to furosemide challenge in these patients has been considered an index of a better prognosis since those who fail to diurese usually do not survive [34].

2.1.2 Effect of Repeated Doses of Furosemide on the Evolution of ATN The first controlled study reported in the literature on the influence of furosemide on the course of ATN is that of Cantarovich et al. [35]. Forty-seven patients with oliguric ARF, who had failed to increase urine output after 60 g of mannitol (300 ml of 20 g/dl, 1,098 mmmol/l, mannitol i.v.) and were therefore treated by daily dialysis, were assigned at random to three groups: a control group (13 patients), a group treated with 600 mg furosemide daily (19 patients), and a group receiving 100 mg of furosemide as the initial dose that was then increased in geometric progression in the following days up to 3,200 mg/day (average dose: 1,240 mg/day for 7 days) (15 patients). The best results were obtained in the group of patients treated with progressive doses of furosemide and may be summarized as follows: (a) 73% of patients (against 56% of controls) reached a urine output of at least 400 ml/24 hours; (b) the duration of anuria was greatly shortened (5.7 days against 15 days in controls); (c) serum creatinine normalized more rapidly (17.2 days against 26.6 days of controls); (d) the average number of dialyses required was greatly reduced (2.8 against 8.8 of controls). The group of patients treated with 600 mg of furosemide as a fixed daily dose, when evaluated by the same criteria, did better than controls but not as well as patients on progressive doses. In a further study, the same authors examined retrospectively 58 additional patients, 39 of whom were treated with a fixed dose of 2,000 mg/day of furosemide, the remainder being controls [36]; the results evaluated by the same criteria were similar to those obtained with progressive doses in the controlled study. Despite these good results, however, in neither study was the mortality rate significantly modified by furosemide. However, the improved clinical course resulting from furosemide administration appears to support widespread use of this diuretic in the management of ARF.

Unfortunately another controlled trial by Kleinknecht et al. [37] could not confirm the above favorable effects of diuretic therapy in ATN. When furosemide was given at doses up to 1,200 mg daily, no difference was observed between treated patients and controls concerning not only mortality but also duration of both oliguria and uremia, as well as number of dialyses required before recovery; a normal urine output, however, was more rapidly obtained in treated patients. The substantial difference between these controlled studies does not seem to be accounted for by different doses of furosemide only; further investigation is required.

More recently, when repeated doses of furosemide were given i.v. (2 g daily) for several days in six patients with oliguric ARF secondary to leptospirosis and not requiring dialysis, a profuse diuresis was obtained in all six, but renal function and clinical course were not modified [38].

2.1.3 Guideline for Furosemide Therapy As stated above the main indication for diuretic therapy is prerenal ARF occurring in cardiogenic shock and left ventricular failure. Under such circumstances, combination with dopamine may give even better results (see later in this chapter).

Furosemide may also be useful in those forms of ARF in which tubular obstruction plays an important role in the renal shutdown, such as in ARF secondary to multiple myeloma (myeloma kidney) or in acute uric acid nephropathy.

However, since its toxicity is low, furosemide may be used in all forms of ARF that have not been reversed by correction of hypotension and volume depletion.

Furosemide should be given undiluted by i.v. drip infusion at a rate not exceeding 1,000 mg/hour [30]. We may start with 100 mg i.v.; should a diuretic response not occur in the following few hours, a further dose of 500 mg i.v. may be given. The total daily dosage may reach 2,000 mg. Further attempts may be re-

peated during the course of the oliguric phase in the hope of hastening the diuretic phase. In my opinion, daily diuretic therapy with high doses should be avoided until its efficacy is clearly proved.

It should be stressed that (a) furosemide should never be given in volume-depleted patients; (b) the association of furosemide with nephrotoxic antibiotics (aminoglycosides in particular) may potentiate the nephrotoxicity of the latter (see chapters 1 and 3); and (c) for the same reason furosemide should not be used in those cases where nephrotoxic antibiotics may have been the cause of the renal shutdown.

2.2 USE OF DOPAMINE + FUROSEMIDE IN ARF

The vasodilating effect of dopamine on renal vessels when given in low doses has suggested the use of this catecholamine in the treatment of the early phase of ARF, when renal vasoconstriction appears to favor the induction of ARF (see chapter 1).

Dogs treated with dopamine immediately after injection of uranyl nitrate, however, were not protected against ARF despite a reversal of renal vasoconstriction; protection occurred only with the combination dopamine + furosemide [39] (see chapter 3, section 5).

When the association dopamine + furosemide was used in humans with ATN, an increase in urine output was regularly observed. Thus, Graziani et al. [40] have reported that five oliguric patients who had failed to respond to i.v. infusion of 200 ml 20 g/dl (1,098 mmol/l) mannitol promptly diuresed after dopamine (0.5–3 μg/kg b.w./min) plus furosemide (1–5 mg/kg b.w./day). Similarly, the 11 patients reported by Henderson et al. [41] to exhibit a diuretic response to dopamine hydrochloride (1 μg/kg b.w./min) were still under the influence of furosemide (250–500 mg i.v.) which they had received one to three hours earlier. It has been shown that when renal clearance is less than 15 ml/min, the plasma half-life of furosemide is 260 minutes [42]. More recently, Lindner et al. [43] have observed not only a prompt diuresis after the combination of dopamine (1–3 μg/kg b.w./min) plus furosemide in six patients with ATN who had been unresponsive to furosemide alone, but also improvement of renal function in two of them. These promising results require further investigation.

The combination of dopamine plus furosemide is particularly likely to improve not only urine output but also renal function in patients with prerenal ARF due to cardiogenic shock [34].

2.3 MANNITOL

While most authors agree on the protective effect of mannitol when given prophylactically (see chapter 3, section 4), mannitol efficacy in improving renal function once the renal insult has occurred is still matter of debate.

Controlled studies have failed to demonstrate a definite effect of mannitol in reversing ARF or at least in reducing its severity. Numerous reports have claimed positive effects when mannitol has been given early in the course of ARF, i.e., within 48 hours of the onset of oliguria [44–48]. Thus, in a recent retrospective study of 20 patients with ARF associated with rhabdomyolysis and myoglobinuria, the i.v. infusion of mannitol and sodium bicarbonate (25 g of mannitol and 100 mmol of sodium bicarbonate in 1 liter of 5g/dl, 278 mmol/l dextrose solution, at an infusion rate of 250 ml/hour) resulted in a clear increase in urine output and normalization of renal function in nine patients. No clinical or laboratory differences, which might be recommended for selecting potential responders, were observed between responders and nonresponders [49]. Hence, the renal response to mannitol is unpredictable.

2.3.1 Therapeutic Mechanism of Mannitol The i.v. infusion of mannitol has frequently produced diuresis in patients with ARF refractory to loop diuretics. This has been attributed to a preserved filtration of mannitol, even in the presence of reduced GFR [50]. But the effects of mannitol on central hemodynamics may also play an important role; increase in cardiac output, expansion in ECV, increase in RBF, and inhibition of renal renin release have been reported after mannitol infusion (see chapter 3).

The recent demonstration that mannitol infusion is followed by much greater increase in RBF and fall in renal vascular resistance (particularly at the afferent arteriole level) in conditions of renal hypoperfusion [51] and that this renal effect is mediated, in large part, by an increase in PGI_2 synthesis [52] appears to support the usefulness of treating prerenal ARF (i.e., a typical condition of renal hypoperfusion) with mannitol. Treatment should obviously start as early as possible since prevention of cell necrosis seems to be important; furthermore, once necrosis has occurred, intratubular casts (made of cell debris and proteinaceous material) may solidify with time. In experimental ARF, in fact, application of pressure within the obstructed tubule through micropuncture could flush out the tubular casts soon after the renal insult, but not 24 hours later [23].

2.3.2 Guidelines for Mannitol Therapy
a. Mannitol should never be used in conditions of ECV depletion, only when hypovolemia has been corrected.
b. In conditions of ECV expansion, the use of mannitol may be hazardous and cause pulmonary edema.
c. Mannitol infusion should be started (if possible) within 48 hours after the renal insult at a dosage of 12.5 g to 25 g (62.5 ml to 125 ml of 20 g/dl, 1,098 mmol/l, mannitol solution).
d. Should 12.5 or 25 grams of mannitol be ineffective in causing diuresis, further doses would be not only ineffective but also hazardous since it is retained in the extracellular compartment [50].
e. After 12.5 g of mannitol i.v., should urine output increase to more than 40 ml/hour during the next two hours, mannitol may be continued intermittently. Dosage should not exceed 50 g/24 hours [50].
f. Urinary losses of water and sodium should be adequately replaced by i.v. infusion of glucose and saline solutions.

3 Conservative Treatment of ATN

With the exception of the effects claimed for mannitol or loop diuretics in reversing renal impairment, treatment of ARF is nothing more than symptomatic care while awaiting spontaneous reparative processes.

3.1 SALT AND WATER BALANCE

In all patients with ATN, the daily external balance of salt and water should be carefully calculated, taking into consideration insensible loss and sweating. Thus, fluid losses should be divided in different categories (urine, vomitus, or nasogastric suction, intestinal drainage, etc.) and their electrolyte content carefully monitored. Similarly the volume of fluid administered intravenously (including blood and plasma), and their electrolyte content should be carefully recorded together with any oral intake of salt and water.

Daily measurement of body weight and clinical examination (recording blood pressure and pulse rate) help in evaluating the fluid balance. Patients with ARF are catabolic; therefore, they should lose body weight (between 0.2 and 0.4 Kg daily) because of loss of endogenous fat and protein. If they gain or even if they only maintain their weight, they are accumulating fluid; fluid overload may cause life-threatening pulmonary edema.

Sometimes, monitoring of central venous pressure may be necessary, such as when the state of hydration is not readily apparent and/or cardiac failure is suspected.

Obviously, the tendency in recent years to use early and frequent dialysis in patients with ATN has greatly reduced the problem of fluid overload. Despite this fact, fluid intake should be limited to avoid the need for excessive fluid removal during dialysis. In patients able to eat who do not have losses of fluid, it has been suggested that a water intake of 400 ml should be allowed plus a volume of water equal to the urine output of the previous day (taking into account that as much as 750 ml of water are introduced with food itself) [53].

Patients with extrarenal losses of fluid (vomiting, diarrhea, intestinal drainage, etc.) may be dehydrated. This ECV depletion should be corrected by saline infusions. As mentioned on chapter 7, usually hyponatremia in oliguric patients does not reflect a salt depletion but a relative water excess that is frequently iatrogenic. Under such circumstances fluid restriction and

dialysis ultrafiltration may correct the condition of fluid excess. Only when serum sodium concentration is less than 120 mmol/l and/or the patient has neurologic symptoms of hyponatremia, may hypertonic saline be given as an emergency measure; the amount of sodium chloride necessary for such correction may be calculated as follows:

$$Na^+ \text{ requirement} = TBW \times ([NA^+]_d - [Na^+]_p),$$

where TBW = total body water which is 50 to 54% of body weight in adult men and 43 to 48% in adult women [4]; $[Na^+]_d$ is the desired serum sodium concentration (in mmol/l) and $[Na^+]_p$ is the patient's present serum sodium concentration (in mmol/l) to be corrected. Thus, for instance, should a 40-year-old patient, with 80 Kg b.w., have a serum sodium concentration of 105 mmol/l with neurologic signs of hyponatremia, the amount of sodium required to raise the serum sodium to 120 mmol/l would be as follows: $40 \times 15 = 600$ mmol (being 0.50×80 Kg = 40 liters and $120 - 105 = 15$ mmol). If we decide to use hypertonic saline, 855 mmol/l (5 g/dl) NaCl solution, 700 ml of such solution should be infused i.v. in a 12-hour period or so.

The above calculation of sodium required to correct hyponatremia assumes that sodium is distributed in total body water. Actually, sodium is distributed in extracellular fluid, but water is diffusible intra- and extracellularly. Thus, when a condition occurs in which water exceeds sodium (with resulting hyponatremia), water moves into cells (because of the osmotic gradient) until osmotic pressure is equal intra- and extracellularly; this process will reduce the hyponatremia by raising sodium concentration in the extracellular fluid. The final serum concentration of sodium, therefore, will be equivalent to that which would be observed if sodium were distributed in total body water [4]. For this reason, correction of severe hyponatremia should be based on TBW rather than on extracellular water.

However, should hyponatraemia reflect severe ECV contraction (see chapter 7), saline infusion is indicated even if there are no neurologic signs of hyponatremia. Under such circumstances, (a) the above calculation of sodium requirements will underestimate the real need for sodium; (b) isotonic saline solution (0.9 g/dl, 154 mmol/l NaCl) is preferred; and (c) the adequacy of saline infusion will be assessed by clinical evaluation of the patient (see chapter 7). Physical examination (including determination of body weight, systemic blood pressure, etc.) and blood-chemistry determinations performed daily indicate the patient's fluid status and dictate, day to day, any changes necessary in parenteral therapy.

Patients with ATN may have a low serum-protein concentration because of accelerated catabolism and/or protein loss (as in burns, for instance). Under such circumstances, the reduced serum oncotic pressure should be corrected by i.v. infusion of plasma or human albumin, thereby correcting abnormalities in fluid distribution in intra- extracellular compartments. When hematocrit (or hemoglobin concentration) is low, whole blood transfusion should be preferred.

3.2   ACID BASE BALANCE

3.2.1   Treatment of Metabolic Acidosis Once renal shutdown has occurred, acid resulting from catabolism of tissue (and dietary) proteins will be retained, invariably leading to metabolic acidosis, with increasing anion gap (see chapter 7). Since the daily endogenous production of acid is approximately 1 mmol/Kg b.w./ day, serum bicarbonate concentration is expected to decrease by 1 to 2 mmol/l day [53]. Any condition in which overproduction of organic or inorganic acids occurs (hypercatabolic states, lactic acidosis, diabetic ketoacidosis) will worsen metabolic acidosis.

It should be stressed that i.v. infusion of amino acids or protein hydrolysates for parenteral nutrition will represent a further acid load.

Mild metabolic acidosis does not require correction. Severe acidosis may decrease myocardial contractility, increase pulmonary vascular resistance, and cause peripheral vasodilation, thus leading to pulmonary edema and shock in addition to severe metabolic disorders [4]. Thus severe metabolic acidosis must be treated.

Alkalinizing solutions for clinical use include sodium bicarbonate, sodium lactate, sodium acetate, and TRIS (or THAM) (table 21–1).

Sodium bicarbonate is undoubtedly the alkali of choice for the treatment of metabolic acidosis since its alkalinizing effect is immediate. Sodium lactate and sodium acetate (the latter is used for dialysate solutions) do so only after conversion of lactate or acetate ions to bicarbonate ion. Lactate was introduced in clinical practice because of technical difficulties in manufacturing bicarbonate solutions for i.v. infusion. It also had the advantage of not forming insoluble salt with calcium (as bicarbonate does), so that calcium can be added to lactate solutions when calcium infusion is needed. Lactate is metabolized in the liver; but in severe acidosis, the liver capacity for metabolizing it is greatly reduced. Thus, lactate is contraindicated in conditions of impaired liver function but also during hypotension, shock, hypoxia, severe anemia, and lactic acidosis [4]. Since the technical problems in preparing bicarbonate solutions have been largely solved, sodium bicarbonate is now preferred for i.v. therapy.

TRIS (tris-[hydroxymethyl] - aminomethane), or THAM, is an organic amine buffer suggested for the treatment of severe metabolic acidosis in patients in whom sodium loading (which would result from sodium bicarbonate or lactate administration) should be avoided; it is a much stronger base than bicarbonate. Furthermore, THAM can combine with carbonic acid and release bicarbonate [4]. A great disadvantage is its tendency to cause respiratory depression and severe hyperkalemia [54]. Furthermore, extravasation during i.v. infusion may cause necrosis of neighboring tissues; its alkalinity (a solution 0.3 M has a pH of 8.6) may cause phlebitis or thrombosis. It has been suggested that THAM should be used in patients with respiratory distress syndrome in which a combined respiratory and metabolic acidosis is observed, provided that facilities for mechanical ventilation are available [54]. Since its excretion is mainly renal, THAM is contraindicated in renal failure [4].

In treating metabolic acidosis with i.v. infusion of sodium bicarbonate, care should be taken to avoid iatrogenic hypervolemic hypernatremia (see chapter 7).

The amount of bicarbonate necessary for the correction of metabolic acidosis may be calculated with the following formula in which bicarbonate space is considered as 50% of body weight [4] (some authors use 40% of body weight as bicarbonate space) [53]:

HCO_3^- requirement
$$= ([HCO_3^-]_d - [HCO_3^-]_p) \times (0.50 \times Kg\ b.w.),$$

where $[HCO_3^-]_d$ is the desired serum bicarbonate concentration (in mmol/l), and $[HCO_3^-]_p$ is the patient's present serum bicarbonate concentration (in mmol/l). Thus, a 40-year-old man, 80 Kg b.w., with 15 mmol/l of serum bicarbonate will require 400 mmol of sodium bicarbonate to obtain a serum bicarbonate level of 25 mmol/l. Fifty percent of the calculated requirement may be given in three to four hours, the remainder later. It is preferable to avoid a rapid complete correction of metabolic acidosis. The equilibration of bicarbonate concentration between blood and cerebrospinal fluid, in fact, is slow, so that a rapid rise in plasma bicarbonate is not associated with a simultaneous rise in brain bicarbonate. The increase in blood pH, however, is responsible for a reduction in ventilation and consequent rise in blood pCO_2. Since CO_2 is readily diffusible, the higher blood pCO_2 is quickly transmitted to the cerebrospinal fluid and brain where the increased pCO_2, in the presence of a continuing low bicarbonate concentration, will result in a further drop in the already low pH. This sharp fall in the pH of the cerebrospinal fluid may cause nausea, vomiting, giddiness, and disturbances of consciousness [55] and even convulsion and coma.

Rapid correction of metabolic acidosis in hypocalcemic patients, by reducing ionized calcium, may cause tetany; it is advisable to give calcium to these patients.

Changes in acid-base balance modify the serum concentration of potassium by redistributing potassium ions between intra- and extracellular fluid. It is usually stated that metabolic acidosis will increase serum potassium concentration by 0.6 mmol/l for every 0.1 unit change in arterial pH. Actually, the correlation between serum potassium and arterial pH is present in patients with metabolic acid-base disturbances but not in those with respiratory disturbances. Furthermore, the hyperkalemic effect of metabolic acidosis is very marked when acidosis is due to mineral acid (such as sulphuric acid and phosphoric acid) retention; under such circumstances, the rise in serum potassium will be much greater than 0.6 mmol/l per 0.1 unit change in pH [3]. In patients with metabolic acidosis due to retention of organic acids (such as lactic acidosis), the increase in serum potassium is much smaller. Only the hyperkalemia of diabetic ketoacidosis may be severe; but this is due partly to the hypertonicity created by hyperglycemia [3] (see below).

Physicians should take into careful consideration the redistribution of potassium that occurs between extra- and intracellular fluid when correcting metabolic acidosis. A patient with a normal serum concentration of potassium and severe metabolic acidosis has a potassium deficiency and will experience dangerous hypokalemia when the metabolic acidosis is corrected unless potassium supplements are given [56].

3.2.2 Treatment of Metabolic Alkalosis

Metabolic alkalosis also may occur in ATN, usually as a result of continuous nasogastric drainage in surgical patients. The use of cimetidine has been suggested to correct this condition [57]. In some patients with severe metabolic alkalosis, however, the i.v. infusion of hydrochloric acid may become necessary [58]. Hydrochloric acid will react with plasma bicarbonate as follows:

$$HCl + HCO_3^- = CO_2 + H_2O + Cl^-,$$

so that chloride will replace bicarbonate. Since this reaction occurs as soon as hydrochloric acid enters the blood vessel, it may leave pure water and cause hemolysis; that is why some authors suggest that i.v. hydrochloric acid should be given in 5 g/dl (278 mmol/l) dextrose solution or in normal saline [59].

The amount of acid required to correct metabolic alkalosis may be calculated as follows [53]:

H^+ requirement
$$= ([HCO_3^-]_p - [HCO_3^-]_d \times (0.40 \times Kg\ b.w.).$$

However, Kopple and Blumenkrantz [4] suggest that acid requirement should be evaluated on calculated chloride deficit:

Chloride deficit
$$= ([Cl^-]_d - [Cl^-]_p) \times (0.20 \times Kg\ b.w.),$$

where $[Cl^-]_d$ is the desired serum chloride concentration (in mmol/l), $[Cl^-]_p$ is the patient's present serum chloride concentration (in mmol/l), and 0.20 indicates the extracellular fluid space (in liters/Kg b.w.), which is the main compartment for chloride. Half of the calculated chloride deficit should be replaced by an equivalent amount of HCl during the first 24 hours; obviously, an additional amount of HCl should replace continuing chloride losses, which must be carefully calculated [4]. Thus, a 40-year-old man, 76 Kg b.w., with ARF and severe metabolic alkalosis due to nasogastric suction of 1.500 ml/day of gastric fluid (with 100 mmol/l of chloride) will lose 150 mmol of chloride daily. If his serum chloride concentration is 80 mmol/l, chloride deficit will be $(150 - 80) \times (0.20 \times 76) = 380$ mmol. Thus, he should receive, in the first 24 hours, 340 mmol of hydrochloric acid (150 mmol to replace the daily chloride loss in gastric juices plus $380:2 = 190$ mmol in order to correct the chloride deficit in part). Hydrochloric acid may be given as a slow i.v. infusion of 0.1N HCl solution (100 mmol/l of HCl possibly in normal saline or dextrose solution) into a large-diameter, high-flow vein since it may cause coagulation of blood at catheter tip and necrosis of tissue at the infusion site [4].

The correction of metabolic alkalosis causes an increase in serum potassium concentration that is, however, less than 0.6 mmol/l per 0.1 unit change of pH [58].

Arginine hydrochloride cannot be used to correct metabolic alkalosis in oliguric patients since it may cause life-threatening hyperkalemia [60]. Ammonium chloride is also contraindicated in ARF since the dissociation of NH_4^+ into H^+ and NH_3 will increase plasma urea level.

3.3   POTASSIUM BALANCE

3.3.1   Treatment of Hyperkalemia   The main danger of death in ARF derives from severe hy-

perkalemia (see chapter 7), which must be treated immediately. The quickest method of lowering serum potassium is not dialysis. Emergency therapy of life-threatening hyperkalemia includes the following.

3.3.1.1 CALCIUM GLUCONATE INFUSION.   This is the emergency therapy of life-threatening cardiac conduction disturbances secondary to hyperkalemia. Hyperkalemia, in fact, may impair membrane excitability by reducing the resting potential; since membrane excitability is defined by the difference between resting and threshold potentials, when resting potential is reduced (as in hyperkalemia), the normal membrane excitability may be restored by reducing the membrane threshold potential; this is obtained by increasing extracellular calcium concentration through calcium gluconate infusion [61]. For this purpose, 10 to 30 ml of 10g/dl (232 mmol/l) calcium gluconate solution may be infused intravenously in three to five minutes under continuous ECG monitoring; conduction abnormalities will reverse in a few minutes. The infusion may be repeated after five to seven minutes if no effect is observed or if conduction abnormalities recur [61]. Calcium infusion is contraindicated in digitalized patients [53].

This emergency treatment has only transient effects since calcium is taken up by bone; it helps, however, in gaining time to prepare other therapeutic measures.

Hypertonic sodium solutions may have similar beneficial effect in hyperkalemic hyponatremic patients since hyponatremia may exaggerate the effects of hyperkalemia on myocardial conduction [61].

3.3.1.2 SODIUM BICARBONATE INFUSION.   This treatment will lower the serum concentration of potassium by promoting entry of potassium into cells, thereby restoring the transcellular gradient of potassium. In severe hyperkalemia, it has been suggested that 50 to 100 ml of 1M (8.4 g/dl) $NaHCO_3$ (i.e., 50–100 mmol of $NaHCO_3$) should be infused i.v. over 5 to 10 minutes [53, 62]; this, however, will be an osmotic load (1M $NaHCO_3$ solution has an osmolality of 2,000 mOsm/Kg H_2O) (table 21–1), which may be partly counterproductive to the treatment of hyperkalemia (hypertonicity, in fact, may cause a shift of potassium from cells to extracellular fluid) [3]. A less concentrated sodium bicarbonate solution may be preferred, such as 1/6M (1.4 g/dl) NaHCO₃ solution (an i.v. infusion of 500 ml will give 83 mmol of NaHCO₃). It should be stressed that the i.v. infusion of sodium bicarbonate may represent a problem in oliguric patients, especially in the presence of congestive heart failure. In patients with life-threatening hyperkalemia, i.v. infusion of sodium bicarbonate may be lifesaving even when metabolic acidosis is not present. The alkalosis induced by bicarbonate may precipitate tetany and even seizure by lowering ionized calcium level; the i.v. infusion of at least 10 ml of 10g/dl (232 mmol/l) calcium gluconate prior to alkali therapy may prevent this complication. It should be stressed that calcium gluconate cannot be added to the solution of sodium bicarbonate because of the precipitation of calcium salts.

3.3.1.3 GLUCOSE-INSULIN INFUSION. The i.v. infusion of insulin (plus glucose) may lower serum potassium concentration within 15 to 20 minutes since potassium will move into the cells with glucose.

The efficacy of insulin in treating hyperkalemia is well known; it stimulates potassium uptake by skeletal muscle and hepatic cells. This hypokalemic effect is dose related, reaching a maximum at blood concentrations of insulin 20 to 40 times the basal levels [63, 64]. It is therefore advisable to give insulin as an intravenous bolus to have the maximal hypokalemic effect, followed by i.v. infusion of glucose to avoid hypoglycemia [3].

It has been suggested that hyperkalemia should be treated by i.v. injection of 50 to 100 ml of 50g/dl (2.775 mmol/l) dextrose with 5 to 10 units of soluble insulin (i.e., 1 unit of soluble insulin every 5 grams of glucose) [53, 62]. The resulting sudden hyperglycemia, however, with the consequent hypertonicity may worsen hyperkalemia by causing a shift of potassium from cells to extracellular fluid (hypertonicity will cause cellular dehydration, an increase in intracellular concentration of potassium, and then passive diffusion of the cation out of cells) [3].

In my opinion, the following schedule is preferable [3]: i.v. bolus of 5 units of soluble insulin, to be repeated every 15 minutes, while

a 10 g/dl (555 mmol/l) dextrose solution is infused i.v. at an infusion rate of 500 ml/h (or 20g/dl, 1.11 mol/l, dextrose solution is infused at 250 ml/h).

The beneficial effect of glucose-insulin may last two to four hours, but the treatment may be repeated. It has been stated that glucose solution may be given i.v. without insulin in nondiabetic patients since the resulting hyperglycemia will readily stimulate insulin secretion [61]. This is not correct since endogenous insulin secretion will not be enough to obtain the maximal hypokalemic effect [3].

All the above maneuvers are only temporary measures and should be followed by potassium removal. As described above (chapter 7), in oliguric ATN, hyperkalemia is mainly due to potassium retention and will be definitively corrected only by potassium removal.

Potassium may be removed by potassium exchange resins, such as sodium polystyrene sulphonate or Kayexalate (Resonium A). Kayexalate acts by exchanging its sodium for potassium in the colon (it is therefore ineffective in patients who have undergone colectomy) [61]. It may be given orally in doses of 20 grams, three to four times daily: with each dose of resin, 20 ml of 70 g/dl sorbitol should be given orally as an osmotic cathartic in order to prevent fecal impaction. Alternatively, 50 grams of Kayexalate in 50 ml of 70 g/dl sorbitol and 100 ml of tap water may be given as a retention enema. The enema should be retained for at least 30 minutes (an inflated rectal catheter may help). Beneficial effect of the resin is evident one to two hours after oral administration and a half to one hour after enema. Each gram of Kayexalate binds 1 mmol of potassium in exchange for 1 mmol of sodium [53]. Thus, Kayexalate leads to sodium retention. The calcium form of the resin is therefore preferable (calcium resonium) [65].

An efficient measure for removing potassium is dialysis. Hemodialysis is more effective than peritoneal dialysis; as much as 50 mmol of potassium may be removed each hour. Peritoneal dialysis using potassium-free dialysate may remove 15 mmol of potassium per hour; but the extent of potassium removal is extremely variable, depending on peritoneal blood flow, time of intraperitoneal infusion and withdrawal of dialysate, etc.; furthermore, in hypotensive patients, the mesenteric vasoconstriction will greatly impair the exchange process [61].

Beta-adrenergic blocking agents and digitalis glycosides may exacerbate hyperkalemia in acidemic patients with ARF [3].

3.3.2 Treatment of Hypokalemia

Hypokalemia may occur in patients with ARF either as a result of extrarenal loss of potassium ions or in the diuretic (recovery) phase of ARF. Severe hypokalemia requires i.v. infusion of potassium.

When serum potassium is less than 3 mmol/l, an i.v. infusion of 200 to 400 mmol of potassium is required to increase serum potassium level by 1 mmol/l; the same increment of 1 mmol/l is obtained with 100 to 200 mmol if serum potassium is greater than 3 mmol/l [4]. Rapid infusion of potassium should be avoided. It is suggested that the infusion rate should be limited to no more than 10 mmol/hour and no more than 100 to 200 mmol/24 hours, using solutions with potassium concentration no greater than 30 mmol/l.

3.4 PREVENTION AND TREATMENT OF COMPLICATIONS

3.4.1 Infections

Since infections represent the major cause of death in ARF, physicians should use all measures to reduce sources of potential infections.

Usually, these patients are maintained in bed and their activities limited to a minimum. Even though this behavior is understandable because of the patient's critical condition, physicians should always encourage mobilization as much as possible to avoid hypostasis in the lung and decubitus ulcers. Physiotherapy is important; breathing exercises are particularly crucial in preventing pulmonary infections.

An indwelling bladder catheter for measuring urine output is not necessary once the diagnosis of ARF has been established; even closed bladder catheter drainage, in fact, will cause urinary tract infections. These should be avoided. Because of the difficulty in obtaining adequate urinary concentration of antibiotics in renal failure, infections of the urinary tract are difficult to treat and may cause septicemia. Obviously, the patient and nurses should be warned about the importance of complete urine collection obtained by spontaneous voiding.

Indwelling central venous lines for parenteral nutrition may also become infected and should be handled with aseptic technique. Obviously, the patient should be encouraged to take food by mouth (see chapter 22).

In surgical patients, all unnecessary tubes and catheters must be removed.

Should infection occur, early identification of the responsible micoorganism is very important. Thus, urine, blood, and drainage fluid cultures should be obtained very frequently and sensitivity to antibiotics tested in order to select the appropriate antimicrobial agents. Obviously, the dosage should be adjusted to reduced renal function (as suggested in chapter 3), taking into account whether or not the patient is treated by dialysis since dialysis may remove drugs.

Should antibiotic therapy be instituted before identification of the responsible microorganism, it should be borne in mind that tetracycline antibiotics (with the exception of doxycycline) may increase BUN by inhibiting protein anabolism. Doxycycline, a tetracycline active against Gram-positive and anerobic microorganisms, has no catabolic effects, is not nephrotoxic, does not accumulate in renal failure, and so can be used without reduction in dosage [66].

It should be stressed that corticosteroids also increase BUN by enhancing protein catabolism.

Body temperature, blood pressure, and pulse rate should be monitored frequently during the day.

3.4.2 Gastrointestinal Complications

Gastrointestinal abnormalities are frequent in patients with ARF, in the form of anorexia, nausea, retching, and vomiting. These symptoms are partially prevented or reversed by early and frequent dialysis.

Gastrointestinal bleeding is not unfrequent. It may be due to bleeding diathesis (see chapter 6), stress ulcers, gastritis, enterocolitis. It occurred (usually in the first 8 days after the onset of ARF) in 151 of 760 cases of ARF (20% incidence) in a study reported in 1973, causing death in 66 patients; its incidence was decreased significantly by early and frequent dialysis [67]. The presence of blood in the gut will represent urea and potassium loading, resulting in severe increase in BUN and hyperkalemia despite intensive dialysis. Stool should be checked frequently for blood in the course of ARF.

The introduction of H_2-receptor antagonists (cimetidine and ranitidine) in clinical pharmacology has greatly reduced the incidence of gastrointestinal bleeding due to stress ulceration in critically ill patients. Thus, some authors treat all ARF patients with cimetidine, as a preventive measure, in a dosage of 300 mg i.v. every 12 hours [53]. In patients without gastric symptoms, it may be given orally, at reduced dosage since the drug is excreted in the urine. Larsson et al. [68] have suggested that 200 mg of cimetidine should be given thrice daily when GFR is 15–30 ml/min, 200 mg twice daily when GFR is less than 5 ml/min, or the patient is on dialysis treatment (the drug should be given after dialysis).

Significant increases in serum levels of creatinine have been reported after cimetidine administration by several authors. It seems, however, that this rise in serum creatinine does not reflect a fall in GFR, since (^{51}Cr)EDTA clearance remained unchanged during long-term treatment with cimetidine [68].

Ranitidine may replace cimetidine in the prevention of gastrointestinal hemorrhage in ARF, in doses of 50 mg i.v. twice daily, or 150 mg/day per os.

3.4.3 Cardiovascular Complications Systemic hypertension and congestive heart failure may occur in ARF patients as a result of volume overload. This should be treated by dialysis.

Hypertension can be treated by common antihypertensive drugs: beta-blocking agents, clonidine, hydralazine, methyldopa, and prazosin. Obviously, dosages should be adjusted to the hypotensive effect, as usual.

Fibrinous uremic pericarditis may also occur; in these cases, a pericardial friction rub is usu-

ally appreciated. Pericardial effusion is uncommon. Pericarditis is an indication for dialysis.

3.4.4 Neurologic Complications The most frequent neurologic abnormalities in patients with ARF involve intellectual function. Mental concentration and recent memory are reduced, and the ability to focus or sustain attention is impaired. Anxiety, irritability, sleeplessness, or apathy and sluggishness may occur and are frequently followed by lassitude, muscular fatigue, weakness, daytime drowsiness, and insomnia at night. If the patient is not treated by dialysis, further deterioration of cerebral function will occur with disorientation, confusion, hallucination, torpor, myoclonus, and convulsions, which will represent a terminal symptom.

These neurologic abnormalities can be corrected by dialysis.

3.5 RECOVERY PHASE OF ATN

After days or even weeks of oliguria, urine output will start increasing in a stepwise fashion, sometimes reaching values greater than normal (polyuria). The improved management of water and salt balance by frequent dialysis in ATN patients has frequently reduced the incidence of postanuric polyuria. Even when polyuria occurs, however, both serum creatinine and BUN continue to increase for one to three days; despite the increase in GFR, in fact, the rate of production of creatinine and urea still exceeds the excretion rate. Then, serum creatinine and BUN level off for a further two to three days (excretion rate equals production rate). Finally, they start to decline (excretion rate exceeds production rate). The fall of serum creatinine will be progressive in the following days, reaching and then exceeding 70.7 μmol/l/day (0.8 mg/dl/day) [69].

During most of the recovery phase, U/P_{Cr}, U_{Osm}, U_{Na}, FE_{Na}, and renal failure index remain within the specific limits of ATN (see chapter 7) [69].

In some patients, recovery of tubular function occurs more slowly than that of GFR. Polyuria will ensue (as mentioned) with salt and water loss. Should this loss not be replaced, volume depletion would result. This may be mirrored by serum creatinine not maintaining its rate of decrease, stabilizing at high levels, or even increasing again; this condition is obviously reversed by correcting volume depletion with i.v. saline solutions.

In the case of polyuria, therefore, urinary losses of water, sodium, and potassium should be replaced. Replacement should be complete during the first days in order to maintain an high urine output and favor the excretion of retained solutes (nitrogen compounds in particular). In the following days, fluid and electrolyte infusion should be gradually reduced, monitoring the state of hydration of the patient. Defect in urine concentration may persist for years.

Even during the diuretic phase, infections may occur and should be prevented.

Obviously, during the diuretic phase the prognosis is improved in comparison with the oliguric phase of ATN. In a series of 276 cases of ARF, however, in which 102 patients died, 30 of these deaths (29%) occurred during the diuretic phase [70].

3.6 PROGNOSIS

When reviewing the 949 patients dialyzed for ARF at the University of Minnesota Hospitals between 1968 and 1979, Kjellstrand et al. [71] found that ARF occurred after renal transplantation in 264 cases; among the remaining 685 cases, ATN was the primary disease in 432 cases (63%), obstruction in 35 (5%), primary glomerulopathy in 75 (11%).

The highest mortality rate (68%) was observed in patients with ATN; there was no difference in the mean age between patients who survived (mean age: 48 years) and those who died (mean age: 47 years). When patients with ATN were subdivided into different basic disease groups, the mortality rate was 63% in the group of medical diseases, 73% in the group of cardiovascular surgery, and 78% in the group of gastrointestinal surgery [71]. Thus, postsurgical ARF has a high mortality rate, especially when surgery involves the abdomen [71–73]. Unfortunately, despite the improvement in dialysis equipment and procedures, better blood access, hyperalimentation, and more efficient antibiotics, the mortality rate of patients with ARF has not decreased over the years.

Thus, the mortality rate reported by Kjellstrand et al. [71] is no better than those reported by Balslow and Jorgensen [72] and by Kennedy et al. [73].

Undoubtedly, gastrointestinal bleeding and infections are the most important complications of ARF that adversely affect the prognosis [71].

It has been stated that neglected surgical complications may contribute to the severe prognosis of ARF [71]. This would suggest a more careful evaluation of the patients operated on by surgeons since early reoperation for surgical complications may decrease the mortality in postsurgical ARF.

Only 140 out of 432 cases of ATN reviewed by Kjellstrand et al. [71] survived (i.e., 32% survival rate), but only four survivors (3% of survivors) had no return of renal function and were maintained on RDT; 87% of survivors regained renal function (enough to go off dialysis) within a month, 9% within two months; in one patient only return of renal function sufficient to stop dialysis occurred after 88 days. ATN following transplantation was characterized by a mean time of 11 days to regain renal function [74].

References

1. Andreucci VE, Dal Canton A. Can acute renal failure in humans be prevented? Proc EDTA 17: 123–132, 1980.
2. Kleeman CR, Narins RG. Diabetic acidosis and coma. In Clinical Disorders of Fluid and Electrolyte Metabolism, Maxwell MH, Kleeman CR (eds). New York: McGraw-Hill, 1980 (3rd ed), pp. 1339–1377.
3. Sterns RH, Cox M, Feig PU, Singer I. Internal potassium balance and the control of the plasma potassium concentration. Medicine 60: 339–354, 1981.
4. Kopple JD, Blumenkrantz MJ. Total parenteral nutrition and parenteral fluid therapy. In Clinical Disorders of Fluid and Electrolyte Metabolism, Maxwell MH, Kleeman CR (eds). New York: McGraw-Hill, 1980 (3rd ed) pp. 413–498.
5. Feest TG. Low molecular weight dextran: A continuing cause of acute renal failure. Brit Med J 2: 1300, 1976.
6. Phillips SF. Water and electrolytes in gastrointestinal disease. In Clinical Disorders of Fluid and Electrolyte Metabolism, Maxwell MH, Kleeman CR (eds). New York: McGraw-Hill, 1980, (3rd edition) pp. 1267–1290.

7. Orloff MJ, Chandler JG. Fluid and electrolyte disorders in burns. In Clinical Disorders of Fluid and Electrolyte Metabolism, Maxwell MH, Kleeman CR (eds). New York: McGraw-Hill, 1972, (2nd edition) pp. 1043–1062.

8. Hartford CE. Burns. In 1983 Current Therapy, Conn Hf (ed). Philadelphia: WB Saunders, 1983, pp. 913–922.

9. Planas M, Wachtel T, Frank H, Henderson LW. Characterization of acute renal failure in the burned patient. Arch Intern Med 142: 2087–2091, 1982.

10. Arieff AI. Principles of parenteral therapy. A Principles of parenteral therapy and parenteral nutrition. In Clinical Disorders of fluid and electrolyte metabolism, Maxwell MH, Kleeman CR (eds). New York: McGraw-Hill, 1972, (2nd ed) pp. 567–589.

11. Eble JN. A proposed mechanism for the depressor effect of dopamine in the anesthetized dog. J Pharmacol Exp Ther 145: 64–70, 1964.

12. Andreucci VE, Dal Canton A, Corradi A. Gli effetti della Norepinefrina sulle pressioni idrodinamiche corticali nei nefroni superficiali di ratti normali ed in ipotensione emorragica. Ateneo Parmense, Acta Bio-Med, 45: 113–129, 1974.

13. Andreucci VE, Dal Canton A, Corradi A, Stanziale R, Migone L. Role of the efferent arteriole in glomerular hemodynamics of superficial nephrons. Kidney Int 9: 475–480, 1976.

14. Hardaker WT Jr, Wechsler AS. Redistribution of renal intracortical blood flow during dopamine infusion in dogs. Circ Res 33: 437–444, 1973.

15. Goldberg LI. Cardiovascular and renal actions of dopamine: Potential clinical applications. Pharmacol Rev 24: 1–29, 1972.

16. Goldberg LI. Dopamine. Clinical uses of an endogenous catecholamine. N Engl J Med, 291: 707–710, 1974.

17. Neiberger RE, Passmore JC. Effects of dopamine on canine intrarenal blood flow distribution during hemorrhage. Kidney Int 15: 219–226, 1979.

18. Reid PR, Thompson WL. The clinical use of dopamine in the treatment of shock. Johns Hopkins Med J 137: 276–279, 1975.

19. Chan L, Ledingham JGG, Dixon JA, Thulborn KR, Waterton JC, Radda GK, Ross BD. Acute renal failure: A proposed mechanism based upon [31]p nuclear magnetic resonance studies in the rat. In Acute Renal Failure, Eliahou HE (ed). London: John Libbey, 1982, pp. 35–41.

20. Chan L, Ledingham JGG, Clarke J, Ross BD. The importance of pH in acute renal failure. In Acute Renal Failure, Eliahou HE (ed). London: John Libbey, 1982, pp. 58–61.

21. Bore PJ, Chan L, Sehr PA, Thulborn KR, Ross BD, Radda GK. Protection of kidney from ischemic acidosis: A new approach to renal preservation. Eur Surg Res 12 (Suppl 1): 20–21, 1980.

22. Bore PJ, Sehr PA, Chan L, Thulborn KR, Ross BD, Radda GK. The importance of pH in renal preservation. Transpl Proc 13: 707–709, 1981.

23. Schrier RW: Acute renal failure. JAMA 247: 2518–2525, 1982.

24. Henrich WL, Anderson RJ, Berns AS, McDonald KM, Paulsen PJ, Berl T, Schrier RW. Role of renal nerves and prostaglandins in control of renal hemodynamics and plasma renin activity during hypotensive hemorrhage in the dog. J Clin Invest 61: 744–750, 1978.

25. van Ypersele de Strihou C. Acute oliguric interstitial nephritis. Kidney Int 16: 751–765, 1979.

26. Minuth AN, Terrell JB Jr, Suki WN. Acute renal failure: A study of the course and prognosis of 104 patients and of the role of furosemide. Am J Med Sci 271: 317–324, 1976.

27. Anderson RJ, Linas SL, Berns AS, Henrich WL, Miller TR, Gabow PA, Schrier RW. Nonoliguric acute renal failure. N Engl J Med 296: 1134–1138, 1977.

28. Bichet DG, Burke TJ, Schrier RW. Prevention and pathogenesis of acute renal failure. Clin Exper Dial Apheresis 5: 127–141, 1981.

29. Kjellstrand CM. Ethacrynic acid in acute tubular necrosis. Nephron 9: 337–348, 1972.

30. Muth RG. Furosemide in acute renal failure. In Proceedings of Acute Renal Failure Conference, Friedman EA, Eliahou HE (eds). Washington, DHEW Publication No (NIH) 74–608, 1973, pp. 245–263.

31. Brown CB, Cameron JS, Ogg CS, Bewick M, Stott RB. Established acute renal failure following surgical operations. In Proceedings of Acute Renal Failure Conference, Friedman EA, Eliahou HE (eds). Washington, DHEW Publication No (NIH) 74–608, 1973, pp. 187–208.

32. Epstein M, Schneider NS, Befeler B. Effect of intrarenal furosemide on renal function and intrarenal hemodynamics in acute renal failure. Am J Med 58: 510–516, 1975.

33. Levinsky NG, Bernard DB, Johnston PA. Enhancement of recovery of acute renal failure; Effects of mannitol and diuretics. In Acute Renal Failure, Brenner BM, Stein JH (eds). New York: Churchill Livingstone, 1980, pp. 163–179.

34. Barcenas CG, Jones P, Salomon S, Van Reet R, Cooley DA. Cardiogenic acute renal failure (CARF) following open-heart surgery. Cardiov Dis 6: 298–307, 1979.

35. Cantarovich F, Locatelli A, Fernandez JC, Perez Loredo J, Cristhot J. Frusemide in high doses in the treatment of acute renal failure. Postgrad Med J (Suppl) 47: 13–17, 1971.

36. Cantarovich F, Galli C, Benedetti L, Chena C, Castro L, Correa C, Perez Loredo J, Fernandez JC, Locatelli A, Tizado J. High-dose frusemide in established acute renal failure. Brit Med J 4: 449–450, 1973.

37. Kleinknecht D, Ganeval D, Gonzales-Duque LA, Fermanian J. Furosemide in acute oliguric renal failure. A controlled trial. Nephron 17: 51–58, 1976.

38. Borirakchanyavat V, Vongsthongsri M, Sitprija V. Furosemide and acute renal failure. Postgrad Med J 54: 30–32, 1978.

39. Lindner A, Cutler RE, Goodman WG. Synergism of dopamine plus furosemide in preventing acute renal failure in the dog. Kidney Int 16: 158–166, 1979.

40. Graziani G, Cairo G, Tarantino F, Ponticelli C. Dopamine and frusemide in acute renal failure. Lancet II: 1301, 1980.

41. Henderson IS, Beattie TJ, Kennedy AC. Dopamine hydrochloride in oliguric states. Lancet 2: 827–828, 1980.

42. Lucas A, Meignan M, Le Gall Jr, Tillement JP, Rapin M. Caractéristiques pharmacocinétiques d'une forte dose de furosémide dans l'insuffisance rénale aiguë. Biomédicine 24: 45–49, 1976.

43. Lindner A, Sherrard DJ, Shen F, Cutler RE. Dopamine and furosemide in acute renal failure. In Acute Renal Failure, Eliahou HE (ed). London: John Libbey, 1982, pp. 174–175.

44. Barry KG, Malloy JP. Oliguric renal failure. JAMA 179: 510–513, 1962.

45. Eliahou HE. Mannitol therapy in oliguria of acute onset. Brit Med J 1: 807–809, 1964.

46. Luke RG, Linton AL, Briggs JD, Kennedy AC. Mannitol therapy in acute renal failure. Lancet 1: 980–982, 1965.

47. Luke RG, Kennedy AC. Prevention and early management of acute renal failure. Postgrad Med J 43: 280–289, 1967.

48. Luke RG, Briggs JD, Allison MEM, Kennedy AC. Factors determining response to mannitol in acute renal failure. Am J Med Sci 259: 168–174, 1970.

49. Eneas JF, Schoenfeld PY, Humphreys MH. The effect of infusion of mannitol-sodium bicarbonate on the clinical course of myoglobinuria. Arch Intern Med, 139: 801–805, 1979.

50. Warren SE, Blantz RC. Mannitol. Arch Intern Med 141: 493–497, 1981.

51. Johnston PA, Bernard DB, Donohoe JF, Perrin NS, Levinsky NG. Effect of volume expansion on hemodynamics of the hypoperfused rat kidney. J Clin Invest 64: 550–558, 1979.

52. Johnston PA, Bernard DB, Perrin NS, Levinsky NG. Prostaglandins mediate the vasodilatory effect of mannitol in the hypoperfused rat kidney. J Clin Invest 68: 127–133, 1981.

53. Ng RCK, Suki WN. Treatment of acute renal failure. In Acute Renal Failure, Brenner BM, Stein JH (eds). New York: Churchill Livingstone, 1980, pp. 229–273.

54. Irvine ROH. Diet and drugs in renal acidosis and acid-base regulation. In Drug Affecting Kidney Function and Metabolism, Edwards KDG (ed). Basel: Karger, 1972, pp. 146–188.

55. de Wardener HE. The Kidney. An Outline of Normal and Abnormal Structure and Function. Edinburgh: Churchill Livingston, 1973.

56. Andreucci VE. Chronic renal failure. In The Treatment of Renal Failure, Castro JE (ed). Lancaster: MTP Press Limited, 1982, pp. 33–167.

57. Barton CH, Vaziri ND, Ness RL, Saiki JK, Mirahmadi KS. Cimetidine in the management of metabolic alkalosis induced by nasogastric drainage. Arch Surg 114: 70–74, 1979.

58. Abouna GM, Veazy PR, Terry DB. Intravenous infusion of hydrochloric acid for treatment of severe metabolic alkalosis. Surgery 75: 194–202, 1974.

59. Garella S, Chang BS, Kahn SI. Dilution acidosis and contraction alkalosis: Review of a concept. Kidney Int 8: 279–283, 1975.

60. Bushinsky DA, Gennari FJ. Life-threatening hyperkalemia induced by arginine. Ann Intern Med 89: 632–634, 1978.

61. Kunis CL, Lowenstein J. The emergency treatment of hyperkalemia. Med Clin North Am 65: 165–176, 1981.

62. Lee HA. The management of acute renal failure. In Acute Renal Failure, Chapman A (ed). Edinburgh: Churchill Livingstone, 1980, pp. 104–124.

63. Cox M, Sterns RH, Singer I. The defense against hyperkalemia: The roles of insulin and aldosterone. N Engl J Med 299: 525–532, 1978.

64. De Fronzo R, Felig P, Ferrannini E, Wahren J. Effects of graded doses of insulin on splanchnic and peripheral potassium metabolism in man. Am J Physiol 238: F421–F427, 1980.

65. Berlyne GM, Janabi K, Shaw AB. Dangers of Resonium A in the treatment of hyperkalemia in renal failure. Lancet 1: 167–170, 1966.

66. Whelton A, Schach von Witenau M, Twomey TM, Gordon Walker W, Bianchine JR. Doxycycline pharmacokinetics in the absence of renal function. Kidney Int 5: 365–371, 1974.

67. Kleinknecht D, Ganeval D. Preventive hemodialysis in acute renal failure. Its effect on mortality and morbidity. In Proceedings of Acute Renal Failure Conference, Friedman EA, Eliahou HE (eds). Washington, DHEW Publication No (NIH) 74–608, 1973, pp. 165–185.

68. Larsson R, Bodemar G, Kagedal B. Effect of cimetidine, a new histamine H_2-receptor antagonist, on renal function. Acta Med Scand 205: 87–89, 1979.

69. Oken DE. On the differential diagnosis of acute renal failure. Am J Med 71: 916–920, 1981.

70. McMurray SD, Luft FC, Maxwell DR, Hamburger RJ, Futty D, Szwed JJ, Lavelle KJ, Kleit SA. Prevailing patterns and predictor variables in patients with acute tubular necrosis. Arch Intern Med 138: 950–955, 1978.

71. Kjellstrand CM, Gornick C, Davin T. Recovery from acute renal failure. Clin Exper Dial Apheresis 5: 143–161, 1981.

72. Balslow JT, Jorgensen HE. A survey of 499 patients with acute anuric renal insufficiency. Am J Med 34: 753–764, 1963.

73. Kennedy AC, Burton JA, Luke RG, Briggs JD, Lindsay RM, Allison MEM, Edward N, Dargie HJ. Factors affecting the prognosis in acute renal failure. Quart J Med 42: 73–86, 1973.

74. Kjellstrand CM, Casali RE, Simmons RL, Shideman JR, Buselmeier TJ, Najarian JS. Etiology and prognosis in acute posttransplant renal failure. Am J Med 61: 190, 1976.

22. THE ROLE FOR NUTRITION IN ACUTE RENAL FAILURE

Joel D. Kopple

Bruno Cianciaruso

1 Metabolism in Acute Renal Failure

Patients with acute renal failure (ARF) have widely varying metabolic and nutritional status. Most patients with ARF have some degree of net protein breakdown (synthesis minus degradation) and have altered fluid, electrolyte, or acid-base status. Commonly, there is water overload, azotemia, hyperuricemia, hyperkalemia, hypocalcemia, hyperphosphatemia, and metabolic acidosis with large anion gap. However, there are patients who show no evidence for negative-nitrogen balance and who have normal water balance, plasma electrolyte concentrations, and acid-base status. These latter patients usually have no severely catabolic underlying illnesses. Generally, they are not oliguric, and, typically, the cause of their ARF is an isolated, noncatabolic event, such as administration of radiocontrast drugs or other medicines.

Patients with ARF can sustain massive net protein degradation, with net losses of 150 to 200 g/day or more [1, 2]; by comparison, the total protein mass of a 70 kg man is about 6 to 10 kg [3]. When ARF is caused by shock, sepsis, or rhabdomyolysis, patients are more likely to be catabolic. Feinstein et al. [2] observed that the mean urea nitrogen appearance (UNA, net urea nitrogen production) in patients was 12.0 ± 7.9 (SD) g/day when ARF was caused by hypotension and/or sepsis and 12.3 ± 7.9 g/day when it was due to rhabdo-

myolysis. These values were significantly greater ($p < 0.001$ and $p < 0.05$, respectively) than the UNA of patients with ARF due to other causes, 3.8 ± 2.4 g/day.

When patients with ARF have marked net protein breakdown, there is usually an accelerated rise in plasma potassium, phosphorus, and nitrogen metabolites, and in acidemia. In nonuremic humans, wasting and malnutrition can impair normal wound healing and immune function [4, 5] and enhance morbidity and mortality. Thus, patients with ARF who are very catabolic may also be at increased risk for delayed wound healing, infection, prolonged convalescence, and increased mortality.

1.1 FACTORS PROMOTING WASTING IN ARF

Many factors cause wasting in ARF. In animals, several studies suggest that acute uremia itself may cause disorders in amino acid and protein metabolism and promote wasting. Lacy [6] observed increased uptake of several amino acids and enhanced urea production in liver from acutely uremic rats. Fröhlich et al. [7] examined net glucose and urea output from perfused liver in rats with bilateral nephrectomy and in sham-operated and nonoperated controls. They found that in comparison to controls, the acutely uremic rats had increased hepatic release of glucose, urea, and the branched chain amino acids—valine, leucine, and isoleucine—which are not well metabolized by the liver. These findings indicate that acute uremia in rats stimulates both gluconeogenesis and protein degradation in the liver.

The response of protein synthesis and degradation to acute uremia may vary independently of each other and according to the organ studied. McCormick et al. [8] found increased incorporation of ^{14}C-leucine into TCA-precipitable material in liver homogenates from acutely uremic rats, suggesting enhanced hepatic protein synthesis. Shear [9] reported that protein synthesis was increased in liver and heart and decreased in skeletal muscle of acutely uremic rats. Flügel-Link et al. [10] and Pan and co-workers [11] studied protein synthesis and degradation in perfused posterior hemicorpus of rats made acutely uremic by bilateral nephrectomy and in sham-operated control rats. There was increased UNA in the acutely uremic rats, indicating enhanced hepatic gluconeogenesis and net protein degradation; plasma and intracellular muscle concentrations of most amino acids were significantly decreased. Muscle protein synthesis was reduced and protein degradation was increased in the acutely uremic animals. These animals also manifested increased release of tyrosine, phenylalanine, alanine, total nonessential amino acids, and total amino acids from the perfused hemicorpus. Clark and Mitch [12] also reported increased degradation and decreased synthesis of muscle protein in acutely uremic rats.

The mechanisms responsible for increased gluconeogenesis and net protein degradation in rats with ARF are not well defined. Sapico and associates [13, 14] report that activity of glutamic oxaloacetic aminotransferase, which catalyzes the transamination of glutamate, is increased in the liver of acutely uremic rats. In addition, there is reported to be increased activity of two enzymes involved with metabolism of urea cycle amino acids, ornithine transaminase, which catalzyes the conversion of glutamate to ornithine, and arginase, which catalyzes formation of urea and ornithine from arginine. In addition, Sapico et al. [15] report that in liver of acutely uremic rats, phenylalanine hydroxylase activity is not increased while tyrosine aminotransferase is elevated; these enzymes catalyze the initial reactions along the major degradative pathway for phenylalanine and tyrosine.

Acute uremia may alter glycogen metabolism. Bergström and Hultman [16] reported decreased muscle glycogen content in catabolic acutely uremic patients. Hörl and Heidland [17] observed reduced muscle glycogen in bilaterally nephrectomized rats in comparison to sham-operated controls. In muscle from these rats, they also found increased activity of phosphorylase a, which catalyzes glycogenolysis, and decreased activity of glycogen synthetase I, which catalyzes glycogen synthesis. It is not known whether these alterations contribute to protein wasting in acute uremia. It is of interest that Hörl and Heidland [17] found that muscle glycogen synthetase I activity increased in these rats when their low-protein diet was supplemented with serine.

The contribution of altered endocrinological function (vide infra) or retention of toxic metabolic products to these metabolic changes in acute uremia is not known. There is also the possibility that the surgical procedures utilized for making rats uremic (e.g., bilateral nephrectomy) may be a greater catabolic stress to the animal than is the sham surgery. If it is, then the enhanced net protein catabolism in these animals might be due to surgical stress rather than to the influence of uremia. However, since almost every study indicates that acute uremia is a catabolic stress in rats, it seems most likely that enhanced catabolism in these animals is due to uremia per se rather than to the methods of creating renal failure.

The wasting that frequently occurs in ARF may be caused by several factors (table 22–1): First, metabolic products that accumulate in uremia may be toxic [18]. Although there have

TABLE 22–1. Potential causes of catabolism in patients with acute renal failure

1. Accumulation of toxic metabolic products.
2. Increased plasma concentrations of catabolic hormones or resistance to the anabolic hormone, insulin.
3. Increased protease activity.
4. Release of endogenous leukocyte mediators.
5. Inadequate nutrient intake.
6. Underlying or superimposed illnesses.
7. Nutrient losses in draining fistulas.
8. Nutrient losses from dialysis.
9. Blood sampling or blood loss.

Note: Although there is evidence that each of these factors contributes to wasting in patients with acute renal failure, the evidence is not always definitive.

been many studies of the potential toxicity of these compounds [18], there are still no definitive studies demonstrating that these compounds may promote wasting in acute or chronic uremia.

Second, increased plasma concentrations of catabolic hormones may also promote wasting. Eigler et al. [19] showed that healthy dogs infused with cortisone, epinephrine, and glucagon in quantities sufficient to raise plasma concentrations to levels found in acutely catabolic patients demonstrated a sustained increase in glucose production. Since much of the glucose formed was probably derived from amino acids, particularly alanine and glutamine, it is likely that these endocrine disorders also promoted protein wasting. There is less information concerning the effects of these hormones in ARF. Serum glucagon levels are increased in ARF [20]. In chronic uremia, there appears to be increased sensitivity to the actions of glucagon [21]; however, Mondon and Reaven [22] were unable to demonstrate enhanced sensitivity to glucagon in acutely uremic rats. Although there is resistance to the action of insulin in chronic renal failure (CRF) [23, 24], there are less data concerning insulin resistance in ARF. Glucose intolerance is common in patients with ARF [2]. Parathyroid hormone, another potentially catabolic agent [25], may be increased in ARF [26, 27].

A third factor, recently reported by Hörl and Heidland [28], is that proteolytic activity is increased in the sera of patients with ARF who are very catabolic. These observations suggest that in sera of such patients, there may be a rise in the quantity of proteases (i.e., enzymes that catalyze the degradation of proteins), a reduction in protease inhibitors, or an increase in factors that enhance protease activity. Increased activity of certain muscle proteases has been reported in nonuremic patients with net protein catabolism [29]. To our knowledge, increased muscle or liver protease activity has not been described in uremic patients. In the acutely uremic rats who have increased muscle protein degradation, Flügel-Link et al. [10] found that muscle activity of the proteases—cathepsin B_1, cathepsin D, and alkaline protease—were not different from controls. The role of protease ac-

tivity in uremia should be an important area for further investigation.

A fourth factor has recently been suggested: that acutely stressed nonuremic catabolic patients have circulating compounds that stimulate muscle protein degradation, possibly by activation of prostaglandins and muscle proteases [30, 31]. The compounds may be structurally related or identical to interleukin-I. Whether these compounds are also active in catabolic patients with ARF is not known.

Other potential causes for wasting and malnutrition in ARF include a fifth factor, that many patients are unable to eat adequately because of anorexia or vomiting. These symptoms may be caused by acute uremia, underlying illnesses, or the anoretic effects of dialysis treatment. Other causes for poor food intake include medical or surgical disorders that impair gastrointestinal function and the frequent employment of diagnostic studies that require the patient to fast for several hours. A sixth factor, the patient's underlying or superimposed medical disorders, frequently is a major cause of wasting. Chief among these catabolic conditions are infection, hypotension, surgical or nonsurgical trauma, and rhabdomyolysis.

Nutrient losses in draining fistulas and losses of nutrients during dialysis therapy, the seventh and eighth causes, may also lead to wasting and malnutrition. Approximately 6 to 7 g of free amino acids are removed during a four-hour hemodialysis [32–34]. During intermittent peritoneal dialysis for approximately 24 to 32 hours, about 5 g of amino acids are lost [35, 36]. With continuous ambulatory peritoneal dialysis (CAPD), about 1.5 to 3.5 g of free amino acids are lost each day [37, 38]. Not much protein is removed during hemodialysis; however, during acute intermittent peritoneal dialysis for about 36 hours, approximately 22 g of total protein and 13 g of albumin are lost [39]. During maintenance intermittent peritoneal dialysis for about 10 hours, about 13 g of total protein and 8 to 9 g of albumin are removed [39]. Much of these losses are from ascitic fluid washout. With CAPD, the 24-hour losses of total protein and albumin are about 9 g and 6 g, respectively. In patients undergoing chronic intermittent peritoneal dialysis who have acute peritonitis, protein losses can increase markedly. We have observed one such patient who lost 106 g of protein during a 24-hour period. With treatment of acute peritonitis, protein losses may fall quickly but may not return to normal for many weeks.

Patients undergoing hemodialysis with glucose-free dialysate may lose 20 to 50 g of glucose during a four- to six-hour procedure. Glucose losses are directly related to the dialyzer used and to the blood glucose levels. There is net glucose absorption with peritoneal dialysis because the dialysate contains glucose monohydrate, 1.5 to 4.25 g/dl. Glucose absorption varies directly with the concentration of glucose in dialysate or the total quantity of glucose instilled. During CAPD, glucose absorption (y, g/day) is related to the quantity instilled each day (x, g/day) as follows [40]: $y = 0.89x - 43$, $r = 0.91$, $p < 0.001$. In the experience of Grodstein et al. [40], about 180 g/day of glucose was absorbed during CAPD. Water-soluble vitamins and probably other biologically active substances are also lost during both hemodialysis and peritoneal dialysis. Losses of the water-soluble vitamins during dialysis are readily replaced with oral or peritoneal vitamin supplements.

A ninth cause of protein depletion in ARF is blood loss; blood drawing, gastrointestinal bleeding, which may be occult, and blood sequestered in the hemodialyzer are the major sources of blood loss. A person with a hemoglobin of 12.0 g/dl and a serum total protein of 7.0 g/dl will lose approximately 16.5 g of protein in each 100 ml of blood removed.

2 Previous Experience With Nutritional Treatment of ARF

There are three major goals for which nutritional therapy has been advocated in ARF: (a) to reduce uremic toxicity and improve metabolic derangements; (b) to maintain or improve overall nutritional and clinical status, particularly with regard to wound healing, immunological function, and host resistance; and (c) to facilitate healing of the injured kidney.

In this section, we will review the published literature concerning nutritional therapy in ARF, particularly with regard to its effects on nutritional and metabolic status, metabolism of the kidney, recovery of renal function, and survival.

2.1 EARLY EXPERIENCE WITH NUTRITIONAL THERAPY FOR PATIENTS WITH ARF

Before the mid-1960s, the primary goal of nutritional therapy was to reduce accumulation of nitrogenous products of protein metabolism that were considered to be toxic. Many clinicians advocated severe or total restriction of protein intake for patients with ARF [41–43]. To reduce the rate of protein degradation, small amounts of energy (e.g., 400 to 800 kcal/day) were given as candy, butterballs, or intravenous infusions of concentrated glucose. This therapy was based on Gamble's studies of lifeboat rations for healthy young men. Gamble [44] found that administration of 100 g/day of sugar could substantially reduce net protein breakdown; 200 g/day of sugar could spare more protein although the protein sparing was not twice as great as with 100 g/day of sugar. However, these latter studies were carried out in healthy volunteers who were clinically stable, whereas acutely uremic patients are often severely catabolic and may have extra losses of nutrients from dialysis, wound drainage, and blood drawing. Hence, the ability of such small quantities of calories to reduce net protein wasting in stressed patients with ARF may have been markedly limited or negligible.

Anabolic steroids were frequently employed because they transiently decreased the UNA, the rate of rise of serum urea nitrogen (SUN) or nonprotein nitrogen, and the development of acidosis. In the 1960s, the Giordano-Giovannetti diet was developed, which provided about 20 g/day of protein. About 12 to 14 g of the protein was usually supplied by two eggs, which provided the recommended daily allowances for essential amino acids (again for healthy young adults). Although this diet was derived for patients with CRF, some clinicians advocated the diet for the acutely uremic patient who was able to eat. These clinicians believed that the diet could be utilized efficiently and, hence, would minimize the degree of protein wasting while it reduced accumulation of nitrogenous metabolites [45].

These techniques for nutritional therapy were developed at a time when dialysis treatment was not readily available. Hence, the primary goal of treatment was to reduce uremic toxicity and other complications of renal failure and thereby to maintain life until renal function recovered. Maintenance of good nutrition was a secondary aim. When dialysis became available, it usually was employed only to treat specific sequelae of renal failure, such as uremic symptoms, congestive heart failure, or hyperkalemia, and great efforts were often made to avoid the need for dialysis therapy. It is now generally accepted that early and frequent dialysis should be employed prophylactically in patients with ARF to prevent uremic signs and symptoms and morbidity as well as mortality [46].

2.2 DEVELOPMENT OF TOTAL PARENTERAL NUTRITION (TPN) FOR ARF

With the development of modern techniques for TPN and more widespread availability of dialysis therapy, many physicians employed this former treatment in patients with ARF who were unable to eat even though it increased the need for dialysis therapy. In 1967, Lee and coworkers [47] described their results in several patients with acute or chronic renal failure; patients were infused solutions containing casein hydrolysate, fructose, ethanol, and soya bean oil emulsion (Intralipid®) into a peripheral vein. Despite the severity of the patients' illnesses, marked loss of weight did not occur and convalescence was shortened.

In 1969 and 1970, Dudrick and associates [48, 49] reported treating 10 acutely or chronically uremic patients with intravenous infusions of essential amino acids and hypertonic glucose into the subclavian vein. They described weight gain, improved wound healing, and stabilization or reduction in SUN levels. Decreased serum potassium and phosphorus and positive nitrogen balance were often observed. They also reported that anephric beagles who received intravenous infusions of essential amino acids and 57% glucose had a lower rise in SUN and longer survival than anephric beagles who were given food or infusions of glucose (5% or 57%) alone [50].

Abel and coworkers [51–55] reported a series of studies in patients with ARF who were treated with hypertonic glucose and eight essential amino acids, excluding histidine. They found that the serum potassium, phosphorus, and magnesium fell and that SUN often stabilized or decreased. They carried out a prospective double-blind study in 53 patients with ARF who were randomly assigned to receive infusions of either essential amino acids and hypertonic glucose or hypertonic glucose alone [51]. Total calorie intake averaged 1,426 and 1,641 kcal/day with the two solutions. Mean amino acid intake with the former preparation was about 16 g/day. It was not stated whether patients ate food during the study. The patients receiving the essential amino acids and glucose had a higher incidence of recovery of renal function. However, overall hospital mortality was only slightly and not significantly improved in this group. The essential amino acid solution appeared to be particularly effective in patients with more severe renal failure, such as those who needed dialysis therapy or who sustained serious complications such as pneumonia and generalized sepsis. Among these latter patients, hospital survival was significantly greater in those who received essential amino acids and glucose than in those infused with glucose alone.

Baek and coworkers [56] compared 63 patients treated with a fibrin hydrolysate and hypertonic glucose with 66 subjects who received varying quantities of glucose. The rate of rise in SUN in the two groups was not different, but the incidence of hyperkalemia, morbidity, and mortality was lower in the patients given the hydrolysate and glucose. However, it is not clear whether the patients were randomly assigned to the two treatment regimens or whether the two groups of patients were even treated concurrently.

McMurray et al. [57] and Milligan and associates [58] studied patients with acute tubular necrosis (ATN) who received either hypertonic glucose alone (200 to 400 kcal/day) or a mixture of essential and nonessential amino acids and hypertonic glucose which provided 12 g nitrogen/day and greater than 2000 kcal/day. In patients with no complications, there was no difference in survival between the two treatment groups. However, in those with three or more complications or with peritonitis, the patients who received 12 g/day of amino acid nitrogen and hypertonic glucose had significantly greater survival in comparison to the individuals receiving low quantities of glucose alone.

Blackburn, Etter and MacKenzie [59] described studies in 11 patients with ARF who were given, in a crossover design, infusions providing 1.2% essential amino acids and 37% glucose, 2.0% essential and nonessential amino acids and 37% glucose, or 2.1% essential and nonessential amino acids and 52% glucose. Patients were not severely ill at the time of the study. Infusion with greater quantities of glucose was associated with a significant fall in SUN and creatinine, whereas there was a slight but not significantly greater decrease in SUN in patients receiving the essential amino acids as compared to those given essential and nonessential amino acids which provided more nitrogen. When nitrogen intake was increased to 4 to 5 g/day, nitrogen balance improved and became almost neutral. Patients did not appear to be assigned in random fashion to their treatment group.

Abitbol and Holliday [60] infused, in sequential order, glucose alone and glucose with essential amino acids to four anuric children who had the hemolytic-uremic syndrome and to two children with systemic lupus erythematosus or congenital nephrosis. Nitrogen balance was negative with glucose alone and positive with glucose and essential amino acids; SUN rose more slowly with the latter solution. As energy intake increased from 20 to 70 kcal/kg/day, nitrogen balance became less negative. The children were malnourished at the onset of the study, and they were given first the glucose infusion and then the infusion of glucose and amino acids; the latter was also higher in calories. These factors could account for the greater anabolic response to both the higher energy intake and the amino acid therapy.

Several studies indicate that nitrogen requirements are high in patients with ARF who are hypercatabolic and that nitrogen balance is difficult to attain with low-nitrogen diets. Leonard, Luke, and Siegel [1] carried out a prospective study in patients with ARF who were randomly assigned to receive infusions of 1.75% L-essential amino acids and 47% dextrose or 47% dextrose alone. Patients who were able to eat or tolerate tube feeding were excluded from the study, and many had severe complicating illnesses. Most patients required dialysis frequently. The rate of rise in SUN was significantly less in the group receiving essential amino acids. However, mean nitrogen balance was negative by approximately 10 g/day in both groups, and there was no difference in the rate of survival or recovery of renal function in the two groups.

Spreiter, Myers, and Swenson [61] carried out 32 studies in 14 patients with ARF who were infused with various quantities of amino acids and hypertonic glucose. Nitrogen balance became positive in only four subjects and at a time when the mean amino acid and glucose intake was 1.03 g/kg/day and 50 kcal/kg/day, respectively. These studies may have underestimated nutrient requirements because patients often were not able to tolerate the fluid and nitrogen loads associated with the higher intakes until some days had passed, and by that time their clinical condition may have improved. Thus, the patients may have received the higher nitrogen and energy intakes at a time when they were less ill and possibly more able to become anabolic.

Lopez-Martinez et al. [62] evaluated the effects of parenteral nutrition for 12 days in 35 septic patients with ARF. At the time of study, the patients were in the polyuric phase and were not very uremic; none had received dialysis therapy. Patients were given 4.4 g/day of nitrogen from essential amino acids and 2,000 kcal/day (group 1), or 15 g/day of nitrogen from essential and nonessential amino acids and 3000 kcal/day provided either from glucose and fat (group 3). Nitrogen balance, apparently estimated from the difference between nitrogen intake and UNA, was initially negative in all three groups and became more positive with time, particularly in groups 2 and 3. During the 12-day period of study, the grand means of nitrogen balances in groups 2 and 3 were each significantly more positive than in group 1.

Hasik et al. [63] fed diets varying in protein content to nine patients with ARF at a time when they were polyuric. The authors concluded that these patients, who were probably not severely ill at the time of study, required 0.97 g protein/kg/day. Since patients were neither very uremic or ill in these last two studies, the results may be more applicable to the patient who is not very catabolic and is recovering from ARF.

Feinstein et al. evaluated 30 patients with ARF who were unable to be adequately nourished through the enteral tract. Patients were randomly assigned to receive parenteral nutrition with glucose alone (n = 7), glucose and 21 g/day of the essential amino acids (n = 11), or glucose and 21 g/day of essential amino acids and 21 g/day of nonessential amino acids (n = 12). They did not receive enteral nutrition during the study [2]. Mean energy intake varied from 2,300 to 2,700 kcal/day and did not differ significantly among the groups. Patients were studied in a prospective double-blind fashion; mean duration of study in the three groups was 9.0 ± 7.7 days. Many patients were markedly catabolic throughout the course of study as determined from the UNA, nitrogen balances, serum total protein, albumin, transferrin levels (table 22-2), and plasma amino acid concentrations (figure 22-1). Mean nitrogen balance, estimated from the difference between nitrogen intake and UNA, which underestimates nitrogen losses, was -10.4 ± 5.7 g/day with glucose alone, -4.4 ± 7.3 g/day with glucose and essential amino acids, and -8.5 ± 7.9 g/day with glucose and essential

and nonessential amino acids. Although the estimated nitrogen balance was not different with the three infusates, in a few patients who received essential or essential and nonessential amino acids balance was only slightly negative or, in one patient, possibly neutral or positive. Serum potassium, phosphorus, and SUN often stabilized or decreased in all three treatment groups; these changes in serum levels were probably related to dialysis therapy, recovering renal function, or the natural history of the underlying metabolic disorders. Of the seven patients who received glucose, two recovered renal function and two survived. Of the 11 patients given glucose and essential amino acids, seven recovered renal function and six survived. Of the 12 patients who received glucose and essential and nonessential amino acids, four recovered renal function and three survived. The slight and not significant tendency for greater recovery and survival in patients who received glucose and essential amino acids may be due to the fact that renal failure was caused by shock or sepsis in a lower proportion of these patients as compared to the other groups [2]. In all patients in whom renal failure was attributed to hypotension and/or sepsis, there was a significantly lower rate of recovery of renal function (17%) and survival (17%) as compared to patients with renal failure from other causes.

The findings from this study, therefore, indicate that there is a high incidence of wasting and malnutrition in patients with ARF who are unable to receive adequate nourishment through the gastrointestinal tract, particularly if shock or sepsis is the cause of their renal failure. None of the nutritional treatments led to defi-

TABLE 22-2. Serum protein concentration at termination of parenteral nutrition in patients with acute renal failure.

Serum proteins	Normal	Glucose	Glucose + EAA	Glucose + ENAA
Number of subjects	49	5	7	9
Total protein (g/dl)	7.43 ± 0.63^a	6.1 ± 1.0^b	5.7 ± 0.9^c	5.0 ± 0.6^c
Albumin (g/dl)	5.06 ± 0.35	2.8 ± 0.7^c	2.8 ± 0.4^c	2.8 ± 0.7^c
Transferrin (mg/dl)	309 ± 39	127 ± 53^c	131 ± 62^c	161 ± 44^c

[a]Mean ± standard deviation. Probability that serum concentrations are not different from normal values;
[b]$p < 0.005$.
[c]$p < 0.001$.
Source: Adapted from Kopple and Feinstein [64].

430

nite clinical improvement. Moreover, the high UNA, negative nitrogen balance, and low serum protein values and plasma amino acid concentrations indicate that with each treatment regimen the patients were often hypercatabolic and wasted.

As a result of these studies, Feinstein and coworkers [64, 65] investigated whether TPN with larger quantities of essential and nonessential amino acids could improve nutritional status, recovery of renal function, and survival in patients with ARF. Patients with ARF who could not be nourished through the enteral tract were randomly assigned to receive one of two intravenous treatments: 21 g/day of the nine essential amino acids (2.3 g amino acid nitrogen/day) or a quantity of essential and nonessential amino acids that varied according to the UNA. With the latter therapy, the daily nitrogen intake was adjusted every two or three days in an attempt to exceed the UNA by 2.0 g N/day. Nitrogen intake, however, was not allowed to increase above 15 g/day. During the study, patients did not receive any nutrition through the enteral tract. The ratio of essential to nonessential amino acids with the latter therapy was 1:1; at the time they commenced, commercially available mixed amino acid solutions that provided a higher ratio of essential to nonessential amino acids were not available. Patients were given hypertonic glucose, minerals, and vitamins with both therapies.

Preliminary data are available in 11 patients; five received the essential amino acid solutions for 12 ± 3 days, and six were treated with the essential and nonessential amino acid regimen for 18 ± 5 days. ARF was attributed to shock in 10 patients. The average daily energy intake was similar with the two treatments, 2542 ± 130 and 2563 ± 137 kcal/day, respectively. Three patients given essential amino acids recovered renal function and two survived. Two patients treated with essential and nonessential amino acids recovered renal function, but non survived. Mean daily nitrogen intake was less in the essential amino acid group than in the essential and nonessential group (2.3 ± 0.3 g/day vs 11.3 ± 1.9 g/day, p < 0.001). UNA was significantly less in patients receiving essential amino acids (7.5 ± 1.4 vs 14.3 ± 1.9 g/day, p < 0.02). Nitrogen balance, estimated

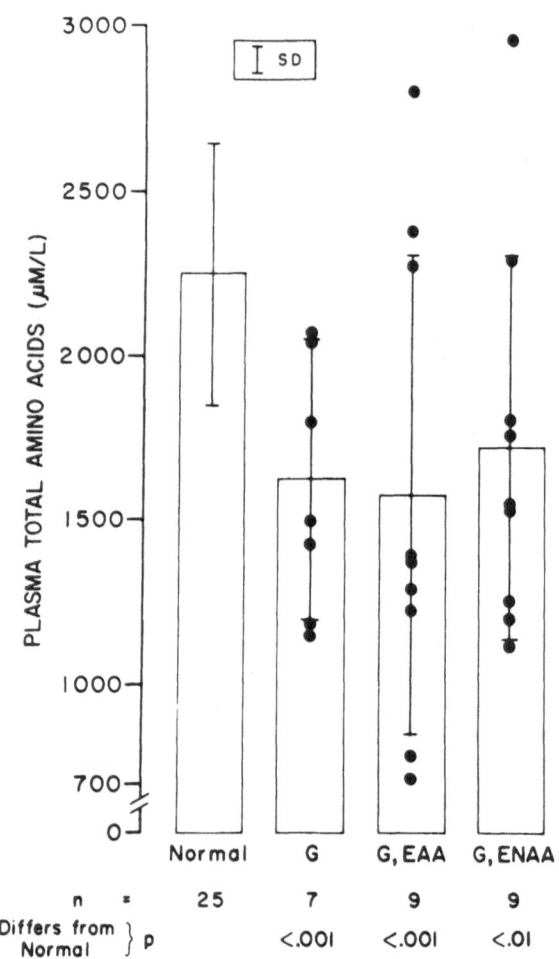

FIGURE 22–1. Plasma total free amino acid concentrations in normal subjects and patients with acute renal failure who received parenteral nutrition, which provided glucose (G); glucose and the nine essential amino acids (G,EAA); or glucose, the nine essential amino acids, and six nonessential amino acids (G,ENAA). The circles are values in individual patients at the end of their treatment with parenteral nutrition. The bars represent the mean values for each group, and the brackets indicate one standard deviation. The uremic patients treated with glucose and essential amino acids or glucose and essential and nonessential amino acids were receiving intravenous amino acids at the time of blood sampling; blood was obtained from normal controls after an overnight fast. From Kopple and Feinstein [64], with permission of the editors.

from the difference between nitrogen intake and UNA, was −2.9 ± 4.0 g/day with the essential amino acids and slightly but not significantly greater with the essential and nonessential amino acids, −5.2 ± 2.9 g/day. This calculation underestimates nitrogen balance by about 2 g/day.

These preliminary results suggest that parenteral nutrition providing larger quantities of essential and nonessential amino acids, with an essential-nonessential ratio of 1 : 1, is associated with increased UNA, no marked improvement in nitrogen balance, and no greater survival in comparison to intravenous therapy with about 21 g/day of essential amino acids. The increased fluid load and UNA with these larger amounts of essential and nonessential amino acids may also increase the dialysis requirements.

2.3 EFFECT OF NUTRITION ON RECOVERY OF RENAL FUNCTION

Several studies suggest that nutritional therapy might facilitate healing of the acutely failed kidney. In rats with acute tubular necrosis caused by injection of mercuric chloride, the proximal tubular cells undergo increased synthesis of protein, nucleic acids, and phospholipids and accelerated replication; these changes are apparent as early as the second day after injection [66–69]. Toback [70] has pointed out that this regrowth should increase the requirements for nutrients and that this greater demand occurs at a time when food intake is often depressed and the organism is developing uremic toxicity. An increased need for nutrients by the injured kidney could be further accentuated by the low plasma amino acid concentrations that are present in many patients with ARF [2]. Moreover, in rats with mercuric chloride-induced ATN, Toback et al. [71] found that free leucine concentrations in regenerating renal cells were 17% below normal. Cells deficient in a single amino acid may have a reduction in protein synthesis, and a deficiency of leucine, which has a special ability to stimulate protein synthesis, might be particularly inhibitory of protein anabolism. Finally, Abel and coworkers [51] found that in patients with ARF who received intravenous glucose and essential amino acids as compared to glucose alone, there was a tendency for serum creatinine concentrations to decrease sooner and to lower levels. The difference between these two treatment groups, however, were not statistically significant.

Toback and coworkers [71–73] carried out a series of studies on the effects of administering essential and nonessential amino acids and glucose to rats with ATN caused by intravenous injection of mercuric chloride. Since cellular membranes are composed in large part of phospholipids and protein, these investigators assessed new membrane formation in regenerating cells of renal cortical slices by the rate of incorporation of ^{14}C-choline into phospholipids. Choline is a precursor of phosphatidylcholine, which is the major phospholipid in membranes of renal cells [74]. During each of the first four days of ARF, the rats who received intravenous infusions of essential and nonessential amino acids and glucose had higher rates of ^{14}C-choline incorporation into phospholipids as compared to those receiving glucose alone.

Preincubation of cortical slices from these rats with amino acids without glucose also increased synthesis without changing breakdown of phospholipids; this finding suggests that amino acids themselves may increase phospholipid synthesis in regenerating renal tubular cells [73]. The amino acids increased the accumulation of ^{14}C-choline in renal cortical cells and Vmax of the choline kinase and cholinephosphotransferase reactions, which catalyze the formation of phosphatidylcholine. Infusion of amino acids also raised the low leucine concentrations in renal cortical cells and increased protein synthesis, as measured by incorporation of ^{14}C-leucine into protein [71]. Toback [72] observed that rats with mercuric chloride-induced ATN who received infusions of amino acids and glucose had a significantly lower serum creatinine level than those who received glucose alone or no infusion. Thus, the rats with ATN who were given amino acids and glucose had greater rates of phospholipid and protein synthesis and decreased severity or enhanced recovery of renal function.

Oken and coworkers [75] were unable to confirm beneficial effects of infusions of amino acids and glucose in rats with ARF. The rats were made acutely uremic by injection of mercuric chloride or glycerol. They were then infused with varying quantities of essential and nonessential amino acids and glucose, essential amino acids and glucose, or glucose alone. The uremic rats infused with large amounts of amino acids had very high SUN levels and much higher morbidity as compared to those given glucose alone or no infusion. The rats with glycerol-induced renal failure who received large quantities of amino acids were the only group receiving amino acids who had a significantly lower serum creatinine. However, this could have been due to the high mortality rate in this group; the ones who died might have had more severe renal failure and higher serum creatinine levels.

2.4 LACK OF CONCLUSIVENESS OF PUBLISHED RESEARCH

Although the foregoing studies, taken together, suggest that treatment of ARF with glucose and essential or nonessential amino acids as compared to glucose alone or no nutrition will improve the rate of recovery of renal function, nutritional status, or survival, the data do not demonstrate this thesis conclusively. There are probably several reasons why it has been difficult to show a beneficial effect for such therapy. They may include the following reasons:

a. The clinical course of patients with ARF is so variable and often so complex that it may be necessary to study scores or possibly hundreds of patients in a randomized prospective study to define accurately the advantages of a specific nutritional therapy. For example, in most groups of patients with ARF, there are some patients who will die despite the most sophisticated medical treatment. Conversely, others will recover without special medical care. For another large segment of patients, survival may depend much more on the types of antibiotics, drainage procedures, or medical interventions than on nutritional therapy. Thus, it might be anticipated that even if nutritional therapy is available, it may affect recovery of renal function or survival in only a small proportion of patients. Hence, to demonstrate its effectiveness on recovery or survival, it may be necessary to study large numbers of patients. Alternatively, one may choose other outcome measurements that may vary more closely with adequacy of nutritional support (e.g., tissue amino acid concentrations,

nitrogen balance, immune function, or wound healing). The limitation to this latter approach is that one must also demonstrate that improvement in such outcomes will, in fact, be associated with a more ultimate benefit, such as better survival and rehabilitation or lower hospital costs.

b. All prospective studies of parenteral nutrition in patients with ARF have evaluated different types of nutritional therapy (e.g., hypertonic glucose with amino acids versus hypertonic glucose without amino acids); none of these studies has compared the response of nutritional therapy to administration of no energy or amino acids.

c. As the foregoing discussion has indicated, the metabolic response to ARF and catabolic stress is very complex. There is increased protein degradation and reduced protein synthesis in muscle. Activity of certain catabolic enzymes in liver and hepatic gluconeogenesis are increased. Most amino acid concentrations in plasma and, in rats, in muscle are decreased; these observations suggest that despite the increased release of amino acids from the liver, the propensity for the liver to catabolize circulating amino acids is so great that the plasma and muscle intracellular amino acids are decreased. When amino acids are infused intravenously in this setting, it is not surprising that they are readily catabolized, raising the UNA.

These and other processes promoting catabolism are, almost certainly, mediated by many factors; these may include increased plasma concentrations of catabolic hormones, resistance to anabolic hormones, enhanced proteolytic activity, interleukin, and uremic toxins (vide supra). Indeed, these catabolic processes may be viewed as formerly a beneficial adaptive response. Until only the last few years, animals or humans who were injured or severely ill were unable to procure, ingest, digest, or assimilate exogenous nutrients. The body's own reserves of protein, fat, and, to a lesser extent, carbohydrate were virtually the only source of energy or amino acids for synthesis of new proteins for antibody formation, cell replication, fibrin and collagen deposition, and a host of other processes.

Now that man can be nourished completely by intravenous infusions, this complex adaptive response for mobilizing and catabolizing the body's nutrients may no longer be of value. Indeed, possibly, the adverse consequences of these processes may now outweigh their former benefits. Not only can they induce profound wasting, but the organism is so organized metabolically that it avidly catabolizes infused amino acids and carbohydrates.

If this hypothesis is correct, then the catabolic patient with ARF may need both techniques for suppressing catabolic processes and enhancing anabolic reactions and provision of nutrients. Infusion of amino acids and glucose without such metabolic intervention may not be sufficient to improve the morbidity or mortality of these patients.

d. Also, the nutrient composition of the infusates is probably not optimal, and this might reduce the clinical benefits of nutritional therapy. For example, there may be advantages to raising or lowering the proportions of certain amino acids in parenteral solutions (vide infra).

Despite the foregoing concerns, intuitively it seems that patients who are very ill should fare better if they are nourished than if they are allowed to starve. The need for nutritional therapy may be particularly great for patients who are wasted, who cannot eat for extended periods, or who are very catabolic. We therefore believe that until more definitive information is available, patients with ARF, in general, should be administered sufficient oral or parenteral nutrition to attain the most optimal nutritional status, provided that the nutritional therapy does not jeopardize the patients' clinical status.

3 Current Recommendations for Nutritional Therapy for Patients with ARF

From the available data, it is not possible to recommend definitive protocols for nutritional treatment of patients with ARF. The following

therapeutic approach is based on our analysis of the literature and our personal experience.

3.1 USE OF UREA NITROGEN APPEARANCE (UNA)

The quantity of nitrogen given to patients with ARF is often dictated by the patients' UNA. UNA is a simple, inexpensive, and accurate measure of net protein breakdown (degradation minus synthesis). The usefulness of the UNA is based on the fact that urea is the major nitrogenous product of protein and amino acid metabolism, and the UNA usually correlates closely with total nitrogen output. UNA is calculated as follows:

$$UNA \text{ (g/day)} = \text{urinary urea nitrogen (g/day)} \quad (22.1)$$
$$+ \text{ dialysate urea nitrogen (g/day)}$$
$$+ \text{ change in body urea nitrogen (g/day);}$$

$$\text{Change in body urea nitrogen (g/day)} \quad (22.2)$$
$$= (SUN_f - SUN_i, \text{ g/L}) \times BW_i(\text{Kg/day})$$
$$\times (0.60 \text{ L/Kg}) + (BW_f - BW_i, \text{ Kg/day})$$
$$\times SUN_f(\text{g/L}) \times (1.0 \text{ L/Kg});$$

where i and f are the initial and final values for the period of measurement; SUN is serum urea nitrogen (grams per liter); BW is body weight (kilograms); 0.60 is an estimate of the fraction of body weight that is body water; and 1.0 is the volume of distribution of urea in the weight gain or loss.

The estimated proportion of body weight that is water may have to be increased in patients who are edematous or lean and decreased in individuals who are obese or very young. Changes in body weight during the one-to-three-day period of measurement of UNA are assumed to be due entirely to changes in body water. In patients undergoing hemodialysis or intermittent peritoneal dialysis, the urea concentration in dialysate is low and difficult to measure accurately, and UNA is usually calculated during the interdialytic interval. The term UNA is used rather than urea production because some urea is degraded in the gastrointestinal tract. Virtually all of the ammonia released from hydrolyzed urea seems to be converted back to urea [76], and this recycling will not affect the accuracy of the UNA as an indicator of net urea production or net protein breakdown. Also, it is not possible to measure the magnitude of urea recycling without isotopic studies.

In our experience, the relationship between UNA and total nitrogen output in chronically uremic patients not undergoing dialysis is as follows:

Total nitrogen output (g/day)
$$= 0.97 \text{ UNA (g/day)} + 1.93. \quad (22.3)$$

If the individual is more or less in neutral nitrogen balance, the UNA also will correlate closely with nitrogen intake. Equation 22.4 describes our observed relationships between UNA and dietary nitrogen intake in clinically stable nondialyzed chronically uremic patients:

Dietary nitrogen intake (g/day)
$$= 0.69 \text{ UNA (g/day)} + 3.3. \quad (22.4)$$

Moreover, if both nitrogen intake and UNA are known, nitrogen balance can be estimated from the difference between nitrogen intake and nitrogen output estimated from the UNA. Pregnancy or large protein losses (for example, nephrotic syndrome or peritoneal dialysis) can alter the relation between UNA and total nitrogen intake or output [77]. Similarly, acidosis in individuals with sufficient kidney function to excrete large quantities of ammonia may change these relationships.

Sargent and Gotch [78] have proposed an ingenious technique for assessing UNA in hemodialysis patients, which they refer to incorrectly as urea generation. Their calculations are based on the SUN and body weight at the beginning of two consecutive hemodialyses and at the end of the dialysis, the residual renal function, the mass transfer characteristics of the dialyzer employed, the blood and dialysate flow rates, and the duration and other aspects of the hemodialysis procedure. Although this technique is useful, it requires a somewhat complicated computer program for calculation, and, in our preliminary experience, it does not appear to be more accurate than the method described here.

3.2 COMPOSITION OF AMINO ACID PREPARATIONS

Currently, most essential amino acid formulations for nutritional therapy in renal failure are based largely on the recommended daily dietary intake for essential amino acids as proposed by Rose from his studies in healthy young adults [79]. Histidine is added because it is considered an essential amino acid in both normal men and in chronically uremic patients [80][1]. Some workers have proposed adding tyrosine and arginine. Tyrosine can be derived in vivo only from phenylalanine or from catabolized peptides or proteins. Since the conversion of phenylalanine to tyrosine is impaired in uremia [81] and plasma, red cell, and muscle tyrosine are usually decreased in uremic patients [81–84], it has been suggested that tyrosine may be essential for uremic patients. Wurtman [85] has suggested that there are pharmacological properties of tyrosine in stressed patients that argue for including tyrosine in amino acid formulations.

Arginine is normally released by the kidney [86], and in renal failure, there also may be a dietary requirement for this amino acid. However, there is not yet convincing evidence that uremic patients receiving low quantities of essential amino acids (e.g., 20 to 30 g/day) benefit from addition of either tyrosine or arginine to the diet.

Several lines of evidence suggest that the patient with renal failure might benefit from a different formulation of amino acids. First, in patients with acute or chronic renal failure, there is an abnormal pattern of plasma amino acids, and concentrations of both essential and nonessential amino acids are altered [2, 18]. In CRF, there tend to be low concentrations of plasma leucine, valine, and tyrosine, and high levels of cystine, citrulline, N^{I}-methylhistidine, and N^{II}-methylhistidine. Also, in chronically uremic patients, abnormal amino acid concentrations have been described in muscle by Bergström and coworkers [84], in blood cells by Ganda et al. [87], in leukocytes by Metcoff and associates [88], and in red cells by Flügel-Link, Jones, and Kopple [83].

In ARF, alterations in plasma amino acid

levels may be more pervasive. Feinstein and co-workers [2] observed low plasma concentrations of histidine, isoleucine, leucine, lysine, threonine, valine, arginine, citrulline, and tyrosine. There were low normal to normal levels of alanine, asparagine, glutamine, serine, ornithine, and cystine and normal to increased concentrations of methionine, phenylalanine, aspartic acid, glutamic acid, and glycine. Tissue amino acid concentrations have not been described in humans with ARF.

Fürst, Alvestrand and Bergström [89] fed nondialyzed chronically uremic patients low-protein diets that were supplemented with a special formulation of essential amino acids and tyrosine, which was designed to normalize plasma and muscle amino acid concentrations. The proportions of the essential amino acids were changed from the Rose formulation so that threonine and valine were increased, tryptophan remained the same, and the other essential amino acids were reduced. Plasma and muscle concentrations of essential amino acids did become more normal with this formulation. Whether similar types of preparations will improve amino acid levels and, more importantly, the clinical status of patients with ARF is not known.

The finding that the branched-chain amino acids—valine, leucine, and isoleucine—are decreased in plasma from patients and in plasma and muscle from rats with ARF suggests that such patients may have a greater nutritional requirement for these amino acids. The branched-chain amino acids, particularly leucine, may stimulate protein anabolism in vitro [90, 91], and recent data suggest that intravenous infusions in which 40% of the total amino acids are branched-chain may ameliorate the hypercatabolic response in severely stressed nonuremic patients [92, 93].

Whether nonessential amino acids should be included in amino acid formulations is controversial. When chronically uremic patients are given very low nitrogen diets (i.e., 2.0 to 3.0 g N/day) containing virtually only essential amino acids, nitrogen balances and plasma amino acid concentrations generally seem to be as well maintained as when such patients are fed isocaloric low-protein diets similar in nitrogen content [94]. At higher nitrogen intakes, the argument for inclusion of nonessential amino acids in oral and parenteral preparations is much stronger. Both animal and human studies indicate that diets providing both essential and nonessential amino acids may be nutritionally superior to those that provide essential amino acids alone. Both the rat and the chick seem to grow better when a mixture of nonessential amino acids is the source of nonspecific nitrogen [95–97]. Moreover, normal humans who eat low nitrogen diets may maintain more positive nitrogen balance when nonspecific nitrogen is provided as a combination of nonessential amino acids rather than as diammonium citrate, glycine, or a mixture of glycine and glutamic acid [98, 99]. Pennisi, Wang, and Kopple [100] tube-fed chronically uremic rats diets providing essential amino acids, essential and nonessential amino acids, or casein. Growth was greater in the rats fed the latter two diets as compared to the ones providing essential amino acids, even when comparisons were between isonitrogenous diets.

Nonessential amino acids are as necessary for protein synthesis as essential amino acids, and a deficiency of a nonessential amino acid inside the cell could disrupt protein synthesis [101]. The metabolic costs of synthesizing nonessential amino acids are not known. Also, since many amino acids share common transport mechanisms and compete for intracellular transport, a selective infusion of essential amino acids that might lead to high extracellular concentrations of some amino acids might impair intracellular movement of others. Conversely, a low extracellular concentration of an amino acid could lead to decreased intracellular movement of that amino acid and accelerated cellular transport of others.

The paper of Motil, Harmon, and Grupe [102], on two children with acute renal failure is pertinent in this regard. The children, who were very ill, had been infused with a relatively large dose per kg of eight essential amino acids without histidine. They had very low plasma concentrations of histidine and the urea cycle amino acids—ornithine, citrulline, and arginine. Plasma methionine and blood ammonia were increased, and the patients developed a metabolic acidosis. When the children received an infusion of essential and nonessential amino acids, the amino acid pattern was more normal. We have also observed striking elevations in plasma lysine, methionine, phenylalanine, and threonine in a man and a woman with ARF who received intravenously about 60 to 75 g/day of essential amino acids and no nonessential amino acids; one patient did not receive histidine. During infusion of these large quantities of essential amino acids, the patients remained severely ill or deteriorated further, and both ultimately died. Both patients had severe underlying illnesses, which could account for their poor outcome. Nonetheless, these findings suggest that large doses of essential amino acids only can disrupt amino acid metabolism and possibly cause clinical deterioration.

In comparison to the daily dietary requirements for proteins or amino acids, the dietary need each day for essential amino acids is quite small. Rose [79] recommended 12.7 g/day as a safe intake for the eight essential amino acids excluding histidine. The difference between the dietary requirements for essential amino acid nitrogen and for total nitrogen is referred to as the need for nonspecific nitrogen. Thus, in a patient who recieves 40 to 100 g/day of amino acids, there may be no advantage to providing only those that are essential.

The foregoing considerations suggest that patients with ARF who receive larger amounts of amino acids (i.e., more than 35 to 40 g/day) should be given both essential and nonessential amino acids. These should probably include arginine, tyrosine, alanine, glycine, proline, and serine. There are little data concerning the optimal ratio of essential to nonessential amino acids for patients with ARF. In standard intravenous solutions, the ratio of essential to nonessential amino acids is about 1:1 with histidine considered essential and arginine, nonessential. For acutely uremic patients, a more effective formulation might be 3:1 or 4:1, with perhaps 40% of the essentials provided as branched-chain amino acids. Patients who are administered small amounts of essential amino acids (e.g., 2 to 3.5 g N/day) should probably also re-

cieve a high proportion of the branched-chain amino acids. Further studies are clearly necessary to examine these questions.

When administering mixtures of essential and nonessential amino acids, it is preferable to use solutions of free L-amino acids rather than protein hydrolysates. There may be compounds in the latter solutions that may not be well-utilized and may accumulate in renal failure [103]. Also, the latter preparations may contain hazardous concentrations of aluminum [104].

3.3 SELECTION OF NITROGEN INTAKE

The decision concerning the quantity and type of amino acids or proteins given to the patient is influenced by a number of factors. In patients who have low rates of UNA (e.g., equal to or less than 4 to 5 g N/day) and who are not very wasted, we may prescribe a dietary or intravenous intake low in nitrogen.

The amount of nitrogen administered also depends on the SUN, residual renal function, anticipated time until renal function recovers, and projected needs for dialysis therapy. If renal function is anticipated to begin recovering imminently, or the patient is about to develop uremic symptoms, and there are indications to postpone or avoid dialysis treatment, we may use 0.3 to 0.5 g/kg/day of high-quality protein or 0.3 to 0.4 g/kg/day of essential amino acids with or without arginine. This regimen will usually maintain neutral or only slightly negative balance and should minimize the rate of accumulation of nitrogen metabolites. Hence, the need for dialysis therapy may be minimized or avoided. On the other hand, in patients who are frankly uremic, highly catabolic and either are or will be needing dialysis therapy, we may provide a higher nitrogen intake, up to 1.0 to 1.2 g/kg/day of protein or amino acids.

As a result of the study of Feinstein and associates that indicated that large quantities of essential and nonessential amino acids (i.e., 11.3 g N/day with an essential-nonessential ratio of 1:1) did not improve the clinical course or nutritional status of patients with ARF, we are inclined to use somewhat lower nitrogen intakes. For patients with UNA rates larger than 4 to 5 g/day, we generally feed or infuse about

0.80 to 1.0 g/kg/day of protein or amino acids.

In comparison to small quantities of essential amino acids, these large nitrogen intakes may reduce the magnitude of negative nitrogen balance. However, the UNA will almost invariably rise, and the large volume of fluid necessary to provide this amount of amino acids may increase the requirements for dialysis. Patients with greater residual renal function, higher fluid tolerance, and a healthy cardiorespiratory system are usually more tolerant of these large nitrogen intakes. With appropriate dialysis or continuous arterial venous hemofiltration, the high-nitrogen intakes are well tolerated by most patients. When renal failure persists for more than two to three weeks and patients undergo regular dialysis treatment, they are treated as with maintenance dialysis patients with about 1.0 to 1.2 g/kg/day of protein or amino acids for hemodialysis or 1.2 to 1.5 g/kg/day for maintenance intermittent or continuous ambulatory peritoneal dialysis.

3.4 NUTRITION VIA THE GASTROINTESTINAL TRACT

For patients who can receive nutrition by eating, enteral tubes, or gastrostomy, it is generally preferable to administer nutrition in this way rather than intravenously. The latter is more hazardous, provides greater fluid loads, and is more costly. There are very little experimental data concerning enteral nutrition for patients with ARF, and the treatment regimens are to a large extent based on experience derived from chronically uremic patients [105].

When the patient requires a low nitrogen diet (vide supra), one may give 0.30 to 0.40 g/kg/day of the nine essential amino acids (approximately 20 to 30 g/day). An additional 0.04 to 0.14 g/kg/day of protein of miscellaneous quality (about 3 to 10 g/day) is contained in the high-calorie, low-nitrogen foodstuffs that provide most of the energy intake. In clinically stable, chronically uremic patients who are not receiving dialysis treatment and who have a low UNA, these diets should maintain neutral or near neutral nitrogen balance [105]. Where available, ketoacid or hydroxyacid analogues may be substituted for several essential amino acids. If the patient has a resid-

ual GFR of about 4 to 10 ml/min, one may add more protein or give diets providing 0.55 to 0.60 g/kg/day of protein. About 20 to 24 g/day of this protein should be of high biological value.

If patients undergo regular dialysis therapy for at least two or three weeks and they are able to eat, they should be prescribed the same protein intake as is recommended for patients undergoing maintenance dialysis (vide supra) [106]. Approximately 50% of this protein should be of high biological value.

For patients who must be fed by an enteric tube or gastrostomy, there are many liquid protein or defined formula (elemental) diets available. The composition and the clinical effects of these diets in nonuremic patients have been reviewed recently [107, 108]. Experimental evidence indicates that when patients receive large quantities of amino acids (e.g., more than 30 to 40 g/day), they should be given nonessential amino acids (vide supra).

3.5. TOTAL PARENTERAL NUTRITION (TPN)

Patients who are unable to receive enteral nutrition, have a UNA of 4 to 5 g/day or less, and are not very wasted are given 0.30 to 0.40 g/kg/day of essential amino acids intravenously (vide supra). With a higher UNA, both essential and nonessential amino acids are given; the quantity and proportions of individual amino acids to be infused are determined as described above. A typical formulation for TPN in acutely uremic patients is shown in table 22–3.

3.6 ENERGY, VITAMINS, AND MINERALS

Since patients with ARF are usually in negative nitrogen balance, large quantities of calories are probably indicated to reduce negative nitrogen breakdown. There is no easy way to estimate the energy expenditure or requirement in these patients, and we empirically administer 35 to 50 kcal/kg/day. Indirect calorimetry has been used to estimate energy expenditure in stressed uremic patients. However, the current studies do not indicate the level of energy intake that will optimize utilization of amino acids or proteins for such patients.

If nitrogen balance, as determined by the difference between observed nitrogen intake

TABLE 22–3. Typical composition of TPN infusate for adults with acute renal failure[a,b,c]

Volume	liters	1.0
70% dextrose (d-glucose) (500 ml)	g/liter	350
Essential and nonessential free crystalline amino acids (≤500 ml)	g/liter	25–40
or essential amino acids (≤500 ml)	g/liter	10–14
Energy (approx.)[d]	kcal/liter	1225-1330
Electrolytes[e]		
Sodium[f]	mmol/liter	50
Chloride[f]	mmol/liter	25-35
Potassium	mmol/day	35
Acetate	mmol/day	35-40
Calcium	mmol/day	5
Phosphorus	mmol/day	8
Magnesium	mmol/day	4
Iron	mg/day	2
Vitamins		
Vitamin A	USP units/day	See text[g]
Vitamin D	USP units/day	See text[j]
Vitamin K[h]	mg/week	4
Vitamin E[i]	IU/day	10
Niacin	mg/day	20
Thiamin HCl (B_1)	mg/day	2
Riboflavin (B_2)	mg/day	2
Pantothenic acid	mg/day	10
Pyridoxine HCl (B_6)	mg/day	10
Ascorbic acid (C)	mg/day	100
Biotin	mg/day	200
Folic acid[h]	mg/day	1
Vitamin B_{12}[h]	μg/day	4

[a]In general, when the UNA is greater than 4–5 g N/day, 1.0 g/day of essential and nonessential amino acids are given. If the UNA is 4–5 g N/day or less, 0.3 to 0.5 g/kg/day of essential amino acids with arginine are administered. See text for a more detailed discussion of indications for different amounts and type of amino acid preparations. Nitrogen content of 42.5–50 g of essential and nonessential amino acids is approximately 6.5–7.9 g, depending on the preparation. The prescribed amino acids often may be provided in less than 500 ml of solution, and the volume of 70% dextrose may be increased to bring volume up to one liter and to provide additional calories. Energy intake is usually maintained at 35–50 kcal/kg/day. Sufficient 70% dextrose may be given to attain this energy intake. A total of 1.5–2.5 L/day of TPN solution may be necessary to provide sufficient amino acids and energy. The fluid load necessary to provide this quantity of amino acids and energy may increase the need for dialysis or continuous arterial venous hemofiltration. During dialysis treatment, amino acid and glucose losses can be replaced by increasing infusions (see text). Administration of 250–500 g of lipid emulsion daily can be used in place of some glucose and will prevent essential fatty acid deficiency. It is particularly indicated in long-term TPN. The 20% lipid emulsion will provide the most fat calories per ml water (2kcal/ml).
[b]These nutrients are included in each bottle containing crystalline amino acids and 70% dextrose. An exception is the vitamins and trace elements that should be added to only one bottle per day.
[c]Composition and volume of infusate may have to be changed if patients are very uremic, acidotic, or volume overloaded, if serum electrolyte concentrations are not normal or relatively constant, or if dialysis therapy is not readily available.
[d]Approximate caloric value of dextrose monohydrate, 3.4 kcal/g; amino acids, 3.5 kcal/g.
[e]When adding electrolytes, the amounts intrinsically present in the amino acid solution should be taken into account.
[f]Refers to final concentration of electrolytes after any extra 70% dextrose has been added.
[g]Vitamin A is best avoided unless TPN is continued for more than several weeks.
[h]Should be given orally or parenterally and not in solution because of antagonisms.
[i]May need to be increased with use of lipid emulsions.
[j]Currently, 1,25-dihydroxycholecalciferol is not commercially available for parenteral administration.
Source: Adapted from Kopple, JD Nutrition and the Kidney, in Hodges RE Human Nutrition. A Comprehensive Treatise (New York: Plenum Publishing Corp., 1979), vol. 4, pp. 409–457.

and nitrogen output calculated from the UNA (equation 22.3), is negative, we try to provide an energy intake closer to 50 kcal/kg/day. Many researchers believe that there is little advantage to administering more than 4,000 to 5,000 kcal/day to catabolic patients. In fact, in patients with higher energy intakes, the large quantity of carbon dioxide produced from the infused carbohydrate and fat can cause hypercapnia if pulmonary function is impaired [109]. Since most acutely uremic patients are intolerant of large water intakes, glucose is generally provided in 70% solution; this preparation is mixed with the amino acid solution so that amino acids and energy are provided concurrently (table 22–3). Patients receiving TPN for more than five to seven days should receive an infusion of 250 to 500 g of lipid emulsions, preferably daily but no less than twice weekly to prevent essential fatty acid deficiency. Both 10% and 20% lipid emulsions are available; they are essentially isotonic and provide 1.1 and 2.0 kcal/ml, respectively. In contrast, 70% dextrose (d-glucose monohydrate) yields about 2.38 kcal/ml and is the parenteral solution that gives the greatest calories per ml. Dextrose is well utilized by virtually all tissues and provides needed calories for those organs that consume glucose as the primary energy source. In catabolic patients, glucose has been reported to promote more positive nitrogen balance than does isocaloric quantities of lipids [110, 111], although more recent evidence disputes this finding. Per calorie, 70% dextrose is far less expensive than a lipid emulsion. For these reasons, in acutely uremic patients receiving parenteral nutrition, glucose is used as the major source of calories, and lipids are given daily but in lesser amounts.

The vitamins and minerals employed with TPN are shown in table 22–3. Vitamin requirements have not been well defined for patients with ARF, and much of the recommended intake is based on information obtained from studies in chronically uremic patients or normal individuals. Vitamin A is probably best avoided because in chronic renal failure, serum vitamin A levels are elevated. Even small doses of vitamin A have been reported to cause toxicity in chronically uremic patients [112]. Also, since most patients with ARF receive TPN for only a few days to weeks, it is unlikely that deficiency of this fat-soluble vitamin will occur.

Although vitamin D is fat-soluble and vitamin D stores should not become depleted during a few days or weeks of TPN, the turnover of its most active form, 1,25-dihydroxycholecalciferol, is much faster. However, the requirement for this vitamin D analogue in ARF has not yet been defined. Furthermore, at the present time, a parenteral preparation of 1,25-dihydroxycholecalciferol is not commercially available. Although vitamin K is a fat-soluble vitamin, deficiencies have been reported in nonuremic patients who were postoperated, not eating, and receiving antibiotics [113]. Vitamin K supplements are therefore given routinely to patients receiving TPN. Ten mg/day of pyridoxine hydrochloride is recommended because studies in patients undergoing maintenance hemodialysis indicate that this amount may be necessary to prevent or correct vitamin B_6 deficiency [114].

The recommended concentrations for minerals with TPN are tentative. If the serum concentration of an electrolyte is increased, it may be advisable to reduce the concentration or not to administer it at the onset of parenteral nutrition. The patient must be monitored carefully, however, because hormonal and metabolic changes that often occur with initiation of TPN may cause serum electrolytes to fall rapidly. This is particularly likely for serum potassium and phosphorus. Conversely, a mineral deficit may indicate a need for greater than usual intake of that element. Again, metabolic changes can lead to a rapid rise in serum levels.

It must be emphasized that the nutrient content of solutions for TPN in acutely uremic patients must be carefully re-evaluated each day and sometimes more frequently. This is particularly important because these patients may undergo rapid changes in their metabolic and clinical status. The actual techniques, complications, and methods for assessing nutritional and clinical status in patients receiving TPN have been described previously [115].

3.7 PERIPHERAL AND SUPPLEMENTAL PARENTERAL NUTRITION

Peripheral parenteral nutrition has been advocated as an alternative to TPN. The solutions are infused into a peripheral vein, and the risks and expenses of inserting a central catheter are avoided. A limitation to peripheral parenteral nutrition is that osmolality of the infusate must be restricted to about 600 milliosmols to prevent thrombophlebitis; even then, the needles or catheters must be changed frequently, usually every 18 to 48 hours. Isaacs et al. [116]

report that addition of heparin, 500 U/L, and cortisol, 5 mg/L, allowed solutions of 900 mosmols to be infused into a peripheral vein for an average of 114 hours before local inflammation required changing the infusion site. In contrast to these infusates, a typical solution for TPN via a central vein has a tonicity of about 1,800 mosmols. Thus, with peripheral parenteral nutrition, less nutrients can be infused per liter, and it has little or no role in the treatment of the hypercatabolic patient, the wasted patient who needs added nutrients for repletion, the patient with oliguria or fluid intolerance, and the patient who will need parenteral nutrition for extended periods of time.

For patients with ARF who are able to ingest some nutrients or tolerate some tube feedings, peripheral infusions may enable them to receive adequate nutrition without resorting to TPN. In these latter cases, it is often most practical to infuse 8.5 to 10% amino acids or 20% lipid emulsions into a peripheral vein and administer as much as possible of other essential nutrients, including carbohydrates through the enteral tract.

Peripheral vascular accesses used for hemodialysis can also be used for TPN [117, 118]. However, this technique probably increases the hazard of infection, and it should not be done in patients who will need a hemodialysis access for extended periods.

In patients who have marginally adequate intakes, supplemental amino acids and glucose may be given during hemodialysis treatment. Some nephrologists infuse 20 or 30 g of the nine essential amino acids at the end of dialysis therapy [119]. However, since most patients who need nutritional supplements have decreased intake of energy and total nitrogen, we give 40 to 42 g of essential and nonessential amino acids and 200 g of d-glucose (150 g of d-glucose if dialysate contains glucose). This preparation is infused into the blood leaving the dialyzer at a constant rate throughout the dialysis procedure in order to minimize disruption of amino acid and glucose pools that occurs with hemodialysis [120]. Patients who have low serum concentrations of phosphorus or potassium at the start of the dialysis treatment may need supplements of these minerals. With

such infusions, plasma amino acids and glucose do not fall during dialysis and over 85% of the infused amino acids are retained [120]. If the dialysate is glucose free, the infusion is not stopped until the end of hemodialysis in order to prevent reactive hypoglicemia. Also, the patient should eat some carbohydrate 20 to 30 minutes before the end of the infusion. Otherwise, the infusion must be tapered or a peripheral infusion of glucose must be started.

3.8 CONTINUOUS ARTERIAL-VENOUS HEMOFILTRATION (CAVH)

CAVH is a new and potentially valuable technique for fluid control in critically ill patients with renal failure [121]. With CAVH, there is a continuous flow of blood through a hemofilter. Up to 10 to 15 ml of ultrafiltrate is formed per minute, and CAVH can prevent or correct fluid overload. Hence, it can obviate the problem of overhydration from parenteral nutrition. Also, since the ultrafiltrate contains the same concentration of the small molecules (e.g., urea, creatinine) as in plasma, it can clear up to 10 to 15 ml/minute of these compounds from plasma, thus allowing patients to readily tolerate higher nitrogen loads.

When sufficient fluid has been removed from the patient, CAVH may be temporarily stopped by clamping the arterial and venous lines, or patients can be infused with replacement solutions. These solutions can be infused into a vein or into the arterial line prior to the hemofilter. In the latter case, the dilution of the blood will decrease the ratio of the solute clearance to the volume of ultrafiltrate.

Arterial and venous catheters can be inserted into a peripheral artery and vein in the arm or leg or into a Scribner shunt.

The resistance through the system is low enough to avoid the need for blood pumps. Thus, monitoring the blood pressure and bleeding can be less stringent. Intensive care unit nurses can be taught to perform CAVH, and the cost for a trained dialysis nurse can be avoided.

Because, with CAVH, fluid removal is slow and continuous and possibly because acetate is not administered, blood pressure is well maintained. CAVH has been employed successfully in hypotensive patients receiving pressor medications [122]. If the ultrafiltration rate is low, it can often be increased with application of continuous suction to the ultrafiltrate outflow tube [123]. Patients are generally given heparin, and CAVH may be more hazardous in patients who are actively bleeding. Amino acid losses into ultrafiltrate are not great [121]. Less is known about the quantity of protein removed with CAVH, but it does not appear to be massive [123].

CAVH may reduce the need for dialysis treatment in sick patients with renal failure, possibly from five to seven times per week to three or four times weekly. However, current experience indicates that will not entirely prevent the need for dialysis treatment unless (a) it is employed virtually constantly with a high rate of ultrafiltrate formation (10 to 15 ml/minute) and infusion of large volumes of replacement fluid, or (b) the patient has substantial residual renal function.

4 Newer Directions for Nutritional Therapy

Several pharmacological techniques may have a role in facilitating anabolic processes or reducing catabolic rates in patients with renal failure. Preliminary results with each of these techniques in sick patients or experimental animals have been promising, although further studies are necessary to define their potential role in patients with ARF. These techniques involve the use of insulin, anabolic steroids, protease inhibitors, and adenine nucleotides.

Since insulin is the most potent known anabolic hormone, it is natural to question whether this compound could reduce protein wasting in sick patients. Two studies have now indicated that in nonuremic patients who have catabolic illnesses, insulin can reduce nitrogen output and negative nitrogen balance [124, 125]. Serum glucose concentrations greater than 460 mg/dl occurred in approximately half our patients with ARF who received parenteral nutrition [2]. Moreover, Clark and Mitch [12] reported that insulin enhances synthesis and reduces degradation of muscle protein from the hindquarter of acutely uremic rats. These observations suggest that there may be value to administering insulin routinely to catabolic patients with ARF.

Anabolic steroids can also promote anabolism and have been used to treat catabolic patients with acute or chronic renal failure [126–130]. These compounds can decrease UNA and the rise in SUN, enhance positive nitrogen and potassium balance, retard the development of acidosis, and delay the need for dialysis therapy [128–131]. In recent years, the use of anabolic steroids for treatment of catabolic patients with renal failure has been largely neglected because its effects last only several days to weeks and dialysis therapy is readily available. However, dialysis treatment does not reduce catabolism and is often hazardous in severely ill patients. Since the period of critical illness in patients with ARF is often only a few days to weeks, anabolic steroids might still be beneficial, even if they reduce net catabolism and UNA only transiently. Recently Pan and associates [11] found improved muscle protein synthesis in perfused hemicorpus from acutely uremic rats when they were given the anabolic hormone oxandrolone prior to the perfusion.

Anabolic steroids are not always effective, particularly in severe catabolic stress, and they can have masculinizing effects in women and children. These compounds may be ineffective unless the patient also receives nourishment. Many anabolic steroids can cause cholestatic jaundice although this is not observed with testosterone or its esters (enanthemate or propionate). Commonly used anabolic steroids include testosterone enanthemate, testosterone proprionate, methandrostenolone, nondrolone decanoate, norandrolone phenylproprionate, and norethandrolone.

Two therapeutic procedures that show exciting promise but have not yet been employed in patients are the use of protease inhibitors and of adenine nucleotides. Hörl and associates [28] described increased protease activity in ultrafiltrates of plasma from patients with ARF who were catabolic. The protease inhibitor alpha$_2$-macroglobulin was undetectable in plasma from some of these patients. Addition of alpha$_2$-macroglobulin, in vitro, to plasma ultrafiltrate inhibited the proteolytic activity

[132]. These findings suggest that in patients with ARF who are catabolic, enhanced activity of proteases in plasma and possibly other tissues may be a cause of accelerated protein wasting. If this is confirmed, eventually such patients may be treated with specific inhibitors of these proteases.

Siegel and coworkers [133] studied the effects of infusion of magnesium chloride with either ATP, ADP, or AMP into rats with ARF caused by ischemia. The rats who received one of these adenine nucleotides with magnesium chloride had less impaired insulin clearance, renal blood flow and osmolar clearance, a low fractional excretion of sodium, and less histological evidence of renal injury as compared to rats who received no infusion or ATP, magnesium chloride, or adenosine alone. Although the mechanism for these effects is unknown, it is tempting to speculate whether adenine nucleotides and magnesium chloride may act by altering glomerulotubular or vascular dynamics or by improving energy metabolism in the injured and regenerating cells.

Note

1. Essential amino acids are histidine, isoleucine, leucine, lysine, methionine, phenylalanine, threonine, tryptophan, and valine.

References

1. Leonard CD, Luke RG, Siegel RR. Parenteral essential amino acids in acute renal failure. Urology VI(2): 154–157, 1975.
2. Feinstein EI, Blumenkrantz MJ, Healy H, Koffler A, Silberman H, Massry SG, Kopple JD. Clinical and metabolic responses to parenteral nutrition in acute renal failure. A controlled double-blind study. Medicine 60(2): 124–137, 1981.
3. Cahill GF. Starvation in man. N Eng J Med 282: 668–675, 1970.
4. Bozzetti F, Terno G, Longoni C. Parenteral hyperalimentation and wound healing. Surg Gynecol Obstet 141: 712–714, 1975.
5. Law DK, Dudrick SJ, Abdou NI. Immunocompetence of patients with protein-calorie malnutrition. The effects of nutritional repletion. Ann Int Med 79: 545–550, 1973.
6. Lacy WW. Effect of acute uremia on amino acid uptake and urea production by perfused rat liver. Am J Physiol 216(6): 1300–1305, 1969.
7. Frölich J, Schölmerich J, Hoppe-Seyler G, Maier KP, Talke H, Schollmeyer P, Gerok W. The effect of acute uremia on gluconeogenesis in isolated perfused rat livers. Europ J Clin Invest 4: 453–458, 1974.
8. McCormick GJ, Shear L, Barry KG. Alteration of hepatic protein synthesis in acute uremia. Proc Soc Exp Biol Med 122: 99–102, 1966.
9. Shear L. Internal redistribution of tissue protein synthesis in uremia. J Clin Invest 48: 1252–1257, 1969.
10. Flügel-Link RM, Salusky IB, Jones MR, Kopple JD. Enhanced muscle protein degradation and urea nitrogen appearance (UNA) in rats with acute renal failure. Am J Physiol 244: E615–E623, 1983.
11. Pan CS, Inadomi D, Laidlaw SA, Jones MR, Kopple JD. Oxandrolone enhances muscle protein synthesis in acutely uremic rats. Abstract. Kidney Int (in press).
12. Clark AS, Mitch WE. Muscle protein turnover and glucose uptake in acutely uremic rats. Effect of insulin and the duration of renal insufficiency. J Clin Invest 72: 836–845, 1983.
13. Sapico V. Enzyme alterations and subcellular translocation of inducible tyrosine aminotransferase in acute uremia. Fed Proc 32: 506A, 1973.
14. Shear L, Sapico V, Litwack G. Induction of hepatic enzymes and translocation of cytosol tyrosine amino transaminase (TAT) in uremic rats. Clin Res 21: 707A, 1973.
15. Sapico V, Shear L, Litwack G. Translocation of inducible tyrosine aminotransferase to the mitochondrial fraction. J Biol Chem 249(7): 2122–2129, 1974.
16. Bergström J, Hultman E. Glycogen content of skeletal muscle in patients with renal failure. Acta Med Scand 186: 177–181, 1969.
17. Hörl WH, Heidland A. Glycogen metabolism in muscle in uremia. Am J Clin Nutr 33: 1461–1467, 1980.
18. Kopple JD. Nitrogen metabolism. In Clinical Aspects of Uremia and Dialysis, Massry SG, Sellers AL (eds). Springfield, Ill: Charles C Thomas, 1976, pp. 241–273.
19. Eigler N, Saccà L, Sherwin RS. Synergistic interactions of physiologic increments of glucagon, epinephrine and cortisol in the dog. A model for stress-induced hyperglycemia. J Clin Invest 63: 114–123, 1979.
20. Bilbrey GL, Faloona GR, White MG, Knochel JP, Borroto J. Hyperglucagonemia of renal failure. J Clin Invest 53: 841–847, 1974.
21. Sherwin RS, Bastl C, Finkelstein FO, Fisher M, Black H, Hendler R, Felig P. Influence of uremia and hemodialysis on the turnover and metabolic effects of glucagon. J Clin Invest 57: 722–731, 1976.
22. Mondon CE, Reaven GM. Evaluation of enhanced glucagon sensitivity as the cause of glucose intolerance in acutely uremic rats. Am J Clin Nutr 33: 1456–1460, 1980.

23. DeFronzo RA, Tobin JD, Rowe JW, Andres R. Glucose intolerance in uremia. Quantification of pancreatic beta cell sensitivity to glucose and tissue sensitivity to insulin. J Clin Invest 62: 425–435, 1978.

24. DeFronzo RA. Pathogenesis of glucose intolerance in uremia. Metabolism 27(12): 1866–1880, 1978.

25. Kopple JD, Cianciaruso B, Massry SG. Does parathyroid hormone cause protein wasting? Contr Nephrol 20: 138–148, 1980.

26. Massry SG, Arieff AI, Coburn JW, Palmieri G, Kleeman CR. Divalent ion metabolism in patients with acute renal failure: Studies on the mechanism of hypocalcemia. Kidney Int 5: 437–445, 1974.

27. Pietrek J, Kokot F, Kuska J. Serum 25-hydroxyvitamin D and parathyroid hormone in patients with acute renal failure. Kidney Int 13: 178–185, 1978.

28. Hörl WH, Heidland A. Enhanced proteolytic activity—Cause of protein catabolism in acute renal failure. Am J Clin Nutr 33: 1423–1427, 1980.

29. Lundholm K, Bylund A-C, Holm J, Schersten T. Skeletal muscle metabolism in patients with malignant tumor. Europ J Cancer 12: 465–473, 1976.

30. Clowes GHA Jr., George BC, Villee CA Jr, Saravis CA. Muscle proteolysis induced by a circulating peptide in patients with sepsis or trauma. N Eng J Med 308: 545–552, 1983.

31. Baracos V, Rodemann HP, Dinarello CA, Goldberg AL. Stimulation of muscle protein degradation and prostaglandin E_2 release by leukocytic pyrogen (Interleukin-1). N Eng J Med 308: 553–558, 1983.

32. Giordano C, DePascale C, DeCristofaro D, Capodicasa G, Balestrieri C, Baczyk K. Protein malnutrition in the treatment of chronic uremia. In Nutrition in Renal Disease, Berlyne GM (ed). Williams & Wilkins, 1968, pp. 23–34.

33. McGale EHF, Pickford JC, Aber GM. Quantitative changes in plasma amino acids in patients with renal disease. Clin Chim Acta 38: 395–403, 1972.

34. Kopple JD, Swendseid ME, Shinaberger JH, Umezawa CY. The free and bound amino acids removed by hemodialysis. Trans Am Soc Artif Intern Organs 14: 309–313, 1973.

35. Berlyne GM, Lee HA, Giordano C, DePascale C, Esposito R. Amino acid loss in peritoneal dialysis. Lancet 1: 1339–1341, 1967.

36. Young GA, Parsons FM. The effect of peritoneal dialysis upon the amino acids and other nitrogenous compounds in the blood and dialysates from patients with renal failure. Clin Sci 37: 1–10, 1969.

37. Giordano C, De Santo NG, Capodicasa G, Di Leo VA, Di Serafino A, Cirrillo D, Esposito R, Fiore R, Damiano M, Buonadonna L, Cocco F, Di Iorio B. Amino acid losses during CAPD. Clin Nefr 14(5): 230–232, 1980.

38. Kopple JD, Blumenkrantz MJ, Jones MR, Moran JK, Coburn JW. Amino acid losses during continuous ambulatory peritoneal dialysis (CAPD). Kidney Int 19(1): 152A, 1981.

39. Blumenkrantz MJ, Gahl GM, Kopple JD, Anjana VK, Jones MR, Kessel M, Coburn JW. Protein loss during peritoneal dialysis. Kidney Int 19: 593–682, 1981.

40. Grodstein GP, Blumenkrantz MJ, Kopple JD, Moran JK, Coburn JW. Glucose absorption during continuous ambulatory peritoneal dialysis. Kidney Int 19: 564–567, 1981.

41. Borst JGG. Protein catabolism in uremia. Effects of protein-free diet, infections, and blood-transfusions. Lancet 1: 824–828, 1948.

42. Bull GM, Joekes AM, Lowe KG. Conservative treatment of anuric uremia. Lancet 2: 229–234, 1949.

43. Blagg CR, Parsons FM, Young BA. Effects of dietary glucose and protein in acute renal failure. Lancet 1: 608–612, 1962.

44. Gamble JL. Physiological information from studies on the life-raft ration. Harvey Lect 42: 247–273, 1946–47.

45. Berlyne GM, Bazzard FJ, Booth EM, Janabi K, Shaw AB. The dietary treatment of acute renal failure. Quart J Med 141: 59–83, 1967.

46. Teschan PE, Baxter CR, O'Brien TF, Freyhof JN, Hall WH. Prophylactic hemodialysis in the treatment of acute renal failure. Ann Int Med 53: 992–1016, 1960.

47. Lee HA, Sharpstone P, Ames AC. Parenteral nutrition in renal failure. Postgrad Med J 43: 81–91, 1967.

48. Wilmore DW, Dudrick SJ. Treatment of acute renal failure with intravenous essential L-amino acids. Arch Surg 99: 669–673, 1969.

49. Dudrick SJ, Steiger E, Long JM. Renal failure in surgical patients—treatment with intravenous essential amino acids and hypertonic glucose. Surg 68: 180–186, 1970.

50. Van Buren CT, Dudrick SJ, Dworkin L, Baumbauer E, Long JM. Effects of intravenous essential L-amino acids and hypertonic dextrose on anephric beagles. Surg Forum 23: 83–84, 1972.

51. Abel RM, Beck CH, Jr, Abott WM, Ryan JA, Jr, Barnett GO, Fischer JE. Improved survival and acute renal failure after treatment with intravenous essential L-amino acids and glucose. N Eng J Med 288: 695–699, 1973.

52. Abbott WM, Abel RM, Fischer JE. Treatment of acute renal insufficiency after aortoiliac surgery. Arch Surg 103: 590–594, 1971.

53. Abel RM, Abbott WM, Fischer JE. Intravenous essential L-amino acids and hypertonic dextrose in patients with acute renal failure. Am J Surg 123: 631–638, 1972.

54. Abel RM, Shih VE, Abbott WM, Beck CH, Jr, Fischer JE. Amino acid metabolism in acute renal failure. Ann Surg 180: 350–355, 1974.

55. Abel RM, Abbott WM, Beck CH, Jr, Ryan JA, Jr, Fischer JE. Essential L-amino acids for hyperalimentation in patients with disordered nitrogen metabolism. Am J Surg 128: 317–323, 1974.

56. Baek SM, Makabali GG, Bryan-Brown CW, Kusek

J, Shoemaker W. The influence of parenteral nutrition on the course of acute renal failure. Surg Gynec Obstet 141: 405–408, 1975.

57. McMurray SD, Luft FC, Maxwell DR, Hamburger RJ, Futty D, Szwed J, Lavelle KJ, Kleit SA. Prevailing patterns and predictor variables in patients with acute tubular necrosis. Arch Int Med 138: 950–955, 1978.

58. Milligan SL, Luft FC, McMurray SD, Kleit SA. Intra-abdominal infection and acute renal failure. Arch Surg 113: 467–471, 1978.

59. Blackburn GL, Etter G, MacKenzie T. Criteria for choosing amino acid therapy in acute renal failure. Am J Clin Nutr 31: 1841–1853, 1978.

60. Abitbol CL, Holliday MA. Total parenteral nutrition in anuric children. Clin Nephrol 3: 153–158, 1976.

61. Spreiter SC, Myers BD, Swenson RS. Protein-energy requirements in subjects with acute renal failure receiving intermittent hemodialysis. Am J Clin Nutr 33: 1433–1437, 1980.

62. Lopez-Martinez J, Caparros T, Perez-Picouto F, Lopez-Diez F, Cereijo E. Nutrición parenteral en enfermos sépticos con fracaso renal agudo en fase poliúrica. Rev Clin Esp 157(3): 171–177, 1980.

63. Hasik J, Hryniewiecki L, Baczyk K, Grala T. An attempt to evaluate minimum requirements for protein in patients with acute renal failure. Pol Arch Med Wewn LXI(1): 29–36, 1979.

64. Kopple JD, Feinstein EI. Current problems in amino acid therapy for acute renal failure. In Proceedings of the European Dialysis and Transplant Association, Davidson Am, Guillou PJ (eds). New York: Pitman Press, 1983, pp. 129–140.

65. Feinstein EI, Kopple JD, Silberman H, Massry SG. Kidney Int Suppl., Dec. 1983.

66. Nicholls DM, Ng K. Regeneration of renal proximal tubules after mercuric chloride injury is accompanied by increased binding of aminoacyl-transfer ribonucleic acid. Biochem J 160: 357–365, 1976.

67. Cuppage FE, Cunningham N, Tate A. Nucleic acid synthesis in the regenerating nephron following injury with mercuric chloride. Lab Invest 21(5): 449–457, 1969.

68. Cuppage FE, Chiga M, Tate A: Cell cycle studies in the regenerating rat nephron following injury with mercuric chloride. Lab Invest 26(1): 122–126, 1972.

69. Toback FG, Havener LH, Dodd RC, Spargo BH. Phospholipid metabolism during renal regeneration after acute tubular necrosis. Am J Physiol 232(2): E216–E222, 1967.

70. Toback FG. Amino acid treatment of acute renal failure. In Acute Renal Failure, Brenner BM, Stein JH (eds). New York: Churchill Livingstone, 1980, pp. 202–228.

71. Toback FG, Dodd RC, Maier ER, Havener LJ. Amino acid enhancement of renal protein synthesis during regeneration after acute tubular necrosis. Clin Res 27, 432A, 1979.

72. Toback FG. Amino acid enhancement of renal regeneration after acute tubular necrosis. Kidney Int 12: 193–198, 1977.

73. Toback FG, Tegarden DE, Havener LJ. Amino acid-mediated stimulation of renal phospholipid biosynthesis after acute tubular necrosis. Kidney Int 15: 542–547, 1979.

74. Rouser G, Simon G, Kritchevsky G. Species variations in phospholipid class distribution of organs: Kidney, liver and spleen. Lipids 4(6): 599–606, 1969.

75. Oken DE, Sprinkel FM, Kirschbaum BB, Landwehr DM. Amino acid therapy in the treatment of experimental acute renal failure in the rat. Kidney Int 17: 14–23, 1980.

76. Walser M. Urea metabolism in chronic renal failure. J Clin Invest 53: 1385–1392, 1974.

77. Blumenkrantz MJ, Kopple JD, Moran JK, Grodstein GP, Coburn JW. Nitrogen and urea metabolism during continuous ambulatory peritoneal dialysis. Kidney Int 20(1): 78–82, 1981.

78. Sargent JA, Gotch, FA. Mass balance: A quantitative guide to clinical nutritional therapy. J Am Diet Ass 75: 547–555, 1979.

79. Rose WC. The amino acid requirements of adult man. Nutr Abstr Rev 27: 631–647, 1957.

80. Kopple JD, Swendseid ME. Evidence that histidine is an essential amino acid in normal and chronically uremic man. J Clin Invest 55: 881–891, 1975.

81. Jones MR, Kopple JD, Swendseid ME. Phenylalanine metabolism in uremic and normal man. Kidney Int 14: 169–179, 1978.

82. Pickford JC, McGale EHF, Aber GM. Studies on the metabolism of phenylalanine and tyrosine in patients with renal disease. Clin Chim Acta 48: 77–83, 1973.

83. Flügel-Link RM, Jones MR, Kopple JD. Red cell and plasma amino acid concentrations in renal failure J. Parent and Enteral Nutr. 7: 450–456, 1983.

84. Bergström J, Fürst P, Norrée L-O, Vinnars E. Intracellular free amino acids in muscle tissue of patients with chronic uremia: Effect of peritoneal dialysis and infusion of essential amino acids. Clin Sci Mol Med 54: 51–60, 1978.

85. Wurtman RJ. Implications of parenteral and enteral amino acid mixtures in brain function. In Amino Acids Metabolism and Medical Application, Blackburn GL, Grante JP, Young VR (eds). John Wright-PSG, Inc. 1983, pp. 219–224.

86. Tizianello A, De Ferrazi G, Garibotto G, Gurreri G, Robaudo C. Renal metabolism of amino acids and ammonia in subjects with normal renal function and in patients with chronic renal insufficiency. J Clin Invest 65: 1162–1173, 1980.

87. Ganda OP, Aoki TT, Soeldner JS, Morrison RS, Cahill GF, Jr. Hormone-fuel concentrations in anephric subjects. Effect of hemodialysis with special reference to amino acids. J Clin Invest 57: 1403–1411, 1976.

88. Metcoff J, Lindeman R, Baxter D, Pederson J. Cell

metabolism in uremia. Am J Clin Nutr 30: 1627–1634, 1978.

89. Furst P, Alvestrand A, Bergström J. Effects of nutrition and catabolic stress on intracellular amino acid pools in uremia. Am J Clin Nutr 33: 1387–1395, 1980.

90. Fulks RM, Li JB, Goldberg A. Effects of insulin, glucose, and amino acids on protein turnover in rat diaphragm. J Biol Chem 250 (1): 290–298, 1975.

91. Buse MG, Reid SS. Leucine. A possible regulator of protein turnover in muscle. J. Clin Invest 56: 1250–1261, 1975.

92. Daly M, Mihranian MH, Kehoe JI, Brennan MS. Effects of postoperative infusion of branched-chain amino acids on nitrogen balance and forearm muscle substrate flux. Surgery 94: 151–159, 1983.

93. Cerra FB, Upson D, Angelico R, Wiles C, Lyons J, Faulkenbach L, Paysinger J. Branched-chain support post-operative protein synthesis. Surgery 92: 192–200, 1982.

94. Kopple JD, Swenseid ME. Nitrogen balance and plasma amino acid levels in uremic patients fed an essential amino acid diet. Am J Clin Nutr 27: 806–812, 1974.

95. Stucki WP, Harper AE. Importance of dispensable amino acids for normal growth of chicks. J Nutr 74: 377–383, 1961.

96. Ranhotra GS, Johnson BC. Effect of feeding different amino acid diets on growth rate and nitrogen retention of weanling rats. Proc Soc Exp Biol Med 118: 1197–1201, 1965.

97. Rogers QR, Chen DM, Harper AE. The importance of dispensable amino acids for maximal growth in the rat. Proc Soc Exp Biol Med 134: 517–522, 1970.

98. Swendseid ME, Harris CL, Tuttle SG. The effect of sources of nonessential nitrogen on nitrogen balance in young adults. J Nutr 71: 105–108, 1960.

99. Anderson HL, Heindel MB. Effect on nitrogen balance of adult men of varying source of nitrogen and level of calorie intake. J Nutr 99: 82–90, 1969.

100. Pennisi AJ, Wang M, Kopple JD. Effects of protein and amino acid diets in chronically uremic and control rats. Kidney Int 13: 472–479, 1978.

101. VanVenrooij WJW, Henshaw EC, Hirsch CA. Effects of deprival of glucose or individual amino acids on polyribosome distribution and rate of protein synthesis in cultured mammalian cells. Biochim Biophys Acta 259: 127–137, 1972.

102. Motil KJ, Harmon WE, Grupe WE. Complications of essential amino acid hyperlimentation in children with acute renal failure. JPEN 4(1): 32–35, 1980.

103. Jonxis JHP, Huisman THJ. Excretion of amino acids in free and bound form during intravenous administration of protein hydrolysate. Metabolism 6: 175–181, 1957.

104. Klein GL, Alfrey AC, Miller NL, Sherrard J, Hazlet TK, Ament ME, Coburn JW. Aluminum loading during total parenteral nutrition. Am J Clin Nutr 35: 1425–1429, 1982.

105. Kopple JD. Treatment with low protein and amino acid diets in chronic renal failure. In Proceedings VIIIth International Congress of Nephrology, Borcelo R, Bergeron M, Carriere S, Dirks JH, Drummond K, Guttman RD, Lemieux G, Mongeau JG, Seely JF (eds). S Karger, 1978, pp. 497–507.

106. Kopple JD. Nutritional therapy in kidney failure. Nut. Rev 39(5): 193–206, 1981.

107. Young EA, Heuler N, Russell P, Weser E. Comparative nutritional analysis of chemically defined diets. Gastroenterology 69: 1338–1345, 1975.

108. Russell RI. Progress report: Elemental diets. Gut 16: 68–79, 1975.

109. Askanazi J, Elwyn DH, Silverberg BS, Rosenbaum SH, Kinney JM. Respiratory distress secondary to a high carbohydrate load: A case report. Surgery 87(5): 596–598, 1980.

110. Long JM, Wilmore DW, Mason AD, Jr, Pruitt BA: Fat-carbohydrate interaction: Effects on nitrogen-sparing in total intravenous feeding. Surg Forum 25: 61–63, 1974.

111. Milne CA, MacLean LD, Shizgal HM. Casein hydrolysate and intralipid vs casein hydrolysate and 25% glucose for hyperalimentation. Surg Forum 25: 52–54, 1974.

112. Farrington K, Miller P, Varghesez, Baillod RA, Moorhead JF. Vitamin A toxicity and hypercalcemia in chronic renal failure. Br Med J 282: 1999–2002, 1981.

113. Udall JA. Human sources and absorption of vitamin K in relation to anticoagulant stability. JAMA 194: 127–129, 1965.

114. Kopple JD, Mercurio K, Blumenkrantz MJ, Jones MR, Tallos J, Roberts C, Card B, Saltzman R, Casciato DA, Swendseid ME. Daily requirement of pyridoxine supplements in chronic renal failure. Kidney Int 19(5): 694–704, 1981.

115. Kopple JD, Blumenkrantz MJ. Total parenteral nutrition and parenteral fluid therapy. In Clinical Disorders of Fluid and Electrolyte Metabolism, Maxwell MH, Kleeman CR (eds). New York: McGraw-Hill, 1980, pp. 413–498.

116. Isaacs JW, Millikan WJ, Stackhouse J, Hersh T, Rudman D. Parenteral nutrition of adults with a 900 milliosmolar solution via peripheral veins. Am J Clin Nutr 30: 552–559, 1977.

117. Shils ME, Wright WL, Turnbull A, Brescia F. A long-term parenteral nutrition through an external arteriovenous shunt. N Engl J Med 283: 341–344, 1970.

118. Zincke H, Hirsche BL, Amamoo DG, Woods JE, Andersen RC. The use of bovine carotid grafts for hemodialysis and hyperalimentation. Surg Gynecol Obstet 139: 350–352, 1974.

119. Heidland A, Kult J. Long-term effects of essential amino acids supplementation in patients on regular dialysis treatment. Clin Nephrol 3: 234–239, 1975.

120. Wolfson M, Jones MR, Kopple JD. Amino acid

losses during hemodialysis with infusion of amino acids and glucose. Kidney Int 21: 500–506, 1982.

121. Kramer P, Böhler J, Kehr A, Gröne HJ, Schrader J, Matthaei D, Scheler F. Intensive care potential of continuous arteriovenous hemofiltration. Trans Am Soc Artif Intern Organs 28: 28–32, 1982.

122. Kramer P, Kaufhold G, Gröne HJ, Wigger W, Rieger J, Matthaei D, Stokke T, Burchardi H, Scheler F. Management of anuric intensive-care patients with arteriovenous hemofiltration. Int J Artif Organs 3: 225–228, 1980.

123. Kaplan AA, Langhecker RE, Folkert VW. Suction-assisted continuous arterio-venous hemofiltration. Trans Am Soc Artif Intern Organs 29: 408–413, 1983.

124. Hinton P, Allison SP, Littlejohn S, Lloyd J. Insulin and glucose to reduce catabolic response to injury in burned patients. Lancet 1: 767–769, 1971.

125. Woolfson AMJ, Healtley RV, Allison SP. Insulin to inhibit protein catabolism after injury. N Engl J Med 300: 14–17, 1979.

126. Hampl R, Stárka L. Practical aspects of screening of anabolic steroids in doping control with particular accent to nortestosterone radioimmunoassay using mixed antisera. J Steroid Biochem 11: 933–936, 1979.

127. Wilson JD, Griffin JE. The use and misuse of androgens. Metabolism 29: 1278–1295, 1980.

128. Freedman P, Spencer AG. Testosterone propionate in the treatment of renal failure. Clin Sci 16: 11–22, 1957.

129. McCracken BH, Parsons FM. Nilevar (17-ethyl-19-nor-testosterone) to suppress protein catabolism in acute renal failure. Lancet 2: 885–886, 1958.

130. Gjorup S, Thaysen JH. The effect of anabolic steroid (Durabolin)® in the conservative management of acute renal failure. Acta Med Scand 167: 227–238, 1960.

131. Saarne A, Bjerstaf L, Ekman G. Studies on the nitrogen balance in the human during long-term treatment with different anabolic agents under strictly standardized conditions. Acta Med Scand 177: 199–211, 1965.

132. Hörl WH, Gantert C, Auer IO, Heidland A. In vitro inhibition of protein catabolism by alpha-macroglobulin in plasma from a patient with post-traumatic acute renal failure. Am J Nephrol 2: 32–35, 1982.

133. Siegel NJ, Glazier WB, Chaudry IH, Gaudio KM, Lytton B, Baue AE, Kashgarian M. Enhanced recovery from acute renal failure by the post-ischemic infusion of adenine nucleotides and magnesium chloride in rats. Kidney Int 17: 338–349, 1980.

23. TREATMENT OF ACUTE RENAL FAILURE BY HEMODIALYSIS

Victor Parsons

1 The Indications for Starting Hemodialysis

Before hemodialysis is instituted, a thorough assessment must be made of the nature of the renal failure as shown by the signs and symptoms of a failure of water excretion, nitrogenous breakdown products and ions, such as potassium, sodium, and phosphate (see chapter 7).

If the ratios between urine and plasma confirm established acute renal failure (ARF) and resultant measures have been instituted and failed, the patient must be dialyzed. Very often, the situation is complicated by surgery, and dialysis must be fit in around it. Priorities must be decided for obligatory situations and elective ones (table 23–1).

2 Peritoneal or Hemodialysis?

The type of dialysis is determined by the advantages of each procedure, as outlined in table 23–2. In addition to these clinical indications, decisions may have to be made according to the facilities available; often peritoneal dialysis can be started while preparations are being made for hemodialysis or ultrafiltration, which demands access to the circulation.

3 Access to the Circulation

3.1 SUBCLAVIAN VEIN CANNULATION

This is the most rapid form of access [1] and provides adequate flows, irrespective of the blood pressure, the state of peripheral vessels, and the size of the patient; it can be inserted while the surgery of trauma or the limbs is anticipated or underway. The technique requires a "single-needle adaptation," or a peripheral vein can be used for the venous return. In between dialyses, the cannula is kept from clotting by replacing the small dead space by heparin. The risks are infection, often with skin organisms, which seldom give rise to significant morbidity [2]. The risks include vessel perforation and hemorrhage; careful radiological checks should be made if there is the slightest problem of flow [3], and ultrasound can be used to locate the vessel more accurately [4].

3.2 CAVAL CATHETERIZATION

This technique was introduced to achieve adequate dialysis in the patient with ARF where peripheral vessels are exhausted or where the patient is hypotensive and shocked. The technique either involves the introduction of a double lumen catheter into the femoral vein or one

TABLE 23–1. Indications for dialysis

Obligatory
    Uremia with confusion, drowsiness, and vomiting
      (Urea >35 mmol/liter).
    Creatinine >1500 μmol/liter, hyperkalemia (K >6.5
      mmol/liter).
    Metabolic acidosis ($NaCO_3$ <10 mmol/liter).
    Hepatic coma, NH_4 ↑, profound hypoalbuminemia
      (albumin <1.5 g/liter).
    Hypervolemia, pulmonary edema, cerebral edema.
    Rarely for drug intoxication.
Elective
    Preoperatively in the absence of any of the obligatory
      reasons above.
    To accommodate intravenous feeding regimens.
    To accommodate blood or plasma infusions.

V.E. Andreucci (ed.), ACUTE RENAL FAILURE.
All rights reserved. Copyright © 1984.
Martinus Nijhoff Publishing, Boston/The Hague/
Dordrecht/Lancaster.

TABLE 23–2. Peritoneal dialysis, hemodialysis, and ultrafiltration. Preferred techniques.

Condition	Peritoneal dialysis	Hemodialysis	Ultrafiltration and reinfusion
Poor cardiac function	+ + +	0	+ +
Pancreatitis and peritonitis	+ + +	+	0
Hepatorenal failure (HRF)	+ + +	±	+ +
Hematological diseases, e.g., sickle cell, bleeding diathesis	+ + +	+	0
Multiple abdominal drains	0	+ +	+
Pulmonary complications	0	+ + +	+
Hypercatabolic states	0	+ + +	±
Ascites and HRF	0	+ +	+ + +
Poisoning	0	+ +	+
Diabetes with gross edema	0 +	+ +	+ + +

into the femoral artery and femoral vein separately using the Seldinger technique [5, 6].

Catheters are reinserted for each dialysis, and the groin sites are alternated. After dialysis and heparinization are reversed, the catheters are withdrawn and a pressure dressing is applied for ten minutes to arrest any leakage. Review of 700 uses of such catheterizations over a period of seven years revealed that five patients had complications, three had femoral vein thrombosis with a small pulmonary embolus in one, while two had retroperitoneal bleeding due to venous tears [7].

3.3 SHUNT INSERTION

Where dialysis is likely to be prolonged and peripheral vessels are usable, the insertion of straight (Ramirez) silastic shunts into arm or leg vessels is to be preferred; in children, groin shunts inserted into the larger vessels using a Thomas applique shunt with a dacron cuff are necessary. Straight shunts in the acute situation are to be recommended in preference to the moulded reflex Scribner variety for ease of declotting, as this occurs in patients subjected to surgery, hypotension, and tranfusion to high hemoglobin concentrations in contrast to the more chronic patients. Flows in excess of 200 ml/min should be aimed for to achieve satisfactory dialysis. Sudden declotting of arterial shunts run the risk of retrograde embolism as the clot is forced into the main circulation, and urokinase (10,000 units in 5 ml of saline) should be left in situ for a time before declotting is attempted. All access sites should be swabbed regularly, and any persistent sepsis treated appropriately, as repeated septic embolization from infected sites leads to endocarditis in susceptible patients.

3.4 PATIENTS ON BYPASS OXYGENATORS

Occasionally, patients with severe trauma to the chest and heart have to receive dialysis while their circulation is being sustained by cardiac bypass or pulmonary bypass procedures. The most common need is ultrafiltration; in these circumstances it is achieved by inserting an ultrafiltration cartridge in the circuit where three liters/hour of ultrafiltrate can be removed without the use of any dialysis apparatus. We have found that where dialysis is necessary to correct uremia, high clearance rates can be achieved by using two coils in series and clearances of 300 mls/min can be achieved with the high flow rates tapping the bypass circuit.

Once access to the circulation has been gained, a series of decisions must be made on what type of dialysis is best to correct the patient's most severe abnormalities. The decision pathways are illustrated in figure 23–1. Ultrafiltration, either a preliminary therapy or an intervening therapy between hemodialysis, is being used increasingly in the treatment of patients with ARF [8]. The removal of up to six liters of excess fluid can be achieved in three hours by using either a conventional dialyzer with a high transmembrane pressure [9]—best achieved by a positive pressure in the blood compartment and a negative pressure in the dialysate compartment—or an Amicon untrafil-

+ = PRESENT

- = ABSENT

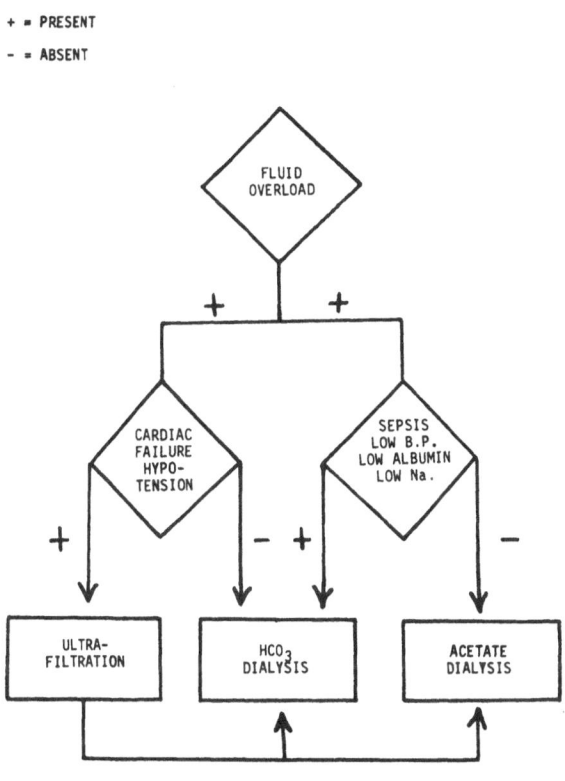

FIGURE 23–1. Choices of treatment for managing the overload high-risk cardiac patient.

tration cartridge containing the XP membrane [10]. Ultrafiltration in the unstable cardiac patient has the advantage of isoosmotic fluid removal without producing severe hypovolemia [11] or pulmonary vascular changes due to hypoxia [12].

4 Choice of Anticoagulant

Once access has been obtained, the choice of anticoagulant is important since in some circumstances further hemorrhage in the patient is likely either from surgical operation sites, tracheostomy, or gastrointestinal ulceration. Various techniques are available to avoid this.

4.1 NO ANTICOAGULANT USED AT ALL

This technique has been used frequently, particularly in patients whose coagulation mechanisms may be reduced by sepsis or liver disease. High flow rates should be aimed at around 300 mls/min, and saline washes can be given into the coil every 15 minutes [13]. Careful monitoring of pressures on either side of the coil will pick up thrombosis within the coil and avoid bursts.

4.2 USE OF REGIONAL HEPARINIZATION

Here heparin at a rate of 1,000 units per hour is introduced using a syringe pump into the arterial line, and protamine at around 1 mg/hour is infused downstream of the coil to neutralize the heparin [14]. Clotting times are estimated rapidly using a Haemochron apparatus incorporating a glass clotting time detected magnetically. One problem is that the heparin protamine complexes may dissociate later to prolong the clotting time [15].

4.3 USE OF PROSTACYCLIN

This agent stops platelet aggregation and indirectly white blood cell sequestration and fibrin deposition within the coil. Given at rates of 5 ng/Kg/minute, dialysis can be achieved without hypotension and flushing within the patients, common signs of prostacyclin administration [16, 17].

4.4 "TIGHT HEPARINIZATION"

This technique is commonly used to achieve the minimum of heparinization consistent with anticoagulation within the coil without overheparinization of the patient. A low dose of heparin (1,000 units for a 70 kg patient) is given to the patient, and small frequent boluses or a constant infusion of small quantities of heparin, often less than 3,000 units, are needed for a four-hour dialysis [18]. Because sudden hemorrhage in an overheparinized patient can provoke massive hemorrhage, particular care is required in patients with pulmonary hemorrhage and Goodpasture's syndrome or pulmonary emboli, and expert help to place bronchial blockers needs to be at hand.

5 Choice of Dialyzer and Techniques

In many circumstances, ultrafiltration and clearance rates should be high in patients with ARF. With subclavian vein catheterization, "single-needle techniques" are often used with

TABLE 23-3. Type of dialyzer with clearances at a dialysate flow of 500 mls per minute and a blood flow of 200 mls per minute

Dialyzer	Thickness of membrane	Area (m^2)	Urea clearance ml/min	B$_{12}$ ml/min	UF ml/hr
Cordis Dow (C Dak 5)	Cellulose 30 μm	2.5	186 ± 2	30	306
HF 130 (Cobe)	Cuprophane 20 μm	1.3	142 ± 3	29	261
Gambro Lundia Major	Cuprophane 13.5 μm	1.5	147 ± 2	25	461
RP6 Rhone Poulenc	Polyacrylonitrile 30 μm	1.2	162.	75	3240

*At 100 mmHg transmembrane pressure.

high pressures developing across the dialyzer membrane. Cuprophane membranes are known to be more likely to activate platelets and white blood cell deposition in the dialyzer and are best avoided in the sensitive patient. Dialyzers are available with cellulose acetate, cellulose hydrate, and polyacrylonitrile membranes (table 23–3).

In the majority of adult patients with high urea generation rates and negligible renal function, a dialyzer will be chosen that will give adequate clearances over a period of time and will not produce disequilibrium or excessive ultrafiltration.

In our experience, machinery designed for chronic hemodialysis is adequate for acute dialysis, particularly where there is an ability to manipulate the sodium concentration. But there is an advantage in the Travenol R.S.P. machine or the Rhone Poulenc fixed-volume dialysate machine, whose composition can be altered at will to contain a dialysate tailored to the patient's needs, which vary according to the situation that led to the patient's needing dialysis (table 23–4).

Such variations are reflected in the large number of commercially concentrated solutions now made available, and certainly some metabolic corrections can be made by ultrafiltration and infusion of the "correct" electrolyte solution to allow for the appropriate excess or deficiency.

Infusion of chelators in the dialysate has been used in the treatment of poisoning with arsenic; the patients are given dimercaprol (BAL), which when mixed with arsenic is di-alyzable. Similarly, EDTA can be used to chelate calcium, and desferrioxamine to chelate iron in the poisoned patient. A series of chelators have been used to remove mercury in similar circumstances, the most effective being acetylcystine [19]. Alcohol has been used to displace ethylene glycol in patients poisoned with the substance [20–21].

In one very restless manic patient who did not warrant paralysis and ventilation, we controlled her mania during dialysis by the use of dialysate containing lithium at 0.85 mmol/liter [22].

6 Acetate or Bicarbonate Dialysate and Acute Dialysis

Acetate was used as an ionic buffer because the introduction of continuously automated, rather than large-batch, mixes of dialysate, which had

TABLE 23-4. Varying dialysate compositions

Corrections required	Dialysate
Overhydration	Na$^+$ 140–145 mmol/l
Hyponatremia	Glucose 12 mmol/l
Hyperkalemia	K$^+$ 1.0 mmol/l
Hypercalcemia	Ca^{++} < 1.0 mmol/l
Cardiac failure and instability	HCO$_3^-$ 20 mmol/l
Dehydration	Na$^+$ 130 mmol/l, Glucose free
Hypocalcemia	Ca^{++} 3.5 mmol/l
Hypokalemia	K$^+$ 3.0 mmol/l, Glucose free
Hyperosmolar states	Na$^+$ 130 mmol/l, Glucose free
Acidosis	HCO$_3^-$ 30 mmol/l

to contain all the constituents, required soluble calcium and magnesium salts that would not precipitate out in cold stored concentrate. At the same time, carbon dioxide was not added to the bath to saturate it. For routine regular dialysis, this was an advance; since automated machines were used for acute dialysis, acetate became the buffer of choice.

Various studies have raised the question that acetate may not be metabolized to bicarbonate as quickly in seriously ill patients as in chronic patients and that as a result certain unwelcome features of acetate as a buffer may hazard the compromised patients [23].

Acetate may not correct the acidosis quickly enough and collect to become cardiodepressant, especially with highly efficient dialyzers [24]. In the chronic situation, high levels of acetate collecting at the end of dialysis have not been associated with any particular hypotensive episode or morbidity [25]; but other evidence has suggested that in the sick patient, acetate may well be vasodilatory, and in children, particularly, hypotensive episodes have been associated with high acetate concentrations [26, 27]. Loss of carbon dioxide in the dialysate may lead to a loss of respiratory function, due either to alterations in pulmonary ventilation perfusion or to depression of the respiratory center [28–30]. Finally, activation of platelet and white blood cell emboli formation and the release of vasoactive substances during membrane dialysate blood interaction within the dialyzer may be heightened in the presence of acetate [12].

For these reasons, a swing back to the use of bicarbonate has been made possible by the adaptation of several machines to deliver from two sources of diluted and heated concentrate a dialysate containing up to 28 mmols/liter of bicarbonate together with up to 12 mmols/liter of acetate required to keep the calcium and magnesium in solution. It is still possible to make up large-bath, single-batch mixes of acetate-free dialysate, adjusting the pH with lactic acid rather than acetate.

Patients who need a long dialysis and yet are hypotensive, have poor cardiac function due to intrinsic heart disease or to exogenous toxins, or who have liver failure are most likely to benefit from bicarbonate dialysis [31, 32], although controlled trials of sequential dialysis

with alternating bicarbonate and acetate dialysis have not shown increased mortality [33]. It must be commented that this trial contained very few children and patients with severe cardiac disease.

7 Complications of Hemodialysis

7.1 PULMONARY COMPLICATIONS

Pulmonary edema is a complex feature of ARF. Studies of pulmonary water in ARF show that it is associated with a high cardiac output and not necessarily with poor ventricular output [34, 35] although after cardiac surgery this may be the dominant cause. Hypoalbuminemia is another contributory factor reflecting increased permeability of capillary beds in many areas. There are a variety of causes of such increased permeability, including septicemia, endotoxemia, and vasoactive substances associated with shock [36]. The pathology of uremic pneumonitis has been reviewed recently and shows that there is evidence for alveolar capillary damage and the formation of a hyaline membrane [37]. It is against this background of pulmonary edema that the added hazard of dialysis hypoxia and hypotension has to be measured. This occurs in the first ninety minutes of connecting the patient to a dialysis circuit and is associated with a series of hematological changes, which include leucopenia, thrombocytopenia, and hypocomplementemia [38], and a loss of fibrin from the blood that is deposited in the dialysis membrane [39]. This activation of the complement and coagulation pathways is associated with local changes in the lungs associated with an alteration in ventilation and perfusion, which mechanical ventilation does not prevent [40].

Pulmonary leucoembolism [41] and platelet activation are probably responsible for these vascular changes and result in hypoxia; and where acetate has been used in the dialysate, the drop of the partial pressure of oxygen may be greater due to the mass transfer of bicarbonate from the plasma to the dialysate, which acetate metabolism is unable to regenerate so quickly [28, 30].

For the majority of patients, such reversible pulmonary changes and hypoventilation are not that dangerous, but where pulmonary reserve is already hazarded, this is an unnecessary risk that can be lessened by the use of membranes that do not activate these embolic and vasoactive changes so readily. Cellulose hydrate and polyacrylonitrile membranes seem less aggregatory in this context [29, 42].

The use of prostacyclin and high-dose methylprednisolone has not been successful in changing the leucopenia and complement activation [12]; even if these changes are minimal as occur in patients with no complement to activate [43], bicarbonate transfer can still account for the hypoventilation, thus making a change to bicarbonate dialysis a further help in this situation.

The interesting effects that temperature may have on this process—and also the fact that during ultrafiltration without dialysate in the compartment these changes are not seen very readily—make ultrafiltration and reinfusion techniques all the more important in the hazarded patient [44].

7.2 CARDIAC COMPLICATIONS

The heart is compromised in various ways during ARF. In the shocked septic patient, acidosis and endotoxins contribute to a depression in cardiac output, pulmonary changes mentioned above only make the situation worse for cardiac function, and the withdrawal of part of the output into the dialysis circuit may make cardiovascular support more important [45, 46].

Hypotension in the first ninety minutes of dialysis may further compromise the pulmonary artery filling, and changing potassium, calcium, and magnesium concentrations render the heart more sensitive to previously administered digoxin. High cardiac outputs are commonplace in ARF and may be altered in either direction by the dialysis procedure [47, 48]. Where tamponade is possible, echocardiographic investigation is helpful and drainage of collections vital [49].

Various techniques are available to support the failing myocardium.

a. *Correction of acidosis.* Myocardial contractility is depressed in the acidotic state. This needs correction not only with dialysis over a pe-

riod of time but also by the active administration of bicarbonate early in dialysis if this is a problem. Inotropes do not work in the presence of metabolic acidosis; this correction is important.

b. *Administration of inotropes,* such as dopamine and dobutamine [50].

c. In the shocked septic patient, naloxone seems to be of use in counteracting endorphine-like substances, which may well depress cardiac and respiratory function [51–53]. Polymyxin has been found in certain circumstances to counteract endotoxin from the pseudomonas pyocyanea; it is useful in patients with hepatorenal failure with this type of septicemia and who have high levels of endotoxemia [54].

d. *Balloon pumping.* This variety of cardiac support has gained increasing use, particularly in patients following cardiac surgery, but it is also being used in patients with overwhelming septicemia to tide them over the period when exo- and endotoxins are at their height and where resuscitation is extremely difficult [55].

e. Finally, the dialysis circuit can be used to aid cardiac output by reversing the flow from venous to arterial so that the dialysis pump provides energy on the left side of the heart. This occasionally has to be resorted to when the patient's blood pressure has rapidly decreased during dialysis and when there is no time to set up a more routine type of caval dialysis [56].

7.3 GASTROINTESTINAL COMPLICATIONS

Many of the factors leading to the establishment of acute tubular necrosis similarly affect the gut, liver, and the mucosa of the gut. Measurements of the partial pressure of oxygen in the venous outflow from the duodenum and pancreas during shock have shown that these areas are even more poorly perfused than the kidney [57]. This is followed in the severe situation by a high incidence of gastrointestinal hemorrhage, perforation of the small and large bowel, pancreatitis, and hepatic cholestasis. Besides perfusion and toxic insults, there are hormonal changes leading to a relative excess of corticosteroids, gastrin, and parathyroid hormone, all factors known to influence the development of gut lesions [58, 59].

"Stress ulcers" are frequently seen after acute cerebral trauma and after multiple surgical operations. Sudden unexplained rises in the serum blood urea concentration often alert the physician to occult bleeding while nasogastric aspiration can suddenly become blood stained. Pancreatitis can also be occult and occur after prolonged hypotension and septicemia [60]. Signs include a deterioration of pulmonary function, rising white blood count, hypocalcemia, and rising amylase concentrations over and above the common rise due to failure of urinary excretion. Benign cholestasis is similarly a complication of prolonged hypotension and sepsis in the portal system.

For these reasons, close attention is paid to the gut to reduce these complications. Gastric acid hypersecretion is countered by the use of alkalis, aluminum hydroxide or carbonate [61], or by the use of H_2 receptor antagonists, cimetidine, [62], or ranitidine [63].

In either case, regular tests for gastric aspirate need to be carried out to make sure that alkalinization has taken place. Prolonged aluminum hydroxide administration can lead to hypophosphatemia and a myopathy [64] while intestinal and colonic overload, especially in these patients with abdominal complications, is to be avoided.

Despite these measures, perforation and gastrointestinal hemorrhage occasionally require surgery, which has to be carried out between dialyses. The anuric transplant patient is particularly prone to peptic and stercoral ulceration and needs immediate surgical intervention. We have also seen multiple ulceration in the gut resulting from treating mercury poisoning with hemodialysis therapy [65]. Pancreatitis is best treated with peritoneal dialysis, but if it accompanies abdominal trauma, total pancreatectomy is the only measure to rescue the patient.

7.4 CENTRAL AND PERIPHERAL NERVOUS COMPLICATIONS

Uremia has a direct effect on cerebral function, but when it is corrected in the acutely ill patient who may have been underdialyzed or di-

alysis has been delayed, the abrupt removal of urea and other metabolites leads to the disequilibrium syndrome [66]. At its simplest, it is accompanied by severe headache and vomiting, and progresses occasionally to semicoma and fits with and without localizing signs. The differential diagnosis of other cerebral lesions must also be made, such as emboli, cerebrovascular accidents, spontaneous hypoglycemia, and, in the dialyzed transplant patient particularly, encephalitis, cerebral abscess, and transplant rejection encephalopathy [67].

In patients with severe pre-existing hypertensive encephalopathy, hypertension may be exacerbated by acute dialysis, and careful control of blood pressure must therefore be achieved.

Occasionally, the fitting may be continuous and difficult to control without paralysis and ventilation; both barbiturates and clonazepam intravenously seem to be the best combination in our experience.

To avoid a recurrence on dialysis due to disequilibration, a high glucose concentration should be used in the dialysate (20 mmol/liter), and mannitol can be infused during or at the end of the shortened dialysis period [33].

In some patients, the main complication is a progressive sensory and motor peripheral neuropathy, probably originating in the same mechanism of neuronal swelling since the intracellular urea gradient has been acutely changed on dialysis [68, 69]. The combination of sepsis, hypotension, and disequilibrium may provoke a more extensive and protracted peripheral neuropathy that is slow to recover and occasionally irreversible.

The differential diagnosis of hypertensive encephalopathic fits, epilepsy due to organic cerebral disease, and disequilibrium needs to be made since patients tend to be given anticonvulsants after a series of fits without the realization that such therapy may complicate further drug therapy such as with vitamin D [70].

8 Dialysis Timing and Strategy

Once the patient has established renal failure and dialysis has been initiated, various criteria determine the length and frequency of dialysis until such function has returned or the patient enters a regular dialysis regimen.

8.1 UREA GENERATION RATE

Protein catabolism depends on a variety of mechanisms, which include the size of the patient; children require a modified time on dialysis according to their body surface area [71]. Patients with obstetric anuria in the absence of sepsis have a slower rise of blood urea than surgical patients with anuria and can be safely dialyzed every other day or every third day. In contrast, higher protein breakdown rates are seen in patients with septicemia, trauma, and hemorrhage into the gut, and after steroid administration; in this group, there is evidence that prophylactic dialysis lessens the urea rise [72]. This is related to the phenomenon that protein catabolism is accelerated at high levels of urea with accompanying metabolites. Another factor is that complications such as septicemia and gastrointestinal hemorrhage are lessened if a deliberate attempt is made to keep the blood urea below 30 mmol/liter [73].

In the hypercatabolic patient who may be breaking down 15 grams of nitrogen a day, the urea rise is greater than 12 mmol/liter/day. In a 70 kg patient with 42 liters of extracellular fluid, this may lead to the collection of 500 mmols urea; and if clearances of 3 to 5 mmols of urea per minute are achieved throughout a dialysis (with a generation rate continuing at the same rate at the same time), the patient will require something of the order of four to six hours dialysis daily on a 1.5 square meter coil [74]. It is possible to construct a mathematical prediction of the "dialysis dose" required to keep the urea concentration within prescribed limits [75].

It is for this reason that peritoneal dialysis has often been abandoned in favor of hemodialysis in the hypercatabolic group. Urea generation rate is depressed in patients with hepatic failure, and dialysis still needs to be carried out while taking more note of the creatinine in these patients [76].

8.2 EDEMA

This condition may be the result of simple fluid overload and is reflected in a high central venous pressure, peripheral vessel engorge-

ment, relative hypertension, and the presence of septal lines on the chest radiograph. Here dialysis with diafiltration or simple hemofiltration is all that is required to correct the situation. With high ultrafiltration rates, the loss of fluid can be predicted with an accurate knowledge of blood flow rates across the membrane in the dialyzer; if fluids and blood are also being administered at the same time, the final fluid loss is best estimated by the use of a bed weighing device.

Not all edema is due to fluid overload, and in septicemic shocked patients, pulmonary edema is due to increased pulmonary leakage of fluid into the interstitial spaces. The shadows on the chest radiograph are much more fluffy and diffuse, and effusions are frequent [77]. The plasma oncotic pressure is low, and the plasma albumin is reduced due to transudation occasionally coupled with low synthetic rates by the liver [36].

In this situation, administration of albumin must be accompanied by dialysis and ultrafiltration—because, occasionally, fluid moved for the periphery by increased oncotic pressure can make central pulmonary edema worse; this can be monitored by transthoracic electrical impedance [78]. Very often until the sepsis is corrected, the albumin will remain low despite adequate replacement and the persistence of an albumin below 2.0 gm/liter is associated with a poor prognosis [79, 80].

8.3 INTRAVENOUS FEEDING— FLUID ADJUSTMENTS

This problem is discussed in greater detail in another chapter, but allowance must be made not only for the volume of fluid required to obtain a sufficient calorie intake but also to calculate the water production from infused carbohydrate and lipid, which may not be lost in the insensible loss fraction of water balance if the patient is on a ventilator with humidified gasses. Once again, bed and patient weighing is important.

8.4 ELECTROLYTE LOADS THAT NEED CORRECTION

Hyperkalemia from tissue breakdown, infused blood, and absorbed gastrointestinal hemorrhage may make daily dialysis necessary for this reason alone. Large quantities of sodium are also given in some salts of carbenicillin; 30 grams may contribute 150 mmol/day and inotropes are often made up in saline. Sodium nitroprusside is occasionally used in the control of severe hypertension and in cardiac failure; cyanide and thyocyanate may collect and need to be dialyzed out, even when the patient is not requiring dialysis frequently.

9 Hemofiltration and Hemoperfusion

Very often, the need for daily dialysis because of uremia is unnecessary owing to the high efficiency of the dialyzers; yet the removal of fluid remains a problem, especially where intensive feeding is required. We have found the use of alternate dialysis and ultrafiltration using one of the high-flux dialyzers (table 23–3) to be a useful additional technique, especially in the patient with an unstable myocardium who responds poorly to dialysis. If a shunt has been inserted, there is no need for a pump in the circuit; and the patient can be "bled" gently over a period of 12 hours with low transmembrane pressures to remove two to six liters of fluid in this time. Reinfusion of 2.78 mol/l (50g/dl) glucose and twice the normal saline (302 mmol/l, 1.8 g/dl) maintains electrolyte balance where fluid loss is excessive [9].

Hemoperfusion using carbon particles or an exchange resin is often carried out at the same time as hemodialysis and has been found of help in hepatic coma with and without paracetamol poisoning [81].

The use of hemoperfusion for the removal of excess drugs and their metabolites is a useful adjunct to hemodialysis, particularly where the drug is protein bound.

Amberlite resins IRA 900, XAD 2, and XAD 4 have achieved clearances of glutethimide approaching 300 mls/minute, methaqualone clearances of 180 mls/minute to 200 mls/minute, and barbiturates from 100 to 250 mls/minute. There is often a lack of close correlation between clinical improvement and the blood concentration of the intoxicant during hemoperfusion. This represents a dynamic relationship between the intracellular compartment, the central nervous system, and the removal rate by the column. It is possible that

intracellular concentration of the drug is mainly responsible for the clinical level of coma and that the measurement of the plasma drug concentration may not be determining all of its physiological effects [82].

Resin columns, particularly XAD 4 and XE 326, have been used to remove excess antibiotics, such as gentamicin and cephalothin. Clearances of between 125 and 190 mls have been achieved in the first hour of the columns' use [82]. Similar clearances have also been achieved with penicillin [83].

10 The Administration of Drugs in Renal Failure and During Dialysis

Renal function profoundly affects the handling of all drugs excreted by the kidney. The first task is to establish how elimination of the drug takes place in the patient with good renal function; there is a quotient of excretion between renal, hepatic, and gastrointestinal routes [84]. Where the main route of excretion is hepatic, alterations in dosage need not take place and are unaffected by dialysis to any extent (see table 23–5). Many of these drugs are not used in the acute situation, but when they are, the drug is best administered after the dialysis procedure is over. With anticonvulsants, regular estimations of blood concentrations are necessary; the same considerations apply to isoniazid and ethambutol and certain antifungals [85].

Where the drug is excreted by glomerular filtration or tubular excretion, the dose is mod-

TABLE 23–5. Drugs whose main route of elimination is hepatic and whose dosage is not affected by acute renal failure and where dialysis should not alter the regime

ANTIBIOTICS	NARCOTICS	SEDATIVES
chloramphenicol	codeine	pentobarbital
clindamycin	methadone	chlordiazepoxide
erythromycin	morphine	diazepam
lincomycin	naloxone	mepobramate
cloxacillins	pentazocine	chlorpromazine

CARDIOVASCULAR DRUGS	OTHERS
lidocaine	warfarin
propranolol	steroids
hydrallazine	diphenylhydantoin
prazosin	trimethadone
minoxidil	chlorpropamide
	isoniazid
	insulin

ified according to the quotient of main renal excretion and increased hepatic excretion in renal failure. Two other features influence therapy: the first is the degree of protein binding of the drug, as in this situation clearance on the hemodialysis is dependent on the degree of binding; the second is that in uremia, drug binding to receptors is altered by the degree of uremia and that dialysis affects such receptor status. The first feature is available for analysis, the second mainly for future investigation [86].

The drugs whose plasma protein binding is decreased in uremia are shown in table 23–6, and as some of the drugs are not excreted normally by the kidney, some loss can be expected on dialysis, for which some allowance should be made over a period of several dialyses.

A full discussion of drug administration in renal failure is not appropriate here and is fully reviewed elsewhere [87, 88] (see also chapter 3). One cardinal feature of the treatment of the ARF patient is to restrict administration to absolutely essential drugs, to give them after the dialysis procedure, intravenously if possible, and to monitor blood concentrations regularly so that effective concentrations are available in the plasma and tissues, avoiding overloading where possible [89].

Drugs that need adjusting because of a period of hemodialysis are shown in table 23–7. Very often, there are alternative drugs that are not excreted either by the kidney or lost across the dialysis membrane. Finally, there are a series of drugs that should not be given to patient with ARF, as shown in table 23–8.

11 The Prognosis in Acute Renal Failure

Every physician involved in the treatment of ARF is concerned in the management of the whole patient, whose renal failure may be the easiest problem to solve, and brings other factors determining the prognosis into relief. Many series of dialysis-treated patients report an overall mortality of 50% or more, depending on the age of the patient and the initial precipitating cause. A careful analysis of the causes of death highlights the problems that must be tackled in reducing the mortality to that of the irreversible damaged organs, such as

TABLE 23–6. Drugs whose plasma protein binding is decreased in uraemic sera (normal binding shown in parentheses)

Barbiturates (20–45%)
Benzylpenicillin (20–60%)
Diazepam (97–98%)
Diazoxide (95%)
Dicloxacillin (94%)
Digitoxin (94%)
Morphine (35%)
Phenytoin (90%)
Warfarin (97%)

TABLE 23–7. Drugs usually requiring supplemental dosage after hemodialysis

ANTIBIOTICS
aminoglycosides, cephalosporins, penicillins, trimethroprim, metromidazole, sulphanamides, 5-fluorocytosine, ethambutol, isoniazid.

ANTICONVULSANTS
phenytoin, barbiturates, phenothiazines, sodium valproate.

H$_2$ RECEPTOR DRUGS
cimetidine, ranitidine

CARDIOVASCULAR DRUGS
procainamide, disopyramide, theophylline, nitroprusside, methyldopa

TABLE 23–8. Drugs best avoided in acute renal failure

Potassium supplements "Slow K"
Potassium-sparing diuretics spironolactone and amiloride
Magnesium trisilicate
Lithium carbonate
Clofibrate
Tetracycline
Prostaglandin synthesis inhibitory drugs
Aminoglycosides, which collect in the renal cortex
Cephalosporins, which will sustain tubular damage

the heart, lungs, and brain. Various clinical scores are available to predict the outcome of a particular illness complicated or precipitated by trauma, surgery, or toxins, and it is the patients with highest risk scores that need particular attention [90, 91]. In a study of patients with multiple systems organ failure, the worse metabolic predictors were the plasma concentrations of urea, glucose, lactate, triglycerides, and free fatty acids, all items reflecting cellular damage and failure of renal homeostasis [92].

Turning particularly to ARF following cardiac surgery, a prospective survey of 500 consecutive patients showed an 88% mortality among those whose creatinine peaked at greater than 450 μmols/liter in contrast to those whose creatinine never rose above 130 μmols/liter (mortality 0.8%). The exact diagnosis of the type of heart disease, the type of operation, the length of time on bypass, the use of balloon pumping postoperatively, and the use of furosemide and nephrotoxic drugs did not correlate positively with a development of ARF. The features of the worst group of patients that could be positively associated with ARF and that had, incidently, a higher mortality are shown in table 23–9 [93]. This characterization of cardiac features, independent of sepsis, shock, and ventilation, illustrates the important effect initial cardiac and renal function play in the development of ARF, particularly in those at high risk. It has been our deliberate policy to prepare patients for dialysis at the time of surgery by the insertion of either a shunt or a peritoneal dialysis catheter so that dialysis can begin immediately. With this regimen, six patients to date have survived ARF postoperatively.

Another group of patients at particular risk are those with ruptured or incipiently rupturing aortic aneurysms. If renal failure develops postoperatively, then mortality is particularly high, ranging from 38 to 88% [94, 96]. Once again, age, cardiac disease, pre-existing renal damage, massive transfusion requirements, prolonged hypotension, and cross-aortic clamping play a part in the development of ARF. Every effort is made with intravenous feeding and prophylactic hemodialysis to keep pace with the hypercatabolic state that characterizes these patients.

Turning to the patients with hepatorenal failure (see chapter 11) whose pathophysiology includes hypovolemia, vasomotor nephropathy, drug toxicity, endotoxemia, hyperbilirubinemia, and sepsis, treatment with both hemodialysis, peritoneal dialysis, and hemoperfusion has led to recovery of renal function determined by the type of hepatic disease and its reversibility and the ability of the liver to regenerate over a period of time following toxic or inflammatory necrosis. Obstructive jaundice, if relieved, holds the best prognosis (>75%) followed by reversible causes of hepatic necrosis (viral hepatitis and a proportion of patients with toxic hepatic damage) where, if dialysis and nutritional support is maintained for weeks, recovery ranges from 30 to 50%; end-stage necrosis holds the worst prognosis (<10%), and here hepatic transplantation seems to offer the only hope for recovery of renal function [76, 81, 97].

In considering ARF developing with trauma, various factors emerge to determine the outcome, however well the electroylyte abnormality and calorie deficit is corrected. Where shock has remained uncorrected with blood and flows for longer than four hours and where transfusion needs have exceeded four times the circulating volume, prognosis is worsened [90]. Trauma to the abdomen with its accompanying sepsis, to the thighs with rhabdomyolysis and to the head and neck—all carry an increased mortality [98]. Combined skin burns and muscle damage carry a worse mortality [99, 100].

In our experience, every patient who did not survive after initially doing well from resuscitation and dialysis was found to be harboring occult collections of sepsis, dead tissue, or un-

TABLE 23–9. Risk factors associated with ARF and eventual mortality

CVS FACTORS	TRAUMATIC FACTORS
Age	Sepsis
Preoperative renal failure	Massive transfusion (>30 units)
Pre- or postoperative cardiac arrest	Major injury to abdomen, thigh, head, and cervical spine
Low preoperative cardiac index (<2.02 liters/ min/sqm)	Presence of skin loss and muscle damage
High LVEDP >17 mmHg[b]	
Long period on bypass or cross-aortic clamping	PULMONARY FACTORS
	Endotoxic and septic edema
HEPATIC FACTORS	Neurogenic edema
Cirrhosis (end-stage)	Gastric aspiration
Massive hepatic necrosis	Massive pneumonic consolidation
Persistent biliary obstruction	

[a]CVS = cardiovascular system.
[b]LVEDP = left ventricular end-diastolic pressure.

suspected bowel perforation. Repeated pressure must be maintained on all the surgical teams to explore and remove all unviable tissue at an early stage [101]. Computerized tomography scanning may now reveal collections of sepsis and cystic gas containing tissue and has been of particular use in the surgical management of acute pancreatitis [102].

One further risk factor, artificial ventilation, adds to the complications of acute renal failure; patients managed in an intensive care area with ventilation have a different prognosis from those managed in a renal unit without ventilation [91]. The degree of shock, pulmonary edema, acute pancreatitis, sepsis, and endotoxemia usually leads to the patient being ventilated despite a full trial of pharmacological measures to combat edema [103]. Dialysis in this situation gives the opportunity to correct fluid overload, raise the oncotic pressure by removal of fluid, and administer albumin. Positive pressure ventilation also helps diminish the collection of edema.

Colonization of the edematous uremic lung is a serious complication and increasing difficulty in maintaining adequate oxygenation a serious prognostic sign. Despite early tracheostomy construction, aspirates of gastric bacteria still take place in antacid-treated patients [104].

Once the pulmonary edema clears, the ventilation can be adjusted, usually by a period of intermittent mandatory ventilation to normal respiration. The nephrologist's task is to reverse the collection of analgesic depressant drugs, to ensure that the patient is not hypophosphatemic from repeated dialysis, and to anticipate rises in potassium as relaxants are withdrawn—which also lead to partial ileus and large quantities of gut fluid being reabsorbed at this time.

The overall mortality of ARF is improving as problems are anticipated, nephrotoxic drugs are avoided, and nephrologists demand more from their colleagues to correct other system failure [105].

References

1. Uldall PR, Woods F, Merchant N, Bird N, Crichton E. Two years experience with subclavian cannula for temporary vascular access for hemodialysis and plasmapheresis. Dial Transplant 8: 963–969, 1979.
2. Uldall PR, Merchant N, Woods F, Yaworski U, Vas S. Changing subclavian hemodialysis cannulas to reduce infection. Lancet 1: 1373, 1981.
3. Fine A, Churchill D, Gault H, Mathieson G. Fatality due to subclavian dialysis catheter. Nephron 29: 99–100, 1981.
4. Petzold R. Ultrasound-guided puncture of the subclavian vein. Intensive Care Medicine 7: 39–40, 1980.
5. Shaldon S, Chain Dussi L, Higgs B. Hemodialysis by percutaneous catherization of the femoral artery and vein with regional heparinization. Lancet 2: 857–859, 1961.
6. Matalon R, Nidus BD, Cantacuzino D, Eisenger RP. Intermittent hemodialysis with repeated femoral vein puncture. JAMA 214: 1883–1855, 1970.
7. Kjellstrand CM, Merino GE, Mauer SM, Casli R, Buselmeier JJ. Complications of percutaneous femoral vein catherizations for hemodialysis. Clin Nephrol 4: 37–40, 1975.
8. Bergstrom J, Asaba H, Furst P, Oules R. Dialysis ultrafiltration and blood pressure. Proc EDTA 13: 293–305, 1976.
9. Ing TS, Wei TC, Daugirdas JT, Kwang HC, Hano JE. Isolated ultrafiltration and new techniques of ultrafiltration during dialysis. Kidney Int 18: 577–582, 1980.
10. Henderson LW. Technical considerations in hemofiltration. Kidney Int 18(Suppl 10): S91–S92, 1980.
11. Asaba H, Bergstrom J, Furst P. Sequential ultrafiltration diffusion as alternative to conventional hemodialysis. Rev Int Radiol 6: 129–135, 1976.
12. Dodd NJ, Turney JH, Fewell MR, Parsons V, Weston MJ. Hemodialysis induced hypoxia: The influence of prostacyclin, methylprednisolone, ultrafiltration and bicarbonate dialysate. J Artif Organs (in press).
13. Casati S, Ponticelli C. Hemodialysis in patient with a risk of bleeding. N Engl J Med 305: 521–522, 1981.
14. Maher JF, La Pierre L, Schreiner GE. Regional heparinization for hemodialysis. N Engl J Med 268: 451–456, 1963.
15. Hampers CL, Blaufox MD, Merrill JP. Anticoagulation rebound after hemodialysis. N Engl J Med 275: 776–778, 1966.
16. Turney JH, Williams LC, Fewell MR, Parsons V, Weston MJ. Platelet protection and heparin sparing with prostacyclin during regular dialysis therapy. Lancet 21: 219–222, 1980.
17. Zusman RM, Rubin RH, Cato AE, Cocchetto DM, Crow JW, Tolkoff-Rubin N. Hemodialysis using prostacycline instead of heparin as the sole antithrombotic agent. N Engl J Med 304: 934–939, 1981.
18. Vogel GE, Kopp KF. Minimal dose heparinization for hemodialysis patients with high bleeding risk. Kidney Int 8: 436–441, 1975.

19. Al-Abbasi AH, Kostyniak PJ, Clarkson TW. An extracorporeal complexing hemodialysis system for the treatment of methyl mercury poisoning. J Pharmacol Exp Ther 207: 249–254, 1978.
20. Harmon WE, Sargent JA. Ethanol during hemodialysis for ethylene glycol poisoning. N Engl J Med 305: 522, 1981.
21. Peterson CD, Collins AJ, Himes JM, Bullock ML, Keane WF. Ethylene glycol poisoning pharmacokinetics during therapy with ethanol and hemodialysis. N Engl J Med 304: 21–23, 1981.
22. Oakly WF, Parsons V, Clarke WF. The use of dialysis bath fluid as a vehicle for a drug with a narrow therapeutic index—Lithium chloride. Postgrad Med J 2: 179–186, 1974.
23. Lewis EJ, Tolchin N, Roberts JL. Estimation of the metabolic conversion of acetate to bicarbonate during hemodialysis. Kidney Int 18 (Suppl 10): S51–S55, 1980.
24. Verman HG, Assomull VM, Kaiser BA, Blaschke TF, Weiner MW. Acetate metabolism and acid base homeostasis during hemodialysis: Influence of dialyzer efficiency and rate of acetate metabolism. Kidney Int 18 (Suppl 10): S62–S74, 1980.
25. Mansell MA, Nunan TO, Laker MF, Boon NA, Wing AJ. Incidence and significance of rising blood acetate levels during hemodialysis. Clin Nephrol 12: 22–25, 1979.
26. Novello A, Kelsch RC, Easterling RE. Acetate intolerance during hemodialysis. Clin Nephrol 5: 29–32, 1976.
27. Schohn DC, Klein S, Mitsuishi Y, Jahn HA. Correlation between plasma sodium acetate concentration and systemic vascular resistances. Proc EDTA 18: 160–168, 1981.
28. Tolchin N, Roberts JL, Lewis EJ. Respiratory gas exchange by high efficiency hemodialysis. Nephron 21: 137–145, 1978.
29. Kraut J, Fafter U, Brautbar N, Miller J, Schinaberger J. Prevention of hypoxemia during dialysis by the use of sequential isolated ulrafiltration diffusion dialysis with HCO₃ dialysate. Clin Nephrol 15: 181–184, 1981.
30. Dolan MJ, Whipp BJ, Davison WD, Weitzman RE, Wasserman K. Hypopnea associated with acetate dialysis carbon dioxide flow dependent ventilation. N Engl J Med 305: 72–75, 1981.
31. Aizawa Y, Ohmori T, Imai K, Nara Y, Matsuoka M, Hirasawa Y. Depressant action of acetate upon the human cardiovascular system. Clin Nephrol 8: 477–480, 1977.
32. Graefe U, Milutinovich J, Follette WC, Vizzo JE, Babb AL, Scribner BI. Less dialysis-induced morbidity and vascular instability with bicarbonate dialysate. Ann Intern Med 88: 332–336, 1978.
33. Borges HF, Fry DS, Rosa AA, Kjellstrand CM. Hypotension during acetate and bicarbonate dialysis in patients with renal failure. Amer J Nephrol 1: 24–30, 1981.
34. Gibson DG. Hemodynamic factors in the develop-ment of acute pulmonary edema in renal failure. Lancet 2: 1217–1220, 1966.
35. Crosbie WA, Snowdon S, Parsons V. Changes in lung capillary permeability in renal failure. Brit Med J 4: 388–390, 1972.
36. George C, Regnier B, Legall JR, Gastinne H, Carlet J, Rapin M. Hypovolemic shock with edema due to increased capillary permeability. Intensive Care Medicine 4: 159–164, 1978.
37. Bleyl U, Sander E, Schindler T. The pathology and biology of uremic pneumonitis. Intensive Care Medicine 7: 193–202, 1981.
38. Craddock PR, Fehr J, Dalmasso AP, Brigham KL, Jacob HS. Pulmonary vascular leucostasis resulting from complement activation by dialyzer cellophane membranes. J Clin Invest 59: 879, 1977.
39. Woods HF, Weston MJ. The use of antiplatelet agents during hemodialysis. Dial Transplant 8: 958–960, 1979.
40. Jones RH, Broadfield J, Parsons V. Arterial hypoxemia during hemodialysis for acute renal failure in mechanically ventilated patients, observations and mechanisms. Clin Nephrol 14: 18–22, 1980.
41. Toren M, Foffinet JA, Kaplon LS. Pulmonary bed sequestration of neutrophils during hemodialysis. Blood 36: 337–340, 1970.
42. Ajama P, Bird PAE, Ward MK, Feest TG, Walker W, Tanboga H, Sussman M, Kerr DNS. Hemodialysis-induced leukopenia and activation of complement, effects of different membranes. Proc EDTA 14: 144–153, 1978.
43. Habte B, Carter R, Shamebo M, Veitch J, Boulton-Jones JM. Dialysis induced hypoxemia. Clin Nephrol 18: 120–125, 1982.
44. Maggiore Q, Pizzarelli F, Zoccali C, Sisca S, Nicolo F, Parlongo S. Effect of extracorporeal blood cooling on dialytic arterial hypotension. Proc EDTA 18: 597–602, 1981.
45. Azancot I, Degoulet P, Juillet Y, Rottembourg J, Legrain M. Hemodynamic evaluation of hypotension during chronic hemodialysis. Clin Nephrol 8: 312–316, 1977.
46. Samii K, Rapin M, Legall JR, Regnier B. Hemodynamic study of patients with severe sepsis during hemodialysis. Intensive Care Medicine 4: 127–132, 1978.
47. Crosbie WA, Parsons V. Cardio-pulmonary function of congested lungs. Quart J Med 43: 215–230, 1974.
48. Hampl H, Paeper H, Volker U, Fischer C, Resa I, Kessel M. Hemodynamic changes during hemodialysis, sequential ultrafiltration and hemofiltration. Kidney Int 18 (Suppl 10): S83–S88, 1980.
49. Westaby S, Westaby D. A simple method for continuous pericardial drainage. Intensive Care Medicine 7: 31–35, 1980.
50. Chamberlain JH, Pepper JR, Yates AK. Dobutamine, isoprenaline and dopamine in patients after open-heart surgery. Intensive Care Medicine 7: 5–10, 1980.
51. Kirksen R, Otten MH, Wood GJ, Verban CJ,

Haalebos MMP, Verdoun PV, Nijhuis GMN. Naloxane in shock. Lancet 2: 1360–1361, 1980.

52. Peters NP, Johnson MW, Freidman PA, Mitch WE. Pressor effect of naloxane in septic shock. Lancet 1: 529–532, 1981.

53. Swinburn WR, Phelan P. Response to naloxane in septic shock. Lancet 1: 167, 1982.

54. Liehr H, Grun M, Brunswig D, Sautter T. Endotoxemia in liver cirrhosis treatment with polymyxin B. Lancet 1: 810–811, 1975.

55. Dhainaut JF, Huet Y, Kahan A, Bricard C, Neveux E, Dallot JY, Bachet J, Carci A, Monsallier FJ. Acute myocardial failure during Yersinia enterocolitica infection. Intensive Care Medicine 8: 49–51, 1982.

56. Connolly JP, Balsys AJ, King EG. Caval catheter hemodialysis. Intensive Care Medicine 6: 129–132, 1980.

57. Haglund U. The small intestine in hypotension and hemorrhage. Acta Physiol Scand (Suppl) 387: 1–37, 1975.

58. Gokal R, Kettlewell M, Drexler E, Oliver DO, Morris PJ. Gastrin levels in chronic renal failure, hemodialysis and renal transplantation. Clin Nephrol 14: 96–97, 1980.

59. Kokot F. The endocrine system in patients with acute renal failure. Proc EDTA 18: 617–632, 1981.

60. Avram MM. High prevalence of pancreatic disease in chronic renal failure. Nephron 18: 68–71, 1977.

61. Priebe HJ, Skillman JJ, Bushneil LS, Long PC, Silen W. Antacid versus cimetidine in preventing acute gastrointestinal bleeding, a randomized trial in 75 critically ill patients. N Engl J Med 302: 420–430, 1980.

62. Jones RH, Lewin MR, Parsons V. Therapeutic effect of cimetidine in patients undergoing hemodialysis. Brit Med J 1: 650–652, 1979.

63. Mc Gonigle RJS, Williams CC, Amphlett GE, England RJ, Parsons V. The pharmacokinetics of ranitidin in renal disease. Brit J Pharmacol (in press).

64. Baker LRI, Ackrill P, Cattel WR, Stamp TCB, Watson L. Iatrogenic osteomalacia and myopathy due to phosphate depletion. Brit Med J 3: 150–152, 1974.

65. Murphy MJ, Culliford EJ, Parsons V. A case of poisoning with mercury chloride. Resuscitation 7: 35–44, 1974.

66. Kennedy AC, Linton AL, Luke RG, Renfrew S, Dunwoodie A. The pathogenesis and prevention of cerebral dysfunction during dialysis. Lancet 2: 790, 1964.

67. Gross MCP, Pearson R, Sweny P, Fernando ON, Moorhead JF. Rejection encephalopathy. Proc EDTA 18: 461–468, 1981.

68. Meyrier A, Fardeav M, Richet E. Acute asymmetrical neuritis associated with rapid ultrafiltration dialysis. Brit Med J, 252–254, 1972.

69. Kjellstrand CM, Evans RL, Peterson RJ, Shideman JR, Hartitzsch B, Buselmeier TJ. The unphysiology of dialysis. A major cause of dialysis side effects?

Kidney Int 7 (Suppl 2): S30–S34, 1975.

70. Kerr DNS, Hoenich NA, Frost TH. Progress in hemodialysis 1974/75. Adv Nephrol 6: 415–452, 1976.

71. Ellis M, Gartiver JC, Galvis AG. Acute renal failure in infants and children, diagnosis, complications and treatment. Critical Care Medicine 9: 607–617, 1981.

72. Congea JD. A controlled evaluation of prophylactic dialysis in post traumatic acute renal failure. J Trauma 15: 1056–1070, 1975.

73. Kleinknecht D, Jungers P, Chanard DJ, Barbanel C, Ganeval D. Factors influencing immediate prognosis in acute renal failure, with special emphasis to prophylactic hemodialysis. Kidney Int 1: 190–196, 1977.

74. Lee HA. The management of acute renal failure. In Acute Renal Failure, Chapman A (ed). Edinburgh: Churchill Livingstone, 1980, pp. 104–124.

75. Wideroe TE. Some special considerations in treating acute renal failure with dialysis, clinical and mathematical evaluations. Scan J Urol Nephrol (Suppl) 57: 43–50, 1981.

76. Parsons V, Wilkinson SP, Weston MJ. Use of dialysis in treatment of renal failure of liver disease. Postgrad Med J 51: 515–521, 1975.

77. Rackow EC, Fein IA. Fulminant non cardiogenic pulmonary edema in the critically ill. Critical Care Medicine 6: 360–363, 1978.

78. Schuster HP, Schuster CJ, Gilfrich HJ, Scholmerich P. Transthoracic electrical impedance during extracorporeal hemodialysis in acute respiratory failure. Intensive Care Medicine 6: 147–154, 1980.

79. Dominguez E, Mosquera JM, Rubio JJ, Galdus P; Balda VD, Serna JL, Tomas MI. Association of a low serum albumim with infection and increased mortality in critically ill patients. Intensive Care Medicine 7: 19–22, 1980.

80. Bradley JA, Cunningham KJ, Jackson VJ, Hamilton DNH, Ledingham I McA. Serum protein levels in critically ill surgical patients. Intensive Care Medicine 7: 291–296, 1981.

81. Silk DBA, Williams R. Sorbents in hepatic failure. In Sorbents and Their Clinical Application, Giordano C (ed). New York: Academic Press, 1980, pp. 415–450.

82. Rosenbaum JL. Poisonings. In Sorbents and Their Clinical Application, Giordano C (ed). New York: Academic Press, 1980, pp. 451–467.

83. Wickerts CJ, Asaba H, Gunnarsson, Bygdeman S, Bergstrom J. Combined carbon hemoperfusion and hemodialysis in treatment of penicillin intoxication. Brit Med J 280: 1239–1286, 1980.

84. Dettli L. Drug dosage in renal disease. Clin Pharmacokinetics 1: 126–134, 1976.

85. Lawson DH. Drug therapy in acute renal failure. In Acute Renal Failure, Chapman A (ed), Edinburgh: Churchill Livingston, 1980, pp. 125–148.

86. Bennett WM (ed). Drugs and Renal Disease. New York: Churchill Livingstone, 1978.

87. Inturrisi CE, Viederman M, Rusk GH, Lowenthal

DT, White RP, Friedman EA, Boris A, David DS, Shahidi NT, Stenzel KH. Combined seminar on the use of drugs in renal failure. Am J Med 62: 527–554, 1977.

88. Maher JF. Principles of dialysis and dialysis of drugs. Am J Med 62: 475–481, 1977.
89. Cheigh JS. Drug administration in renal failure. Am J Med, 62: 555–563, 1977.
90. Civetta J. Selection of patients for intensive care. In Recent Advances in Intensive Therapy. Ledingham I McA (ed). Edinburgh: Churchill Livingstone, 1977, pp. 9–18.
91. Routh GS, Briggs JD, Mone JG, Ledingham I McA. Survival from acute renal failure with and without multiple organ dysfunction. Postgrad Med J 56: 244–247, 1980.
92. Moyer E, Cerra AF, Chenier R, Peters D, Oswald G, Watson F, Yu L, Mc Menamy RH, Border JR. Multiple systems organ failure. VI Death predictors in the trauma septic state. The most critical determinants. J Trauma 81: 862–869, 1981.
93. Abel RM, Buckley MJ, Austen WG. Etiology, incidence and prognosis of renal failure following cardiac operations: Results of a prospective analysis of 500 consecutive patients. J Thorac Cardiovasc Surg 71: 323–353, 1976.
94. Abbott NM, Abel RM, Beck CH, Fischer JE. Renal failure after ruptured aneurysm. Arch Surg 110: 1110–1115, 1975.
95. Chawla SK, Najafi H, Ing TS, Dye WS, Javid H, Hunter JA, Goldin MD, Serry C. Acute renal failure complicating ruptured abdominal aortic aneurysm. Arch Surg 110: 521–528, 1975.
96. Sapir DG, Dandy WE, Whelton A, Cooke CR. Acute renal failure following ruptured abdominal aneurysm: An improved clinical prognosis. Critical Care Medicine 7: 59–62, 1979.
97. NG RCH Suki WN. Treatment of acute renal failure. In Acute Renal Failure, Brenner BM, Stein JH (eds). Edinburgh: Churchill Livingstone, 1980, pp. 229–273.
98. Barsoum RS, Zakareya REB, Baligh O, Hozayen A, Elghoneimi EG, Ramzy MF, Ibrahuim AS. Acute renal failure in the 1973 Middle East War: Experience of a specialized case hospital. Effect of the site of injury. J Trauma 20: 303–307, 1980.
99. Davies DM, Brown JM, Bennett JP, Rainford DJ, Pusey CD. Survival after major burn complicated by gas gangrene, acute renal failure and toxic myocarditis. Brit Med J 1: 718–719, 1979.
100. Davies DM, Pusey CD, Rainford DJ, Brown JM, Bennett JP. Acute renal failure in burns. Scand J Plast Reconstr Surg 13: 184–192, 1979.
101. Ledingham I McA, Mc Ardle CS, Mc Donald RC. Septic shock. In Recent Advances in Surgery, Taylor S (ed). Edinburgh: Churchill Livingstone, 1980, chapter IV.
102. Kestens PJ, Otte JB, Haot J, Reynaert M. Le traitment chirurgical de la pancreatite aigue necrotico-haemorragique. Acta Chiurgica Belgica 6 : 373–385, 1981.
103. Carlet J, Francoual M, Lhoste F, Regnier B, Lemaire F. Pharmacological treatment of pulmonary edema. Intensive Care Medicine 6: 113–122, 1980.
104. du Molin GC, Paterson DG, Hedley Whyte J, Lisbon A. Aspiration of gastric bacteria in antacid treated patients: A frequent cause of post operative colonization of the airway. Lancet 1: 242–245, 1982.
105. Andreucci VE, Dal Canton A. Can acute renal failure in humans be prevented? Proc EDTA 17: 123–136, 1980.

24. TREATMENT OF ACUTE RENAL FAILURE BY PERITONEAL DIALYSIS

Charles M Mion,

Jean-Jacques Béraud

1 Introduction

In 1959, Maxwell et al. [1] introduced a sim-plified technique of peritoneal dialysis using a single disposable peritoneal catheter, commer-cially produced sterile dialysis solutions, and disposable tubing sets. Peritoneal dialysis (PD) became practicable as a clinical routine, and its effectiveness for controlling abnormalities of acute uremia was soon confirmed on a large number of patients. However, a high incidence of peritonitis remained associated with this technique. Effective prevention of peritoneal infection was made possible by the develop-ment of a closed dialysate delivery circuit with an automated cycling machine by Boen in 1962 [2] and was later improved when Tenck-hoff introduced a bacteriologically safe perma-nent peritoneal access in 1968 [3]. These ad-vances were primarily intended for treatment of end-stage renal disease, as was the new mode of PD introduced by Popovich et al. in 1976 [4]. However, these remarkable technological and conceptual innovations have strongly influ-enced the technique and indications of PD in acute renal failure (ARF).

In this chapter, our goal will be to review the technical aspects of PD and also to analyze the advantages and shortcomings of this di-alysis method when it is utilized in patients with ARF.

We wish to express our most sincere thanks to Mrs. M. Elie for her secretarial assistance in the preparation of this manuscript.

V.E. Andreucci (ed.). ACUTE RENAL FAILURE.
All rights reserved. Copyright © 1984.
Martinus Nijhoff Publishing, Boston/The Hague/
Dordrecht/Lancaster.

2 Kinetics of Peritoneal Dialysis

Following the pioneering work of Boen [5], a considerable wealth of knowledge has been gathered on the physiology of the peritoneum and the kinetic of peritoneal transport [6, 7]. A brief overview of the main functional char-acteristics of PD is presented here to emphasize the factors that affect the removal of uremic toxins and/or fluid across the peritoneal mem-brane.

The peritoneal blood flow rate, the dialysate flow rate, and the mass transfer area coefficient are the three dominant parameters determining the peritoneal clearance of urea [6]. The mass transfer area coefficient is a measure of the max-imum possible dialysis clearances that would occur if the dialysate metabolite concentration level was maintained at zero at all times. The relative values of the blood and dialysate flow rates and the mass transfer area coefficient are the limiting factors of peritoneal clearance. At infinite blood and dialysate flow rates, the clearance value will equal the mass transfer area coefficient value and is therefore mass-transfer limited. If the dialysate flow rate is lower than the mass transfer area coefficient, the clearance will become dialysate-flow-rate limited. At lower dialysate flow rate, the clearance will equal the value of dialysate flow rate including ultrafiltration volume, as in continuous ambu-latory peritoneal dialysis (in the range of 5 to 8 ml per minute). The peritoneal clearance of urea increases to a value of 30 to 35 ml/min with increases in dialysate flow rate in the range of 70 to 80 ml/min; at higher dialysate flow rates, very small increments of urea clearance will be observed as mass transfer area coefficient becomes the limiting factor. Therefore, the optimum urea clearance to be expected in clinical PD equals at most one-fifth to one-sixth of the clearance of modern artificial kidneys. In practice, the limited efficiency of PD should always be kept in mind when using PD in the context of acute renal failure. Prolonging the duration of dialysis (i.e,, continuous dialysis) will often be necessary to control adequately uremic abnormalities [8].

The factors affecting the efficiency of PD are listed in table 24–1. Changes in membrane permeability may be permanent, such as reduced effectiveness induced by anatomical factors (e.g., peritoneal adhesions, vascular disease of the splanchnic arterial bed). They may also

TABLE 24–1. Factors affecting the effectiveness of peritoneal dialysis

I. Diffusion
  A. Increasing with
      higher dialysate flow rate (up to 80 ml/min)
      larger dialysate volume per exchange
      ultrafiltration rate
      increased dialysate temperature
      peritonitis (increased permeability of the
        peritoneal membrane)
      use of various drugs (intraperitoneal and/or
        systemic)
  B. Decreasing with
      lower dialysate flow rate
      alterations in permeability of the peritoneal
        membrane (e.g., vascular disease,
        peritoneal sclerosis)
      patients with acute renal failure secondary to
        heat stroke, hemolysis
      low dialysate temperature
      severe hypotension, shock (decreased
        splanchnic blood flow)
      loss of peritoneal surface area (e.g., adhesions
        with loculations of dialysis fluid, extended
        resection of bowel and mesenterium)
      ileus
II. Convection
  A. Increasing with
      osmolality of dialysis solution
      optimal dwell time
  B. Decreasing with
      peritonitis (higher permeability to small
        solutes)
      reduced surface area (adhesions)
      loculation of dialysis fluid
      serum hyperglycemia
      too long a dwell time

be transient as the increase in the permeability of the peritoneum induced by peritoneal inflammation, which improves peritoneal clearances, reduces the capacity of the peritoneum to ultrafiltrate and increases protein losses [9].

Ultrafiltration in PD is accomplished by creating a gradient of osmotic pressure between dialysis solutions and blood [10]. Dialysate is rendered hyperosmolar by its high glucose content (15 g/l to 42.5 g/l; 83 mmol/1 to 233 mmol/1). Dialysate hyperosmolality is the driving force for the transport of water from blood to the peritoneal cavity. This process is self-limited, as glucose concentration in dialysate decreases exponentially with time. The dissipation of the osmotic gradient is explained (a) by the addition of plasma water to dialysis fluid and (b) by the rapid loss of glucose passing into the blood stream. Convective transport has a small but definite influence on urea removal.

The permeability characteristics of the peritoneal membrane also allow the transfer of large molecular species. Proteins, including albumin, transferrin, and immunoglobulin have all been found in the peritoneal fluid following various diffusion times [11]. The resulting protein loss is usually moderate (6 to 15 g/day according to the dialysis schedule), but it may increase to a high level in peritonitis and contributes significantly to the negative nitrogen balance observed in this setting.

In infants and small children, the peritoneal surface area in relation to body weight is greater than in the adults, and PD is more efficient in this group of patients [12].

3   *Technical Aspects of Peritoneal Dialysis*

In this section, an overview of the various techniques of PD will be presented. The reader looking for more detailed information concerning the realization of a dialysis session should refer to the selected references where catheter placement and connect-disconnect procedures, preparation of the dialysate delivery circuit, and automated equipments are described in detail [13–15].

3.1 PERITONEAL CATHETERS

PD requires the creation of a peritoneal access to the peritoneal cavity, which will permit the instillation and drainage of dialysate through repeated cycles.

3.1.1 Catheters Two main types of peritoneal catheters are available; the rigid disposable plastic catheters [16] and soft indwelling silastic catheters [3]. Both types of catheters have an intraperitoneal segment with multiple small holes in the distal 7.5 cm. They are supplied in two sizes, one for adult, the other for children and infants. The rigid nylon catheter intended for acute use only is disposable and should be removed after each dialysis session. The "acute" indwelling catheter developed by Tenckhoff [17] incorporates a dacron felt cuff on its subcutaneous portion: tissue ingrowth into the dacron anchors the tube more firmly in position and minimizes the likelihood of bacterial ingress through the sinus tract around the tubing.

3.1.2 Disposable Versus Indwelling Catheter In our opinion, indwelling silastic catheters should always be preferred except in the following circumstances: (a) acute emergencies (e.g., hyperkalemia, pulmonary edema) where inserting a catheter at the bedside with a stylet method may be life saving; (b) cases of ARF where only one dialysis lasting at most 48 hours is planned; (c) waiting procedure prior to the placement of an indwelling catheter; and (d) in cases of failure to drain with a Tenckhoff catheter due to one-way obstruction. Despite slightly more complex implantation procedures, indwelling silastic catheters offer many advantages: better irrigation characteristics (shorter infusion and drainage times); less abdominal discomfort; possibility to mobilize the patient during dialysis and also to dialyze in the sitting position or ambulatory; easy initiation and discontinuation of PD by nursing personnel, facilitating frequent dialysis; and single permanent peritoneal access in case of protracted anuria.

3.1.3 Catheter Placement Peritoneal catheters can be implanted using a stylet [16], using a trocar [3, 17], or with a surgical technique under local anesthesia. In our unit, the latter is mastered by trained nephrologists and is almost exclusively used, as it permits catheter place-

ment under direct vision control, so eliminating the hazards of blind catheter insertion, particularly bowel perforation or mesenteric vessel wall erosion [18]. Without going into details of placement procedures, we stress here the main rules to be adhered to for a safe implantation. Even in an emergency, adequate psychological (in conscious subjects) and physical preparation is mandatory. To obtain the patient's cooperation during catheter placement, the operator, after a careful physical examination of the abdomen, should give the patient a detailed description of the procedure prior to operation; explanation should be reiterated step by step during implantation. The bladder should be empty, either by asking the patient to void or by urethral catherization. Prevention of infection should be a major concern. The abdomen will be carefully shaved from xyphoid to symphysis; the surgical field, disinfected with povidone iodine widely applied on the abdominal wall with particular attention to the umbilicus, will be carefully draped. The rules of surgical asepsy should be strictly respected by the operator and all bystanders, whether the placement is done at the bedside or in the operating room. Whenever a blind technique is used (stylet or trocar), it is safer to instill two liters of dialysis fluid in the abdomen, either prior to operation using a standard 18-gauge needle or at the time of operation by burying the perforated part of the catheter into the peritoneal cavity. Sites for implantation are the midline of the abdominal wall, 3 to 4 cm below the umbilicus, or either fossa iliaca. For stylet or trocar insertion, a narrow skin incision will ensure postoperative tightness as the surrounding tissues will fit snugly around the catheter. With a surgical technique, a midline incision 4 to 6 cm long will permit an easy dissection down to the peritoneum. During placement, the greatest attention should be given to several steps. Avoiding catheter entanglement in the omentum is essential. When inserted blindly, the catheter should never be pushed in against a resistance; if this happens, the catheter should be withdrawn and insertion attempted at a different angle. When a surgical technique is used, it is easier to pull up the omentum with the index finger or a smooth forceps toward the epigastric fossa to remove it from the lower abdominal cavity. When the catheter is introduced into the peritoneal cavity, the operator should make sure that the metallic stylet or obturator used to stiffen the catheter has its extremity sheathed inside the catheter lumen, to prevent accidental erosion of the peritoneum and/or a mesenteric blood vessel. Before closing the peritoneum, the catheter should be checked for ease of irrigation if adequate return of the infused fluid is not obtained. At the end of the procedure, the peritoneal cavity should be tightly closed around the catheter to prevent postoperative leaks.

In a patient requiring abdominal surgery in whom there is a high probability of acute tubular necrosis (ATN), it is simpler to have the catheter placed at the time of operative closure for use in the immediate postoperative period.

3.1.4 Postimplantation Care After catheter placement, the skin exit site should be protected with a closed dressing made with 10 x 10 cm square gauzes, cut to fit around the tubing. PD should be started as soon as possible using heparinized dialysis fluid. During the first 48 hours, small volumes of dialysate (about 1 l per exchange) should be used to minimize the likelihood of dialysate leakage.

3.2 PERITONEAL DIALYSIS SOLUTIONS

3.2.1 Composition Irrigation of the peritoneal cavity requires sterile apyrogenic solutions, either commercially produced and ready mixed, or prepared at the bedside by proportionate mixing of a concentrate with reverse-osmosis-treated water [19]. To prevent the rapid absorption of dialysate in the vascular compartment and to permit fluid removal, all dialysis solutions are made hypertonic with the addition of glucose. Table 24–2 shows the composition of standard dialysis solutions available on the market. Over the years, guidelines have been proposed to standardize the formulae [20], and commercially produced dialysates have very similar electrolyte content. The three main formulae are characterized by increasing osmolality with the glucose concentrations of 82.5, 137.5, and 233 mmol/l (1.5, 2.5 and 4.25 g/dl), respectively. Calcium and magne-

TABLE 24–2. Composition of the most commonly prescribed peritoneal dialysis solutions

Solution	Compositions available		
Glucose (mmol/l)	83	137	233
Sodium (mmol/l)[a]	135	135	135
Chloride (mmol/l)	105	105	105
Lactate (mmol/l)[b]	35	35	35
Calcium (mmol/l)	1.75	1.75	1.75
Magnesium (mmol/l)	0.75	0.75	0.75
Potassium (mmol/l)[c]	0	0	0
Total osmolality (mOsm/kg)	359.5	414.5	510

[a]Sodium concentrations of 130, 132, 137, and 140 mmol/l are also available.
[b]Acetate is used instead of lactate by certain pharmaceutical companies.
[c]Some formulae include potassium chloride at a concentration of 2 mmol/l.

sium levels of 1.75 and 0.75 mmol/l, respectively, are standard, although a lower magnesium concentration seems commendable to obtain a better control of hypermagnesemia. Potassium-free dialysate is administered in most patients with ATN as potassium removal is slow in PD. However, potassium should be added to prevent myocardial irritability and potentially lethal arrhythmias that could be induced by sudden serum potassium changes in digitalized patients or in malnourished subjects dialyzed continuously for several days. Bicarbonate cannot be included in preparations containing calcium and magnesium. Lactate and/or acetate in a concentration of 35 mmol/l are used instead as a source of bicarbonate: a slightly higher concentration (38 to 40 mmol/l) would permit a more complete correction of metabolic acidosis.

There are two concentrate solutions for use with reverse osmosis machines: a glucose and electrolyte concentrate used for preparing diluted dialysate with 82.5 mmol/l (1.5 g/dl) and 135 mmol/l sodium; a pure glucose concentrate containing 2.75 mol/l (50 g/dl) glucose, used for adjusting the dextrose content of the final dialysate, according to the patient's needs.

3.2.2 Conditioning Today, most dialysis solutions are available in two- to three-liter plastic bags and in ten-liter plastic containers. Plastic bags and containers offer many practical advantages by comparison with the classic one- to two-liter glass bottles. However, it is impossible to guarantee the absolute sterility of their content at the time of use, particularly when they are made of thick translucent plastic material. To obviate the risk of peritoneal infection from a dialysis fluid contaminated during storage, we routinely use an 0.22 μm pore bacteriological filter (Twin 90, Millipore, Bedford, Ma.) placed in the dialysate infusion line [21].

3.2.3 Additives Addition of various drugs to the dialysate is indicated in various circumstances. Heparin (100 to 1,000 I.U./l), prescribed after catheter implantation to prevent plugging of the catheter lumen by clots in case of postoperative bleeding, is also considered as a useful adjunct in the treatment of peritonitis. Systemic blood coagulation was not affected by 1,000 I.U. doses of intraperitoneal heparin [22].

Addition of antibiotics to dialysis solution is an important aspect of the treatment of peritoneal infection. Penicillin G, methicillin, ampicillin, cephalothin, nafcillin, carbenicillin, vancomycin, kanamycin, tobramycin, gentamycin, 5-fluorocytosin, and amphothericin B have all been used in various protocols. However, few studies have demonstrated that these antibiotics retain their full activity with time once added to the dialysate. In one study, the deactivation of kanamycin added to fresh ready-mixed dialysis solutions amounted to 30% of initial dosage at 24 hours [23]. Similar effects were observed in another study when antibiotics were added to commercially produced concentrates: after 24 hours gentamicin retained 80% of its activity, nafcillin 70% activity, cephalothin and penicillin G less than 50% activity [24].

When prescribing several additives in the same solution, the physician should be aware of the possible interference between drugs. For instance, heparin has been shown to have adverse effects on gentamicin activity in blood [25]. However, if the final concentration of heparin and gentamicin in the dialysate is kept at 1 I.U./ml and 10 μg/ml, respectively, the activity of both drugs will be preserved [26]. No

significant deactivation of tobramycin was observed after 48 hours in dialysate containing 10 μg/ml tobramycin and 1 to 2 I.U./ml of heparin [27].

Insulin addition to dialysate has been shown to effectively control hyperglycemia and to obtain excellent control of blood sugar in diabetic patients [28].

Various vasoactive substances have also been added to dialysate in order to modify mass transfer rates across the peritoneal membrane, but the clinical implications of these investigations have not yet been fully elucidated [29, 30].

3.3 IRRIGATION OF THE PERITONEAL CAVITY

3.3.1 Manual Techniques The use of a straight polyvinyl chloride tubing to connect the peritoneal catheter to the dialysate bag from both infusion and drainage, as originally described by Maxwell et al. [1], remains the simplest technique for irrigation of the peritoneal cavity. However, to obtain adequate dialysate flow rates, fresh dialysis solution has to be exchanged at frequent intervals (once or twice an hour). These time-consuming procedures expose the peritoneal cavity to a high risk of bacterial contamination due to the repeated openings of the dialysate delivery circuit.

3.3.2 Automatic Cyclers Several models of automated equipments have been designed for the delivery of dialysis solutions with a closed circuit. They derive from the original concept of Boen [2], and they utilize commercial ready-mixed solutions. Several 2-1 bags or 10-1 containers are assembled in series or in parallel to form a single reservoir, with a total volume of dialysate proportional to the planned duration of dialysis to the expected dialysate flow. Automatic cyclers consist of three electric clocks activating two electric clamps controlling the succession of unlimited number of PD cycles, each cycle comprising three periods, one for infusion, one for diffusion (dwell time), and one for drainage of the dialysis fluid. The delivery circuit, including interconnecting tubings for peritoneal irrigation and drainage, is available in disposable sets specially designed for a given equipment.

3.3.3 Reverse Osmosis Machines

These PD systems use reverse osmosis to produce sterile apyrogenic water from tap water. Dialysis solutions are prepared by a proportioning pump that mixes one volume of glucose electrolyte concentrate to 19 volumes of reverse osmosis treated water; to the mixture, a variable amount of dextrose concentrate is added to modulate the glucose concentration of the final dialysate according to the patient's needs [19]. The safety of this system depends on the perfect quality of the reverse osmosis modules that should be disinfected with 3% formalin after each use and that should be tested every three months for intactness of the membranes. The use of reverse osmosis machines in the intensive care unit necessitates well trained personnel, precisely defined protocols for sterilization and rinsing procedures, and a closely controlled maintenance program to prevent the risk of bacterial contamination of the equipment [31].

3.3.4 Dialysis Schedules

Peritoneal dialysis may be administered according to a wide spectrum of schedules [32]. In practice, the two main modes are periodic PD (improperly termed *intermittent peritoneal dialysis*) and continuous equilibration [33] or low-flow PD [34], both deriving from the concept of continuous ambulatory peritoneal dialysis (CAPD) used in patients with end-stage renal disease [6]. In periodic PD, dialysate flow rate is kept in the high range (between two and six liters per hour) with a dwell time of 2 to 30 minutes. The dialysis session may last 12 hours or be continued without interruption during several consecutive days. The interval between the sessions and the duration of each dialysis are determined according to the patient's catabolic state and the peritoneal urea clearance [5, 6, 8].

In continuous equilibration PD [33, 34], the dwell time is prolonged up to three or six hours (four to eight exchanges per day). In this setting, the peritoneal clearance of urea equals the volume of drained peritoneal fluid (i.e., infused dialysate volume plus ultrafiltration volume).

The volume of dialysate infused at each exchange is standardized at two liters in adults and at 50 ml per kg body weight in infants. The dialysate infusion volume should be reduced soon after catheter implantation, after recent abdominal surgery, and in patients with acute or chronic respiratory insufficiency.

The choice of dialysis solutions will be decided on by considering the type and severity of water and electrolyte imbalances observed in the individual patient. This choice should be adapted daily in case of long-lasting dialysis sessions to prevent the occurrence of hypernatremia or extracellular volume depletion. Dialysis fluid with high-dextrose concentration may also be required to maintain fluid balance in patients receiving large daily volumes of intravenous fluid for parenteral nutrition. Table 24–3 presents rough estimates of ultrafiltration rates that can be expected as a function of dialysate osmolality and duration of dwell times. However, as the capacity of the peritoneum to

TABLE 24–3. Approximate ultrafiltration rates obtained with intermittent (periodic) peritoneal dialysis (IPD) and continuous equilibration peritoneal dialysis (CEPD) using three dialysate formulae and various dwell times

PD technique	Duration of dwell time (minutes)	Dialysate glucose concentration mmol/l (g/dl)		
		83 (1.5)	137 (2.5)	233 (4.25)
IPD[a]	20	300–1000	3000–4000	6000–7000
CEPD[b]	180	200–400	300–500	600–1000
	340	100–300	200–400	600–800

[a] Fluid removal per 24 hours: compiled from [35] and from our personal experience (unpublished data).
[b] Fluid removal per two-liter exchanges: compiled from [36] and [37].

ultrafiltrate varies greatly between patients, the effect of dialysate composition on ultrafiltration rates should be carefully monitored in each patient.

3.3.5 Monitoring In patients with ARF, peritoneal dialysis is in most cases only one aspect of a complex therapeutic approach, including respiratory care, parenteral nutrition, and/or postoperative care. Peritoneal dialysis procedures should be mastered by the nursing personnel of the intensive care units. Nursing protocols should be established with three major aims: (a) prevention and early detection of peritoneal infection; (b) maintenance of an adequate fluid and electroylte balance; and (c) prevention of severe hyperglycemia.

Strict adhesion to sterile procedures by physicians and nursing staff is a must during catheter implantation and whenever manipulations of the dialysate delivery circuit are required. The higher risk of contamination is at the time of bottle or bag exchange of fresh dialysate, particularly when a manual technique and a rewarming bath are used. The drained peritoneal fluid should be checked at frequent intervals to detect without delay the appearance of a cloudy dialysate heralding a peritonitis episode.

Meticulous recording of fluid intake and output is essential. Errors in cumulative fluid balance may occur as a consequence of underestimated leaks around the peritoneal catheter or through peritoneal drains, but also because the dialysate content of commercial containers is often larger than indicated on the label [38]. The physician's prescription should include predetermined levels of positive or negative balances, beyond which the physician should be notified.

In the diabetic patient or in patients in whom the protracted use of high-dextrose-content dialysate is deemed necessary, blood glucose levels should be monitored every three to four hours. Regular insulin should be added to the dialysate or given subcutaneously to maintain blood glucose in a safe range (i.e., below 16.5 mmol/l or 300 mg/dl). Insulin should be witheld four hours before discontin-

uing dialysis to prevent severe postdialysis hypoglycemia.

3.4 HAZARDS AND COMPLICATIONS OF PERITONEAL DIALYSIS
The hazards and complications of PD have been thoroughly reviewed in recent years [39, 40] and are listed in table 24–4. In the following section, we discuss in detail only those problems that are frequently encountered in the context of acute renal failure.

3.4.1 Complications Related to Catheter Placement and Function Most of the complications related to catheter placement can be prevented by careful preparation of the patient and use of a meticulous surgical technique [18].

Bleeding mostly comes from the abdominal wall. The peritoneal fluid, initially pink or grossly bloody during the first exchanges, has a tendency to clear spontaneously. A colorimetric estimation of the degree of bleeding with time is obtained by saving aliquots of drainage fluid every two hours. Attempts to stop persisting bleeding include the following: (a) injection of sterile saline around the plastic catheter to create a high tissue pressure acting as an internal tourniquet; (b) placement of a deep purse string around the catheter; and (c) discontinuation of heparin addition to the dialysis fluid. The latter may result in catheter plugging by clots. Catheter disobstruction may be obtained by the introduction of streptokinase or urokinase (2 500 000 I.U./l) in the catheter lumen.

One way obstruction, the most frequent mode of catheter dysfunction, may be due to organic causes: catheter entanglement in the peritoneum; catheter encasement by surrounding tissues (particularly in case of peritonitis); internal obstruction due to suction of peritoneal fringes into the catheter lumen when wall perforations are too large; dislodgement of the intraperitoneal segment of a silastic catheter from the pelvis gutter. However, catheter failure to drain is most commonly functional and in some way related to bowel function [13]. Bowel stimulation by a suppository or a small enema will often re-establish a satisfactory catheter

TABLE 24–4. Hazards and complications of peritoneal dialysis

I. Related to peritoneal catheter
    Bleeding (intraperitoneal; parietal)
    Dialysate leakage around catheter
    Hollow viscus perforation (bowel, bladder)
    Preperitoneal placement
    Catheter dysfunction:
      two-way obstruction
      one-way obstruction (failure to drain)
    Skin exit infection
    Accidental catheter removal (unconscious agitated patients)
    Dissection of dialysate into the subcutaneous tissue
II. Pain
    Localized
      Permanent or at the end of drainage: pressure of the catheter tip on the peritoneum
      During infusion:
        hypertonic and/or low pH dialysate
        incarceration of tissue inside holes of the catheter
    Diffuse
      During infusion only: high dialysate flow rate and pulsatile flow from roller pump
      At the end of infusion: distention of abdominal cavity from excessive dialysate volume
      Permanent (with rebound tenderness): peritonitis
III. Related to irrigation of the peritoneal cavity
    Peritonitis
      Infectious peritonitis
      Aseptic peritonitis: "chemical peritonitis"; endotoxin containing dialysate
    Pleuropulmonary complications
      Basal atelectasia
      Pneumonia
      Bilateral pleural effusion
      Massive hydrothorax
      Hypoventilation and hypoxemia
    Cardiovascular complications
      Reflex bradycardia
      Arrhythmias
      Hypotension and shock
    Metabolic consequences
      Extracellular volume depletion or excess
      Water deficit (hypernatremia)
      Hypokalemia
      Hyperkalemia (hypercatabolic patients)
      Metabolic alkalosis
      Persisting lactic acidosis in liver-failure patients dialyzed with lactate containing dialysis solutions
      Hyperglycemia
      Protein losses

flow and should always be tried first in order to avoid unnecessary catheter procedures.

3.4.2 Abdominal Pain Pain is more commonly observed with rigid plastic catheters. Persisting localized pelvic pain or intermittent pain occurring when drainage is completed results from pressure of the catheter tip on posterior parietal, rectum, or bladder peritoneum and is promptly relieved by withdrawing the catheter one or two centimeters.

Diffuse abdominal pain occurring at the end of infusion is often associated with respiratory embarrassment. It results from too large a volume of infused dialysate or from the accumulation of fluid in the peritoneal cavity due to incomplete drainage during several successive dialysis cycles. It requires complete evacuation of the peritoneal fluid by prolonged drainage and subsequent adjustment of the volume of infused dialysate and of the duration of drainage time.

When dialysis lasts more than 24 to 36 hours, diffuse permanent abdominal pain, rectus muscle pain at the costal margin, and shoulder pain referred from the diaphragm are frequently present. They do not indicate bacterial peritonitis and vanish in a few hours after dialysis discontinuation.

3.4.3 Peritoneal Infection Bacterial peritonitis remains the most feared complication of peritoneal dialysis. Exogenous contamination of the peritoneum occurs through the catheter lumen or across the abdominal wall through the sinus tract around the catheter. Contaminated dialysis solutions at time of dialysate exchange (particularly when a rewarming bath is used), negligent connect-disconnect procedures, or accidental opening of the dialysate circuit are the main causes of exogenous peritoneal infection. This may also occur from a defective reverse osmosis module when a reverse osmosis machine is used. Endogenous contamination resulting in secondary bacterial peritonitis [41] is due to acute visceral diseases such as appendicitis, cholecystitis, diverticulitis of the colon, or perforation of the bowel.

The diagnostic criteria of peritonitis are both clinical and bacteriological including at least two of the following: (a) symptoms and signs of peritonism; (b) cloudy dialysate effluent; (c) positive cultures of the peritoneal fluid. A cloudy effluent is a constant finding. Diffuse abdominal pain, rebound tenderness, and fever are observed in more than 50% of the cases. Nausea, vomiting, ileus, or diarrhea are less frequent (10 to 30% of the cases).

Peritoneal fluid cultures are the cornerstone of the diagnosis. An adequate methodology should be used to obtain a high percentage of positive cultures [42]. Peritoneal fluid specimens should be transferred without delay to the microbiology laboratory. Appropriate media should be used for aerobic, anaerobic and fungal cultures. Cultures should be kept in the oven for at least one week (aerobic organisms) or two weeks (anaerobic organisms) to allow time for growth of fastidious organisms.

Gram staining of the peritoneal fluid is a useful diagnostic tool when peritonitis is suspected: organisms seen on direct examination in 30 to 40% of smears give a useful clue as to the choice of the initial antibiotic before the results of cultures become available.

Cell numeration in the peritoneal fluid adds little to the diagnosis since an increase in the number of cells is detectable by the naked eye beyond 50 cells per mm^3. A differential cell count showing more than 50% polymorphonuclear and its return to a normal pattern is useful for monitoring the effectiveness of antibiotic therapy.

The most common infectious agents are Gram-positive cocci (i.e. Staphylococcus epidermidis, Staph. aureus, Streptococcus viridans, Enterococcus) and Gram-negative bacteria (i.e., Enterobacteriaceae, Pseudomonas sp., Acinetobacter sp.). Yeasts (Candida sp.), fungi, and anaerobic species are less frequently encountered. The simultaneous identification of several organisms in the same culture (particularly Gram-negative bacteria together with yeasts and/or anaerobic bacteria) is highly suggestive of fecal leakage from the bowel.

To maintain a low incidence of peritoneal infection in patients receiving PD in the intensive care unit, an active prevention program should be established with the nursing staff. Precise protocols should be designed concerning catheter care, connect-disconnect procedures, and preparation of automated equipments. With manual techniques, plastic bags should be preferred and rewarming baths abandoned. A closed-dialysate-delivery circuit should be used whenever possible. The use of inline bacteriological filter on the dialysate infusion line [21, 43] will further reduce the potential risk of peritoneal contamination from infected dialysis fluids. Routine disinfection of reverse osmosis machines with 2 to 4% formalin after each use and frequent checks on membrane integrity are mandatory with this type of equipment [31]. Finally, as the incidence of peritonitis rises with the duration of dialysis (at least with manual techniques), limiting each dialysis session to less than 72 hours is another useful preventive measure [44]. Antibiotic prophylaxis showed no benefit in several studies and adds a potential risk of selecting antibiotic-resistant strains and of facilitating Candida peritonitis.

The management of peritoneal infection includes both intraperitoneal and systemic antibiotic treatment [42]. Peritoneal lavage removing fibrin and cellular debris is instituted after completion of diagnostic procedures. Heparin should be added to the dialysate at a concentration of 500 I.U./1. Continuation of peritoneal lavage has been proposed until negative cultures have been obtained on three consecutive days. The usefulness of this procedure has recently been questioned [45].

Antibiotics are prescribed intraperitoneally, systemically, or by both routes. Addition of antibiotics to the dialysate according to conventional dosages, shown in table 24–5, maintains bactericidal concentration inside the peritoneal cavity. Most antibiotics diffuse readily across the peritoneal membrane and can attain bactericidal serum levels provided their dialysate concentration is adequate. An initial loading dose given intravenously or intramuscularly is recommended to obtain without delay an effective serum concentration. There is a risk of antibiotic accumulation in the serum when intraperitoneal antibiotics are used for several consecutive days. Serial serum concentrations measured at daily intervals are of particular importance to prevent aminoglycoside ototoxicity.

TABLE 24–5. Recommended antibiotic concentrations to be added to dialysis solutions for the treatment of bacterial peritonitis

Antibiotic generic name	Recommended intraperitoneal dose (mg/l)
Penicillin G	50 000 Unit/l
Cloxacillin	100
Ampicillin	50
Cephalothin*	250
Cefuroxime*	50
Carbenicillin	200
Tobramycin*	8
Gentamicin*	8
Kanamycin	150
Amikacin	50
Vancomycin*	30
5-Fluorocytosine	50
Amphotericin B	2–4

*An initial loading dose is recommended to reach serum bactericidal concentration. This dose can be given parenterally or intraperitoneally.

A practical antibiotic regimen includes the addition of 200 mg cephalothin per liter dialysate as initial therapy. If Gram stains and/or cultures show the presence of Gram-negative bacteria in the peritoneal effluent, tobramycin (8 mg/l dialysate) should be added too. Such an antibiotic association has a broad activity spectrum and is effective against most bacteria [42]. Kanamycin [23] or trimethoprim sulfamethoxazole [46] have also be proposed as the initial antibiotic, but this choice should be revised later according to the in vitro sensitivity testing of isolated organisms. In case of staphylococcal infection with a penicillin resistant strain, vancomycin has given excellent results [47].

Fungal peritonitis has been successfully managed with intraperitoneal 5-fluocytosine [48]. Cure has also been obtained with intraperitoneal and/or intravenous amphotericin B [49]. However, catheter removal and discontinuation of PD has also been recommended as a safer therapeutic approach to fungal peritonitis [50].

The resolution of peritonitis should occur promptly. If peritoneal fluid cultures remain positive after three to five days of adequate antibiotic treatment, infection of the sinus tract around the catheter or fecal leakage from the bowel should be suspected. This is an indication for catheter removal and/or abdominal surgery in search of a visceral lesion.

3.4.4 *Pleural and Pulmonary Complications*
Prolonged bed rest, inefficient cough with bronchiolar stasis of mucous secretions, and limitation of diaphragmatic excursion induced by the distension of the peritoneal cavity with dialysate may trigger pulmonary or pleural complications. Bacterial pneumonia with severe hypoxemia may result from latent basal atelectasia or from aspiration of gastric content, particularly in patients with hiatal hernias, and carries a significant mortality. The prevention of these ventilatory disorders necessitates stimulation of frequent coughing, deep breathing, and forced expiration.

More exceptional is the occurrence of acute massive hydrothorax, either spontaneously or in patients with a posttraumatic diaphragmatic rent. This complication, revealed by a severe dyspnea occurring during the first 24 hours of

PD, improves with the cessation of dialysis and may require thoracocentesis [51].

3.4.5 Cardiovascular Complications

Cardiovascular complications consist of reflex bradycardia at time of catheter implantation [52] with the stylet method and arrhythmias observed more commonly in digitalized patients who become hypokalemic during dialysis. The addition of 4 mmol/l potassium chloride to a potassium-free dialysate should maintain an adequate serum potassium level and minimize the likelihood of myocardial irritability.

3.4.6 Fluid and Electrolyte Disorders

Extracellular volume depletion leading to hypovolemia and hypotension may occur as a result of excessive ultrafiltration without compensatory sodium and water intake. Instances of extracellular volume excess have been ascribed to the dissection of dialysis fluid through operative incisions of the peritoneum (posterior or anterior) into the subcutaneous tissue and to its subsequent mobilization [38].

Hypernatremia with serum sodium concentration above 150 mmol/l may lead to obnubilation and hyperosmolar coma. This complication has been observed with the protracted use of hypertonic solutions providing a negative free-water balance. A water allowance equal to half the ultrafiltration volume has been suggested to prevent this disorder [53].

Severe hypokalemia is seldom observed except in patients unable to eat and receiving continuous peritoneal dialysis during several consecutive days. In these circumstances, the addition of potassium chloride (2 to 4 mmol/l) to the dialysate is mandatory.

Acid-base disorders are very unlikely to occur with the usual concentrations of lactate and acetate in dialysis solutions. Metabolic alkalosis has been ascribed to the use of dialysis fluid containing 42 to 45 mmol/l of lactate [38]. Rare instances of persisting metabolic acidosis have been reported in patients with severe liver failure dialyzed with lactate-containing dialysate [54].

3.4.7 Metabolic Complications

Hyperglycemia with blood glucose levels in the range of 10 to 15 mmol/l (180 to 260 mg/dl) is very common. Severe hyperglycemia leading to hyperosmolar nonketotic coma and convulsions may be fatal. It has been observed in patients treated with dialysate containing high dextrose concentration (233 mmol/l, 4.25 g/dl) used continuously for several hours. Alternating "isotonic" (83 mmol/l 1.5 g/dl glucose concentration) and "hypertonic" (233 mmol/l 4.25 g/dl glucose) dialysate formulae prevents this complication. Close monitoring of blood glucose level and a judicious use of insulin as described above (see section on monitoring) will prevent this potentially lethal complication.

Protein losses are obligatory during peritoneal dialysis due to the high permeability of the peritoneal membrane. The amount of protein lost per dialysis is influenced by the nature and type of peritoneal catheter, the duration of dwell time, the osmolality and temperature of dialysis solutions, and the duration of dialysis. It remains in the range of 6 to 12 g/24 hours in the absence of peritoneal infection [11]. Five to 15-fold increases in protein loss have been observed during peritonitis. These losses may induce a hypercatabolic state with negative nitrogen balance, leading ultimately to severe protein malnutrition. In this setting, the use of parenteral nutrition is mandatory to supply the patient with adequate amounts of proteins and calories [55].

4   Indications of Peritoneal Dialysis in Acute Renal Failure

In spite of remarkable improvements in hemodialysis techniques, including high-performance dialyzers and easier blood connections, peritoneal dialysis still remains an essential part of the therapeutic armamentarium in ARF. However, there is a wide range of opinions regarding its value, some clinicians considering peritoneal dialysis as the treatment of choice [56] and others, as a poor substitute of hemodialysis except in special circumstances [57].

4.1   PERITONEAL DIALYSIS VERSUS HEMODIALYSIS IN ACUTE RENAL FAILURE

By comparison with hemodialysis, PD admittedly offers some advantages, such as technical simplicity, safety due to the absence of the extracorporeal circuit, no bleeding risk, excellent cardiovascular tolerance, and lower risk of disequilibrium syndrome. PD has also recognized limitations with a lower effectiveness, the risk of peritoneal infection, the need for an intact peritoneal cavity offering the necessary tightness for intermittent dialysate flow, and an adequate membrane surface area, protein losses and restrictions to early mobilization of the patient.

In routine clinical practice, the preference for PD is often dictated by logistics or by the physician's biases and personal experience. However, ARF is a syndrome observed in patients of all ages, with a wide spectrum of etiological factors and various degrees of severity, depending on the presence or the absence of infection, gastrointestinal bleeding, and/or associated multiple organ involvement. It is our opinion, therefore, that PD and hemodialysis should be seen as complementary to each other. By having both dialysis methods available in the intensive care unit, the nephrologist may provide patients with the most suitable treatment at any given time. This view seems justified because most series comparing the outcome of patients with ARF treated either with hemodialysis or PD show no difference in the success rate with either technique [58]. However, this point should be accepted with caution and should be clarified best by prospective studies reevaluating the incidences of complications during hemodialysis or PD, as a recent study reported a high incidence or arrhythmia and cardiac arrest in peritoneal dialyzed patients with pre-existing heart disease, thus suggesting that PD may not be as safe for such patients as has been previously contended [59].

4.2 GENERAL INDICATIONS

Peritoneal dialysis may be utilized in all varieties of ARF. In obstructive ARF, it is the technique of choice to correct hyperkalemia or pulmonary edema in a patient requiring general anesthesia for urologic or surgical procedures. In cases of prerenal ARF associated with high blood urea levels, PD can be used to permit a faster control of uremia. However, PD finds its main indications in ATN. In adults, PD should be preferred in cases of ARF without hypercatabolism, in patients with bleeding

complications, or in those with predominant extracellular volume excess, hypervolemia, and cardiopulmonary overload. When there is a doubt as to the nature of the renal disease, PD remains the best approach since it allows a rapid correction of the main acid-base and fluid electrolyte disorders, prevents or corrects the bleeding tendency of uremia, and buys time to assess the patient's status and to decide whether to resort to hemodialysis or to continue with PD. Patients with severe cardiac disease or with a disease of the central nervous system will also fare better with PD. In small children, PD is more efficient than in the adult and is preferable in all forms of ARF [60].

4.3 SPECIAL INDICATIONS

4.3.1 Hypercatabolic Acute Renal Failure A hypercatabolic state, defined by a high urea apparition rate with a daily rise in blood urea levels greater than 10 mmol/l, is observed in ATN complicating accidental trauma, postoperative surgery, severe burns, and leptospirosis. In such cases, early institution of dialysis, maintenance of a high nitrogen and caloric intake during the period of illness, and continuation of periodic PD with adequate dialysate flow rates will permit keeping blood urea levels below 30 mmol/l [8]. If the control of uremia remains inadequate despite the abovementioned measures, hemodialysis should be instituted as soon as possible to meet the patient's dialysis needs.

4.3.2 Acute Renal Failure Following Cardiac Operations ARF is a frequent complication of operations utilizing cardiopulmonary bypass. When this complication is severe enough to require dialysis, it is said to be highly lethal [61]. Early institution of dialysis, as little as 24 hours after oliguria, has been recommended to improve the outcome. Although hemodialysis can eventually be conducted without major complications, in such cases the less vigorous peritoneal dialysis will give better results in patients with extremely unstable cardiovascular status [62]. Continuous equilibration peritoneal dialysis was highly successful in a recent series of ARF after open-heart surgery.

Serum urea and creatinine were stabilized at 25 mmol/l and 550 μmol/l, respectively, serum potassium was constant at 4.6 mmol/l, and extracellular volume was controlled satisfactorily with 2.3 liters ultrafiltration per day. Hemodynamic disturbances were avoided in all patients. Depression of respiratory function due to the upward displacement of the diaphragm did not occur [63].

4.3.3 Acute Renal Failure after Major Abdominal Surgery Several reports have confirmed that peritoneal dialysis is technically possible after major abdominal surgery (including abdominal aortic grafts) and that it can obtain satisfactory results [64]. However, the occurrence of specific complications might be expected, particularly when the posterior peritoneum has been opened or when abdominal drains or colostomy are in place. Dissection of dialysis fluid in the subcutaneous tissue of the retroperitoneal space can lead to scrotal edema and pulmonary edema later when the fluid is mobilized into the vascular space. Dialysate leakage around drains and enterostomies are almost unavoidable and results in grossly inaccurate fluid balance. Wound dehiscence from abdominal distention can occur if too large a volume of dialysate is infused with each exchange or if dialysis fluid accumulates due to incomplete drainage during several cycles. In our experience, this complication carries a significant mortality. These potential problems are often seen as strong arguments to recommend hemodialysis in such patients [65].

4.3.4 Secondary Bacterial Peritonitis Complicated with Acute Renal Failure An approach to the management of patients with secondary bacterial peritonitis complicated with ATN is to use PD to treat both peritoneal infection and ARF [41]. At the end of abdominal surgery and after careful peritoneal toilet, a silastic catheter is implanted and peritoneal irrigation is immediately initiated. Heparin and appropriate antibiotic should be added to dialysis solutions. However, this approach is a source of potential danger. The respiratory failure that often accompanies peritonitis may be aggravated, requiring mechanical respiratory assistance via an endotracheal tube during the period of lavage [41]. Peritoneal irrigation per se and the considerable protein loss observed in case of peritoneal inflammation may interfere with wound healing of enterostomies and anastomoses. Finally, a positive fluid balance may result from the decreased capacity of the peritoneum to ultrafiltrate during peritonitis [9].

4.3.5 Acute Renal Failure and Acute Pancreatitis In cases of ATN secondary to acute pancreatitis (see chapter 2), PD offers the potential advantage of washing clear the peritoneum of pancreatic enzymes (and so limiting autodigestion) while correcting uremic waste retention and fluid electrolyte imbalances. Monitoring of blood glucose is mandatory for the early detection of hyperglycemia and immediate institution of insulin therapy.

PD has also been proposed in the management of acute pancreatitis in patients with preserved renal function [66]. In most cases, peritoneal lavage resulted in a marked clinical improvement and a decreased mortality. A recent study of lipase and amylase peritoneal clearances suggests that both enzymes were removed by direct spilling into the dialysate from necrotic pancreatic and surrounding tissues rather than by passive diffusion from peritoneal capillaries to the dialysate [66].

4.3.6 Acute Uric Acid Nephropathy Hyperuricemia complicating acute leukemia may result in intratubular precipitation of uric acid, particularly when the tubular urine is concentrated and highly acid (see chapter 2). When renal failure has set in, only allopurinol and dialysis have resulted in consistent improvement. The use of peritoneal dialysis in several series has been accompanied by a prompt lowering of the serum uric acid concentration and remarkable recoveries [67, 68]. The peritoneal clearance of uric acid is in the range of 10 to 15 ml/min for a dialysate flow rate of 2 to 4 l/hour [5].

4.3.7 Acute Renal Failure after Renal Transplantation Patients with end-stage renal disease treated by maintenance PD may benefit from a renal transplant. With the advent of

CAPD, the number of patients receiving a renal graft while treated with peritoneal dialysis has increased in recent years. Early reports suggest that peritoneal dialysis can be safely resumed in the postoperative period in case of ATN, provided the peritoneal membrane is left intact after transplantation [69, 70]. The usual sterile procedures recommended for the prevention of peritoneal infection should be strictly reinforced for use of PD in such immunocompromised patients.

4.3.8 Acute Renal Failure Following Administration of Radiographic Contrast Material ARF has been reported with an increasing frequency following the administration of large doses of iodinated contrast material (see chapter 2). In these cases, early institution of peritoneal dialysis is recommended for preventing uremia and pulmonary edema and is also an effective method to remove the offending agent. In one study, the peritoneal clearance of iodide was 12 ml/min with two liters 60 min exchanges, and 56% of iodide was removed during 64 hours of intermittent peritoneal dialysis [71].

4.3.9 Acute Renal Failure Complicating Malaria ARF may cause death in falciparum malaria. Hemodialysis, though effective, is not commonly available in endemic malarial areas. PD is eminently suitable for hospitals in the tropics and has been successful in the treatment of ARF following malarial hemoglobinuria [72].

Studies of peritoneal solute clearances in these patients have shown that urea and creatinine clearance values were low during the early acute stage of illness and returned to normal by the time the second dialysis is done 48 hours later. It was suggested that this phenomenon might be explained by the known occurrence of intravascular coagulation deficits and sludging in malaria or by a reduction in splanchnic blood flow during the acute illness [72].

4.4 PERITONEAL DIALYSIS AND PARENTERAL NUTRITION IN ACUTE RENAL FAILURE
During peritoneal dialysis, glucose is readily absorbed; the amount transferred into the blood is related to dialysate blood flow rate and dialysate glucose concentration.

In periodic peritoneal dialysis, an average of 9.5 g and 38 g of glucose was absorbed each hour when dialysate containing 83 mmol/l (1.5 g/dl) and 233 mmol/l (4.25 g/dl), respectively, was used [73]. Thus, the daily glucose load will theoretically vary between 230 to 800 g during a 24 hour dialysis, depending on the amount of hypertonic solution prescribed.

In continuous-equilibration peritoneal dialysis, there is a close relationship between the amount of glucose absorbed each day and the concentration of glucose in the dialysate [74]. The net glucose uptake can be predicted from the concentration of glucose in the inflow using the following equation:

$$\frac{\text{Glucose absorbed}}{\text{Liter of dialysate}} \quad (24.1)$$
$$= 11.3 \text{ (average daily concentration in mg/dl)} - 10.9.$$

For instance, a patient with ATN receiving six exchanges per day with three two-liter exchanges of 1.5 g/dl (83 mmol/l) glucose and three two-liter exchanges of 4.25 g/dl (233 mmol/l) glucose will have an average daily glucose concentration of 3.0 g/dl (165 mmol/l). From equation (24.1), it is therefore possible to predict the amount of glucose absorbed from each liter of inflow as follows:

$$\text{glucose absorbed} = 11.3 \ (3) - 11$$
$$= 22.9 \text{ g/l dialysate inflow;}$$

giving a daily intake of:

$$22.9 \times 12 \text{ liter inflow} = 275 \text{ g/day.}$$

The quantity of glucose absorbed during dialysis is a valuable source of energy provided blood glucose levels are monitored during dialysis and insulin is added in case of hyperglycemia.

The administration of aminoacids through the peritoneal membrane has also been advocated to suppress aminoacid losses and to improve nitrogen balance during peritoneal dialysis [75]. A preliminary work has recently confirmed that the peritoneal cavity may be used safely as a simplified gut for total parenteral nutrition in patients with ARF [76]. This possibility deserves further evaluation.

5 Contraindications

It has been commonly held that there are no absolute contraindications for peritoneal dialysis. Although such a statement might still hold true today in centers where peritoneal dialysis is the only available dialytic method, there are circumstances where hemodialysis (or hemofiltration) should be preferred.

Patients with severe chronic respiratory failure or with postoperative pneumonia are at risk of becoming severely hypoxemic during peritoneal dialysis. The patient with multiple abdominal scars and/or peritoneal adhesions from previous abdominal surgery is also a poor candidate for peritoneal dialysis. In patients with intestinal ileus, drainage problems, or poor respiratory tolerance to the infusion of the adequate dialysate exchange volumes, a low efficiency is to be expected. In patients with enterostomy and colostomy or with peritoneal drains, leakage of dialysis fluid is frequent, rendering it difficult to maintain an accurate fluid balance and increasing the risk of peritoneal infection. Discontinuation of peritoneal dialysis and transfer of the patient to hemodialysis is mandatory in cases of acute massive hydrothorax [51]. Hemodialysis should be resorted to without delay when an inadequate control of uremia (persisting blood urea concentration >25 mmol/l) results either from a hypercatabolic state (daily blood urea increases of 10 mmol/l or more) or from reduced peritoneal clearances due to alteration in the splanchnic arterial bed (e.g., diabetics, scleroderma [77]) or due to heat-stress-induced ARF [78]. Finally, when ARF occurs in the context of acute poisoning, the use of hemodialysis and/or hemoperfusion seems preferable, taking into account the superior effectiveness of poison removal obtained with these two techniques by comparison with PD [79].

References

1. Maxwell MH, Rockney RE, Kleeman CR, Twiss MR. Peritoneal dialysis. I. Technique and application. JAMA 170: 917–924, 1959.
2. Boen ST, Mulinari AS, Dillard DH, Scribner BH. Periodic peritoneal dialysis in the management of chronic uremia. Trans Am Soc Artif Intern Organs 8: 256–262, 1962.
3. Tenckhoff H, Schechter H. A bacteriologically safe peritoneal access device for peritoneal dialysis. Trans Am Soc Artif Intern Organs 14: 181–186, 1968.
4. Popovich RP, Moncrief JW, Decherd JB, Bomar JB, Pyle WK. The definition of a novel portable/wearable equilibrium peritoneal dialysis technique. Abstracts Am Soc Artif Intern Organs 5: 64, 1976.
5. Boen ST. Kinetics of peritoneal dialysis. A comparison with the artificial kidney. Medicine 40: 243–287, 1961.
6. Popovich RP, Pyle WK, Moncrief JW. Kinetics of peritoneal transport. In Peritoneal Dialysis, Nolph KD (ed). The Hague: Martinus-Nijhoff, 1981, pp. 79–123.
7. Nolph KD, Sorkin MI. The peritoneal dialysis system. In Peritoneal Dialysis, Nolph KD (ed). The Hague: Martinus-Nijhoff, 1981, pp. 21–41.
8. Cameron JS, Ogg C, Trounce JR. Peritoneal dialysis in hypercatabolic acute renal failure. Lancet 1: 1188–1191, 1967.
9. Raja RH, Kramer MS, Rosenbaum JL, Bolisay C, Krug M. Contrasting changes in solute transport and ultrafiltration with peritonitis in CAPD patients. Trans Am Soc Artif Intern Organs 27: 68–70, 1981.
10. Henderson LW. Ultrafiltration with peritoneal dialysis. In Developments in Nephrology 2: Peritoneal Dialysis, Nolph KD (ed). The Hague: Martinus-Nijhoff, 1981, pp. 124–145.
11. Blumenkrantz MJ, Gahl GM, Kopple JD, Kamdar AV, Jones MR, Kessel M, Coburn JW. Protein losses during peritoneal dialysis. Kidney Int 19: 53–58, 1981.
12. Kallen RJ. A method for approximating the efficacy of peritoneal dialysis for uremia. Am J Dis Child 3: 156–160, 1966.
13. Tenckhoff H. Home peritoneal dialysis. In Clinical Aspects of Uremia, Massry SG, Sellers AL (eds). Springfield Il: Charles C Thomas, 1976, pp. 583–615.
14. Henderson LW. Hemodialysis. In Strauss and Welt's Diseases of the Kidney (3rd ed) Earley LE, Gottschalk CW (eds). Boston: Little, Brown, 1979, pp. 421–462.
15. Mion CM. Practical use of peritoneal dialysis. In Replacement of Renal Function by Dialysis (2nd ed), Drukker W, Parsons FM, Maher JF (eds). The Hague: Martinus-Nijhoff, 1983, pp. 457–492.
16. Weston RE, Roberts M. Clinical use of a stylet catheter for peritoneal dialysis. Arch Int Med 115: 659–662, 1965.
17. Tenckhoff H. Catheter implantation. Dial Transpl (1) 3: 18–20, 1972.
18. Slingeneyer A, Charpiat A, Balmes M, Mion C. Is an alternative to the Tenckhoff catheter necessary? In Advances in Peritoneal Dialysis, Gahl GM, Kessel M, Nolph KD (eds). Amsterdam: Excerpta Medica, International Congress series 567, 1981, pp. 179–184.
19. Tenckhoff H, Meston B, Shilipetar RG. A simplified automatic peritoneal dialysis system. Trans Am Soc Artif Intern Organs 18: 436–439, 1972.
20. Vidt DG. Recommendations on choice of peritoneal

dialysis solutions. Arch Intern Med 78: 144–146, 1973.

21. Slingeneyer A, Mion C, Despaux E, Perez C, Duport J, Dansette AM. Use of a bacteriological filter in the prevention of peritonitis associated with peritoneal dialysis. Long-term clinical results in intermittent and continuous ambulatory peritoneal dialysis. In Peritoneal Dialysis, Atkins RC, Thomson NM, Farrell PC (eds). Edinburgh, Churchill Livingstone, 1981, pp. 301–312.

22. Furman RL, Gomperts ED, Hockley S. Activity of intraperitoneal heparin during peritoneal dialysis. Clin Nephrol 9: 15–19, 1978.

23. Atkins RC, Mion C, Despaux E, Van Hai N, Jullien C, Mion H. Peritoneal transfer of Kanamycin and its use in peritoneal dialysis. Kidney Int 3: 391–396, 1973.

24. Gutman RA. Automated peritoneal dialysis for home use. Quart J Med New Series 47: 261–280, 1978.

25. Regamey C, Schaberg D, Kirby WM. Inhibitory effect of heparin on gentamycin concentrations in blood. Antimicrob Agents Chemoth 6: 329–332, 1972.

26. Koup JR, Gerbracht L. Combined use of heparin and gentamycin in peritoneal dialysis solutions. Drug Intell Clin Pharm 9: 388–389, 1975.

27. Vas ST. Can heparin and antibiotics be mixed in the same bag? Perit Dial Bull 1: 67, 1981.

28. Crossley K, Kjellstrand CM. Intraperitoneal insulin for control of blood sugar in diabetic patients during peritoneal dialysis. B Med J 1: 269–270, 1971.

29. Nolph KD, Ghods A, Brown P, Miller F, Harris P, Pyle K, Popovich R. Effects of nitroprusside on peritoneal mass transfer coefficients and microvascular physiology. Trans Am Soc Artif Intern Organs 23: 210–217, 1977.

30. Hirszel P, Lasrich M, Maher JF. Augmentation of peritoneal mass transport by dopamine. Comparison with norepinephrine and evaluation of pharmacologic mechanisms. J Lab Clin Med 94: 747–754, 1979.

31. Petersen NJ, Larson LA, Favero MJ. Microbiological capacity of water in an automatic peritoneal dialysis system. Dial Transpl (6) 2: 38–86, 1977.

32. Villaroel F. Future of intracorporeal dialysis. Contribut Nephrol 17: 111–119, 1979.

33. Posen GA, Luisiello J. Continuous equilibration peritoneal dialysis in the treatment of acute renal failure. Perit Dial Bull 1: 6–7 1981.

34. Gastaldi L, Baratelli L, Cassani D, Cinquepalmi M, Frattini GM, Martegani M. Low flow continuous peritoneal dialysis in acute renal failure. Nephron 29: 101–103, 1981.

35. Tenckhoff H. Chronic Peritoneal Dialysis Manual. University of Washington, 1974.

36. Canaud B, Mimran A, Liendo-Liendo C, Slingeneyer A, Mion C. Blood pressure control in patients treated by continuous ambulatory peritoneal dialysis. In Continuous Ambulatory Peritoneal Dialysis, Legrain M (ed). Amsterdam: Excerpta Medica, 1980, pp. 212–219.

37. Pyle WK, Moncrief JW, Popovich RP. Peritoneal transport evaluation in CAPD. In CAPD Update, Continuous Ambulatory Peritoneal Dialysis, Moncrief JW, Popovich RP (eds). Paris: Masson, 1981, pp. 35–52.

38. Gault MH, Fergusson EL, Sidhu JS, Corbin RP. Fluid and electrolyte complications of peritoneal dialysis. Ann Int Med 75: 253–262, 1971.

39. Vaamonde CA, Michael UF, Metzger RA, Carroll KE. Complications of acute peritoneal dialysis. J Chron Dis 26: 637–659, 1975.

40. Oreopoulos DG, Khanna R. Complications of peritoneal dialysis other than peritonitis. In Developments in Nephrology 2: Peritoneal Dialysis, Nolph KD (ed). The Hague: Martinus-Nijhoff, 1981, pp. 309–343.

41. Hau T, Ahrenholz DH, Simmons RC. Secondary bacterial peritonitis: The biologic basis of treatment. Curr Probl Surg 16: 3, 1979.

42. Vas SI, Low DE, Oreopoulos DG. Peritonitis. In Developments in Nephrology 2: Peritoneal Dialysis, Nolph KD (ed). The Hague: Martinus-Nijhoff, 1981, pp. 344–365.

43. Sarles HE, Lindley JD, Fisch JC, Biggers JA, Cottom DL, Cottom JR, Mader JT, Dunaway JE, Remmers AR Jr. Peritoneal dialysis using a Millipore filter. Kidney Int 9: 54–57, 1976.

44. Schwartz FD, Kallmeyer J, Dunea G, Kark RM. Prevention of infection during peritoneal dialysis. JAMA 199: 115–117, 1967.

45. Williams P, Khanna R, Oreopoulos DG. Treatment of peritonitis in patients on CAPD: No longer a controversy. Dial Transpl 10: 272–275, 1981.

46. Rottembourg J, Jacq D, Singlas D, Nguyen M. Medical management of peritonitis. In Continuous Ambulatory Peritoneal Dialysis, Legrain M (ed). Amsterdam: Excerpta Medica, 1980, pp. 248–257.

47. Atkins RC, Humphery T, Thomson N, Hooke D, Davidson A. Efficacy of treatment in CAPD peritonitis—The problem of staphylococcal antibiotic resistance. In Peritoneal Dialysis, Atkins RC, Thomson NP, Farrell PC (eds). Edinburgh: Churchill Livingstone, 1981, pp. 333–342.

48. Holdsworth SR, Atkins RC, Scott DG, Jackson R. Management of Candida peritonitis by prolonged peritoneal lavage containing 5-fluorocytosine. Clin Nephrol 4: 157–159, 1975.

49. Bayer AS, Blumenkrantz MJ, Montgomerie GZ, Galpin JE, Coburn JW, Guze LB. Candida peritonitis. Report of 22 cases and review of the English literature. Am J Med 61: 832–839, 1976.

50. Khanna R, Oreopoulos DG, Vas SI, McCready W, Dombros N. Fungal peritonitis in patients undergoing chronic intermittent or continuous ambulatory peritoneal dialysis. Proc Eur Dial Transpl Assoc 17: 291–296, 1980.

51. Rudnick MR, Coyle JF, Beck LH, McCurdy DK. Acute massive hydrothorax complicating peritoneal dialysis, report of 2 cases and review of the literature. Clin Nephrol 12: 38–44, 1979.

52. Rutsky EA. Bradycardic rhythms during peritoneal dialysis. Arch Int Med 128: 445–448, 1971.
53. Nolph KD, Hano E, Teschan PE. Peritoneal sodium transport during ultrafiltration peritoneal dialysis. Ann Intern Med 70: 931–941, 1969.
54. Burns RO, Henderson LW, Hager EB, Merrill JP. Peritoneal dialysis. Clinical experience. N Engl J Med 267: 1060–1066, 1962.
55. Grodstein GP, Blumenkrantz MJ, Kopple JD. Effect of intercurrent illnesses on nitrogen metabolism in uremic patients. Trans Am Soc Artif Intern Organs 25: 438–441, 1979.
56. Merrill JP. Dialysis in acute renal failure. In Replacement of Renal Function by Dialysis, Drukker W, Parsons FM, Maher JF (eds). The Hague: Martinus-Nijhoff, 1978, pp. 322–333.
57. Kerr DNS. Acute renal failure. In Renal Disease, Sir Douglas Black (ed). Oxford: Blackwell Scientific Publications, 1972, pp. 417–461.
58. Stewart JH, Tuckwell LA, Sinnett PF, Edwards KDG, Wayte HM. Peritoneal and hemodialysis: A comparison of their morbidity and of the mortality suffered by dialysed patients. Quart J Med New Series 35: 407–420, 1966.
59. Swartz RD, Valk TW, Brain AJP, Hsu CH. Complications of hemodialysis and peritoneal dialysis in acute renal failure. ASAIO J 3: 98–101, 1980.
60. Ellis D, Gartner JC, Galvis AG. Acute renal failure in infants and children: Diagnosis, complications and treatment. Critical Care Med 9: 607–617, 1981.
61. Abel RM, Buckley MJ, Austen WG, Barnett GO, Beck CH, Fischer JE. Etiology, incidence and prognosis of renal failure following cardiac operations. J Thorac Cardiovasc Surg 71: 323–328, 1976.
62. Gailunas P Jr, Chawca R, Lazarus JM, Cohn C, Sanders J, Merrill JP. Acute renal failure following cardiac operations. J Thorac Cardiovasc Surg 79: 241–243, 1980.
63. Fraedrich G, Scholz R, Mulch J, Leber HW, Hehrlein FW. Continuous ambulatory peritoneal dialysis in acute renal failure after cardiovascular surgery. Thorac Cardiovasc Surgeon 28: 246–248, 1980.
64. Tzamaloukas AH, Garella S, Chazan JA. Peritoneal dialysis for acute renal failure after major abdominal surgery. Arch Surg 106: 639–643, 1973.
65. Berne TV, Barbour BH. Acute renal failure in general surgical patients. Arch Surg 102: 594–597, 1971.
66. Glenn LD, Nolph KD: Treatment of pancreatitis with peritoneal dialysis. Perit Dial Bull 2: 63–68, 1982.
67. Weintraub LR, Penner JA, Meyers MC. Acute anuric acid nephropathy in leukemia. Arch Int Med 113: 111–114, 1964.
68. Maher JF, Rath CE, Schreiner GE. Hyperuricemia complicating leukemia. Treatment with allopurinol and dialysis. Arch Int Med 123: 198–200, 1969.
69. Cardella C. Renal transplantation in patients on peritoneal dialysis. Perit Dial Bull 1: 12–13, 1980.
70. Evans DH, Sorkin MI, Nolph KD, Whittier FC. Continuous ambulatory peritoneal dialysis and transplantation. Trans Am Soc Artif Intern Organs 27: 320–323, 1981.
71. Brooks MH, Barry KG. Removal of iodinated material by peritoneal dialysis. Nephron 12: 10–14, 1973.
72. Donadio JV, Whelton A, Kazyak L. Quinine therapy and peritoneal dialysis in acute renal failure complicating malarial hemoglobinuria. Lancet 1: 375–378, 1978.
73. Nolph KD, Rosenfeld PS, Powell JT, Danforth E Jr. Peritoneal glucose transport and hyperglycemia during peritoneal dialysis. Am J Med Sci 259: 272–281, 1970.
74. Grodstein GP, Blumenkrantz MJ, Kopple JD, Moran JK, Coburn JW. Glucose absorption during continuous ambulatory peritoneal dialysis. Kidney Int 19: 564–567, 1981.
75. Gjessing J. Addition of aminoacids to peritoneal dialysis fluid. Lancet 2: 812–, 1968.
76. Giordano C, De Santo NG, Capodicasa G, Di Iorio B, De Simone V, Capasso G, Arico C, Catellino P, Nuzzi F, Trasente I, Alinei P. CAPD in acute renal failure. The usability of the peritoneal cavity as a simplified gut for total parenteral nutrition. In Acute Renal Failure, Eliahou HE (ed). London: John Libbey, 1982, pp. 186–189.
77. Nolph KD, Stoltz ML, Maher JF. Altered peritoneal permeability in patients with systemic vasculitis. Ann Int Med 75: 753–759, 1971.
78. Nolph KD, Whitcomb M, Schrier RW. Mechanisms for inefficient peritoneal dialysis in acute renal failure associated with heat stress and exercise. Ann Int Med 71: 317–326, 1969.
79. Winchester JF, Gelfand MC, Knepshield JH, Schreiner GE. Dialysis and hemoperfusion of poisons and drugs. Update. Trans Am Soc Artif Intern Organs 23: 762–842, 1977.

25. LONG-TERM FOLLOW-UP OF RENAL FUNCTION AFTER RECOVERY FROM ACUTE TUBULAR NECROSIS

Arthur C. Kennedy

The management of acute renal failure (ARF) was dramatically altered in 1945 by the successful use of hemodialysis by Kolff [1] in a patient with acute postoperative renal failure and by the improved understanding of the basic principles of fluid and electrolyte management [2, 3]. Attention at first naturally focused on the impact of these newer forms of management on the immediate prognosis, particularly since it appeared that if death during the acute phase could be prevented, complete clinical recovery was the rule. Study of the literature, however, shows that even from the late forties it was becoming apparent that recovery, although complete in the clinical sense, was not necessarily complete as regards renal function. Burwell et al. [4] reported a patient who developed ARF following abortion and died three months later after a good clinical recovery. Death was due to serum hepatitis, but at postmortem examination the kidneys showed minor but definite abnormalities, including subcapsular scarring, lymphocytic foci, and some dilated tubules with flattened epithelium. Marshall and Hoffman [5] reported delayed recovery of renal function in three out of four patients, and in four cases of acute tubular necrosis (ATN) due to carbon tetrachloride poisoning, Sirota [6] observed that although renal function usually returned to the lower limit of normal, there might be some residual vascular damage.

All the above reports [4–6] were on small numbers of cases followed up for relatively short periods of time. A more extensive but still preliminary report came from Lowe [7], who found in 14 patients with ARF followed for periods varying from 78 to 38 months that renal function tests tended to remain below normal limits. All the patients were females, and none had received dialysis, a fact that might possibly suggest that the severity of the ARF could have been somewhat less than that of patients in later series, many of whom would have undoubtedly died but for dialysis. Lowe speculated on the possibility of increased frequency of hypertension in the survivors, but the number of patients was insufficient to permit a definite view. Finkenstaedt and Merrill [8] reported on 16 patients studied at periods ranging from 1 month to 76 months after recovery from ARF. The subjects were selected because of the absence of any cardiovascular or renal disease before the acute episode. Some patients were studied on more than one occasion. The findings were similar to those of Lowe [7], namely, that clearance values remained below the lower limit of normal in most patients; they concluded that "these findings are consistent with permanent renal damage of mild degree." Only one patient showed progressive decrease of renal function but this was attributed to the development of periarteritis nodosa with renal involvement.

A more favorable report came from Edwards [9], who found that in 15 patients in Australia followed for periods of up to 76 weeks after recovery from ARF, the glomerular filtration rate (GFR), as measured by endogenous creatinine clearance or urea clearance, returned to normal in 14 out of 15 cases within three months. Edwards, however, comments that he placed the normal range of GFR at "a somewhat lower level than other workers" and that this might account for his more optimistic findings. Certainly, no subsequent authors have reported in such an optimistic fashion. Price and Palmer [10] carried out a functional and morphological follow-up study of 14 patients who had recovered from ARF. Glomerular filtration was assessed by inulin clearance in 10 of the 14 patients; the mean value was 94 ± 27 ml/min., the three lowest values being 79, 73, and 40 ml per minute, respectively. Renal biopsy was performed in eight patients, and it is perhaps unfortunate, from the scientific viewpoint, that they did not include any of the three patients with the lowest glomerular filtration rates. Ward et al. [11] studied maximum urine osmolality in 11 patients some months after recovery from ATN. The response improved to normal values over the months, but a severe defect (maximum urine osmolality of 356 mOsm/kg) was still evident at 10 months in one patient. A comprehensive study of renal function after recovery from ATN was reported by Briggs et al. [12]. Fifty patients were studied, all of them after a previously well-documented episode of ATN. The age of the patients at the time of the ATN ranged from 18 to 67 years. The patients were studied on average at 35 months after the episode of renal failure, and the follow-up period varied from 4 to 75 months. It was less than one year in only 2 of the 50 patients. Some abnormality of renal function was present in 37 (74%) of the patients, the most common defect being a lowered GFR, which was present in 71% of the patients. The mean GFR was 94 ml/min, and in seven patients (17%), the rate was less than 50 ml/min. Tests of tubular function were found to be abnormal in a smaller number of patients, the concentration test being impaired in 31%. No correlation was found between renal function at the time of follow-up and either the severity of the renal failure or the precipitating cause, except that patients in whom the renal failure had been due to antepartum

hemorrhage or postpartum hemorrhage with a preceding pre-eclampsia did have a greater likelihood of residual renal functional impairment. There was no evidence in this study [12] that hypertension developed after the ATN, nor was any alteration in renal size or calyceal change evident on intravenous pyelography nor was there any apparent predisposition to subsequent urinary tract infection. Serial studies in 14 patients suggested that no subsequent deterioration in renal function followed the initial recovery.

Hall et al. [13] published very similar findings from the Mayo Clinic. From an initial population of 186 patients with ARF, 87 survived, and from these 36 patients underwent a study of renal function more than three months after recovery from the episode of ARF. Of the 36 patients, 22 (61%) had incomplete renal functional recovery using the same criteria as Briggs et al. (12), namely, that inulin clearance values were more than one standard deviation below expected values. Patients who failed to regain normal function were on the average nearly two decades older and had experienced a more prolonged period of oliguria. Five patients in the group with incomplete functional recovery were suspected of having prior renal disease, but even when these patients were excluded, the mean clearance values for the group were essentially unchanged. Hall et al. [13] did not find any evidence for an increased occurrence of urinary tract infection after recovery. These authors made serial observations in 22 patients for an average observation period of 42.4 months (range: 2 to 125 months), and nine patients were followed for seven years. In seven of these nine patients, inulin clearance values decreased, the average decline being 17.6%. Rather similar findings were noted by Lewers et al. [14]. Thirty patients who had survived ATN were followed from 2 to 15 years. Although clinical recovery was complete in all patients, endogenous creatinine clearance was abnormal in 37%, and there was a defect of urine concentration power in 47%. There was no correlation of abnormal GFR with interval of follow-up or age at follow-up. No increased prevalence of hypertension or urinary tract infection was noted. In only 30% of the patients were all renal function studies within normal limits, which is almost identical to the findings of Briggs et al. [12]. Long-term prognosis after ARF was also studied by Amerio et al. [15] in 57 ARF survivors. Only 14 of the 57 patients were studied more than two years after recovery. Although some of these patients had attained a normal GFR, the mean values for the group were lower than normal (76.6 ± 24.4 ml/min). Bonomini and his colleagues [16] have recently reported their clinical and renal biopsy findings in a large number of patients with ARF, including 125 patients with ATN. Follow-up studies at one year revealed 62.4% with complete functional recovery, 31.2% with partial recovery, and 6.4% with no recovery. No detail is given of the laboratory investigations used to determine renal function or what "partial recovery" means. Repeat follow-up studies at five years included measurement of GFR although the method is not recorded. Of the 125 patients, 56.8% had a GFR greater than 80 ml/min, 32% a GFR greater than 15 ml/min, and 11.2% a GFR less than 15 ml/min.

Leaving aside the more optimistic report of Edwards [9], it is possible on the basis of several studies [7–16] involving a total of 353 patients who had all survived ATN to define in broad terms a spectrum of the outcome as regards return of renal function:

a. Restoration of normal, or virtually normal, renal function in perhaps 30 to 40% of patients.
b. Complete clinical recovery but with a slight to modest defect of glomerular filtration and or tubular function in perhaps 40 to 50% of patients.
c. Significant impairment of renal function, which may require medical supervision in perhaps 10% of patients.
d. In a small minority of patients, impairment of renal function of such a degree that renal replacement therapy is likely to be required either soon or relatively soon after the acute illness.

A few patients with significant or marked impairment of renal function after ATN are included within some of the larger series [12, 16], but individual clinical details are not recorded.

In the 38-year-old male patient reported by Levin et al. [17], severe ATN developed after a perforated appendix with peritonitis. Although he was oliguric for only a few days, the renal failure was extremely protracted. On the 37th day, when the creatinine clearance was 5 ml/min, a renal biopsy was carried out for diagnostic and prognostic reasons; it revealed ATN with evidence of tubular regeneration and normal glomeruli. The creatinine clearance rose slowly to plateau at 18 ml/min by 30 months. A second renal biopsy, 17 months after the initial illness, showed widespread tubular atrophy with diffuse interstitial fibrosis. Some tubules were well differentiated, indicating that regeneration had occurred. The authors suggest that the antibiotic therapy given to control the peritonitis may have contributed to the renal damage (three of the six antibiotics used were potentially nephrotoxic) and that continuing active pyelonephritis (of which there was evidence on the second biopsy) may have been an additional factor. Siegler and Bloomer [18] reported five patients with presumed ATN who remained oliguric for 31 to 72 days. All recovered from the ARF, but in three patients significant renal failure persisted. No renal biopsies were performed, so it is uncertain whether there was any renal abnormality apart from the presumed ATN. Merino et al. [19] reported 125 patients with postsurgical ATN, of whom 87 died, 34 regained normal renal function (assessed by the level of serum creatinine), and 4 were left with severe permanent renal failure. Preoperatively, these patients had normal renal function. These authors believe that the combination of older age (over 60 years), the use of nephrotoxic antibiotics (particularly cephalothin and gentamicin sulphate), and the use of methoxyflurane anesthesia is particularly liable to produce a very severe form of ATN. Renal histology was obtained (at autopsy) in only one of the four patients: the kidneys showed fibrosis of the renal cortex with multiple small abscesses; so in this patient at least the renal histology was not simply that of ATN. Collins et al. [20] reported the case of a 65-year-old woman with very severe ATN (confirmed by serial biopsies) due to ethylene glycol poisoning. Oliguria persisted for 50 days, and at three and one-half months the creatinine clear-

484

ance had reached its maximum value of 9.5 ml/ min. Irreversible acute oliguric renal failure after methoxyflurane anesthesia was described in three patients by Hollenberg et al. [21]; but renal histology revealed that in addition to ATN, there were severe glomerular damage and marked interstitial edema, fibrosis, and round-cell infiltrate. In arsine-induced acute oliguric renal failure [22, 23], marked tubular necrosis occurs, but it is accompanied by a severe degree of diffuse interstitial nephritis, which is followed by interstitial fibrosis. The importance of acute interstitial fibrosis as a cause of ARF is now well recognized [16, 24, 25]. It may be present as the sole or the dominant lesion, or it may be present in addition to severe ATN. The combination of the two lesions seems likely to have an adverse effect on ultimate recovery of complete renal function. It is apparent, therefore, that in many of the well-documented cases of incomplete recovery, some renal damage in addition to ATN is also present.

Clinical features suggested [13, 18, 19, 21] as likely to be associated with incomplete recovery of renal function include older age, very protracted oliguria, use of nephrotoxic antibiotics and methoxyflurane anesthesia. Harwood et al. [26] have made the interesting suggestion that incomplete recovery of renal function can be predicted early in the illness by renal scanning.

Most nephrologists, understandably, do not carry out renal biopsies as part of the long-term follow-up of patients who have made a complete clinical recovery from ATN and who have regained normal or near normal renal function. Biopsies were performed in 8 of the 14 patients in the study by Price and Palmer [10] but not in the three patients who had the greatest functional impairment. In two patients, the biopsies were performed very close to the acute illness (five and six weeks, respectively), and the other biopsies ranged from six months to four years after the initial illness. Price and Palmer found little correlation between the kidney biopsy findings and the clearance values in these patients. They observed, however, that the small number of patients examined does not permit any real conclusions to be made. Changes observed tended to be particularly in

the glomeruli and consisted of thickening and splitting of the basement membrane of the glomerular tuft and Bowman's capsule as well as thickening of the capillary walls and adhesions between the glomerulus and Bowman's capsule. Such changes were noted in six of eight biopsy specimens. Periglomerular fibrosis was noted in three out of eight patients. An impression was noted of an increase in the number of hyalinized glomeruli. Tubular lesions consisted of tubular atrophy and basement membrane thickening; in almost all cases they were associated with glomeruli that showed mild, moderate, or severe damage. Areas of interstitial fibrosis, often associated with infiltration of chronic inflammatory cells, were noted. Renal biopsy was carried out at long-term follow-up in 11 of the 30 patients reported by Lewers et al. [14]. Four had completely normal renal function. The follow-up biopsy specimens frequently had mild interstitial edema or fibrosis. Vascular changes were not impressive except for occasional atherosclerotic changes, presumably unrelated, and glomerular changes were noted to be "insignificant." Obsolescent glomeruli were occasionally seen but were usually associated with vascular changes. Electron microscopic studies in six patients showed increased intertubular collagen material, with some thickening of the tubular basement membrane in two patients. These authors observe that there was no correlation between the histology and renal function after prolonged follow-up. Renal biopsy was carried out in three of the 57 patients studied by Amerio et al. [15]. The biopsies were taken three years after the ARF; unfortunately, the renal function of these patients at the time of biopsy is not given. Histological abnormalities included chronic interstitial changes, tubular damage sometimes amounting to atrophy, thickening and rupture of basement membranes, sclerosis of glomeruli, and disturbed architecture of the mesangium. These authors suggest that some of these changes might be due to a progressive pyelonephritis, but such evidence is difficult to obtain from their report. Bonomini et al. [16] used renal biopsy to classify 227 patients in their series of ARF. No details are given of the biopsy findings in the 125 patients classified as suffering from ATN, either at onset or on follow-up, although repeat biopsies were clearly carried out. Twelve patients from the series of ARF were classified as suffering from acute interstitial nephritis, but there is no indication whether any of the 125 patients classified as having ATN also had any element of interstitial nephritis.

In summary, in those patients who make a good clinical recovery from ATN and who regain normal renal function or are left with a clinically unimportant slight to modest defect in renal function, the characteristic late biopsy findings range from minimal chronic tubular changes to the loss of a proportion of the original nephron population. In those patients who are left with critically damaged kidneys, the late biopsy will show changes consistent with massive nephron loss and may also indicate that the original ATN was accompanied by interstitial nephritis and possibly by a glomerular lesion.

References

1. Kolff WJ. The Artificial Kidney. (Shortened English version of De Kunstmatige Nier. MD Thesis.) University of Groningen, Kampen (Holland), JH Kok.
2. Borst JGG. Protein katabolism in uremia. Effects of protein-free diet, infections and blood transfusions. Lancet 1: 824–828, 1948.
3. Bull GM, Joekes, AM, Lowe KG. Conservative treatment of anuric uremia. Lancet 2: 229–234, 1949.
4. Burwell EL, Kinney TD, Finch CA. Renal damage following intravascular hemolysis. N Engl J Med 237: 657–665, 1947.
5. Marshall D, Hoffman WS. The nature of the altered renal function in lower nephron nephrosis. J Lab Clin Med 34: 31–39, 1949.
6. Sirota JH. Carbon tetrachloride poisoning in man. I. The mechanisms of renal failure and recovery. J Clin Invest 28: 1412–1422, 1949.
7. Lowe KG. The late prognosis in acute tubular necrosis: Interim follow-up report on 14 patients. Lancet 1: 1086–1088, 1952.
8. Finkenstaedt JT, Merrill JP. Renal function after recovery from acute renal failure. N Engl J Med 254: 1023–1026, 1956.
9. Edwards KDG. Recovery of renal function after acute renal failure. Aust Ann Med 8: 195–199, 1959.
10. Price JDE, Palmer RA. A functional and morphological follow-up study of acute renal failure. Arch Intern Med 105: 90–98, 1960.
11. Ward EE, Richards P, Wrong OM. Urine concentration after acute renal failure. Nephron 3: 289–294, 1966.
12. Briggs JD, Kennedy AC, Young LN, Luke RG, Gray Mary. Renal function after acute tubular necrosis. Brit Med J 3: 513–516, 1967.
13. Hall JW, Johnson WJ, Maher FT, Hunt JC. Immediate and long-term prognosis in acute renal failure. Ann Intern Med 73, 515–521, 1970
14. Lewers DT, Mathew TH, Maher JF, Schreiner GE. Long-term follow-up of renal function and histology after acute tubular necrosis. Ann Intern Med 73: 523–529. 1970.
15. Amerio A, Vercellone A, De Benedictis G, Linari F, Piccoli G, Coratelli P, Vacha G, Ragni R, Mastrangelo F, Pastore G. Long-term prognosis in acute renal failure of primarily tubular origin. Minerva Nefrol 19: 7–17, 1972.
16. Bonomini V, Vangelista A, Frasca GM. Value of renal biopsy for long-term prognosis in acute renal failure. In Acute Renal Failure, Seybold D and Gessler U (eds). Basel: Karger, 1982, pp. 207–213.
17. Levin ML, Simon NM, Herdson PB, Del Greco F. Acute renal failure followed by protracted slowly resolving chronic uremia. J Chron Dis 25: 645–651, 1972.
18. Siegler RL, Bloomer HA. Acute renal failure with prolonged oliguria. JAMA 225: 133–136, 1973.
19. Merino GE, Buselmeier TJ, Kjellstrand CM. Postoperative chronic renal failure; a new syndrome? Ann Surg 182: 37–44, 1975.
20. Collins JM, Hennes DM, Holzgang CR, Gourley RT, Porter GA. Recovery after prolonged oliguria due to ethylene glycol intoxication. Arch Intern Med 125: 1059–1062, 1970.
21. Hollenberg NK, McDonald FD, Cotran R, Galvanek EG, Warhol M, Vandam LD, Merrill JP. Irreversible acute oliguric renal failure. A complication of methoxyflurane anesthesia. N Engl J Med 286 (16): 877–879, 1972.
22. Muehrcke RC, Pirani CL. Arsine-induced anuria. A correlative clinicopathological study with electron microscopic observations. Ann Intern Med 68: 853–866, 1968.
23. Uldall PR, Khan HA, Ennis JE, McCallum RI, Grimson TA. Renal damage from industrial arsine poisoning. Brit J Indust Med 27: 372–377, 1970.
24. Pasternack A, Tallqvist G, Kuhlback B. Occurrence of interstitial nephritis in acute renal failure. Acta Med Scand 187: 27–31, 1970.
25. Pusey CD, Saltissi D, Bloodworth L, Rainford DJ, Christie JL. Drug-associated acute interstitial nephritis: Clinical and pathological features and the response to high-dose steroid therapy. Quart J Med, New Series LI1, 206: 194–211, 1983.
26. Harwood TH, Hiesterman DR, Robinson RG, Cross DE, Whittier FC, Diederich DA, Grantham JJ. Prognosis for recovery of function in acute renal failure. Value of the renal image obtained using iodohippurate sodium I 131. Arch Intern Med 136: 916–919, 1976.

INDEX